Prescription for
DIETARY
WELLNESS

SECOND EDITION

PHYLLIS A. BALCH, CNC

AVERY

a member of PENGUIN GROUP (USA) INC.   *New York*

Most Avery books are available at special quantity discounts for bulk purchase for sales promotions, premiums, fundraising, and educational needs. Special books or book excerpts also can be created to fit specific needs. For details, write Penguin Group (USA) Inc. Special Markets, 375 Hudson Street, New York, NY 10014.

a member of
Penguin Group (USA) Inc.
375 Hudson Street
New York, NY 10014
www.penguin.com

Library of Congress Cataloging-in-Publication Data

Balch, Phyllis A., date.
Prescription for dietary wellness / Phyllis A. Balch.—2nd ed.
p.   cm.
Includes bibliographical references and index.
ISBN 1-58333-147-6 (alk. paper)
1. Nutrition.   2. Health.   3. Vitality.   I. Title.
RA784.B2492   2003   2002043600
613.2—dc21

Printed in the United States of America

10   9   8   7   6   5   4   3   2   1

This book is printed on acid-free paper. ∞

Acknowledgments

There are many people who have come and gone in my life and have contributed to my books in many different ways, but I want to dedicate this one to these loyal and true friends who are no longer with me:

Judge Wendell W. Mayer

Charles R. Cripe

Skeeners Balch

Last but not least, my mother, Mary Henning

I also wish to acknowledge the following people, who both advised and supported me as I prepared and wrote the second edition of this book: my daughters, Ruby Hines and Cheryl Keene; my grandchildren, Lisa, Ryan, and Rachel; my brother, Al Henning; my researcher and editor, Betty Lou Thiersmann; researcher Sheila Arp; my publisher's editor, Amy Tecklenburg; and the manufacturers and suppliers who allowed me to evaluate their products before recommending them to my readers. Finally, I would like to thank all the readers who have remained loyal throughout the years.

One cannot be happy if not healthy; may this book bring you both happiness and health for many years to come.

Contents

Part Five   Super Foods

Part Six   Proceed with Caution

Part Seven   Unique Nutritional Needs

Preface to the Second Edition

As I see it, every day you do one of two things: build health or produce disease in yourself.

—*Adelle Davis, nutritionist and author*

In the United States, which uses 50 percent of the drugs produced in the world, infectious diseases are on the rise. In the past twenty years, more than thirty new diseases, including AIDS, toxic shock syndrome, flesh-eating bacteria, and the Ebola virus, have emerged for which there are no cures or vaccines. Chronically ill children have grown up to be chronically ill adults. Type 2 diabetes and coronary artery disease, once almost exclusively diseases of later adulthood, are appearing in people at younger and younger ages. The cost of health care in the United States is the highest in the world, and it is increasing at a galloping 17 percent a year. The unchecked use of antibiotics in humans and animals has resulted in antimicrobial resistance that can make certain strains of tuberculosis, malaria, and pneumonia, to name a few, deadly diseases again. Doctors documented the first large-scale U.S. outbreak of an antibiotic-resistant strain of strep throat when forty-six children failed to respond to treatment with erythromycin, a widely used antibiotic. The U.S. Centers for Disease Control and Prevention (CDC) has launched a campaign aimed at slowing the growth of "super-germs," powerful bacteria that develop resistance to overused antibiotics. "The bugs are developing resistance faster than we can develop drugs to combat them. They keep one step ahead of us," according to Dr. Julie Gerberding, CDC disease expert.

Meanwhile, the "wonder" drugs and vaccines that are prescribed to heal us often harm and even kill us. Who can forget thalidomide, a drug used in the late 1950s that caused severe birth defects? What is a sure cure for a disease on Monday may be taken off the safe-drug list on Friday. The information from health "experts" changes with such regularity that we wonder how it can possibly be reliable, or how we can continue to pay exorbitant prices for what may turn out to be misinformation.

There has never been a more crucial time to take charge of our own health. The good news is that the resources to make sound decisions on many of the issues surrounding our well-being are now available to everyone. *Prescription for Dietary Wellness* provides inexpensive, natural, time-proven nutritional information about how "pharmafood" can be used as medicine for many of the illnesses that plague us from childhood to old age, *including* aging itself.

Nearly every ancient culture used remedies created from plants for the prevention and cure of disease. Throughout history, a partnership of nature's pharmacopoeia and the body's inherent wisdom worked together to restore health. No scientific explanation was available for how or why plants worked. However, plants did work, and folks kept on using what our Creator had provided. For thousands of years, this was not "alternative" healing. It was the only healing there was. More than 60 percent of the world still relies on this proven traditional type of medicine.

Plant-formulated treatments were widely used in the United States until the late 1800s, when science, led by Pasteur's germ theory of disease, took a distinct turn. Chemical manufacturers started to extract and synthesize the active components in plant remedies and physicians began to rely solely on these pharmaceutical drugs. This method, called allopathic medicine, aggressively attacked bacteria and viruses—and, many times, the body's own defense system. Today, modern allopathic medicine fights the "enemy" with a combination of drugs, surgery, and radiation. This approach, however, does not always uncover or address the underlying *cause* of illness and disease or why the physical system is declining.

When we ingested the "whole" plant, built-in natural buffers and regulators minimized the side effects and aided in assimilating the "medicine." Prescription drugs, on the other hand, isolate or synthesize a part of the plant in exceptionally high amounts that may produce undesirable side effects. When overused or incorrectly prescribed or dispensed, these drugs can be fatal.

Misuse of certain herbs may also cause occasional side effects. Kava kava is one example. There were six reported cases of problems with kava kava (from people who were also using prescription drugs), and almost at once there were calls to take it off the market. In contrast, the negative effects of prescription drugs kill an estimated 106,000 people each year, and yet very few are taken off the market. Certainly, prescription drugs are very necessary at times. However, if health-conscious people choose alternative remedies, when appropriate and with the approval of their health-care professional, they should get the same considerations and access to products as do those who turn to mainstream medicine. The appropriate use of herbs can be safer and more effective than many drugs when people educate themselves properly to avoid misuse.

Once allopathic medicine had a foothold, the old (but proven) practice of using plants and diet to heal the body was ignored and even discredited by many orthodox medical practitioners. Science had not yet uncovered the secrets of "holistic" healing, and without this proof, physicians relied more and more on prescription drugs. Today, that proof exists. Through new technologies, research, and clinical trials, scientists have been able to isolate the key components from plants that cured, and more important, *prevented*, illness for centuries. The exact therapeutic applications to heal health disorders have been identified. This information is the basis of *Prescription for Dietary Wellness*.

These powerful prescription foods that support health and cure disease are readily available to everyone. A diet of fresh vegetables, fruits, sea vegetables, whole grains, nuts, seeds, beans and legumes, soybean products, and herbs pave the road to optimum health. The rate of obesity, which is linked to diabetes, arthritis, stroke, heart disease, and some cancers, doubled in the 1990s. It has never been more important to eliminate [unhealthy] fat and sugar from the diet. Instead, fill up on delicious meals from a variety of healthy foods that can be eaten raw, fresh, steamed, boiled, baked, poached, or sautéed. Eating nutritionally rich food, properly combined, can also detoxify the body by helping it to eliminate cancer-causing chemicals. The simple foods recommended in this book have all the vitamins, minerals, enzymes, fiber, protein, and other nutrients needed for a healthy body. Many of the "power" foods have specific immune-boosting and curative potential.

Those of us who are new to the idea of diet as medicine will learn exactly what organic foods to buy or grow in our gardens, how to store and prepare them for maximum benefit, and how to use diet to heal particular problems with health.

NEW INFORMATION

Several sections have been added to this newly revised edition of *Prescription for Dietary Wellness* that reflect current findings from extensive research and studies. These parts explain, in scientifically accurate but easy-to-understand terms, why diet plays such a key role in the quest for optimum health, and how to use it to prevent disease and aging. Remember, unhealthy diet is the number-one cause of illness in the United States.

Antioxidants

Antioxidants are the powerful nutritional allies that fight disease, cancer, and even the aging process. They are certain nutrients, minerals, phytochemicals, herbs, and enzymes that counteract the harmful effects of free radicals on the body. As the cells in your body burn fuel (food) for energy, they also burn oxygen, a process that creates atoms, molecules, and portions of molecules known as free radicals. These toxic molecules contain unpaired electrons that bind to and destroy healthy cells, creating more free radicals to attack other healthy cells. This results in oxidative damage to cells and tissues—similar to the formation of

rust on your car. Free radicals also destroy and cause mutations in cells that render them unable to absorb the nutrients you need. This "cell starvation" results in an inability to fight off disease. To gain an understanding of how to use the remarkable dietary tool that antioxidants are, and to learn which foods contain abundant amounts of antioxidants, read this very important chapter.

Phytochemicals

For years, researchers have recognized that diets high in fruits, vegetables, grains, and legumes reduce the risk of a number of diseases, including cancer, heart disease, diabetes, and high blood pressure. A group of nutrients beyond the realm of traditional nutrients (like carbohydrates, proteins, fats, vitamins, and minerals) called *phytochemicals* (*phyto* is the Greek word for "plant") are powerful ammunition in the war against cancer, aging, and other illnesses. These nutrient-rich chemicals are formed by nature to work *with* the human body, not against it, as drugs often do. The role of phytochemicals in plants is to protect the plant against biological and environmental hazards. Fortunately, if humans consume plants rich in these chemicals, tremendous health benefits can be achieved as well. Major research on phytochemicals is being undertaken all over the globe, with new discoveries being made every day. This expanded edition of *Prescription for Dietary Wellness* includes the most important current information on phytochemicals, their curative powers, and which foods contain this powerful medicine.

Women Have Special Needs

Because of their physical ability to reproduce the human species, women have special nutritional needs. The delicate hormonal balance that fluctuates throughout women's lives greatly affects their health. Today, the hand that rocks the cradle is also bringing home the bacon, and all kinds of new problems with health are starting to affect women in greater numbers. Hormone replacement therapy, osteoporosis, cancer, and heart disease (surprisingly, the number-one killer of women) are all addressed from a nutritional viewpoint, along with dietary suggestions for continuing health.

Threats to Health

There is so much information—both valid and invalid—about the myriad ways in which food, water, and environment may be harmful to health. It is difficult to understand how food additives, irradiation, preservatives, pesticides, herbicides, and soil depletion affect health. Will we learn fifty years from now, after irreparable damage has already been done, that bioengineered crops and microwave rays are unsafe? Do the tons of antibiotics fed to livestock adversely affect humans? Are there ways to protect your family from bioterrorism? Is lead poisoning still an issue?

Chapter 26 separates fact from myth on all these scary subjects and then suggests safety measures that will help protect hearth and home. This chapter is a *must read* for inhabitants of the third planet from the sun.

A Vegetarian Diet

There are many different reasons to consider a vegetarian diet. Some of us are concerned about the use of hormones and antibiotics in livestock (also sprayed on feed), as well as diseases passed on to humans. Health, animal welfare, religion and spirituality, and a concern for the planet's resources are just a few reasons why people consider trying a vegetarian diet. The big question is, "Can I get all the nutrition I need to be healthy if I become a vegetarian?" The answer is a resounding "Yes!" In truth, studies show that with the proper diet, many vegetarians are healthier and even live longer than their meat-eating counterparts.

Deciding to adopt a vegetarian diet leaves room for different interpretations and choices. This section explains types of vegetarianism, which foods need to be combined to replace meat proteins, and the simple precautions that should be taken to ensure that all of your nutritional needs are met.

HOW TO PROCEED

All individuals should take an active part in the maintenance of their health and in the treatment of disorders with the guidance of a health-care professional. The more we take it upon ourselves to learn about nutrition, the better prepared we will be to take an active role. The realization that body (lifestyle), spirit (desire), and mind (belief) work together is the first step to health.

It is important to stress that the suggestions offered in this book are not intended to replace appropriate medical investigation and treatment. The dietary remedies recommended for a particular disorder should be approved and monitored by a trained health-care professional. And if surgery or other conventional medical interventions are crucial and cannot be avoided, the proper diet can shorten healing time.

Preface

*When health is absent, wisdom cannot reveal itself, art cannot manifest,
strength cannot fight, wealth becomes useless, and intelligence cannot be
applied.*

—Herophilus

Prescription for Dietary Wellness is a nutritional guidebook designed to show, precept-by-precept, a method to attain optimum health. It explains how proper nutrition, partnered with the God-given *healing power within,* will help to maintain, rejuvenate, rehabilitate, and heal our bodies.

One out of three Americans will get some form of cancer in his or her lifetime. Breast cancer is an epidemic, affecting one in eight women. One out of ten of us will develop heart disease. More than half of us will die from one or the other of these ailments. In the most affluent, physician-riddled country in the world, chronic and deadly diseases continue to grow at an alarming rate. *How is this possible? It's simple.* One out of every ten deaths is directly related to diet! The majority of chronic and deadly illnesses stem from preventable causes.

A typical American diet consists of 90 percent cooked, processed, packaged, adulterated, irradiated, and even genetically engineered foods. What we eat is sprayed with poison, chock-full of chemicals and preservatives, grown in nutrient-depleted soil, and then stored on shelves indefinitely. This "dead-food diet" results in a massive nutritional deficit. We subsist largely on meals high in fat, sugar, and salt, and then become overweight as our bodies demand more and more food to fill vital nutritional gaps. The Big Mac has spawned the Big Butt. We are dying of obesity and malnutrition *at the same time.* As living, growing, fuel-burning organisms, we cannot build strong new cells and maintain a healthy immune system on dead matter. Simply put, "lifeless" food cannot sustain life.

For thirty years, I have been preaching what evolving research and the latest statistics prove: Nutrition plays a major role in the prevention, treatment, and cure of most disease and sickness. The vitamins, minerals, and antioxidants found in our food are the front-line defense against premature aging, cancer, diabetes, high blood pressure, heart disease, allergies, and most other illnesses. While conventional medicine was trying, and often failing, to heal with an ever-expanding grab bag of drugs, I decided to explore the road less traveled—a holistic route to vital health using nature's remedies, remedies that do not have the life-threatening side effects of prescription drugs.

Prescription for Dietary Wellness is a resource and guide that advocates using superlative nutrition to heal existing health problems, provide protection against further disease, and halt the premature aging process in its tracks. The information in this book can help people to make crucial choices that will lead to vigorous health—safely, naturally, and inexpensively, as our Creator provided and intended. Included is vital evidence of inherent dangers from the way food is farmed, processed, transported/ imported, and prepared, and how to fight the growing effects on health.

Growing research and evidence support what I have been asserting all along—food fights disease. I predict that nutrition will emerge as the cornerstone of preventative medicine and be recognized as the key to health and longevity in the very near future. For my readers, the future is right now.

PART ONE

===

NUTRITIONAL ROADS TO HEALTH

INTRODUCTION

Each day, scientists and researchers worldwide seek cures for the growing number of diseases, including infectious diseases, that plague the human, animal, and plant species of planet Earth. At the same time, strains of infectious organisms that cause diseases for which there had been cures, such as tuberculosis, pneumonia, and gonorrhea, have mutated into "super" bugs that are now resistant to those remedies. Viruses and bacteria travel around the world daily, transported by unsuspecting hosts—returning tourists. Young children, older adults, and people with certain chronic diseases are the most susceptible. If that information isn't enough to send you looking for a face mask, then consider even newer threats from bioterrorism, plus the increasing number of environmental hazards that we all must face.

Miraculously, the human body has built-in tools to fend off these microscopic invaders and to fight or prevent many disorders, including cancer and heart disease. We know that when serious outbreaks of potentially deadly infectious diseases hit, not everyone gets sick, and among those who are stricken, not everyone dies. Acquired immunodeficiency syndrome (AIDS) is a prime example. From the beginning of the epidemic, there have been some individuals who, though infected with HIV, the virus that causes AIDS, nevertheless remained healthy for many years.

The body's ability to fight off offending organisms is determined by the functioning of the immune system, our front-line defense against biological invasion. This brilliantly responsive system may be weakened or strengthened, depending, in part, on some of the lifestyle choices we make. Sleep deprivation, stress, drug use, poor diet, and emotional trauma are just a few things that weaken the immune system. A healthy diet that is packed with phytochemicals, proper exercise, and certain nutritional supplements and herbs, on the other hand, can greatly strengthen it.

In Part One, we will examine the threshold that leads to optimum health. A properly functioning immune system is the vital foundation on which we build all physical well-being. In it, I provide a simple explanation of how this intricate network of organs, glands, and cells functions together for maximum efficiency. You will learn the symptoms of a failing or depressed immune system and, more important, ways to maintain, restore, and repair it in times of crisis. Simply put, good health starts here.

CHAPTER ONE

THE IMMUNE SYSTEM: THE FOUNDATION OF HEALTH

Clearly, if disease is manmade, it can also be man-prevented. It should be the function of medicine to help people die young as late in life as possible.

—*Dr. Ernst Wunder, President, American Health Foundation (1975)*

The entire physical healing process is engineered by the immune system. It is truly the healing power within. This complex network of cells and biochemicals is the front-line defense system against viruses, fungi, and bacteria. The immune system is the key to fighting every insult to the body, from a little shaving nick to a deadly virus like the human immunodeficiency virus (HIV).

Poor diet, daily stress, and exposure to toxins in food, water, and the environment all cause a decline in immune system activity.

A healthy immune system not only defends against infectious diseases, but also can prevent dreaded diseases such as cancer. Scientists have known for years that, regardless of a person's individual genetic makeup, if the body's toxic load is kept under control and the immune system is strong, cancer is unlikely to develop. According to an article by Lorna Vanderhaeghe that was published in edition 6 of *Healthy Immunity*, "Our immune system is the body's most powerful defense against cancer. Treatments should focus on enhancing our immune system's ability to seek and destroy cancerous cells, keeping DHEA at adequate levels, and regulating cortisol. No one nutritional supplement can cure cancer; a multifaceted approach including a diet high in vegetables, fresh fish, and juicing, along with many well-researched nutritional supplements, is the key to ensuring our body can fight cancer from within. Viruses are a known factor in the risk of getting some cancers. [The bacterium] *Helicobacter pylori* is now thought to be a causative agent for stomach cancer; human T-cell lymphoma virus is responsible for T-cell lymphoma; human papillomavirus is involved in cervical cancer; and hepatitis virus is linked to liver cancer."

It is possible that the immune system even extends influence over how people age. Current research suggests that aging may be more closely related to the functioning and effectiveness of the immune system than it is to the passage of time.

It is obvious that understanding how the immune system works and what can be done to keep it functioning at maximum efficiency is a top priority if your goal is optimum health.

IMMUNODEFICIENCY

A weakened immune system results in an increased susceptibility to virtually every type of illness. Common signs of impaired immune function include fatigue, listlessness, repeated colds and infections, inflammation, allergic reactions, slow wound healing, and chronic diarrhea. Infections caused by an overgrowth of some normally present organism, such as oral thrush, systemic candidiasis, or vaginal yeast infections, becomes problematic when immunity is low. Some cases of weakened immunity are a result of immunodeficiency disorders, such as HIV/AIDS, or chronic or prolonged health problems like leukemia, diabetes, mononucleosis, and chronic hepatitis.

AUTOIMMUNITY

Proper immune function is an intricate balancing act. While inadequate immunity predisposes one to infectious illnesses of every type, it is also possible to become ill as a result of an immune response that is too strong or directed at an inappropriate target. Many different disorders, including allergies, lupus, pernicious anemia, rheumatic heart disease, rheumatoid arthritis, and, possibly, diabetes, have been linked to inappropriate immune system activity. Consequently, they are known as autoimmune, or "self-attacking-self," disorders.

Researchers are discovering that an overactive immune system just might be one of the causes of severe depression. Levels of the neurotransmitter serotonin are often lower than normal in depressed people, and immune-boosting substances can deplete tryptophan, a precursor the body uses to make serotonin. If this process goes on for too long, it may affect moods and cause depression.

HOW THE IMMUNE SYSTEM WORKS

The basic task of the immune system is to identify what is "self" (naturally belonging in the body) and what is "nonself" (foreign or otherwise harmful material), and then neutralize or destroy that which is nonself. The immune system is not a physical structure, but a complex of interactions involving many different organ structures and substances. Among them are white blood cells, bone marrow, appendix, tonsils, thymus, spleen, lymphatic vessels and organs (specialized cells found in various body tissues), and substances called serum factors present in the blood. All of these components work together to protect the body against infection and disease. From birth, immunity develops as the body matures and learns to identify and defend itself against foreign invaders, called antigens. The immune system learns to identify and then remember specific antigens as they are encountered.

Now let us look more closely at some of the important parts of the immune system and what they do.

The Lymphatic System

A main component of immunity is the lymphatic system. This is composed of a number of different organs (including the spleen, the thymus, the tonsils, and the lymph nodes) and fluid, called lymph, that circulates through the lymphatic vessels in the body and also bathes the body's cells. The lymphatic system provides a kind of continuous cleansing that operates at the cellular level. It is through the lymphatic system that fluid from the spaces between cells is drained, taking with it waste products, toxins, and other debris from the tissues. As it passes through the lymphatic vessels, the lymph flows through the lymph nodes, where macrophages (a subgroup of white blood cells that "eat" invaders) filter out the undesirables. From there, the lymph returns to the bloodstream.

The Spleen

The spleen is an organ located on the left side of the upper abdomen that filters the blood and removes and breaks down old red blood cells that need replacing. Present in the spleen are an assortment of immune cells, including macrophages, dendritic cells, red blood cells, killer cells, and B and T lymphocytes (often referred to simply as B and T cells). Antigens, which are usually proteins, are brought to the spleen through the bloodstream and are held in place by dendritic cells while B or T cells learn to manufacture the appropriate antibodies in response to them. People whose spleens have been removed tend to be more prone to illness because these important functions are no longer performed.

The Thymus

The thymus is a small glandlike organ located behind the top of the breastbone. It is in the thymus that T cells mature. T cells help the immune system by secreting a number of body chemicals—namely interleukin 1, interleukin 2, and interferon—and by activating B cells so that they produce antibodies. Also in the thymus, maturing T cells that might cause harm by responding to the body's tissues as nonself are destroyed, while those that appropriately recognize antigens are allowed to mature and then enter the bloodstream.

Bone Marrow

The soft, spongy tissue found in the center of the bones, bone marrow produces a variety of immune cells, including new white blood cells, platelets, B cells, killer cells, granulocytes, and thymocytes. All white blood cells are made from stem cells. Stem cells branch out and have the capacity to become many different types of cells. Some of the white blood cells made in the bone marrow leave the bone marrow and mature elsewhere in the body, while others mature in the bone marrow and support the immune system. Once mature, white blood cells are larger than red blood cells. They can move independently in the bloodstream, and are able to pass through cell walls. This enables them to travel quickly to the site of an injury or infection.

The Appendix and Tonsils

The appendix, also known as the *vermiform appendix,* is a tiny tubelike structure attached to the large intestine. The tonsils are two small masses of lymphatic tissue located in the throat. Although their precise functions are not well understood, it is now generally accepted that both the appendix and the tonsils also support the immune system.

PROPER CARE OF THE IMMUNE SYSTEM

As marvelous as it is, the immune system can safeguard health only if it is cared for properly. This means getting all the right nutrients, providing a healthy environment, and avoiding those things that tend to depress immunity. Many elements of the environment today compromise our immune systems' defensive abilities. The chemicals in household cleaners; the overuse of antibiotics and other drugs; the antibiotics, pesticides, and myriad additives present in the foods we eat; the exposure to environmental pollutants; and even the air we breathe all place a strain on the immune system. (These subjects will be discussed in detail in Chapter 26.) In 1987, the National Academy of Sciences reported that "fifteen percent of the U.S. population has an increased allergic sensitivity to chemicals commonly found in household products such as detergents, solvents, pesticides, metals and rubber, thus placing them at increased risk of disease."

Another factor that adversely affects the immune system is stress. Stress results in a sequence of biochemical events that ultimately suppresses the normal activity of white blood cells and places undue demands on the endocrine system, as well as depletes the body of needed nutrients. The result is impaired healing ability and lowered defense against infection.

The food and herbs outlined throughout this book are designed to strengthen the immune system, whether it is damaged as a result of disease, stress, inadequate nutrition, poor living habits, alcohol or drug use, chemotherapy, or a combination of one or more of these factors. Each of the foods and herbs will be discussed in more detail in later sections; however, following is a brief preview of some of the most important items in each of these categories.

Immune-Boosting Foods

Supply your immune system with adequate amounts of nutrients that promote proper immune function. Compounds known as antioxidants—particularly vitamins A, C, and E; selenium; and zinc—as well as other vitamins and minerals, help to maintain a powerful immune response. Selenium is lacking in most of our soils, so it may be necessary to take supplements to get enough.

All fresh fruits and berries are beneficial for the immune system, but particularly good choices include apricots, kiwis, avocados, blueberries, blackberries, and strawberries. Among the best vegetables are broccoli, Brussels sprouts, spinach, kale, watercress, turnip greens, collards, carrots, squash, sweet potatoes, red and orange sweet peppers, and (for selenium) onions and garlic. Barley, a grain, is also good. If possible, try to eat at least half of your fresh fruits and green leafy vegetables raw.

Lactobacillus acidophilus is a type of friendly bacteria that normally resides in the intestinal tract. A good way to maintain or replenish your body's stores of this bacteria is to eat plain yogurt (preferably nondairy yogurt such as soymilk yogurt) labeled "live culture." Yogurt also contains vitamin A, vitamin D, and the B-complex vitamins. Acidophilus is also available in capsules that may be taken orally or blended into juices. Natren is one company that makes quality acidophilus products; Wakunaga of America Company has a dairy-free acidophilus supplement that is good for vegetarians and dairy-sensitive people. (See the RESOURCES section for more information about the companies mentioned in this book.) Take acidophilus capsules on an empty stomach, in the morning and before each meal. Do not take them at the same time as antibiotics, because antibiotics will kill off the good bacteria along with the bad.

Garlic and yogurt are foods that stimulate macrophages. Zinc-rich foods, which are also important for immune function, include brewer's yeast, fish, legumes, mushrooms, oysters, pecans, all types of seeds, soybeans, soy lecithin, and whole grains.

Additional beneficial foods are chlorella and pearl barley. These foods contain germanium, a trace element beneficial for the immune system. It is also a good idea to include kelp in your diet in the form of giant red kelp or brown kelp. Kelp contains protein as well as the nutrients carotene, calcium, iodine, iron, vitamin B_2 (riboflavin), and vitamin C, all of which are necessary for the immune system's functional integrity.

Chinese herbalists have long considered mushrooms to be the most beneficial of all medicinal foods; however, the ordinary culinary mushrooms found at the supermarket are not as advantageous to the immune system as the more exotic reishi, maitake, or shiitake mushrooms. Modern research has determined that these mushrooms can support immune function. Extracts of these mushrooms can be purchased in capsule form.

Herbs for Immunity

Aloe vera has been found to "turn on" the immune system by activating macrophages. It also provides enzymes, vitamins, and minerals the immune system needs to function properly.

Astragalus boosts the immune system and generates anticancer cells in the body. It also stimulates the activity of T-helper cells (the type of immune cell depleted by HIV/AIDS), acts as an antioxidant, protects the liver from toxins, and boosts energy. You should not use this herb if you have a fever, however, as it can make fever worse.

Bayberry, fenugreek, hawthorn, horehound, licorice root, and red clover all enhance the immune response. A word of caution, though: If overused, licorice root can elevate blood pressure. Do not use this herb on a daily basis for more than seven days in a row. Avoid it entirely if you have high blood pressure.

Black radish, burdock root, dandelion, milk thistle, and red clover help to cleanse the liver and the bloodstream. The liver is the body's primary organ of detoxification and must function optimally for the immune system—indeed, for the entire body—to be healthy.

Boxthorn seed, ginseng, suma, and wisteria are herbs that contain germanium, a trace element that aids immune function and has anticancer properties. You should not use ginseng if you have high blood pressure, however.

Cat's claw boosts immune function, fights infection, and reduces inflammation.

Echinacea boosts the immune system and enhances lymphatic function. You should not use it have an autoimmune disorder, however.

Ginkgo biloba is good for brain cells, aids circulation throughout the body, and is a powerful antioxidant. You should not take ginkgo if you are taking blood-thinning medication or if you have a clotting disorder.

St. John's wort is a natural blood purifier and has been found in laboratory studies to have antiviral activity that fights HIV and viruses in the herpes family, including the Epstein-Barr virus. It is also used as a treatment for mild to moderate depression; depressed mood can lower immunity.

Ligustrum (known in Chinese herbology as *nu zhen zi*) increases the production of lymphocytes in the bone marrow as well as their maturation into T cells. It is beneficial for thymus and spleen health and inhibits tumor growth.

Picrorrhiza, an Indian herb used in Ayurvedic medicine, is a powerful immunostimulant that boosts all aspects of immune function.

In addition to individual herbs that aid immunity, there are a number of combination herbal supplement products that may be beneficial. Esberitox from Enzymatic Therapy is one. ImmunoCare from Himalaya USA is an Ayurvedic remedy containing herbs that may protect white blood cells.

Nutrients Vital to Immune Health

Even the best regimen of food and herbs may not be able to bolster a failing immune system that is under attack. For that reason, along with food sources, certain nutrients should be taken in supplement form during crisis or to help rebuild faulty or depressed immunity. For detailed information on recommended supplements and the dosages to use for specific problems or during times of physical crisis, refer to the book *Prescription for Nutritional Healing* (Avery/Penguin Putnam, 2000). Information about pharmafoods—healing foods—that are rich in these nutrients can be found in chapters 6 and 7.

Following is a summary of some of the individual nutrients and other substances that are most important for healthy immunity:

- Vitamin A and the carotenoids, a group of related nutrients, are anti-infection vitamins. Vitamin A is a cell-signaling vitamin that supports immunity by helping to maintain the surfaces of the body's mucous membranes. If used properly and in moderate doses, vitamin A is rarely toxic and is a very important part of the body's frontline defense system. However, pregnant women should not take large doses (usually defined as more than 5,000 international units daily), as some studies suggest vitamin A may cause cancer in a developing fetus. Rather than using vitamin A, a pregnant woman should take 10,000 international units of beta-carotene or a carotenoid complex daily. The body converts beta-carotene into vitamin A only as needed, and it has no known side effects. Food sources of these nutrients include animal livers, fish liver oils, and green and yellow fruits and vegetables. Significant amounts can be found in apricots, asparagus, beet greens, broccoli, cantaloupe, carrots, collards, dandelion greens, dulse, garlic, kale, mustard greens, papayas, peaches, pumpkin, red peppers, spinach, spirulina, sweet potatoes, Swiss chard, turnip greens, watercress, and yellow squash. Animal sources of vitamin A are up to six times as strong as vegetable sources. Beta-carotene, the best known of the carotenoids, is converted into vitamin A by the body. It may be beneficial for the body's surveillance to detect viruses and tumors. Research has shown it to have a powerful effect in boosting the activity of the class of immune cells known as natural killer cells in older men. Red, orange, and yellow vegetables generally contain high levels of carotenes.

- Alpha-lipoic acid is a substance that is involved in the production of energy from glucose. It is a more potent antioxidant than vitamins C and E. It is both water and fat soluble, so it can protect cells from toxins both inside and outside. People with diabetes should note that it can lower glucose levels, improve insulin sensitivity, and help the body burn glucose. Good food sources are spinach, broccoli, beef, yeast, kidney, and heart.

- Pyridoxal-5-phosphate, a form of vitamin B_6, is involved in more bodily functions than almost any other single nutrient. It affects both mental and physical health and plays a role in the body's defenses against cancer. Food sources include brewer's yeast, carrots, chicken, eggs, fish, meat, peas, spinach, sunflower seeds, walnuts, and wheat germ.

- Beta-1,3-D-glucan is a polysaccharide (a complex type of carbohydrate molecule) that stimulates the activity of macrophages, immune cells that destroy cellular debris by surrounding and digesting them. It interacts with immune system cells and turns on their anticancer activity. Oats, barley, mushrooms, and yeast contain beta-glucans.

- Vitamin C may be the single most important vitamin for the immune system. It is essential for the formation of adrenal hormones and the production of lymphocytes. It also has a direct effect on bacteria and viruses. Vitamin C cannot be manufactured or stored by the body, so daily dietary sources or supplements are mandatory for good immune function. When taken in supplement form, vitamin C should be combined with bioflavonoids, natural plant substances that enhance the absorption and reinforce the action of this vitamin. Vitamin C is found in berries, citrus fruits, and green vegetables. Good sources are asparagus, avocados, beet greens, broccoli, Brussels sprouts, cantaloupe, collards, dandelion greens, dulse, grapefruit, kale, lemons, mangoes, mustard greens, onions, oranges, green peas, pineapple, radishes, rose hips, spinach, strawberries, Swiss chard, tomatoes, turnip greens, and watercress.

- Calcium D-glucarate, a natural substance in apples, grapefruits, grapes, sprouts, and cruciferous vegetables (broccoli, cauliflower, and cabbage), increases the production of key enzymes and helps to bind estrogen in the liver so that excesses of this hormone can be excreted, thus helping with the body's detoxification process.

- Coenzyme Q_{10} is a powerful antioxidant with antibacterial, antitumor, and antiviral properties. It is found in high concentrations in heart muscle, so it is an important nutrient for people with cardiovascular disorders. Coen-

Eternal Youth Laws

Dietary wellness is the foundation for having a healthier, happier, more youthful life, and actually reversing aging and disease. Do you really care enough about yourself to gain optimum health? Staying young for life is a choice!

Obey the following rules to stay well, to keep your immune system functioning properly, to prevent disease, and to add life to your years and years to your life:

- Be aware that maintaining a healthy diet must be a lifelong endeavor.
- Chew your food well. Digestion starts in the mouth.
- Avoid ice-cold beverages. Do not drink beverages with meals.
- Do not eat heavy foods upon rising or before retiring.
- Eat only when you are very hungry, then just until you are no longer hungry.
- Do not consume saturated fats. (See Chapter 28.)
- Consume a diet consisting of 50 percent raw foods. Purchase organic foods when possible.
- Avoid precooked and processed foods. These processes destroy the natural enzymes and nutrients in food. Consuming precooked and processed foods overworks the organs.
- Steam, broil, or bake foods, and cook vegetables very lightly—they should still be crunchy.
- Omit from your diet white flour, white sugar, white rice, and iodized table salt.
- Cleanse your system periodically by fasting with pure, fresh juices. (See Chapter 4.)

- Consume foods free of toxic insecticides, chemicals, preservatives, and additives.
- Avoid tobacco, caffeine, drugs, stress, and excessive consumption of alcohol.
- Take a quality multivitamin and mineral supplement daily.
- Drink six to eight glasses of quality water daily. (See Chapter 15.)
- Exercise daily. Include walking, stretching, and enjoying fresh air and sunshine.
- Keep active both mentally and physically, and get plenty of rest.
- Maintain a positive state of mind and be grateful for who and where you are.
- Actively nourish your spiritual side, through prayer, meditation, or whatever practice is meaningful to you. Be thankful for everything.
- Do not expect the impossible. Set realistic goals and achieve them.

zyme Q_{10} is present in fatty fish and organ meats, but it is hard to obtain enough from these sources, so a supplement is recommended. The body's storehouse of coenzyme Q_{10} declines with age, so people age fifty or older produce only half the amount they did at age twenty. The best food sources are mackerel, salmon, and sardines. Small amounts are present in beef, peanuts, and spinach.

- Colostrum is a thin, yellowish fluid secreted by mammals after giving birth, and before the true milk comes in. It sets the stage for the immune system at the beginning of life, and studies indicate it possesses micronutrients that are beneficial throughout life. Bovine (cow) colostrum is available in supplement form.

- Vitamin E, a primary antioxidant and scavenger of toxic free radicals, interacts with vitamins A and C and the mineral selenium. Its antioxidant activity is crucial to cardiovascular health. Thus, vitamin E is an integral part of the body's defense system. Vitamin E is found in cold-pressed vegetable oils, dark green leafy vegetables, legumes, nuts, seeds, whole grains, brown rice, cornmeal, dulse, eggs, kelp, desiccated liver, milk, oatmeal,

organ meats, soybeans, sweet potatoes, watercress, wheat, and wheat germ.

- Essential fatty acids (EFAs), particularly the class of EFAs designated omega-3, are essential for a healthy immune system. Good food sources include marine fish, fish oil, and flaxseed oil.

- Manganese is a mineral that is important to the immune system and is necessary for healthy growth. It can be found in dried beans, blueberries and blackberries, carrots, bran, some types of nuts, oatmeal, peanuts, peas, seaweed, spinach, and whole grains.

- Zinc boosts the immune system and promotes the healing of wounds when consumed at appropriate doses (100 milligrams or less daily). It also helps to protect the liver. More than 100 milligrams per day may actually depress immune function, however. Food sources are brewer's yeast, fish, oysters, legumes, lima beans, mushrooms, pecans, all seeds, soy lecithin, soybeans, and whole grains.

- A number of amino acids also aid in proper immune function. *Glutathione* is a powerful antioxidant produced in the liver that protects the cells from damage by free radicals. *Methionine* neutralizes the most dangerous types of free radicals. Food sources of methionine are beans, eggs, lentils, fish, garlic, meat, onions, soybeans, seeds, and yogurt. *Taurine* is necessary for the production of white blood cells. Food sources of taurine are eggs, fish, meat, and milk.

Other Considerations

Take an inventory of the factors that may be compromising your immune system, then take steps to correct them. Two of the most common immune suppressors include stress and an improper diet, especially a diet high in fat and refined processed foods.

As much as possible, avoid stress, and learn techniques to help you cope with stress you cannot avoid. "Stress is one of the biggest suppressors of our immune system," according to Amy Turnbull, N.D., of Seattle's Bastyr Center for Natural Health. "It increases the level of adrenal gland hormones, including adrenaline and corticosteroids and inhibits immune function." It has long been known that your mental state can affect your immune response. A positive frame of mind is important in building up the immune system.

Consume "green drinks" to build or boost your immune system (more about these in Chapter 5). Avoid overconsuming animal products, processed foods, sugar, and soft drinks. Avoid overeating in general.

Follow a fasting program once a month to rid your body of toxins that can weaken your immune system. (See Chapter 4.) Use spirulina and/or wheat grass, especially while fasting. Spirulina is a naturally digestible food that aids in protecting the immune system. It supplies many nutrients plus protein needed for cleansing and healing.

Be sure to get sufficient sleep. Much of the regeneration and healing of the body happens during sleep.

Get regular moderate exercise (but don't overdo it). Exercise reduces stress and elevates mood, which has a positive effect on immune response. It also helps to maintain the immune system by promoting blood circulation and ensuring a plentiful supply of oxygen to every part of the body.

Do not smoke or consume beverages containing alcohol or caffeine, and do not take any drugs except those prescribed by your physician. The recreational drug MDMA (ecstasy), which is chemically related to amphetamines, has been shown to cause a dramatic fall in the level of immune system T cells, which are needed to help fight infections. Marijuana use weakens the immune system. Delta-9 tetrahydrocannabinol (THC), the most active compound in marijuana, alters the normal immune response, making white blood cells 35 to 40 percent less effective than normal.

Toxic metals suppress the immune system. A hair analysis can be used to check for heavy metal intoxication. (More information about this can be found in Part Six.)

An underactive thyroid usually results in immune deficiency. A thorough physical examination should include a blood test to evaluate your thyroid function. Food allergies and adverse food reactions also can place stress on the immune system.

Research has shown that the hormone dehydroepiandrosterone (DHEA) may enhance immune function. Another hormone, melatonin, which is produced by the pineal gland, stimulates the immune system. Human growth hormone (HGH) strengthens the immune system as well. This hormone is naturally produced by the body, but levels decline with age. Treatment with supplemental HGH requires the supervision of a physician.

The information in this chapter is some of the most important in this book. Without a strong immune system, your ability to fight illness and disease will be greatly compromised.

CHAPTER TWO

BASIC DIETARY GUIDELINES

My mother's menu consisted of two choices: Take it . . . or leave it.

—*Buddy Hackett, comedian*

The purpose of this book is to help you understand how and why the choices you make concerning the food you eat affect every single area of your life. Deciding what to eat may be the single most important choice you make each day. Food affects how you look; how you feel; how much energy you have; how healthy (or ill) you are, including your odds of developing cancer, heart disease, and other chronic illnesses; how much you weigh; how much "brain power" you have; how healthy any future children will be; how strong your sex drive is; and whether you will age with vitality or with diminished capacity.

Research has shown, at a molecular level, why you are indeed what you eat. Using that information, I have devised some simple basic dietary guidelines that form the basis of recommendations on using nutrition to fuel, nurture, and heal your body. This chapter serves as an introduction to basics that underlie the more detailed information that follows in the rest of the book.

First, it is wise to always to eat a variety of food. This helps to minimize the possibility of repeated exposure to the same pesticide residues and other toxins and unnatural, harmful things that may be attached to foods or introduced during the growth cycle. It also ensures that you will be getting a wide range of necessary nutrients. Foods are handled and grown differently in different parts of the country. Foods rich in valuable nutrients, phytochemicals, and antioxidants work synergistically with one another to create maximum healing potential.

Second, try to introduce "live foods," such as raw fruits and vegetables and freshly made fruit and vegetable juices, into your diet as much as possible for maximum nutritional benefit. Cooking greatly reduces the vitamin and mineral content of foods. Use raw fruits and vegetables for snacks (these are great for children) instead of processed and junk foods.

Foods that can be eaten plentifully are fresh fruits and vegetables, steamed vegetables, nuts (except for peanuts,

seeds, beans, legumes), and whole grains. Avoid or strictly limit sugar, salt, dairy products, red meat, white-flour products, caffeine-containing drinks, and eggs. Especially avoid processed foods and foods that contain or have been fried in hydrogenated oils. One easy rule of thumb is simply not to eat white foods (except for cauliflower) as much as possible. Color in food is a sign of vitamin content, so avoid bleached celery and bleached endive; choose yellow turnips over white, sweet potatoes over white potatoes, dark green vegetables over light green ones. Use a mixture of colors to get a variety of nutrients.

Purchase organic food whenever possible. This, too, helps to keep down potential exposure to toxins. In commercial agriculture, some food plants are treated with dangerous pesticides, and the resulting food can be laced with pesticide residue. If food is cosmetically perfect, odds are that it has encountered high amounts of pesticides in the growing cycle. The occasional imperfections found in organic fruits and vegetables may mean that even insects are smart enough to choose food that is free from harmful substances, so don't be alarmed if you find a few signs of pests in your organic grains and produce. You will never find these in highly processed or chemically treated foods. If you choose to have meat in your diet, try to buy organically or range-fed meat and poultry. The antibiotics and hormones used in conventionally produced meat, eggs, and milk can have a multitude of adverse affects on the human body.

Eat plenty of foods that are rich in fiber, which speeds the elimination of dangerous toxins through the intestinal tract, binding and neutralizing them before they can do any harm. Fiber should be part of every meal. It is found in whole grains, beans, legumes, vegetables, and fruits. Processed foods often lack fiber, so be sure to include fresh food in every meal. In addition to preventing constipation, fiber also cuts down on allergic reactions to food and on fluctuations in blood sugar levels. Fiber is the internal "broom" that sweeps the colon. It is particularly important to eat fiber if you have diabetes.

Reduce your consumption of foods that are high in fat. Toxins are concentrated in the fat of animals and in the saturated fats used in commercial cooking. Eating out in restaurants or consuming fast foods generally introduces unhealthy fats into meals. Toxins are also concentrated in the liver. Do not consume liver or other organ meats.

Avoid highly processed foods like ketchup, beef jerky, luncheon meats, and hot dogs, potato chips, and French fries. All of these are more likely than other types of foods to contain potentially dangerous concentrations of toxins. Recent studies have shown that eating processed foods, including potato chips, French fries, some types of breakfast cereals, breads, and other fried or baked starchy foods can lead to a buildup of high levels of acrylamide, a substance that has been found to cause cancer in laboratory animals. While dangers to humans have not yet been proven, some Swedish scientists have said they believe that foodborne acrylamide may be responsible for several hundred cases of cancer annually in their country. The U.S. Food and Drug Administration (FDA) and similar agencies in several other countries have made the study of acrylamide in foods a top priority. To be on the safe side, either remove these foods from your diet or strictly limit them, and instead eat plenty of fruits and vegetables.

Avoid stale food. Buy the freshest food your market has. Ask on what days they receive the fresh produce. Even better, start a garden and grow your own organic food. If you cannot always purchase fresh vegetables, choose frozen over canned. Food that is flash-frozen retains more nutrients than canned food.

Eating food in the correct combinations is important. (This will be discussed in detail in Chapter 19.)

Choose cooking methods that minimize losses of vitamins and minerals. For vegetables, the best method is to steam the vegetables lightly and eat them while they are still crunchy. When steaming vegetables, use as little water as possible and save the water once they are finished cooking—use the vegetable water for soup stock so that you get the benefit of all the nutrients dissolved in the water. Avoid frying (with the exception of stir-frying) entirely. Always remember that every cooking method has its drawbacks and may destroy vitamin value to a certain extent. Cook vegetables, except for dried peas and beans, as lightly as possible. Vegetables taste, keep their color, and retain their nutrients better when not overcooked.

As long as you are eating organic produce, do not discard the edible green outer leaves of vegetables like cabbage, broccoli, and lettuce. Encourage the grocer to leave the outer green leaves on. The outer leaves have been kissed with sunlight and are filled with vitamins and minerals. Do, however, wash all fresh foods thoroughly, especially melons. There have been several documented cases of Salmonella poisoning that resulted from cutting melons before washing them—the knife transferred the bacteria from the exterior rind to the fruit within. Wash the knife blade used to cut the rind before cutting the fruit, as it may have picked up harmful bacteria, mold, or pesticides from the rind. Washing will also help to eliminate waxes and the bacteria encountered in the supermarket from handling.

Refrigerate all fresh foods or cooked foods quickly, before bacteria and mold can form. Taking food directly from the store to the refrigerator is the best way to prevent foodborne illness. Your refrigerator and microwave oven can be breeding grounds for bacteria—be sure to keep surfaces clean in both. Do not use the same cutting board for poultry or meat as for vegetables. This is important; Salmonella bacteria can be transferred if you fail to do this. Be careful with all canned foods. If the top is not tight, if there are noticeable dents or bulges, throw it away.

Store grains in a cool, dry place. Place bay leaves in containers to deter insects but accept the fact that food without insecticides might have a few bugs. A healthy bug is less dangerous than poisonous chemicals. If you find a bug in grains or flours, do not panic. Instead, pay more attention to insects and all other life forms. They can tell us a lot. Insects usually do not choose food that is laced with chemicals. They seem always to pick the organically grown grains over others.

Avoid eating burned foods. Burning can cause the formation of carcinogens (cancer-causing substances). There are studies that indicate it is best to limit our intake of charcoal-grilled food as well.

Buy only frozen fish unless you know and trust the source. "Fresh fish" in a grocer's case may have been around several days. Not only does it have the potential to make you sick, but it also has lost its nutritional value. Do not eat raw fish.

Avoid foreign-made dinnerware, glassware, and other tableware. They may contain leaded glasses and glazes that may leach lead into your food. Also, avoid antique crystal dishes and other dinnerware made in the United States before 1971, when the lead-based paint poisoning prevention act was passed. This act prohibited the application of lead-based paints to any cooking, eating, or drinking utensil; any toy or article of furniture; and any residential structure constructed or rehabilitated by or with the assistance of the federal government.

If you must use a microwave oven to heat food, do not use plastic wrap or plastic containers to do so. Use glass containers instead. Also, use only glass for food storage. Using plastic, especially for heating or reheating, can result in petrochemicals leaching into your food.

Eat lightly. Eating too much at one time overloads the stomach and the resulting pressure can force acid to back up into the esophagus, leading to heartburn, gas, and bloating. Eating too much in general results in obesity and all of the health problems that come with it. These foods are high in fat and, therefore, calories. Also, high fat content or spicy foods put stress on the gallbladder and the liver, often resulting in heartburn and indigestion.

Dietary Changes That Promote Wellness

Even among basically healthy foods, some individual items are better for you than others. Use the following table as a guide when deciding which types of food to include in your diet and which ones to avoid in order to maintain good health.

Type of Food	Avoid	Enjoy!
Beans	Canned pork and beans, canned beans with salt or preservatives, frozen beans.	All beans cooked without animal fat or salt.
Beverages	Alcoholic drinks, coffee, cocoa, pasteurized and/or sweetened juices and fruit drinks, sodas, tea (except herbal tea).	Herbal teas, fresh vegetable and fruit juices, cereal grain beverages (often sold as coffee substitutes), mineral or distilled water.
Dairy products	All soft cheeses, all pasteurized or artificially colored cheese products, ice cream.	Raw goat cheese, nonfat cottage cheese, kefir, unsweetened yogurt, goat's milk, raw or skim milk, buttermilk.
Eggs	Fried or pickled.	Boiled or poached (limit of four weekly).
Fish	All fried fish, all shellfish, salted fish, anchovies, herring, fish canned in oil.	All freshwater white fish, salmon, broiled or baked fish, water-packed tuna.
Fruits	Canned, bottled, or frozen fruits with sweeteners added; oranges.	All fresh, frozen, stewed, or dried fruits without sweeteners (except oranges, which are acidic and highly allergenic), unsulfured fruits, home-canned fruits.
Grains	All white flour products, white rice, pasta, crackers, cold cereals, instant types of oatmeal and other hot cereals.	All whole grains and products containing whole grains: cereals, breads, muffins, whole-grain crackers, cream of wheat or rye cereal, buckwheat, millet, oats, brown rice, wild rice. (Limit yeast breads to three servings per week.)
Meats	Beef; all forms of pork; hot dogs; luncheon meats; smoked, pickled, and processed meats; corned beef; duck; goose; spare ribs; gravies; organ meats.	Skinless turkey and chicken, lamb. (Limit meat to three 3-oz servings per week.)
Nuts	All salted or roasted nuts; peanuts (if suffering from any disorder).	All fresh raw nuts (peanuts in moderation only).
Oils (fats)	All saturated fats, hydrogenated margarine, refined processed oils, shortenings, hardened oils.	All cold-pressed oils: corn, safflower, sesame, olive, flaxseed, soybean, sunflower, and canola oils; margarine made from these oils; eggless mayonnaise.
Seasonings	Black or white pepper, salt, hot red peppers, all types of vinegar except pure natural apple cider vinegar.	Garlic, onions, cayenne, Spike, all herbs, dried vegetables, apple cider vinegar, tamari, miso, seaweed, dulse.
Soups	Canned soups made with salt, preservatives, MSG, or fat stock; all creamed soups.	Homemade (salt- and fat-free) bean, lentil, pea, vegetable, barley, brown rice, onion.
Sprouts and seeds	All seeds cooked in oil or salt.	All slightly cooked sprouts (except alfalfa, which should be raw and washed thoroughly), wheatgrass, all raw seeds.
Sweets	White, brown, or raw cane sugar, corn syrups, chocolate, sugar candy, fructose (except that in fresh whole fruit), all syrups (except pure maple syrup), all sugar substitutes, jams and jellies made with sugar.	Barley malt or rice syrup, small amounts of raw honey, pure maple syrup, stevia, unsulfured blackstrap molasses.
Vegetables	All canned or frozen with salt or additives.	All raw, fresh, frozen (no additives), or home-canned without salt (undercook vegetables slightly).

Last, but most important, eat all natural foods that do not contain additives and chemicals. Most processed foods are simply empty calories that add to weight gain and provide little to no nutritional value. Fresh fruits, vegetables, legumes, nuts and seeds, and unrefined grains (no white bread or rice!) are always the best selections. The chapters that follow will help you to choose a diet that nurtures and heals, and to understand how to achieve the many and varied benefits of eating for health.

PART TWO

THE FASTEST PATHS TO HEALING

INTRODUCTION

Most of us already know that if the body is not properly maintained, it will break down. Just like an automobile or any other internal combustion engine, we need the right mixture of fuel and oxygen (food, water, and air), generous lubrication (dietary fats), and electrical energy (vitamins and minerals). Without proper maintenance, our health will eventually fail, leaving us the option to rejuvenate, rehabilitate, or set our affairs in order.

Part Two gives you the best methods to use nutrition to keep your body "tuned up" for maximum efficiency, vitality, and healing. It reveals proven powerhouse techniques available to achieve optimum health. We know that juices made from fresh fruits and vegetables are potent healing resources. They make concentrated nutrients and enzymes available instantly to nourish and regenerate cells, tissues, glands, and organs. Some diseases or disorders can even be arrested or healed using live juice therapy.

Consuming raw foods provides the body with live disease-fighting phytochemicals and fiber. Cooking depletes vitamins and phytochemicals, destroys enzymes necessary for easy digestion, and damages fats and protein. Raw food explodes with life and provides the natural balance of fiber, nutrients, and the water we need. Incorporating raw foods into your diet plus some delicious recipes will make it easy for you to utilize this powerful tool for dietary wellness.

In addition to the finest nutritional fuel, it is vitally important to cleanse the body internally and externally to rid it of toxins and accumulated wastes. These built-up toxins contribute to nearly every type of illness and disease. Cleansing is therefore a necessary step on the path to vital health. My recommended cleansing program is a combination of fasting, cleansing enemas, nutritional therapy, and dry-scrubbing of the skin that have been used for centuries to heal illness. Even if cleansing is a new concept to you, this section will give you enough information to successfully incorporate this necessary ingredient into your health regimen.

CHAPTER THREE

THE RAW FOODS STORY:
A PLANET- AND ANIMAL-FRIENDLY PATH

Recent years have seen a renewed interest in incorporating raw foods into the diet, and some people are even making raw foods their entire diet. Eating raw foods has a number of health benefits. The process of cooking food depletes vitamins, destroys enzymes that help digestion, and damages vital fats and proteins. It also results in the creation of free radicals, which are a major contributor to cancer and many other illnesses.

Raw food has a natural balance of the fiber, nutrients, and water that your body needs. It is exploding with life. Fingers, mouths, and tongues never get burned during preparation or consumption. Eating a diet of raw foods provides powerful healing nutrition that can limit or even reverse some chronic diseases. Raw foods are unprocessed, so fat, processed sugar, and additives are not a worry. Vegetarians and others concerned about the unhealthy aspects of eating meat do not have to worry about any such moral or physical implications with a raw-foods diet. And finally, raw food enthusiasts say the diet is earth-friendly because the use of paper and plastic for processing is minimal.

TIPS FOR GOING RAW

At the end of this chapter, you will find a number of raw foods recipes designed to help with specific health conditions. All of these recipes are excellent for making fresh juices as well. When using these or other raw foods recipes, there are a number of general principles to keep in mind.

Shred vegetables either in a food processor or by hand, fresh for each meal. Use a blender for soft foods such as fruits. Do not store them for later use. Raw foods contain live enzymes needed for healing as well as many nutrients, proteins, and substances that speed the healing process and the longer you keep them, the less "life" and nutrients they contain. If it is necessary to store them, keep them in an airtight container in the refrigerator for no more than twenty-four hours.

Do not go overboard on spinach or Swiss chard. These foods contain oxalic acid, which inhibits the absorption of the essential minerals calcium, magnesium, and zinc. Do not omit them from your diet entirely, however, because they do contain important nutrients. Do not eat more than one raw beet and its top daily. Use parsley sparingly; it is a strong diuretic.

If at all possible, eat only fresh organic vegetables. If you are unable to do that, soak all nonorganic vegetables in a mixture of 1 teaspoon of chlorine bleach (Clorox) and 1 gallon of water for five minutes and rinse well. Some newer bleach products may contain a lye mixture. Be sure to use a product that contains chlorine only. Or try using a vegetable and fruit cleanser, available in health food stores. Either treatment helps to removes bacteria and pesticide residues. Scrub root vegetables well with a stiff brush that you use just for food.

If you are on a weight-loss program, omit salad dressings. Instead, squeeze the juice of a fresh lemon on salads—it brings out the flavor of the vegetables. Lemon juice is a great blood purifier and healer.

If you have a lung disorder such as asthma or bronchitis, add grated fresh horseradish to each serving of salad. Add onion for sinus conditions and colds.

Grated raw potatoes, which are high in potassium, are good for people with peptic ulcers, diabetes, and heart disorders. Cut out the center of the potato and discard it. Grate the potato or cut slices about one-inch thick, including the peel.

Raw broccoli can be added to any recipe, or try using any of the other vegetables in the section on cruiferous vegetables in Chapter 9. Be creative with all raw foods; there are so many to choose from.

Another Good Reason to Go Raw

In April 2002, researchers in Sweden announced findings that a substance known as acrylamide was present in certain processed foods. The exact mechanism by which acrylamide forms during commercial food processing is not well understood, but its formation is believed to be related to cooking at high temperatures and/or for long periods of time. Acrylamide is a known carcinogen (cancer-causing agent) and neurotoxin. The Swedish research has been furthered by studies in Norway, Switzerland, United Kingdom, and the United States. All have found acrylamide in starch-based foods subjected to high temperatures, including potato chips, french fries, cookies, cereals, donuts, baked potatoes, and bread. Other foods have not been studied yet to determine their acrylamide content, if any.

The World Health Organization (WHO) collaborated with the Food and Agriculture Organization (FAO) of the United Nations to address the issue of acrylamide in food. Using the limited amount of data available, it concluded that the presence of acrylamide in food is a major concern for the world population. Researchers are further studying how acrylamide forms and exactly which foods are affected. Because so few foods have been studied so far, it is impossible to know for sure which levels of acrylamide are safe and which are not. In the meantime, the WHO and FAO give this advice:

- Do not cook food for extended periods of time or at excessive temperatures. However, certain foods, especially meat products, must still be cooked thoroughly enough to destroy foodborne pathogens.

- Eat a balanced and varied diet, including plenty of fresh raw fruits and vegetables.

- Reduce your consumption of fried and fatty foods.

RAW FOOD RECIPES

Raw Foods Salad No. 1

This combination is good for treating gallbladder problems, cancer, liver disorders, heartburn, indigestion, and all colon disorders.

    1 medium beet
    1 medium carrot
    ¼ head cabbage
    ½ medium apple

Shred the beet, carrot, and cabbage, and slice the apple into bite-sized pieces. Toss all of the ingredients together. Top with salad dressing (see page 21) if desired and serve.

Raw Foods Salad No. 2

This combination is good for people recovering from surgery. It's also good for those with infection and inflammation of the colon, skin disorders, tuberculosis of the bones and lungs, and diabetes.

    1 carrot
    1 stalk celery
    1 turnip
    ½ onion
    ¼ head cabbage

Grate or shred all the ingredients into a medium bowl. Toss together to mix. Top with salad dressing (see page 21) if desired and serve.

Raw Foods Salad No. 3

This combination helps rid the body of toxins and is good for people with intestinal disorders, heart disorders, and high blood pressure. Onions and garlic calm the nerves, and improve the condition of skin, nails, and hair. Celery and cucumbers are very low in calories and are good for weight loss.

    1 stalk celery
    1 green or red bell pepper
    ¼ cucumber
    ¼ onion
    ¼ jicama
    1 clove garlic, crushed

Chop the celery, pepper, cucumber, onion, and jicama into bite-sized pieces and place in a medium bowl. Add the garlic, then toss all of the ingredients together to mix. Top with salad dressing (see page 21) if desired and serve.

Raw Foods Salad No. 4

This is a very effective mix for relieving hemorrhoids. It's also a good general tonic.

    2 carrots
    1 turnip
    ¼ bunch spinach or chicory
    ¼ bunch watercress

Chop the carrots and turnip and tear the spinach or chicory and watercress into bite-sized pieces. Toss all of the ingredients together in a medium bowl. Top with salad dressing (see page 21) if desired and serve.

What You Eat Affects Your Temperament

Research into brain function reveals evidence that the emotions of love, faith, joy, fear, and sadness—and even our sense of purpose in life—are not merely attitudes created through the mind's thought processes. They are actually produced and reinforced by biochemical activity within the brain, which in turn is affected by nutrients supplied by the food we eat. Raw foods contain nutrients needed for proper brain function. Cooking and, especially, processing of foods destroy nutrients needed to avoid anxiety, depression, mood swings, and many other mental and psychological disorders. Until we know more about the connections between food and our emotions, the purest, safest, most animal- and planet-friendly source of nutrition is raw plant foods.

RAW FOODS SALAD NO. 5

This combination is good for people who have anemia or other blood disorders. It can also be processed in a juicer and enjoyed as a juice.

    ½ bunch beet greens
    ½ bunch dandelion greens
    1 leaf kale or mustard greens, or ½ bunch spinach
    1 turnip
    1 clove garlic

Tear the greens and chop the turnips into bite-sized pieces. Mince the garlic. Toss all of the ingredients together in a medium bowl. Top with salad dressing (see page 21) if desired and serve.

RAW FOODS SALAD NO. 6

This combination improves kidney function by reducing water retention. It aids in weight loss and digestion, cleanses the system and the liver, and helps to correct many vitamin deficiencies.

    4 asparagus spears
    ½ bunch dandelion greens (8 leaves)
    ½ jicama
    ¼ cucumber
    ¼ medium bunch parsley
    ¼ medium bunch watercress
    ½ turnip or one stalk of celery

Chop all of the ingredients finely and toss them together in a medium bowl. Top with salad dressing (see page 21) if desired and serve.

RAW FOODS SALAD NO. 7

This combination is good for people with chronic liver disorders, blood disorders, gallbladder problems, and glandular problems.

    1 medium apple
    1 medium beet
    ¼ black radish
    ¼ head red cabbage

Grate or shred all of the ingredients and toss them together in a medium bowl. Top with salad dressing (see page 21) if desired and serve.

RAW FOODS SALAD NO. 8

This recipe is good for growing children and anyone suffering from any form of bone softening. Turnips are high in vitamins A and C, the B-complex vitamins, and the minerals copper, iodine, iron, magnesium, and sulfur. This combination can also be processed in a juicer. The resulting juice is high in usable calcium, magnesium, and potassium.

    1 handful dandelion leaves
    1 large kale leaf
    1 turnip, with 2 of the leaves
    1 carrot

Tear the greens and chop the carrot and turnip into bite-sized pieces. Toss all of the ingredients together in a medium bowl. Top with salad dressing (see page 21) if desired and serve.

RAW FOODS SALAD NO. 9

This combination is good for treating water retention, colon disorders, vitamin deficiencies, cancer, and digestive problems.

    3 radishes
    1 carrot
    1 stalk celery, with the leaves
    ½ cucumber
    ½ medium bunch spinach
    ⅛ medium bunch parsley

Slice the radishes; chop the carrot, celery, and cucumber; and tear the greens into bite-sized pieces. Toss all of the ingredients together in a medium bowl. Top with salad dressing (see page 21) if desired and serve.

RAW FOODS SALAD NO. 10

Use this combination for all chronic diseases, blood disorders, colon cancer, colon disorders, and obesity. It cleanses all the glands and the bloodstream. It is also good, with the addition of a small amount of grated raw horseradish (it is quite strong, so try using a teaspoon at first and then increase if desired), for the lungs and for those with asthma and bronchitis.

1 bunch beet greens
½ bunch romaine lettuce
¼ bunch turnip greens
½ bunch watercress
2 carrots
1 sprig wheatgrass (optional; it has an earthy taste,
    so use it sparingly)

Tear the greens into bite-sized pieces. Grate or shred the carrot and, if using wheatgrass, chop the wheatgrass. Toss all of the ingredients together in a medium bowl. Top with salad dressing (see page 21) if desired and serve.

RAW FOODS SALAD NO. 11

This salad is good for people with cancer, heart disorders, high blood pressure, and viral disorders—virtually any type of illness. If you are very sick, steam the ingredients lightly and use fresh lemon juice in place of salad dressing.

½ cup chopped broccoli
½ cup chopped cauliflower
¼ cup chopped onion
½–1 parsnip
½ carrot

Place the broccoli, cauliflower, and onion in a medium bowl. Grate or shred the parsnip and carrot and add. Toss all of the ingredients together. Top with salad dressing (see page 21) if desired and serve.

RAW FOODS SALAD NO. 12

This combination is excellent for improving thyroid function and treating mineral dysfunctions. It is also good for people with cancer.

1 cup chopped broccoli
½ cup chopped cauliflower
¼ medium bunch parsley
⅛ medium bunch watercress
6 drops World Organic liquid kelp or fresh kelp or
    1 stalk fresh kelp or 1 tablespoon dried kelp
    soaked in quality water

Place the broccoli and cauliflower in a medium bowl. Tear the greens into bite-sized pieces and add. Add the kelp and toss to mix. Top with salad dressing (see page 21) if desired and serve.

POWER FRUIT SALAD

This salad is good for treating inflammation, arthritis, colon disorders, ulcers, stiff muscles, enzyme deficiencies, and heart disorders. It also helps to detoxify the body and aids digestion. Children love this salad; for them, throw in some walnuts or sunflower seeds.

½ fresh papaya
½ banana
½ peach
¼ cup pineapple juice
½ cup chopped fresh pineapple
½ cup seedless grapes
¼ cup blueberries (in season)

Slice the papaya, banana, and peach and place in a medium to large bowl. Pour the pineapple juice over the fruit. Add the pineapple, grapes, and blueberries, and toss gently to mix. Serve.

SALAD DRESSING

Prepare this dressing ahead for use on any of the vegetable salads in this chapter.

1 cup pure virgin olive or canola oil
¼ cup pure apple cider or balsamic vinegar
¼ cup quality water
1 tablespoon honey
1 teaspoon chopped parsley
¼ teaspoon barley malt concentrate or brown rice
    syrup or sweetener of your choice
1 dash garlic powder
1 dash onion powder
1 dash powdered kelp (optional)

Add all of ingredients to a jar or bottle with a tightly fitting lid. Shake well to mix. Shake again before using.

CHAPTER FOUR

CLEANSING AND HEALING: PREVENT TOXIC OVERLOAD

Fasting can restore health where other methods fail.

—*Paavo Airola, N.D., nutritionist and author*

A buildup of toxins in the body contributes to nearly every type of illness. Toxic overload is also the primary cause of liver damage. The best way to reduce the body's load of toxins is with a cleansing and healing program. A combination of internal and external body cleansing has been used for centuries to help heal the sick.

The first step in any cleansing and healing program is to rid the body of toxins and the waste accumulated primarily in the colon. The cleansing program recommended in this chapter—a combination of fasting, enemas, nutritional therapy, and dry-scrubbing the skin—is most beneficial if it is repeated on a regular basis, or at least once every two months.

FASTING

You can add years to your life by periodic fasting. Even a one-day liquid fast is beneficial. Fasting gives the organs a much-needed rest and helps the body to heal more quickly. When the liver, kidneys, and bloodstream have been cleansed, the body is better able to flush out the toxins that have built up in the colon. Harmful bacteria and parasites flourish in a toxic colon and cause malabsorption of nutrients, skin eruptions, bad breath, and even body odor. Some of the other possible effects are mental confusion, liver spots, stiffness of the joints, and headaches.

Juice or Water Fasting?

The digestive process consumes a large amount of energy. Taking in only liquids while fasting allows more of the body's energy to go to the healing process. There are several different approaches to fasting. Some people advocate consuming only water while on a fast. I have found that fasting on a combination of fresh juices and quality water is superior to plain-water fasting as it rejuvenates and nour-

ishes the body as well as the mind. It is also a gentle, easy method to shed pounds quickly. Fasting on fresh juices and quality water for three to five days once a month will maintain a healthy body and help keep the pounds off. (For juice combinations designed to treat specific ailments, see Chapter 5.)

For first-time cleansing, it is wise to make a vegetable broth. (See the recipes on page 29). With either version of vegetable broth, be sure to strain out the vegetables before drinking it. Do not eat the vegetables at this time, as taking even the smallest amount of solid food will ruin the fast. Fasting brings about a total change in the body's metabolism. If you prefer, you can process the vegetables in either broth recipe in a juicer (omitting the water). Do not cook the vegetables before juicing. Consume half of the juice immediately and the rest an hour later. When preparing fresh juice, make only as much as you will consume that day and keep any unused juice refrigerated in a jar with a tightly fitting lid until you drink it.

Finally, some words of caution for people with certain conditions. If you are pregnant or nursing, or if you have kidney dysfunction or advanced heart disease, you should not fast. If you have diabetes, do not fast on juices or water only. Add fresh vegetables without seasonings or dressings and nonsweet fruits such as green apples, grapefruit, or kiwi fruit. If you want to use sweet fruit in juices, dilute the juice with an equal amount of quality water. Water with lemon juice added is cleansing and helps to balance the body's pH. Plain vegetable broth and herbal teas can be used on "liquid" days. If you have hypoglycemia, always use a quality protein supplement when fasting. Spirulina is a good choice. It keeps blood-sugar levels from dropping too quickly, helps to get rid of hunger pangs and supplies chlorophyll—it is good even when you're not fasting. Fiber and spirulina should not be taken at the same time as or with other supplements.

Getting Started

There are a few items you will need to obtain before starting on any fast. Make sure to have on hand the following:

- Plenty of steam-distilled or other quality water, never tap water.

- Sugar-free "live" juices. (More about fresh juices in Chapter 5.)

- The fruits and vegetables used in the fasting recipes at the end of this chapter.

- Powdered buffered vitamin C.

- Pure, unprocessed virgin olive oil.

- Fresh coffee (not instant or decaffeinated). Organic coffee, available in health food stores and organic markets, is best.

- A fiber source such as psyllium seed powder or oat bran.

- Three of the following herb teas: alfalfa, burdock, dandelion, echinacea, goldenseal, milk thistle, pau d'arco, red clover, or rose hip. Houston Enterprises has a good formula called Daily Detox that can be drunk at any time to keep toxins from building up. It contains a combination of eleven herbs to detoxify the body, blood, and lymphatic system.

- Spirulina (optional).

If you have colon problems, add to the above list fresh or powdered wheatgrass, which is loaded with nutrients, including vitamins, minerals, amino acids, and chlorophyll and other phytonutrients. A fresh "green drink" made from any green, leafy vegetable is an excellent detoxifier. Chlorophyll, in the form of alfalfa, which is available in health food stores, helps the body to rid itself of toxins and is particularly good for arthritis. Another good detoxifier is garlic. Liquid Kyolic, which is an odorless aged garlic extract produced by Wakunaga of America Company, can be added to fresh juices. You can also use it in retention enemas. (More about that subject later in this chapter.)

Why the Emphasis on Quality Water?

Continual hydrating and rehydrating of the body is very important. If the body becomes dehydrated, it is thrown into "crisis mode" and many vital functions shut down or cease to work effectively. For this reason, it is important to select the best sources of water available and drink at least eight glasses a day.

Distilled water is excellent, but the distillation process also removes beneficial minerals that are important for health and well-being. Reverse osmosis purification is a technology that produces pure water from which almost all the sodium has been removed. However, you should not rely on drinking water as a significant source of minerals in any case. The minerals found in live foods are in natural, ionic electrolyte solutions, just as minerals in the body are. They are also the same as many of the elements in pure, natural drinking water. They are very similar to, and completely compatible with, the body's fluids.

If you choose to use distilled water, you can remineralize it to the consistency of natural spring water by adding ¼ to ½ teaspoon of a mineral supplement such as ConcenTrace trace mineral drops to each gallon of distilled water. This is a product that can add a host of important trace minerals to your diet if used on a regular basis. One 8-ounce bottle will remineralize up to 192 gallons of distilled water at a cost of only about five cents per gallon. Add more—up to 2 teaspoonfuls per gallon, or to taste—to remineralize water to the same levels as those expensive bottled mineral waters.

One-Day Fast

For first-time fasters concerned about how they will feel on a liquid-only diet, a one-day fast is an easy introduction. This fasting routine, similar to one developed by the Kripalu Center for Yoga and Health in Lenox, Massachusetts, has an interesting variety and a combination of fruit and vegetable juices that help detoxify the entire body.

The simple procedure is as follows:

- Upon waking, drink 1 cup of fresh Lemon Quality Water. (See the recipe on page 29.) You can take this either warm or cold, as you prefer, but body or room temperature is best.

- At 10:00 A.M., drink 1 cup of Apple-Cranberry Juice. Freshly made juice is best. (See the recipe on page 29.)

- At 12:00 noon, take 1 cup Carrot-Aloe-Ginger Juice. (See the recipe on page 29.)

- At 2:00 P.M., have 1 cup of Cucumber-Apple Juice. (See the recipe on page 29.)

- At 4:30 P.M., drink 2 cups vegetable broth. (See the recipe on page 29.)

- Throughout the day, drink warm or cold plain or Lemon Quality Water at any time during the day and herbal teas as desired. For detailed information on healing herbs, you may wish consult *Prescription for Herbal Healing* (Avery/Penguin Putnam, 2002).

If organic fruits and vegetables are not available to make the juices, remove peels before juicing. To bolster the fast, add protein powder and omega-3 and omega-6 essential fatty acid supplements to supply nutrients the body needs. If you have symptoms of low blood sugar, taking a rounded teaspoon of spirulina in an 8-ounce glass of fruit juice or water as needed is recommended.

THE SIX-DAY CLEANSING WELLNESS DIET

Following a six-day cleansing diet once a month will help you to balance your metabolism and keep your weight stable. The simple procedure for this diet follows, with day-by-day instructions.

Day 1

This first day's diet prepares the body for cleansing.

Breakfast

Immediately upon rising, drink a glass of quality water to flush your kidneys.

Eat one serving of any kind of fresh fruit (except oranges). If you have diabetes or hypoglycemia (low blood sugar), you should also avoid sweet fruits like grapes, pears, papaya, melon, or grapefruit.

Drink a glass of any kind of unsweetened juice (except orange juice) with 1,000 milligrams of vitamin C powder and 1 tablespoon of a fiber supplement (oat bran, glucomannan, or psyllium seed) added. Be sure to drink this quickly, as it thickens and can lodge in the throat. Follow it with a full glass of quality water. Take the fiber supplement three times a day, every day during the six-day cleansing period.

Lunch

Eat a fresh vegetable salad. (See the recipes on pages 19–21 for suggestions.) Make a dressing of 1 cup virgin olive oil; the juice of one lemon; ¼ teaspoon of barley malt, rice syrup, or blackstrap molasses; a pinch of dried parsley; and a dash of garlic powder or fresh garlic juice. Stevia is a good sweetener and has many health benefits, and can be used in place of the barley malt, rice syrup, or blackstrap molasses if you wish.

Take 1 tablespoon of a fiber supplement such as oat bran, glucomannan, or psyllium seed. Follow it with a full glass of quality water.

Dinner

Eat a serving of any type of steamed or boiled vegetable or have a raw salad. Do not have any salt, sugar, or other seasonings except for the salad dressing described above. To flavor your vegetables, you can use cold-pressed sesame seed or pure virgin olive oil, chopped chives, and a little pure garlic powder. A small amount of kelp adds minerals and aids weight loss.

Take 1 tablespoon of a fiber supplement such as oat bran, glucomannan, or psyllium seed. Follow it with a full glass of distilled water.

Throughout the Day

If you feel hungry between meals, eat a piece of fresh fruit or drink a cup of herbal tea. Combine herbal teas and one-third cup unsweetened fruit or vegetable juice for speed-healing. Drink at least six glasses of liquid during the day. Do not drink liquids with meals, only before or after.

Before Retiring

Give yourself a lemon cleansing enema. (See page 27.) If you normally take calcium supplements, continue taking them. You can also take vitamin E, but you should omit other vitamin supplements while cleansing.

Day 2

The second day's program helps the body to begin flushing out toxins and accelerate the healing process.

Breakfast

Immediately upon rising, drink a glass of steam-distilled water to flush your kidneys. The juice of a fresh lemon may be added for additional cleansing.

Use a coffee retention enema. (See page 27.)

Drink a glass of unsweetened fruit juice with 1,000 milligrams of powdered vitamin C and your fiber supplement added.

If you have diabetes or hypoglycemia, you may drink a green drink for speed-healing. Spirulina is particularly good for hypoglycemia. Kyo-Green from Wakunaga of America Company is also good. All green drinks tend to be strong and bitter-tasting, so it is best to add them to apple or carrot juice.

Lunch and Dinner

Consume only fresh apples or homemade applesauce made without sugar on this day for solid food. You can use any variety of apple—all are good because they have a high fiber content. Eat them alone while on this diet.

When making fresh apple juice, remove the stem and juice the whole fruit, including the skin. Remove the seeds if you are juicing more than one apple. To make homemade applesauce, leave the skins on and place the apples in a food processor or blender. Add a small amount of lemon juice to fresh applesauce mixture to keep it fresher longer, and do not add any sweeteners. Do not use canned applesauce.

Take 1 tablespoon of a fiber supplement such as oat bran, glucomannan, or psyllium seed. Follow it with a full glass of distilled water.

Throughout the Day

Make the following drink to have as often as desired throughout the day: Add the juice of four lemons to 4 cups of quality water. Sweeten it with 2 tablespoons of blackstrap molasses or barley malt sweetener. Or use stevia, following the directions on the product label (stevia is very concentrated). Consuming herbal teas mixed with fresh juice (three parts herbal tea to one part juice) throughout the day is also good. You can also drink fruit juices alone, unless you have diabetes or hypoglycemia. Do not drink liquids with meals, only before or after.

If you are using wheatgrass or some other source of chlorophyll, add it to juice. If you are using spirulina, take three tablets or 1 teaspoon of the powdered form three times a day.

Before Retiring

Give yourself a lemon cleansing enema. (See page 27.) If you normally take calcium supplements, continue taking them. You can also take vitamin E, but you should omit other vitamin supplements while cleansing.

Day 3

This is a liquid day.

Breakfast

Immediately upon rising, drink a glass of steam-distilled water to flush your kidneys. The juice of a fresh lemon may be added for additional cleansing.

Use a coffee or wheatgrass retention enema. (See page 27.) It is a good idea to alternate between coffee and wheatgrass retention enemas.

Drink a glass of grapefruit juice or Lemon Quality Water with 2 tablespoons of pure cold-processed olive oil added. This aids in cleansing and healing the gallbladder. Repeat the oil and lemon juice drink just after rising in the morning and just before retiring at night for the next three days.

Drink a glass of unsweetened fruit juice with 1,000 milligrams of powdered vitamin C and your fiber supplement added.

Throughout the Day

Drink all the herbal tea, distilled water with lemon juice added, vegetable broth, and fresh juices as desired. Be sure to dilute any juices you drink with quality water. Make the fresh vegetable broth or juice to sip throughout the day. Do not have any applesauce on this day, only liquids.

Twice during the day, take 1 tablespoon of a fiber supplement such as oat bran, glucomannan, or psyllium seed. Follow it with a full glass of distilled water.

Before Retiring

Drink another glass of grapefruit juice or Lemon Quality Water with 2 tablespoons of pure cold-processed olive oil added.

Use a cleansing enema, if you are constipated or having symptoms of toxicity such as lethargy or headaches. This is especially helpful if this is your first fast. If you prefer, you can use an herbal laxative such as Naturalax 2 from Nature's Way. These work well when used occasionally.

Decision Point 1

At this point, you can continue with the six-day plan or repeat Day 3 on Days 4, 5, and 6 before going on. Staying on liquids for only three consecutive days will promote faster weight loss and speed healing. If you have special dietary needs—for instance, if you have diabetes—consult a doctor before continuing a fast for longer than three days.

DAY 4

This day's program adds modest amounts of whole live foods to the cleansing liquids.

Breakfast

Immediately upon rising, drink a glass of quality water to flush your kidneys. The juice of a fresh lemon may be added for additional cleansing.

Use a coffee or wheatgrass retention enema. (See pages 27–28.) It is a good idea to alternate between coffee and wheatgrass retention enemas.

Drink a glass of grapefruit juice or Lemon Quality Water with 2 tablespoons of pure cold-processed olive oil added. Or, if you prefer, simply add the oil to the juice of half a lemon.

Drink a glass of unsweetened fruit juice with 1,000 milligrams of powdered vitamin C and your fiber supplement added.

Drink a glass of unsweetened cranberry juice, available in health food stores and natural foods markets. This promotes cleansing and healing of the bladder and the rest of the urinary tract.

Lunch

Shred two beets and dress them with a mixture of 1 tablespoon olive oil and the juice of one lemon.

Take 1 tablespoon of a fiber supplement such as oat bran, glucomannan, or psyllium seed. Follow it with a full glass of quality water.

Dinner

Shred two beets, two carrots, one-quarter head of cabbage, or a combination of these vegetables. Dress them with a mixture of 1 tablespoon olive oil and the juice of one lemon.

Take 1 tablespoon of a fiber supplement such as oat bran, glucomannan, or psyllium seed. Follow it with a full glass of distilled water.

Throughout the Day

Drink all the herbal tea, distilled water with lemon juice added, vegetable broth, and fresh juices as desired. Be sure to dilute any juices you drink with quality water. Make the fresh vegetable broth or juice to sip throughout the day. Do not drink liquids with meals, only before or after.

Drink pear juice on this day, mixed with an equal amount of quality water. (If you have sugar problems, substitute diluted apple juice.) Drink as much pear juice as you like, but do not have it at the same time as the beets. Drinking beet juice, which is made by putting the beets and the tops into a juicer or blender with distilled water, is another good option. If a juicer or beets are not available, beet juice can be found in most health food stores. This is beneficial for the gallbladder and liver.

Before Retiring

Drink a glass of grapefruit juice or Lemon Quality Water with 2 tablespoons of pure cold-processed olive oil added.

DAY 5

Your body should now be flushing toxins from all the major organs. Using only live foods and liquids accelerates the healing process. Be sure to drink plenty of liquids to help with elimination and speed healing.

Breakfast

Immediately upon rising, drink a glass of quality water to flush your kidneys.

Eat one serving of any kind of fresh fruit (except oranges). If you have diabetes or hypoglycemia, you should also avoid sweet fruits like grapes, pears, papaya, melon, or grapefruit.

Drink a glass of any kind of unsweetened juice (except orange juice) with 1,000 milligrams of vitamin C powder and 1 tablespoon of a fiber supplement (oat bran, glucomannan, or psyllium seed) added.

Drink a glass of grapefruit juice or Lemon Quality Water with 2 tablespoons of pure cold-processed olive oil added. This aids in cleansing and healing the gallbladder.

Lunch and Dinner

Shred 1 beet, 1 carrot, 1 turnip, ¼ head of cabbage, and ¼ onion, all raw. Toss with a dressing made from 1 cup virgin olive oil; the juice of one lemon; ¼ teaspoon of barley

malt, rice malt sweetener, or blackstrap molasses; a pinch of dried parsley; and a dash of garlic powder or fresh garlic juice.

Take 1 tablespoon of a fiber supplement such as oat bran, glucomannan, or psyllium seed. Follow it with a full glass of distilled water.

Throughout the Day

Drink all the herbal tea, distilled water with lemon juice added, vegetable broth, and fresh juices desired. Be sure to dilute any juices you drink with quality water. Make fresh vegetable broth or juice to sip throughout the day. Do not drink liquids with meals, only before or after.

Before Retiring

Drink a glass of grapefruit juice or Lemon Quality Water with 2 tablespoons of pure cold-processed olive oil added. This aids in cleansing and healing the gallbladder.

Decision Point 2

At this point, you can choose to repeat the entire regimen for the preceding five days for more dramatic results. Or you can continue with the program for Day 6 if you are satisfied with the weight-loss and healing results you have achieved thus far.

Day 6

This day reintroduces your body to regular solid foods. It is a gentle way to break the fast and introduce easily digested foods. Do not come off the program (or any liquid fast) with heavy meals or foods that contain saturated or hydrogenated fats, refined flours, added salt, or sugar. Keep your food light and fresh as much as possible for an easier transition, or you may erase many of the healing benefits of this program.

Breakfast

Have a bowl of fresh fruit or prunes or a bowl of wholegrain cereal. Do not eat the cereal and the fresh fruit at the same time. Wait at least a half-hour between them. Drink a glass of any kind of unsweetened juice (except orange juice) with 1,000 milligrams of vitamin C powder and 1 tablespoon of a fiber supplement (oat bran, glucomannan, or psyllium seed) added. Follow it with a full glass of distilled water.

Drink a glass of grapefruit juice or Lemon Quality Water with 2 tablespoons of pure cold-processed olive oil added. This aids in cleansing and healing the gallbladder. Repeat this drink just after rising in the morning and just before retiring at night for the next three days.

Lunch

Eat a fresh raw vegetable salad (shred the vegetables if desired) topped with avocado, raisins, and sunflower seeds. Be sure to chew the food until it is almost liquid. You can now use an olive oil and balsamic vinegar dressing. (See the recipe on page 21.)

Take 1 tablespoon of a fiber supplement such as oat bran, glucomannan, or psyllium seed. Follow it with a full glass of quality water.

Dinner

Eat a meal of steamed broccoli, carrots, and cauliflower over brown rice. Add onions and other vegetables if desired, and season them with lemon juice and a small amount of garlic. Do not eat any processed foods or breads, only freshly prepared foods.

Take 1 tablespoon of a fiber supplement such as oat bran, glucomannan, or psyllium seed. Follow it with a full glass of distilled water.

Throughout the Day

Drink all the herbal tea, distilled water with lemon juice added, vegetable broth, and fresh juices as desired. Be sure to dilute any juices you drink with quality water. Make the fresh vegetable broth or juice to sip throughout the day. Do not drink liquids with meals, only before or after.

Before Retiring

Drink a glass of grapefruit juice or Lemon Quality Water with 2 tablespoons of pure cold-processed olive oil added.

After Day 6

Once you have completed the six-day program, do not return to eating meals heavy in protein or laden with processed foods. Doing so will reverse the results you worked so hard to achieve! If you wish, make these six days a routine once each month. This will help you to stabilize your weight and keep your system clean.

ENEMAS

Gentle infusions of warm water or lemon water enemas are easier on the colon than laxatives or drugs and should be part of a monthly cleansing program, but not used in between the monthly fasts. Clinics around the world use this procedure to treat many different ailments.

There are two types of enemas: cleansing enemas and retention enemas. Cleansing enemas are used to flush out and clean the colon. Retention (or suppository) enemas are held in the colon for a specified period, and are designed to aid the absorption of necessary nutrients and antitoxin substances, like coffee, through the colon wall. The water should not be uncomfortably hot or cold for either type of enema.

Cleansing Enemas

A cleansing enema that can be used daily during a cleansing routine is administered as follows: In an enema bag, mix the juice of two lemons with two quarts of lukewarm water. Lubricate the tip of the tube with a tiny bit of pure virgin olive oil, vitamin E oil, or aloe vera gel, and gently insert the tip into your rectum. The best position for inserting the fluid is on your knees with your head down and rear up. Introduce the fluid slowly. If you start to feel discomfort, squeeze the tube with your fingers to shut off the flow of liquid and take a few deep breaths. Then try releasing your fingers to start the flow again. Once the liquid has been inserted, roll first onto your back and then onto your left side while using your fingers to massage your abdomen, starting on the right side and moving in a circle up and over to the left side. After three or four minutes, expel the liquid.

It is always best to take any type of enema after a natural bowel movement if possible. If you find yourself unable to insert all of the liquid before expelling it, just release and try again. It will become easier after a couple of enemas.

Retention Enemas

For effective detoxification, I recommend using coffee retention (suppository) enemas during the fasting portions of the cleansing and healing program. Only 1½ cups of solution is required, so it is easy to retain. In the treatment of degenerative diseases, coffee enemas stimulate the liver to secrete toxins and help to loosen months' and years' worth of fecal matter that has built up on the colon walls. Open two acidophilus capsules and add the contents to enhance the detoxification and replace friendly bacteria. Or you can crush two tablets of an acidophilus tablet such as Probiata, produced by Wakunaga of America Company, and add the crushed tablets to cooled coffee. You can also add ¼ cup of food-grade aloe vera juice to soothe the lining of the colon and supply many beneficial nutrients.

To make a coffee retention enema, in a saucepan, put 6 heaping tablespoons of fresh (not instant or decaffeinated), preferably organic, ground coffee and 2 quarts of quality water. Bring to a boil over high heat and boil for fifteen minutes. Remove it from the heat, allow the mixture to cool, and strain out the coffee grounds. Use only 1 to 1½ cups at a time and save the rest in the refrigerator. If you are adding acidophilus and/or aloe vera juice, wait until the coffee is cool before adding them. Use this enema once a day (mornings are best) while detoxifying to relieve headaches that may be caused by the release of built-up toxins. Do not overuse coffee enemas—when not detoxifying use them only occasionally, as needed. If you want to use coffee enemas for longer periods of time than this program, use them after a natural bowel movement to avoid the risk of weakening bowel muscle function. If you have hemorrhoids, add a dose of white oak bark extract, as directed on the product label, to a retention enema.

Wheatgrass suppository enemas are used in many clinics and are beneficial for people who have cancer or virtually any other disorder. To make the enema, add ¼ cup of fresh wheatgrass juice to 1 cup of warm quality water. If fresh wheatgrass juice is not available, a freeze-dried product called Sweet Wheat, available in health food stores, is a good substitute. Place 1 teaspoon in quality water and mix well. If you wish, you can add 1 tablespoon to your cleansing enemas as well.

For additional detoxifying power, you can add 6 drops of Liquid Kyolic to retention (suppository) enemas.

Enema Hygiene

To get the maximum cleansing benefit from enemas, and to avoid introducing new health problems, it is very important to maintain scrupulous enema hygiene, including the following:

- Always rinse the enema bag and let hot water run through the hose before and after each use. Wash the entire apparatus in hot soapy water and rinse, then hang it up to dry, between uses.

- Once a month, soak the enema bag in a solution made from 1 gallon of water and 1 tablespoon of bleach to destroy mold, bacteria, and other potentially harmful microorganisms. Rinse the bag well after soaking.

- Keep a small jar of pure olive oil by the enema bag to use on the tip for easy insertion. Olive oil will not turn rancid. As an alternative, liquid vitamin E oil is good for soothing the anus and for hemorrhoids. Pure aloe vera gel works well also and is healing to hemorrhoids. Do not use petroleum jelly (Vaseline), which is a petrochemical product and contains potentially toxic substances. Un-petroleum, a plant-based product that can be found at most health food stores, looks and feels the same but is not toxic.

- Do not abuse enemas. Prolonged use can result in a dependency on enemas for normal bowel movements.

DRY-BRUSH MASSAGE

Dry-brush massage is important for detoxifying because it rids the body of dead cells so that healthy new cells can form. Dead skin cells prevent skin from breathing. The massage increases circulation, bringing more blood to the surface of the skin. The body actually breathes through the skin, absorbs oxygen, and helps to throw off toxins. Each morning, just before showering, use a natural bristle brush and brush your entire body, starting with your feet and moving up your legs and torso. Always brush toward the heart. Your skin will glow and begin to look years younger.

People with severe circulatory problems (even those who have difficulty standing for prolonged periods) can improve their circulation with dry-brush massage. It also helps to rejuvenate the nervous system by stimulating the nerve endings. Researchers have found that many nutrients could be absorbed through the skin system, so be careful about what you apply to your skin after massaging—read labels on skin-care products thoroughly!

EXERCISE

While on a detoxifying program, it is good to get some form of exercise, such as walking, swimming, or stretching. If you already have a regular exercise program, continue it, but reduce the duration of exercise sessions. If not, take a gentle walk and do some basic stretches each day, but be careful not to overdo it if you are an exercise novice.

Additional Cleansing Measures

Fasting, using enemas, and skin brushing are vital parts of the cleansing and healing program. There are also other things you can do that are important for helping your body to achieve and maintain internal detoxification—while you are on the program and even when you are not.

Get some fiber in your diet every day. If you are trying to lose weight, take a fiber supplement just before meals to decrease your appetite. Rice bran, oat bran, apple pectin, agar, psyllium, and flaxseeds are recommended sources. Wheat bran also is a source of fiber, but it may be too irritating for an inflamed colon wall. If you are using any type of fiber in capsule form, be sure to take it with a large glass of water and follow that with another glass because fiber capsules expand. Aerobic Bulk Cleanser (ABC) from Aerobic Life Industries is an excellent fiber supplement. You must drink it immediately after mixing and follow it with another glass of water.

Take spirulina, in tablet or powder form, daily. Take five tablets or 1 teaspoon of powder dissolved in juice three times a day. Spirulina is a perfect food. It is high in protein and contains virtually all the vitamins and minerals the body needs, plus chlorophyll for cleansing. Make sure the spirulina you buy is of high quality. Earthrise Spirulina from Earthrise Nutritionals is a good choice. Kyo-Green from Wakunaga is another excellent choice that contains additional nutrients.

Drink only quality water and plenty of it. You can dilute juices with it, but use only unsweetened juices with no additives. Do not use tomato or orange juice because of their high acidity. If you feel you need a little sweetener, use blackstrap molasses, which is rich in minerals and B vitamins. It is a good source of usable iron because it is easily assimilated. It has the least sugar of any type of sweetener.

THE RECIPES

LEMON QUALITY WATER

2 quarts quality water
Juice of 3 lemons
½ teaspoon stevia or blackstrap molasses (optional)

Place the water in a pitcher. Stir in lemon juice and add stevia or molasses for sweetness. Serve at room temperature.

APPLE-CRANBERRY JUICE

1 apple (everything but the stem)
½ cup cranberries
quality water

Place ingredients in a juicer and process until pureed. Add water until the desired consistency is achieved. Drink immediately.

CARROT-ALOE-GINGER JUICE

3 large carrots
2 tablespoons fresh ginger
½ cup food-grade aloe vera juice

Place all of the ingredients in a juicer and process until puréed. Drink immediately.

CUCUMBER-APPLE JUICE

1 cucumber
1 green apple (including skin and seeds)
1 handful parsley
Food-grade aloe vera juice or quality water
    (optional)

Place all of the ingredients in a juicer and process until puréed. If desired, add aloe vera juice or water until the desired consistency is achieved. Drink immediately.

VEGETABLE BROTH I

4 cups quality water
½ well-scrubbed potato, chopped
½ cup grated beets
½ cup sliced carrots
½ cup chopped celery
½ cup sliced onion
2 cloves garlic, minced
1 bay leaf
1 pinch dried thyme
1 pinch powdered cayenne pepper

1. Place all of the ingredients in a soup pot and bring to a boil over high heat.
2. Lower the heat to simmering temperature and allow the soup to simmer for one hour.
3. Remove from heat and strain out the vegetables (discard the bay leaf), reserving them for another use. Drink a large glass of broth while fasting as needed to suppress feelings of hunger.

VEGETABLE BROTH II

4 cups quality water
2 beets, with greens, chopped
2 carrots, chopped
2 stalks celery, chopped
2 cloves garlic, minced
1 turnip, chopped
½ head cabbage, shredded
½ onion, chopped
¼ bunch parsley, minced

1. Place all of the ingredients in a soup pot or large saucepan. Bring to a boil over high heat.
2. Lower the heat to simmering temperature and allow the soup to simmer for one hour.
3. Remove from heat and strain out the vegetables, reserving them for another use. Drink a large glass of broth while fasting as needed to suppress feelings of hunger.

POTATO PEELING BROTH

3 potatoes (*Note:* It is very important to use
    potatoes that have *no* green tint.)
1 carrot, sliced
1 celery stalk, sliced
1 onion, sliced and/or 3 cloves garlic, peeled
2 quarts quality water

1. Scrub the potatoes well and cut out any eyes. Cut the potatoes in half and cut the peel from the potatoes, making sure to keep about ½ inch of the potato with the peel. Set aside the potato centers for another use.
2. Scrub the carrots and celery, peel the onion and/or garlic, and slice them into ½-inch pieces.
3. Place the potato peelings, carrot, and celery in a large pot. Cover with the water. Add the onion and/or garlic. Bring to a boil and cook for about 30 minutes.
4. Remove from heat and allow the broth to cool to the desired temperature. Strain out and discard the vegetables. Drink hot or cold, as desired.

BARLEY WATER

1 cup barley
3 quarts steam-distilled water
½ teaspoon or the contents of 3 capsules of
    powdered slippery elm bark (optional)

1. Place the barley and the water and slippery elm bark, if desired, in a large pot.
2. Bring to a boil, then reduce the heat and allow to simmer for three hours.
3. Remove from heat and allow the broth to cool to the desired temperature. Strain out and discard the barley. Drink hot or cold, as desired.

CHAPTER FIVE

JUICING: MAXIMIZED NOURISHMENT FOR HEALING

Juicing is one of the most powerful healing tools available. Fresh, "live" juices supply the body with the concentrated nutrients and enzymes needed for the nourishment and regeneration of the body's cells, tissues, glands, and organs. There have been numerous accounts of people who have healed themselves of degenerative diseases using live juice as a therapy.

Juicing also is an easy way to ensure that your diet includes the five to seven daily servings of raw fruits and vegetables that are necessary to maintain health. If you are in reasonably good health, you should benefit from at least a pint of fresh juice a day; if you are trying to treat a specific disorder, you will need to drink more.

When you extract juice from fruits and vegetables, leaving behind the pulp, fiber is lost, so you need to include other sources of fiber in your diet. (See Chapter 16.) Fiber is essential to proper digestion and optimal health; however, when you are juicing, it is actually a good thing that it is removed. Without the fiber, all of the nutrients, enzymes, and phytochemicals extracted from fresh, raw produce can be quickly digested and absorbed by the body.

The digestive process absorbs a large percentage of the nourishment in whole raw fruits and vegetables. The body's rapid absorption of raw juices quickly provides cells and tissues with the nutrients and enzymes needed to heal and regenerate. There is no limit to how much live juice can be consumed safely. Two 8-ounce glasses a day will help maintain good health. When you are fasting and/or speed-healing, you should drink at least four 8-ounce glasses a day. Drinking live juices helps the body to rid itself of toxins rapidly while providing needed nutrients.

CHOOSING A JUICER

There are a variety of juicing machines on the market today, manufactured by a number of different companies. Prices range from eighty dollars to more than two thousand dollars, depending on the make and model. All juicers, however, use one of three basic methods of extraction: centrifugal, masticating, or triturating.

Centrifugal juicers essentially cut the fruits and vegetables fed into them into tiny pieces and spin them in a basket at high speeds. This separates the juice from the pulp. Because of the way in which centrifugal juicers extract the juice, a certain amount of oxygen is introduced into the final product, which can compromise the quality of the juice to some extent. If you are considering buying this type of juicer, look for one that has a pulp ejector. This eliminates the need to stop the machine to empty pulp.

Masticating juicers grind vegetables and fruits into a paste, then spin the pulp at high speed, squeezing the juice through a screen at the bottom. The friction involved in this process generates heat, which may affect the nutrient content of the resulting juice.

Triturating, or hydraulic press, juicers cut and grind vegetables and fruits, then extract the juice by applying great pressure. This extraction method yields the most juice, and also provides juice with the highest nutritional value, because the least amount of oxygen is introduced during processing.

Whatever type of juicer you are considering, you should keep in mind the following factors before choosing one:

- Ease of use and cleaning. A juicer that is easy to clean and operate will get more use.

- Juice quality. Good machines produce juice that is abundant in nutrients and enzymes. The quality of fresh juice also depends on the extraction method. Oxidation and heat destroy nutrients. The more oxygen introduced (as with the centrifugal method) or heat generated (the masticating method) during processing, the less nutrients survive in the juice.

- Yield. How many ounces of juice does the machine produce from each pound of fruit or vegetables?

- Reliability. Most low-priced juicers are not built for daily operation—the cutting blade and motor soon wear out. If you are planning to juice regularly, look for a machine for which the power of the motor and durability are comparable to specifications for the more expensive juicers. Also, get one with a multiple-year warranty.

PREPARING JUICES FOR SPEED-HEALING

The benefits of juicing, obviously, are influenced not only by the quality of the equipment you use, but also by the ingredients you use and how you prepare them. It goes without saying, of course, that you should use only freshly made juices, never canned or frozen ones. Following are guidelines to keep in mind when preparing your fresh live juices.

Whenever possible, buy fresh organic produce. Not only is it free of toxic chemical pesticides, but some research indicates that it is more nutritious. If organic produce is not available, use one of these other methods to prepare produce for juicing:

- Scrub produce with a natural bristle vegetable brush. Remove any bruised or wilted portions.

- Place fruits or vegetables in a dishpan filled with pure water to which the juice of a fresh lemon (or a few drops of grapefruit seed extract) and ¼ cup of salt have been added for each 2 gallons of water. Soak the produce for ten to fifteen minutes, then rinse the produce in fresh water.

- Place fruits or vegetables in a dishpan filled with pure water to which 1 teaspoon of bleach has been added for each gallon of water. Be sure to use chlorine bleach that has not had any lye added to it. Allow the produce to soak for ten minutes, then drain and soak for an additional ten minutes in fresh water. While this method may seem odd, it destroys virtually all types of germs, chemical residue, and heavy metals, and is well supported by many nutritionists and naturopathic physicians. It even intensifies the color of the vegetables. Place the vegetables or fruits on a drainboard for twenty minutes before juicing. Bleach vaporizes when it comes in contact with air. If you are allergic to chlorine, you can purchase organic liquid vegetable wash at a health food store that will remove unwanted substances.

- Whatever type of juicer and produce you use, follow the manufacturer's directions regarding the chopping and peeling of the fruit and/or vegetables.

Fresh juice should be consumed as soon as it is made, especially if you use a centrifugal extractor. Light, air, and heat initiate the process of oxidation (chemical reaction with oxygen), which causes juice to lose precious enzymes, vitamins, and minerals. If you cannot consume all the juice

Commonsense Juicing Precautions

Because fresh juice is unpasteurized, it can contain harmful microorganisms, even potentially dangerous strain of *Escherichia coli* (*E. coli*) bacteria. Be wary of drinking unpasteurized fresh-squeezed juices that are sold in restaurants or prepackaged. When juicing at home, wash fruits and vegetables thoroughly before slicing them to prevent transferring any bacteria or fungi that may be present on the peel or rind to the pulp. And keep the knife and cutting board you use to slice produce for juicing scrupulously clean—knives and cutting boards can carry bacteria or pesticide residue.

you have made at once, keep it as cold as possible without freezing it (35°F to 38°F). Do not store it in a big container for repeated servings; instead, decant it into prechilled, single-serving-size, amber-colored glass bottles. Fill the bottles as close to the top as possible to prevent air from coming into contact with the juice and refrigerate them quickly. Properly stored juice will maintain its nutritional value for up to twenty-four hours.

A vacuum bottle or other temperature-retaining vessel, such as a Thermos, also is a good way to store juice, and it's convenient when traveling.

Fruits that have been imported from tropical regions should be peeled before juicing, since many countries in such regions of the world do not have protective laws governing the use of potentially carcinogenic chemicals such as fertilizers and pesticides.

Pits—such as those found in peaches, plums, cherries, and apricots—should be removed prior to juicing. Seeds from grapes, melons, and citrus fruits are okay to juice; however, apple seeds contain small amounts of cyanide. You should not juice more than one apple with the seeds each day. Remove the seeds if you are juicing more than one apple.

Dilute juices with quality water and sip them slowly. Drink fruit juices in the morning for quick energy. Strong-flavored vegetables such as turnips, rutabaga, broccoli, and onions should be juiced in small amounts. For example, one-quarter of a turnip would be sufficient per glass of juice. Foods that have a high water content, such as carrots, cabbage, apples, and grapes, should be the base juice. Leafy greens can add many powerful healing elements to juices. (More information about them can be found in Chapter 9.) Carrot tops and rhubarb greens should be removed before juicing, as they contain toxic compounds.

Juices can be combined to treat specific ailments. For example, juicing carrots, celery, garlic, and parsley yields a healing drink that helps to treat the flu and other infectious diseases. Parsley is a good source of zinc, which promotes healing and bolsters the immune system. Garlic acts as a natural antibiotic, although you should not juice more than a single clove for one serving, as raw garlic may irritate the stomach lining. Both carrots and celery are high in potassium and sodium, nutrients that can be lost if you have a fever or diarrhea. Carrots also provide energy and are a delicious, sweet base for many healing combinations.

Fruits and vegetables are not ordinarily juiced together because of food-combining rules (see Chapter 19). Food-combining theories have been developed in recent years in response to the apparently growing incidence of food allergies and digestive problems. Because apples contain malic acid, a compound that plays a role in the generation of energy at the cellular level, they are frequently included in juice combinations.

Acidic fruits, such as citrus fruits, are best juiced alone or with other acidic fruits. Grapefruit juice is both sweet and sour, so it can be used either way. The essential oil in the peel of oranges and grapefruits contains toxins that should not be consumed in large quantities. (Lemons are okay, but they may be waxed—see the inset "Waxed Fruits and Vegetables" on page 37.) Do juice the white, pithy part just under the peel because it contains a high concentration of beneficial flavonoids and vitamin C.

Herbs can be added to juice combinations for health benefits. Use fresh herbs such as dandelion greens, fennel, ginger root, and mint. Other herbs, such as echinacea and dong quai, are not as readily available fresh and may give juice a bitter taste. To add such herbs, purchase them in capsule or liquid extract form, then stir the contents of a capsule or a few drops of extract into the juice. If you are pregnant or nursing, or have a liver or heart disorder or high blood pressure, consult with a health-care professional before using any herbs. Detailed information on individual herbs, their medicinal uses, and precautions to be aware of when using them may be found in *Prescription for Herbal Healing* (Avery/Penguin Putnam, 2002).

Alternate juices made from the foods and herbs from the tables in Appendix D: Live Juice Therapy every day to receive all their healing and prevention benefits. Gradually work through the entire list—each has a specific role in restoring and balancing the metabolism.

TYPES OF JUICES

Juices can be divided into three basic categories: cereal grass and algae juices, vegetable juices, and fruit and melon juices.

Cereal Grass and Algae Juices

Cereal grasses are the young plants of cereal grains. They are at their nutritional peak about twenty days after germination of the seed, when the grass begins to form a stem. This is referred to as the *jointing* stage. Harvested at this young age, cereal grasses are chemically and nutritionally different from the fully developed grain they would even-

tually produce. For instance, 100 grams (about 3½ ounces) of wheatgrass has 32 grams of protein, whereas the same amount of wheat flour contains only 13 grams of protein.

Cereal grass juices cleanse and detoxify the system and provide the body with energy. Their powerful cleansing may produce nausea, however, so it is a good idea to dilute them with quality water. Some are also bitter-tasting; adding a small amount of carrots or apples will help to sweeten the taste.

Powerhouses of nutrition, green superfoods such as cereal grasses and algae contain high concentrations of protein, vitamins, minerals, antioxidants, and phytochemicals. They are nature's most protective medicine. They detoxify the organs, reduce tumors, and act to overcome all toxic substances in the body. They have in common an abundance of chlorophyll, the substance that helps plants convert sunlight into energy—and gives them their green color. On the molecular level, chlorophyll has virtually the same structure as hemoglobin, the substance that transports oxygen in the bloodstream, and is therefore known as the "blood" of plant life. The only difference is the central atom: At the center of a molecule of chlorophyll is magnesium, while the center of hemoglobin is iron. The beneficial effects of chlorophyll include:

- It can reverse the mutagenic capacity of some cancer-causing chemicals.

- It slows cellular damage caused by radiation.

- It aids wound healing by stimulating new cell growth.

- It builds up the blood and neutralizes toxins such as pesticides.

- It binds with heavy metals, removing them from the body.

- It fights infections.

- It improves liver function.

- It helps eliminate mouth and body odors.

- It is good for all degenerative disorders.

Fresh cereal grasses can be juiced only by the triturating method. However, you can buy dehydrated forms, known popularly as green drinks, in health food stores and add them to any vegetable juices or to quality water.

Alfalfa Juice

Alfalfa juice is rich in vitamins A, B_6, C, D, and K; bioflavonoids; and the minerals calcium, magnesium, and manganese, as well as many trace elements, including boron, chromium, molybdenum, and selenium. Its high chlorophyll content relieves respiratory disorders and many degenerative disorders, such as arthritis; and it may lower cholesterol and help guard against atherosclerosis. Classified by some as a legume rather than a cereal grass, alfalfa also contains eight essential amino acids that the body needs to build protein.

Barley Grass Juice

Barley grass juice, also known as green barley juice, is rich in vitamins C, B_1, B_2, B_3, B_6, and C, as well as biotin, folate, and beta-carotene. It also contains a form of vitamin E called alpha-tocopherol succinate, which, in clinical trials, has demonstrated a significant ability to block the growth of cancer cells. This form of vitamin E also helps to regulate human growth hormone and hormones that are crucial for reproductive health. It is rich in calcium, iron, phosphorus, potassium, sulfur, zinc, and superoxide dismutase (SOD), a powerful antioxidant enzyme. Green barley juice can be used to treat many ailments, including hepatitis, arthritis, peptic ulcers, hypoglycemia, sexual dysfunction, cardiovascular disease, asthma, gastrointestinal disorders, and possibly cancer.

Wheatgrass Juice

Wheatgrass juice has been called the king of all juices. It has the highest beta-carotene and chlorophyll content of all the cereal grasses. It is one of the best detoxifiers and blood purifiers available. It contains many vitamins, minerals, enzymes, proteins, and trace minerals, but is especially rich in the antioxidants selenium and vitamins A and E. Wheatgrass contains virtually all known essential minerals if it is grown in good, rich soil—this makes it superior to virtually all other plant foods. Its ability to work directly on the liver makes it valuable in treating all sorts of disorders, including those of the lung and colon. It is also used to help the body eliminate excess metals, and to control irregularity. Many health clinics use wheatgrass juice to heal a variety of disorders and also use it in retention enemas. Among the thousands of testimonials to the ability of wheatgrass juice to reverse degenerative conditions is the story of Dr. Ann Wigmore, founder of the Hippocrates Health Institute in Boston, who cured herself of gangrene with this treatment and averted the need for amputation of both of her legs—in fact, Dr. Wigmore went on to run the Boston marathon. Her miraculous recovery created renewed interest and research into the value of cereal grasses.

Wheatgrass juice is so potent that it may have a nauseating effect in the beginning, so start with ½ ounce at a time and increase the amount gradually. Sweet Wheat, made by Sweet Wheat, Inc., is a freeze-dried product that is a good substitute if fresh wheatgrass is not available. It can be added to any type of juice.

Pets can benefit from wheatgrass as well. High-protein canned pet food, which has high acidity, can be balanced by adding ½ teaspoon of wheat grass powder per ½ cup of food.

Green Drinks

These are natural food formulas made from dehydrated green super foods, including dark green leafy vegetables. They are good detoxifiers and blood cleansers. Available in health food stores, they are usually sold in powder form (though some companies offer capsules or caplets also) to be mixed into juices just before use. Kyo-Green from Wakunaga of America Company is one such drink. A powdered mix made from barley grass, wheatgrass, chlorella, Pacific kelp, and cooked brown rice, it can be mixed with quality water by itself or added to any juice (fresh is always best!) for extra nutrition.

Green drinks are very powerful and so may cause nausea and headaches at first. To avoid this, add quality water and sip slowly.

Chlorella

Chlorella is a tiny single-celled water-grown green alga that contains the highest chlorophyll level per ounce of any plant, as well as protein (nearly 58 percent), carbohydrates, all of the B vitamins, vitamins C and E, amino acids (including all nine essential ones), enzymes, and rare trace minerals. It contains more vitamin B_{12} than liver, plus a sizable amount of beta-carotene. It is also high in the nucleic acids RNA and DNA. It is virtually a complete food. Chlorella strengthens the immune system, promotes bowel health, helps to detoxify the body, alleviates peptic and duodenal ulcers, fights infection, and helps to counteract fatigue and mood swings associated with premenstrual syndrome (PMS) and perimenopause. It has also been shown to protect against the effects of ultraviolet radiation. Because it has a strong cell wall, which makes it difficult to access its nutrients, chlorella requires factory processing to make it effective.

Spirulina

Spirulina is a blue-green alga found naturally in alkaline, warm-water lakes. It is cultivated for commercial use in specially designed algae farms. Spirulina contains concentrations of nutrients unlike any other single grain, herb, or plant. It has the essential fatty acids gamma-linolenic acid (GLA), linoleic and arachidonic acids; is virtually the only vegetarian source of vitamin B_{12}, which is (needed for healthy red blood cells; and contains significant amounts of iron, protein (60 to 70 percent), essential amino acids, the nucleic acids RNA and DNA, and chlorophyll. Spirulina is a naturally digestible food that helps to protect the immune system, reduce blood cholesterol levels, and boost the absorption of necessary minerals. Taking spirulina in supplement form is beneficial while fasting, as it supplies the nutrients needed to cleanse and heal, while also curbing the appetite. If you have hypoglycemia (low blood sugar), you may benefit from using this food supplement between meals because its high protein content helps to stabilize blood sugar levels. Spirulina comes in tablet and powdered forms to be added to liquids such as juices. Follow the directions on the product label.

Vegetable Juices

Rich in vitamins, minerals, live enzymes, amino acids, and phytochemicals, vegetable juices help to balance the body's metabolism and aid in weight loss. They also help damaged tissues to regenerate and heal. Certain individual vegetable juices also have specific healing properties, which we will look at in this section.

Beet Juice

Beet juice is among the most valuable healing juices available. Be sure to juice the tops also—they contain more nutrients than the beet. Beets and beet tops contain a form of iron that is readily absorbed into the blood, nourishing and toning it and building red blood cells. Beet juice is helpful in the treatment of menstrual irregularities as well as the symptoms of menopause. It helps to strengthen the immune system and detoxify the kidneys, liver, and gallbladder. It also is useful in treating anemia and liver disorders. Beet juice is best combined with other vegetable juices to buffer its powerful cleansing action, which can cause nausea and dizziness because it releases nutrients very quickly. Also, its strong, earthy taste is more palatable if it is combined with other juices. If you do drink pure beet juice, do not consume more than 4 ounces at a time, and dilute the juice with 2 or more ounces of quality water. A combination of 3 ounces each of beet and cabbage juice mixed with 10 ounces of carrot juice furnishes the body with a good balance of nutrients necessary for all physiological functions.

Brussels Sprout Juice

Brussels sprouts can be juiced and used to treat diabetes, as they strengthen pancreatic function and stimulate the production of insulin. Brussels sprout juice may help protect against colon and stomach cancer and estrogen-related cancers such as breast, uterine, and endometrial cancer. It contains considerable amounts of calcium, potassium, phosphorus, folate, and vitamins A and C. Fresh Brussels sprout juice contains twice as much vitamin C as an equal portion of orange juice.

Cabbage Juice

Cabbage juice has a well-earned reputation for healing duodenal ulcers. It is high in calcium, vitamin C, sulfur, vitamin A, and much more. Cabbage juice has also helped people with eczema, seborrhea, and infection. The fresh juice should be consumed immediately since one of the beneficial compounds it contains, methylmethioninesulfonium chloride (popularly known as vitamin U) diminishes upon exposure to air. The juice has a high iodine content, which helps to regulate thyroid function and therefore can help with weight control. Cabbage juice has a cleansing effect on the mucous membranes lining the intestinal tract and the stomach, helps to regulate bowel function, and may aid in preventing stomach cancer. Drinking cabbage juice can cause gas; however, this is a normal response brought on by the cleansing action of the juice as it breaks down waste in the intestines. Excessive and/or painful gas resulting from drinking cabbage juice may be a sign of too many accumulated toxins in the intestinal tract. Always dilute fresh cabbage juice with water, in a ratio of one part juice to one-quarter to one-half part water. Or juice two carrots or one apple with the cabbage to sweeten the strong flavor.

Carrot Juice

Carrot juice, a great source of beta-carotene, is one of the most popular juices, and its versatility makes it a good base for most juice combinations. It has a normalizing effect on the body and is useful in the treatment and prevention of many disorders. Its abundant supply of beta-carotene makes it useful in treating many types of cancer, and helps to protect against macular degeneration. It is a good source of minerals, the B vitamins, and vitamins A and C. Carrot juice is excellent for treating diarrhea (even in infants) and intestinal infections and other disorders. The fresh juice contains sufficient quantities of calcium to help build and maintain strong bones and healthy teeth. It protects the nervous system, increases energy, can help ward off infections, and enrich a nursing mother's milk. Many skin problems, such as eczema and psoriasis, have responded favorably to carrot juice therapy. Even normal skin responds with an improvement in texture.

Consuming large quantities of carrot juice (or whole carrots) may give your skin an orange or yellowish tint. This is harmless. If it happens, simply reduce your consumption of carrot juice, and it should go away within a few days.

Celery Juice

Celery juice is an excellent source of the B vitamins; vitamins A, C, and E; and the minerals calcium, iron, magnesium, and potassium. It has a natural diuretic effect, helps to regulate body temperature, and aids in the elimination of carbon dioxide from the body. It is good for arthritis, appetite, adrenal function, and weight loss. Celery juice is useful for combating dizziness and headaches, aids digestion and weight loss, and stimulates adrenal function.

Juicing Made Simple

Fresh live juices provide live enzymes as well as vitamins, minerals, proteins, carbohydrates, purified water, essential fatty acids, chlorophyll, flavonoids, and powerful healing phytochemicals for superior healing, cleansing, and body maintenance. Use the table below as a quick reference guide to help you get the most out of these wonderful healing drinks. For detailed information about juices for specific health problems, see Appendix D: Live Juice Therapy.

Drink Type	Primary Attribute	Benefits	Comments
Category: Cereal Grass and Algae Top 4: Wheatgrass Spirulina Chlorella Barley	Healers	Stimulate cells Rejuvenate the body Build red blood cells Promote fast energy Act as internal disinfectants Reduce body odor and bad breath Improve blood disorders Cleanse the liver Are excellent for the digestive tract Cleanse drug and metal deposits Combat toxins	Add carrot or apple juice to sweeten and dilute. No fruit juice other than fresh, unsweetened apple juice should be added to cereal grass or algae juices. Cereal grass and algae juices are good for any type of illness. Include them as part of cancer treatment, especially if you are undergoing radiation therapy. Wheatgrass, one of the most potent greens, is loaded with enzymes.
Category: Vegetable Top 4: Beet Cabbage Carrot Garlic	Health restorers	Boost the immune system Remove acid waste Balance metabolism Aid in controlling obesity Slow aging Prevent degenerative disease Are fat- and cholesterol-free Are low in calories Are excellent for all disorders	Combine different-colored vegetables to obtain maximum nutritional variety. Remember to peel waxed cucumbers and apples and thoroughly wash all unpeeled vegetables before juicing. When juicing fresh garlic, place the clove in vinegar for 1 minute to destroy any bacteria or surface mold before processing. Use only 1 fresh clove of garlic per 2 glasses of juice to avoid intestinal irritation. For additional healing benefits, dip fresh reishi or shiitake mushrooms in boiling water to destroy bacteria, purée them in a blender, and add to vegetable juices.
Category: Fruit and melon Top 4: Berry (all kinds) Lemon Grape Apple	Body cleansers	Provide concentrated vitamin C Heal and energize Have powerful antioxidant effects Are rich in phytochemical Lower cholesterol levels Are naturally low in fat and calories Help to regulate blood sugar	Juice most fruit with the skins. Exceptions to this rule are apricots, bananas, citrus fruits, kiwis, melons, mangoes, papaya, peaches, and pineapple. Remove pits from fruits such as apricots and plums but leave small seeds. The exception to this rule is apples: Do not use the seeds from more than one apple per drink; they contain small amounts of cyanide. To use soft fruits that contain little water, such as papaya, banana, and avocado, purée and then add them to other juices. For a refreshing summer delight, freeze fresh melon juice such as cantaloupe, honeydew, or watermelon juice in ice cube trays. Add a few cubes to iced herbal tea. Makes even bitter teas delicious! If you have candida or a blood-sugar disorder, avoid juices made from sweet fruits.

Cucumber Juice

Cucumber juice is one of the best-known diuretics. It is good for the spleen, stomach, and large intestine. It is a blood cleanser and, as such, is good in the treatment of acne. The juice contains an abundance of potassium, which can help to regulate blood pressure. It was once thought that the level of sodium in the body was the key to normal blood pressure; however, it is now known that it is a correct balance between the levels of sodium and potassium that is important. To maintain the necessary balance of sodium and potassium in the body, combine celery or dandelion-green juice with cucumber juice. Cucumber juice also contains silicon, which can help strengthen hair and nails and improve skin conditions.

Dandelion-Green Juice

Dandelion greens yield a juice that is abundant in potassium, calcium, phosphorous, iron, chlorophyll, and sodium. It is the best source of organic magnesium, a key nutrient in many body functions. Fresh, live dandelion juice helps to build healthy cells and tissues, especially lung tissue. It is used as a blood cleanser and liver rejuvenator. Both the leaves and the root can be juiced and taken as a general tonic to restore vitality and energy. It is also helpful in balancing stomach acidity, strengthening the skeletal system, and building the blood. Juice extracted from the dandelion leaves, as well as a tea infused from the leaves, can be taken to ease the symptoms of rheumatoid arthritis. These are powerhouse greens for healing, giving strength, and working as a tonic.

Dandelion greens are increasingly available in farmer's markets and grocery stores, and are also (as anyone with a lawn knows!) easy to grow. However, you should not use any greens that may have come into contact with chemical herbicides or pesticides. If fresh dandelion greens are not available, you can purchase liquid dandelion extract—just add a few drops to each glass of any other kind of fresh vegetable juice.

Parsley Juice

Parsley is a rich source of vitamin C, beta-carotene, and folate, nutrients that help to protect against cancer. It has diuretic properties and helps treat conditions of the genitourinary system, such as kidney stones and other disorders of the kidneys and bladder. Parsley juice helps to regulate the function of the thyroid and adrenal glands, and strengthens and supports the capillaries and arterioles. It is beneficial in the treatment of disorders related to the eyes and optic nerve system. Because it is an herb, parsley's therapeutic powers are concentrated, so only a small amount is needed. Always mix parsley with other vegetables before juicing. Drinking large quantities of pure parsley juice can have a detrimental effect on the nervous system.

Potato Juice

Potato juice is a potassium cocktail that is particularly valuable for people who are convalescing from illness and for those who are sick and unable to eat. It is full of organic minerals and vitamins that will quickly restore energy and help the body to regenerate healthy cells and tissues. Raw potato juice cleanses the system and is helpful in treating gastric disorders. The potassium content makes it a good tonic for the heart. Its cleansing action makes it an effective treatment for skin disorders, especially acne.

Spinach Juice

Spinach juice contains high amounts of vitamins C and E, and is a rich source of minerals and other organic compounds necessary for optimum health. The fresh raw juice has a remarkable cleansing and healing effect on the entire intestinal tract. Because of its high folate content, expectant mothers (and women who plan to become pregnant) would be well advised to include fresh spinach juice in their diets; folate helps to protect against both miscarriage and certain types of birth defects. Spinach juice is also thought to improve the quality of milk of nursing mothers. If you have a history of liver disease, kidney stones, or arthritis, however, you should not consume concentrated spinach juice and should eat raw or cooked spinach sparingly, as it contains significant concentrations of oxalic acid, which interferes with calcium absorption and other metabolic functions.

Turnip Juice

Turnip juice, with twice the amount of vitamin C as oranges or tomatoes, can be extracted from both the root and the leafy greens of the turnip. The greens contain more calcium than any other vegetable and yield a juice that is recommended for growing children and women at risk of developing osteoporosis. The root helps the body eliminate uric acid, making it useful in the prevention of kidney stones and gout. It also helps with weight loss. The juice from the root has expectorant actions and can be used to treat bronchitis and sinusitis.

Watercress Juice

Watercress has been used as a digestive aid for centuries. More recently, it has been shown to benefit the gallbladder and liver ailments. Watercress juice contains high levels of nutrients and should be used sparingly. Adding one-quarter bunch to other vegetables for juicing is appropriate. Watercress juice contains ample amounts of calcium, magnesium, phosphorus, potassium, and vitamins A and C. It is a powerful intestinal cleanser that helps to oxygenate the blood and stimulate the formation of red blood cells. Its high sulfur content helps to kill viruses and maintain

Waxed Fruits and Vegetables

Fruits and vegetables are often coated with a thin layer of wax to enhance their appearance and to preserve them for long-distance shipping. Some of the waxes are derived from natural sources like honeycombs, while others come from petroleum and resins. Waxes used on produce with edible peels (apples, cucumbers, pears, and the like) are categorized by the U.S. Food and Drug Administration as *generally recognized as safe* (GRAS). Waxes used on citrus foods and other fruits with inedible peels, however, do not have to meet this standard, and some may contain substances that are potentially carcinogenic. Another consideration is that waxes may contain animal products (such as tallow) that would violate kosher and strict vegetarian dietary restrictions.

Regardless of their composition, waxes may trap residues from pesticides and other chemicals. Most waxes can be removed by scrubbing the produce with soapy water that is hot enough to melt the wax. Other waxes can be removed only by peeling. To avoid waxes altogether, try to purchase organic, unwaxed produce.

healthy hair, nails, skin, and bones. Watercress juice is also beneficial for people with asthma and emphysema.

Watercress juice is acid-forming. It should not be used alone but in combination with highly alkaline vegetables, such as carrots or celery.

Fruit and Melon Juices

Fruit and melon juices supply carbohydrates and sugars the body needs to produce energy and keep working. Full of vitamins, minerals, and disease-fighting antioxidants, they nourish and help to cleanse the body. Fruit juices have a high sugar content and ferment quickly in the stomach, so you should always dilute them with pure water (one part juice to one part water).

Apple Juice

Apple juice has a high mineral content. It also contains malic acid, which plays an important role in normalizing the intestines, has a detoxifying effect in the body, and is good for treating muscle disorders. Apple juice can lower blood cholesterol and aid liver function, and is good for cleansing and healing internal inflammation. Drinking 12 ounces of apple juice (or eating two whole apples) per day

can reduce the oxidation of low-density lipoprotein (LDL, or "bad") cholesterol, an important factor in the buildup of cholesterol in blood vessels, according to researchers at the University of California at Davis. The lead researcher there, Dianne Hyson, stated, "Apples are packed with antioxidants, potassium, fiber, and other key nutrients, all of which may offer protection." In the Netherlands, another study concluded that the phytochemicals in apples could help cut the risk of death from stroke and heart disease in half. Apple juice has antiviral properties, making it a valuable preventive measure against colds, bronchitis, and other viral infections. The whole fruit helps regulate steep rises in blood sugar levels, while the juice can cause a sharp decrease in blood sugar.

Cantaloupe and Honeydew Melon Juice

Cantaloupe is an excellent source of beta-carotene, which helps to reduce the risk of certain cancers, protects against night blindness and other eye problems, and improves memory function. It is loaded with potassium, which can normalize body fluids, lower blood pressure, and help to reduce the incidence of muscle cramps. Honeydew melons lack the beta-carotene found in cantaloupe, but they do have a good supply of potassium. Both melons contain adenosine, the same anticoagulant compound found in onions and garlic, which can thin the blood and lower the risk of stroke and heart attack.

Cantaloupe and honeydew melons can be juiced with the skins on if they are organically grown and if you are certain they are free of pesticides or waxes. However, you should wash all melons before cutting them, as there can be mold and/or bacteria present on the rind that can be transferred to the pulp if you do not wash them.

Grape Juice

Grape juice is high in potassium and is therefore a good beverage to help lower high blood pressure. Red grapes tend to have the highest levels of potassium. Juice prepared from fresh grapes is nothing like the bottled grape juice in your grocery store. A drink made with fresh grapes and blueberries, both of which contain phytochemicals that can neutralize viruses, helps to combat herpesviruses. Grape juice has antibacterial activity and can help reduce tooth decay. It also contains caffeic acid, a phytochemical that acts as an antioxidant and helps protect against cancer. Researchers at the University of Wisconsin Medical School found that purple grape juice has anticlotting effects, possibly stronger than those of aspirin, which can help keep the heart and blood vessels healthy.

Grapefruit Juice

Grapefruit juice is credited with cancer-fighting capabilities due to its high vitamin C content. Red grapefruit also contains lycopene, a phytochemical that helps lower the risk of prostate cancer. If you prepare the fruit with the white membrane still intact, it contains galacturonic acid, which can lower blood cholesterol by removing plaque from artery walls.

A word of caution: There is a substance in grapefruit juice that significantly increases the body's absorption of some commonly used drugs, especially certain blood pressure medications, immunosuppressive drugs, and sedatives. Having a higher than normal concentration of these drugs in your body can have serious side effects. Consult your health-care provider before combining grapefruit juice with medication.

Lemon Juice

Lemon juice has antibacterial properties and can be used to cleanse the system and purify the blood. Diluted with quality water, it can be used as a cleansing enema to detoxify the system and balance the pH (the level of acidity) in the colon. No drink can compare with the valuable properties of lemon juice, either internally or externally. Taken each morning upon rising, a mixture of lemon juice and quality water helps to detoxify the system and act as a natural antacid. (See the recipe for Lemon Quality Water on page 29.) The juice contains high amounts of vitamin C and has been used by travelers to thwart scurvy and sanitize drinking water. People with ulcers should avoid drinking the juice of lemons and other citrus fruits, however.

Orange Juice

Orange juice that is made from fruit with the white, pithy parts still attached is a frothy beverage high in vitamin C and phytochemicals that fight cancer, strengthen the capillaries, and have antiviral properties. Orange juice can help ward off colds and other viral infections.

Papaya Juice

Papaya juice is an excellent source of vitamin C and beta-carotene. One 8-ounce cup of papaya juice supplies three times the RDA of vitamin C and almost twice the amount of beta-carotene needed per day. It also contains a wealth of proteolytic enzymes, which enable the body to digest protein. Papain, the most important of these enzymes, is used in meat tenderizers. Papaya juice improves digestion and heals ulcers and other gastrointestinal disorders. It contains arginine, an amino acid that stimulates the pancreas to release insulin and plays an important role in male fertility.

If you have a baby, save a tablespoon of the whole papaya, mash it, and add it to your child's formula or soft food to help his or her digestion. You can also save the seeds, rinse them off, allow them to dry, and grind them up and use them in place of pepper. The seeds have a peppery flavor and aid digestion.

PART THREE

HOW FOOD HEALS

INTRODUCTION

Healers around the world have used food and herbs as medicine for centuries. Much of the global population still depends on the plant kingdom as their main source of medicine. It is only recently, however, that scientific research has determined more precisely how it is that nature works in tandem with the body to fight disease.

Articles in health-related publications and even daily newspapers now speak regularly about antioxidants and free radicals. You have probably gotten the basic idea that antioxidants are good and free radicals are bad. That's true, but there is more to it than that. Actually, antioxidants are a class of substances encompassing certain nutrients, minerals, phytochemicals, herbs, and enzymes that counteract the negative effects of free radicals on the body. Free radicals are unstable molecules and fragments of molecules that are toxic to cells and tissues because they attack them at the molecular level, causing destruction and mutations. They are believed to be the driving force behind premature aging and many chronic degenerative diseases. Antioxidants are powerful neutralizers that reduce the harm. In Part Three, you will learn what is going on in your body at a cellular and molecular level, and how these processes affect your health. You will also learn which food, herbs, and supplements are rich in antioxidants and how you can use them to combat illness and aging.

Beyond the realm of our traditional understanding of nutrition and nutrients exists an enormous plant resource for nutritional healing. These are called phytochemicals (or phytonutrients). Found in fruits, vegetables, legumes, grains, and herbs, these "phytos" help to fight cancer, aging, and most health disorders. Research studies on these plant compounds are growing daily. This is the most current, cutting-edge information on phytochemicals, how they heal, where they exist in the plant world, and how they can be used as preventives and cures.

CHAPTER SIX

ANTIOXIDANTS: POWERFUL DISEASE PREVENTION

Since oxygen is essential for life, it's ironic that burning it sets the stage for aging and many diseases. The good news is that antioxidants in foods seem to stave off these effects.

—Foods That Harm, Foods That Heal (Reader's Digest)

Antioxidants are certain nutrients, minerals, phytochemicals, herbs, and enzymes that counteract the harmful effects of free radicals on the body. Thus, to understand antioxidants and what they do, you must first understand free radicals.

As the cells burn fuel (food) for energy, they also burn oxygen, a process that creates atoms, molecules, and fragments of molecules that are called *free radicals*. Exposure to polluted air, toxic chemicals, radiation, ultraviolet rays, and tobacco smoke also results in the formation of free radicals. On the molecular level, free radicals are unstable; they each contain an unpaired electron that, in an effort to pair up and stabilize the substance, will bind to and "steal" electrons from other substances, including healthy cells. This damages cells and tissues and creates even more free radicals that may then attack other healthy cells. This results in oxidative damage to cells that can be compared to rust on a car. Free radicals also destroy and cause mutations in the body's cells, which then become unable to absorb the nutrients needed. This "cell starvation" results in an inability to fight off disease caused by free radicals

Everyday choices in diet, lifestyle, and environment affect the delicate balance of this energy exchange at a molecular level. Left unbalanced, free-radical damage plays a major role in nearly every chronic illness, including cancer and heart disease, and is believed to be the driving force behind premature aging. Antioxidants are the powerful neutralizers that reduce and prevent harm from oxygen-free radicals.

For many years, scientists believed that the quintessential antioxidants were vitamins A (and beta-carotene, which the body uses to make vitamin A), C, and E, and the mineral selenium, with vitamin E generating the most interest among researchers. Newer studies, however, are examining phytochemicals, or phytonutrients, which are naturally occurring compounds found in plants. Some of the groups of phytochemicals that have been the subject of greatest interest are carotenoids, flavonoids, isoflavones, and procyanidolic oligomers, or PCOs (also known as oligo-

meric proanthocyanidins, or OPCs), which are believed to be fifty times stronger than vitamins C and E. *The American Journal of Clinical Nutrition* has reported that the carotenoids lycopene (found primarily in tomatoes), zeaxanthin, and lutein are the true superheroes when it comes to controlling the activity of oxygen free radicals. This is great news, because these super antioxidants are easily and naturally obtained from fruits (oranges, grapefruits, apricots, berries, papayas, cantaloupe, and nectarines), deep-colored vegetables (carrots, spinach, cabbage, kale, yams, squash, and broccoli), nuts, seeds, and wheat germ.

While many antioxidant nutrients are available in supplement form, for the most part it is better to get a combination of food-derived antioxidants. Whole foods also contain fiber, and nutrients from whole foods are probably more readily absorbed than those in pills or supplements. Growing research shows that there is a synergy among dietary antioxidants and that "networking" combinations are more beneficial, as each antioxidant has special protective properties for particular body functions. Foods and products that combine two or more of these vital nutrients provide the most effective balance.

CAROTENOIDS—THE "BIG GUN" ANTIOXIDANTS

A class of phytochemicals, carotenoids are natural fat-soluble pigments found principally in plants, algae, and photosynthetic bacteria, and are responsible for many of the orange, red, green, and yellow hues of leaves, fruits, vegetables, and flowers. They are a potent family of antioxidants numbering more than 600. The most powerful carotenoids known are beta-carotene, lutein, and lycopene.

Beta-Carotene

The liver uses the carotenoid beta-carotene to manufacture vitamin A, so it is sometimes referred to as preformed vitamin A. Beta-carotene is abundant in dark green, yellow, and orange vegetables, such as broccoli, carrots, pumpkin, and sweet potatoes, as well as some fruits. It also is found in some foods, including eggs, fish, fortified milk, and organ meats such as liver. It is best to get beta-carotene from food sources that are easily assimilated by the body. Recent studies indicate that taking excessive doses of beta-carotene supplements may actually work against the body's natural cell division and increase the risk of lung cancer in smokers. A diet rich in beta-carotene may help counter the effect of aging on the eyes, boost the immune system, help prevent heart disease, and work at the molecular level to prevent the formation of carcinogens. While large amounts of vitamin A can be toxic, particularly for pregnant women, the natural beta-carotene in foods is not dangerous because the body converts it into vitamin A only as needed.

Lutein

Lutein is a phytochemical found in broccoli, kale, spinach, and other dark-green leafy vegetables; egg yolks; and peaches and oranges. It is beneficial for the eyes. In a 1995 study conducted by the National Institutes of Health and reported in the *Journal of the American Medical Association*, people who ate large amounts of lutein-containing foods were found to have a lower than average incidence of cataracts and macular degeneration, the leading cause of blindness in older adults. The biologic plausibility for a protective role for lutein and another carotenoid, zeaxanthin, in eye health is quite strong.

Lycopene

Lycopene, the carotenoid that gives tomatoes their red color, is an important quencher of free radicals. Found in high concentrations in the prostate gland, it apparently plays a role in protecting against abnormal cellular proliferation. A study reported in the *Journal of the National Cancer Institute* showed that men with the most lycopene in their blood had the lowest risk of prostate cancer. Lycopene packs an antioxidant punch at least two to three times more potent than that of beta-carotene. Found in tomatoes, guavas, and other red-pigmented fruits and vegetables, lycopene has stirred the interest of the scientific community for its anticarcinogenic effects. Interestingly, tomato juices and sauces are a more concentrated source of lycopene than are fresh, whole tomatoes.

ACETYL-L-CARNITINE, ALPHA-LIPOIC ACID, AND COENZYME Q$_{10}$

Working together, acetyl-L-carnitine, alpha-lipoic acid, and coenzyme Q$_{10}$ support cellular energy throughout the body and protect against age-related degeneration.

Acetyl-L-Carnitine

Acetyl-L-carnitine is a form of the amino acid-carnitine, found in proteins. It increases brain levels of acetylcholine, a main neurotransmitter needed for memory and learning. Several studies have indicated that acetyl-L-carnitine may delay the onset of Alzheimer's disease and improve the performance of those who already have the disease. It is produced in the brain, liver, and kidneys.

Alpha-Lipoic Acid

Alpha-lipoic acid (ALA) is an essential coenzyme involved in the production of energy in every organ of the body and is a powerful antioxidant. It is found primarily in broccoli, spinach, and organ meats. Because ALA is soluble in both water and fat, it is very readily absorbed from our food and is effective at deactivating free radicals in the cells. It can actually recycle other antioxidants, including vitamins C and E, the amino acid compound glutathione, and coenzyme Q$_{10}$, when they are depleted. In Europe, ALA has been prescribed by physicians to lower glucose (blood sugar) levels in people with diabetes. It also detoxifies the liver of metal pollutants, interferes with the formation of cataracts, reduces cholesterol levels, protects nerve tissue, and lessens the effects of aging. Animal studies suggest that ALA may reduce high levels of free radicals and increase energy levels. Human clinical trials are planned.

Coenzyme Q$_{10}$

Coenzyme Q$_{10}$, also known as ubiquinone, is a substance that is produced by the body and that is structurally similar to vitamin E. Some evidence suggests that coenzyme Q$_{10}$ slows the aging process, enhances the immune system, increases circulation, slows the spread of cancer, and aids in the prevention and treatment of cardiovascular disease. Studies have focused on its proven benefits to the heart, and in Japan, it has been approved for treating congestive heart failure. It is especially plentiful in organ meats, such as liver and kidney, as well as avocados, beef, peanuts, soy oil, spinach, and seafood, with mackerel, salmon, and sardines containing the highest amounts.

GLUTATHIONE

Glutathione, a type of protein that is produced in the liver from the amino acids cysteine, glutamic acid, and glycine, is the main water-soluble antioxidant and is essential for maintaining a strong immune system. It is the most powerful intracellular antioxidant (antioxidant that works within individual cells) and scavenges hydroxyl radicals, which are considered by some experts to be the most dangerous kind of free radical.

People with cancer, diabetes, or HIV/AIDS need to maintain a healthy level of glutathione. It also effectively detoxifies heavy metals and toxins and is used to treat blood and liver maladies. In addition to protecting individual cells, it guards tissues of the arteries, brain, eyes, heart, immune system, liver, lungs, and skin, and has been hailed as a cancer-preventing substance that may target carcinogens for eradication. People with autoimmune diseases usually have low levels of glutathione. As people age, glutathione levels drop, resulting in a decreased ability to deactivate free radicals. Researchers think that getting enough cruciferous vegetables, such as broccoli, Brussels sprouts, cabbage, and kale, helps to raise glutathione levels in the body.

METHIONINE

Methionine is a sulfur-rich essential amino acid found in meat, dairy products, fish, eggs, beans, garlic, lentils, onions, yogurt, and seeds. It neutralizes hydroxyl radicals—dangerous free radicals that damage body tissues. Methionine helps to prevent hair, skin, and nail disorders; counteract fatty liver disease; lower cholesterol; protect the kidneys; detoxify the body of heavy metals; prevent bladder irritation; and promote hair growth. People with HIV/AIDS, liver problems, Parkinson's disease, or pancreatitis may benefit from increasing their intake of methionine, as might women who take birth control pills and people diagnosed with schizophrenia. Methionine is also available in supplement form, but you should exercise caution if you are interested in getting it this way—it is advisable to consult a physician about this, as excessive doses may increase levels of blood cholesterol and homocysteine, an amino acid that has been associated with hardening of the arteries.

SELENIUM

Selenium, a trace mineral, is used by the body to produce glutathione peroxidase, a powerful antioxidant enzyme. By fighting cell damage, selenium may lower the risk of cancer and play a crucial role in supporting the overall immune response. All of the body's tissues contain selenium, but it is most plentiful in the liver, kidneys, spleen, pancreas, and testes. Selenium works synergistically with vitamin E to protect tissues and cell membranes, aid in the production of antibodies, and help maintain a healthy heart and liver. In a study at the University of Arizona Cancer Center, researchers discovered a dramatically lower than normal incidence of cancer among people who took supplemental selenium: 66 percent less prostate cancer, 50 percent less colon cancer, and 40 percent less lung cancer. Additional studies have concluded that, when combined with zinc and vitamin E, selenium promotes prostate health. James D. Brooks, M.D., a Stanford University researcher and specialist in prostate cancer, has said that there is a direct connection between selenium intake and

the risk of prostate cancer, with older men who consumed higher levels of selenium at a lower risk than those with lower intake.

You should not exceed an intake of over 800 micrograms of selenium a day, as hair and nail loss may result. Pregnant women should get no more than 40 micrograms daily. Selenium is found in seafood, liver, garlic, onions and leeks, asparagus, broccoli, kelp, wheat germ, brown rice, Brazil nuts, brewer's yeast, and grains. The selenium content of foods can vary widely, however, depending on the soil content of this mineral in the areas in which it is produced. Most of the soil in American farmland is low in selenium, resulting in selenium-deficient produce, so it may be necessary to take supplements to ensure an adequate intake. Two hundred micrograms daily is a typical recommended dose.

SUPEROXIDE DISMUTASE

The enzyme superoxide dismutase (SOD) neutralizes superoxide radicals, which are among the most harmful of all free radicals, and reduces the rate of cell destruction. Working together with catalase, another enzyme found in abundance in the body, SOD destroys harmful hydrogen peroxide, reduces high blood pressure, and helps to prevent cataracts. SOD helps the body to process zinc, copper, and manganese. Barley grass, broccoli, Brussels sprouts, cabbage, wheatgrass, and most green plants are rich in this enzyme.

VITAMIN C

Vitamin C is a nutrient that is prevalent in asparagus, avocados, berries, broccoli, Brussels sprouts, cantaloupe, most citrus fruits (especially grapefruit, lemons, mangoes, papayas, oranges, and pineapples), collards, dandelion greens, kale, onions, potatoes, and turnips. It is also widely available in supplement form, though supplements may not be as effective as the vitamin C found in whole foods. This vitamin is water-soluble, which allows it to dissolve easily in bodily fluids. It also helps other antioxidants keep their potency and aids in their absorption.

A diet high in vitamin C has proven to reduce the risk of heart disease and cancer. It is thought to help stave off osteoarthritis pain in two ways. First, it is necessary for the formation of collagen and proteoglycans—major components of cartilage that act like joint cushions. Second, as an antioxidant, it quenches free radicals that rip through cartilage. The joint inflammation that characterizes rheumatoid arthritis also can be relieved by vitamin C.

Researchers from Cornell University and Seoul National University in South Korea found that vitamin C inhibits the cancer-causing effects of hydrogen peroxide on cell communication. "Vitamin C has been considered one of the most important essential nutrients in our diet since the discovery in 1907 that it prevents scurvy. In addition, vitamin C aids the synthesis of amino acids and collagen, wound healing, metabolism of iron, lipids and cholesterol and others," said Dr. C. Y. Lee of Cornell. The researchers pretreated rat liver cells with vitamin C and saw that hydrogen peroxide could not exert an inhibitory effect, while other antioxidants tested failed to prevent it. Researchers concluded, "A diet rich in phytochemicals and vitamin C will reduce the risk of cancer."

Alcohol, analgesics, antidepressants, anticoagulants, oral contraceptives, and steroids may reduce levels of vitamin C in the body. Smoking causes a serious depletion of vitamin C. In one study, women younger than sixty years old who consumed large amounts of vitamin C were about 57 percent less likely to develop cortical cataracts, which affect the central outer part of the lens.

VITAMIN E

Vitamin E is believed to reduce the risks of heart disease and may also protect the body against cancer, Alzheimer's disease, and Parkinson's disease. Emerging data suggest a definite potential benefit of vitamin E for those considered to be high-risk cardiac patients. Quite by accident, in separate studies on skin and lung cancer, scientists discovered that a combination of vitamin E and selenium greatly decreased the incidence of prostate cancer in men. The National Cancer Institute is conducting a twelve-year study inspired by those findings. Foods rich in vitamin E include cold-pressed vegetable oils, fortified cereals, legumes, nuts (particularly almonds and hazelnuts), spinach and other dark-green leafy vegetables, sunflower seeds, sweet potatoes, wheat germ, and whole grains. Selenium increases the absorption of vitamin E if the two nutrients are consumed together.

ZINC

Zinc is a mineral that is necessary for cell division, growth, wound healing, and proper immune system function. Its main antioxidant function is in the prevention of fat oxidation. Zinc is needed for proper maintenance of vitamin E levels in the blood and aids in the absorption of vitamin A. It plays an important role in the health of the reproductive organs, is essential to prostate function, and boosts testosterone levels. Its effect on prostate health may be due to the fact that it inhibits the production of the enzyme 5-alpha-reductase and reduces the body's production of the chemical dihydrotestosterone (DHT), a form of the male hormone testosterone that is linked to enlargement of the prostate. Zinc also helps the body to excrete excess DHT and assists in shrinking already enlarged prostates. Dietary sources of zinc include animal proteins, such as organ meats, seafood (especially oysters and sardines), milk, poultry, and eggs. Plant sources include mushrooms, soybeans, sunflower seeds, and wheat germ.

Less Inflammation and Soreness after Workouts with Vitamin E

In people who exercise intensively, particularly older people, free-radical production can go into overdrive and break down more tissue than it builds, according to a report from Jennifer Sacheck, Ph.D., a researcher at Tufts University. She hypothesized that giving older exercisers supplements of vitamin E to dampen free-radical activity might help to curtail any muscle damage. Tests showed that older exercisers experienced less inflammation and younger ones had less soreness and muscle damage after dosing with 1,000 international units of vitamin E every day for three months. Vitamin E can cause bleeding problems, however, particularly if it is combined with certain drugs, so you should always consult a health-care professional before taking high amounts of vitamin E.

ANTIOXIDANT HERBS

In addition to food and supplements, some herbs and herbal extracts are highly valued for their antioxidant qualities. Following is an outline of some of the more important antioxidant herbs. More details on using herbs to cure or prevent health problems can be found in *Prescription for Herbal Healing* (Avery/Penguin Putnam, 2002).

Bilberry

Bilberry hails from the same plant family as the blueberry and huckleberry. The part used as an herb is the leaf portion of the plant. Bilberry conditions capillaries and red blood cells, thereby helping to lower blood pressure. It also protects the eyes; inhibits bacterial growth; has anticarcinogenic, anti-inflammatory, and antiaging properties; and helps to lower blood sugar levels. The collagen-stabilizing antioxidant and anti-inflammatory properties of bilberry extract make it helpful for the treatment of arthritis. Bilberry contains phytochemicals known as anthocyanidins, which studies indicate can provide up to fifty times the antioxidant protection of vitamin E and ten times the protection of vitamin C.

Burdock

Burdock, a relative of the sunflower, when taken in combination with vitamin E, is extremely effective for eliminating harmful free radicals. It also helps to prevent cell mutation, which might otherwise lead to cancer. Burdock purifies the blood and, when prepared as a tea, has proven beneficial for treating chronic skin conditions such as acne and eczema, and ridding the body of kidney stones and gallstones. It eliminates toxins, supports digestion, and is a good source of calcium, phosphorus, potassium, and protein. It is reputed to help heal liver damage and offer protection from further damage. In addition, some people with diabetes place great confidence in burdock. It is available in burdock-seed cereals, sold as *gobo* or *goboshi* in Japanese groceries, and is also available as a tea.

Garlic

Garlic is extremely effective at neutralizing the effects of free radicals. Considerable evidence suggests that organosulfurs found in garlic (and onions) may help to prevent atherosclerosis (hardening of the arteries) through its free-radical-scavenging effects and also through its effects on cholesterol buildup, blood pressure, and platelet aggregation. It has been known to protect the body against cholesterol buildup, prevent blood clots, and lower high blood pressure. In one study in *The Journal of Nutrition*, participants were given garlic extract for fourteen days, and blood and urine samples were taken at fourteen and twenty-eight days to measure levels of free 8-iso-prostaglandin F2-alpha, a compound that is an indication of oxidative stress. At the beginning, blood plasma concentrations in smokers were 58 percent higher than in nonsmokers and urine concentrations were 85 percent higher. After fourteen days on aged garlic supplementation, the nonsmokers experienced a 29 percent drop in the plasma concentration of the oxidative stress marker, while smokers experienced a 35 percent drop. Urinary concentrations fell by 37 percent in the non-smoking group and 48 percent in smokers. Researchers noted the confirmation of the increased oxidative stress in smokers as compared with nonsmokers, and concluded that dietary supplementation with aged garlic may help to prevent diseases associated with oxidative stress like atherosclerosis. Garlic is available in capsule and liquid form for those who do not enjoy fresh garlic or worry about the socially unacceptable scent.

Garlic's sulfur compounds have the ability to reduce the formation of carcinogenic compounds, inhibiting the growth of different types of cancer, including colon cancer. Garlic also has antibacterial, antiviral, and antifungal properties. Aged garlic extract provides the greatest concentration of beneficial compounds; however, fresh garlic and garlic oil can be used daily for favorable results. (More information about this powerful herb can be found in Chapter 20).

Ginkgo

Ginkgo biloba has a stabilizing effect on cellular membranes. It also has powerful antioxidant effects in the brain, retina, and cardiovascular system. Widely known as the "smart herb," it is the most widely prescribed drug in Germany, where it is considered an effective treatment for Alzheimer's disease and other severe forms of memory deficit and decline in mental function. Growing evidence suggests that it is helpful for ordinary age-related memory loss, tinnitus (persistent ringing in the ears), balance disorders, impotence, and macular degeneration. Ginkgo is available as an extract in liquid, tablet, and capsule forms.

Green Tea

Green tea leaves are rich in flavonoids and other compounds that may possess potent antioxidant properties. Recent studies lend merit to the already substantial evidence that the polyphenols in green tea have anticarcinogenic and anti-inflammatory properties. Other studies suggest that green tea may also protect against damage done by cholesterol and help prevent blood clots. It shows promise as a weight-loss aid that can promote the burning of fat and help to regulate blood sugar and insulin levels. Tea polyphenols are increasingly being used to treat skin disorders and in skin care products.

Drinking as little as one cup of green tea each day appears to offer some protection against heart disease. Green tea is the dried, unfermented, leaves of the plant. The fermentation process, which produces black tea, destroys most of the polyphenols, making black tea less effective as an antioxidant.

Milk Thistle

Milk thistle and silymarin, a compound extracted from the seeds of milk thistle, have been used for centuries to treat diseases of the liver. This powerful antioxidant guards the liver from oxidative damage; protects the liver from toxins, drugs, and the effects of alcohol (cirrhosis) and the hepatitis B and C viruses; and promotes the growth of new liver cells. In addition, silymarin increases levels of glutathione, a potent antioxidant enzyme produced in the liver. (See page 43.) Milk thistle extract has virtually no known side effects and can be used by most people. Silymarin gelcaps contain the greatest concentration of active ingredients.

Turmeric

Turmeric, which comes from the large, deep-yellow rhizome (underground stem) of the plant *Curcuma domestica*, commands a venerable medicinal position in Asia and in India, where it is considered a tonic for the whole body. Traditional Chinese healers prescribe it for liver problems and colic. American herbalists recommend turmeric for reducing the pain and inflammation of arthritis and preventing gallbladder disease. The active constituent in turmeric is curcumin, a strong antioxidant. Other substances in turmeric help remove toxic byproducts that may contribute to the formation of cancer cells. It soothes inflammation by reducing levels of histamine, a body chemical that is released as part of the immune response. Research raises hope that turmeric may help to prevent blood clots, reduce cholesterol levels, and, possibly, protect against gallbladder disease. It is available as a powdered root, in capsules, and as a liquid tincture.

Grapeseed and Pine Bark Extracts

Grapeseed extract and pine bark extract (also available under the trademarked name Pycnogenol) possess flavonoids known variously as procyanidolic oligomers (PCOs) and oligomeric proanthocyanidins (OPCs). These are naturally occurring substances found throughout plant life, and are concentrated in grapeseed and pine bark extracts. PCOs, which are highly water soluble and are rapidly absorbed by the body, help to promote cardiovascular health, balance body fluids, and strengthen capillaries. They also are believed to provide certain benefits for people with arthritis and allergies. They have a special affinity for the collagen-based tissues of the body, such as the skin. These biologically active compounds support the body's defense mechanisms and fight bacteria. PCOs are also found in red- and blue-colored berries.

CHAPTER SEVEN

PHYTOCHEMICALS: THE BODY'S ARSENAL

Somewhere in the plant kingdom there is a remedy for everything.

—*James A. Duke, Ph.D., ethnobotanist*

Phytochemicals—naturally occurring compounds in plants—are a vast, relatively untapped resource for natural healing. Beyond the realm of traditional nutrients (carbohydrates, proteins, fats, vitamins, and minerals) exists another world of nutritional curatives in fruits, vegetables, grains, legumes, and herbs. These powerful plant compounds are potent agents formed by nature to work *with* the body to fight disease, rather than working *against* it, as drugs often do. Phytochemicals are powerful ammunition in the war against cancer, aging, and most health disorders.

Phyto is the Greek work for "plant." There is a small debate as to whether to call these plant chemicals *phytochemicals* or *phytonutrients*. Some scientists classify them as nonessential, which would disqualify them from being considered nutrients. Thousands of phytochemicals are found everywhere in the plant world, where they often function as natural defenses against biological hazards. Among other things, they give plants their color, flavor, and natural disease resistance. Tomatoes alone are believed to contain an estimated 10,000 different phytochemicals.

The average American diet today, most people would admit, is sorely lacking in plant-derived nutrition. According to the U.S. Department of Agriculture (USDA), only 49 percent of the population consumes the minimum number of servings of vegetables recommended (three servings per day). Only 29 percent consume the minimum number of servings of fruit recommended (two per day). A nutrition-packed dinner would consist of 45 percent vegetables and fruits, 25 percent protein (legumes, soybean products, or fish), and 30 percent whole grains, nuts, and seeds. If you do not eat fish, you can get essential fatty acids from virgin olive oil, fresh nuts, and flaxseeds. The National Cancer Institute has invested well over $20 million in recent years to investigate the anticancer properties of plant foods. In an article published in *The Natural Physician*, renowned cancer researcher Dr. Patrick Quillin, Ph.D., R.D., CNS, said, "Proper nutrition could prevent 50 to 90 percent of all cancers."

It is extremely important to increase your intake of phytochemicals. The best way to obtain the benefits from phytochemicals is through eating a variety of foods. Taking supplements does not have as much benefit; however, if it is not possible to consume large amounts of phytochemical-rich food, supplementation may be necessary. Phytochemicals also have a synergistic effect. For example, carotenoids work best in the presence of flavonoids when they are eaten together in the same foods. Phytochemicals react biochemically to one another within the plant, so the same probably holds true in the body. Eat a variety of fruits and vegetables of all colors—the more colorful, the better.

Different phytochemicals have different reactions in the body. One may neutralize a carcinogen, while another might carry it away. Still another might act as an antioxidant to handcuff a free radical and keep it from roaming. Most important are the phytochemicals that stimulate the body's own enzymes to destroy carcinogens before they have a chance to begin their damage.

The primary benefits of phytochemicals lie in their abilities as antioxidants and in aiding the body's resistance to cancer. Antioxidants block the action of free radicals, which can damage cell contents and membranes. (See Chapter 6.) Antioxidants are also a powerful aid to the immune system. With their help, the body is far better equipped to defend itself. Not all free radicals come from inside the body—there are outside sources as well. Some of these invading molecules are known carcinogens (cancer-causing substances). Tobacco smoke, radiation, and air pollution are all known sources of free radicals that invade the body.

Cancer is just one example of a disease caused by free radical damage; heart disease is another. Inflammation in the body can be hard to detect, yet it slowly attacks healthy tissues in the brain, arteries, and joints, leading to a large number of different illnesses and diseases. There are about twenty known anti-inflammatory phytochemicals, including apigenin (found in celery stalks and seeds), which can help reduce pain and inflammation from a variety of disorders, including gout. Other important foods that contain inflammation-fighting phytochemicals are blackberries, cherries, raspberries, and strawberries. Phytochemicals in

Color Your Plate: Fight Disease and Aging with "Colorful" Food

Eat one serving daily from each of these phytonutrient-rich color groups to prevent disease and premature aging:

- Red. Choose apples, beets, cherries, cranberries, kidney or adzuki beans, plums, red bell peppers, radishes, raspberries, red cabbage, red grapes, strawberries, tomatoes, and/or watermelon.

- Orange or yellow. Enjoy apricots, cantaloupe, carrots, mangoes, nectarines, oranges, pineapple, pumpkin, squash, sweet potatoes, yams, and yellow or orange bell peppers.

- Green. Have some asparagus, avocado, broccoli, Brussels sprouts, green cabbage, celery, kale, kiwi, okra, spinach, watercress—virtually any leafy green vegetable.

- Other mixed colors, including white and purple. Add to your diet foods such as cauliflower, celery, eggplant, kohlrabi, parsnips, rutabaga, and turnips.

For each of the vegetables and fruits mentioned above, one serving is equivalent to:

- One medium-sized fruit, such as an apple, pear, or orange.
- ½ cup raw, cooked, frozen, or canned fruit or vegetable.
- 1 cup raw, leafy greens, such as spinach, kale, or lettuce.
- ¾ cup 100 percent fruit or vegetable juice.
- ½ cup cooked or canned beans or peas.
- ¼ cup dried fruit, such as raisins or dates.

---

blueberries help the body to repair damage already caused by inflammation.

Cancer is a category of disorders characterized by cells that have mutated and begin to reproduce themselves in an uncontrolled fashion. Under normal circumstances, the body's natural defense system would attack such cells and, hopefully, destroy them. If the body's natural killer cells are not successful, however, cancerous cells continue to reproduce wildly and, eventually, spread to other parts of the body. Phytochemicals like the catechins found in green tea act to prevent cell mutation and keep cells reproducing normally. Allyl sulfides, found in garlic and onions, trigger enzymes that help to rid the body of carcinogens before damage to the cell can be done.

Where are all the phytochemicals? Carotenoids are the most common. They are responsible for the red, orange, and yellow pigments found in fruits and vegetables. The heavy hitters of the family are alpha-carotene, beta-carotene, and lycopene. These carotenoids are found in carrots, broccoli, pumpkin, tomatoes, watermelon, guava, and pink grapefruit, to name a few. Another fine family of helpful phytochemicals is the phenols. These are further classified as flavonoids or nonflavonoids. The flavonoids include substances known as catechins, flavanones, and isoflavones, among others. They can be found in apples, lemons, green tea, and red wine or red grapes. Nonflavonoids, such as coumarins, can be found in strawberries, blueberries, raspberries, or soybeans.

Some of the best phytonutrient-rich foods are:

- Blueberries (All berries are good, but blueberries are the highest source.)
- Broccoli and other cruciferous vegetables
- Chili peppers
- Citrus fruits
- Dark-green leafy vegetables
- Flaxseeds
- Garlic
- Melons
- Pink grapefruit
- Soybeans and other soy foods
- Sweet potatoes

PHYTOCHEMICAL CLASSES

The biochemistry of phytochemicals is amazingly complex, and although thousands of them have been isolated, science has not yet discovered all of the phytochemicals that exist. Isolated phytochemicals are grouped into classes based on the number, type, and basic structure of their atoms. The classes are further categorized into subclasses, types, and subtypes according to chemical composition and function.

Class: Isoprenoids/Terpenes

Isoprene units are the basis of the largest class of phytochemicals known so far. Approximately 22,000 isoprenoids are currently known. Terpenes, built on isoprene units, are found throughout the plant kingdom and protect plants from attack by free radical oxygen species.

Subclass: Carotenoids

Carotenoids, which are fat soluble, are found in fatty tissues throughout the body. They are transported in the blood by lipoproteins.

Type: Carotenes

Carotenes are carotenoids that contain only carbon and hydrogen.

Alpha-carotene slows the growth of cancer cells, helping to protect against oral, pancreatic, lung, liver, and skin cancers. It is an extremely powerful antioxidant and cell protector. Food sources include asparagus, avocado, bananas, blueberries, broccoli, cantaloupe, carrots, cauliflower, dates, grapefruit, grapes, kale, mangoes, oranges, palm oil, peppermint, pumpkin, raspberries, red and yellow peppers, sea vegetables, tangerines, and yellow corn.

Beta-carotene acts as an antioxidant and reduces the risk of heart disease, strokes, and eye disorders. It stimulates the immune system, lowers serum cholesterol, and is converted into vitamin A in the body as needed. Food sources include apples, apricots, avocado, bananas, berries, broccoli, cantaloupes, carrots, cherries, citrus fruits, currants, dates, dill, figs, grapes, honeydew melons, hot and sweet red peppers, kiwi, leafy greens, mangoes, nectarines, papayas, parsley, peaches, pears, persimmons, pineapple, plums, pomegranates, pumpkin, squash, sweet potatoes, watermelon, and yams.

Lutein protects against age-related macular degeneration and guards against cell damage. Food sources include beet greens, broccoli, cilantro, collard, dill, honeydew melon, kale, kiwi, mangos, marigolds, mustard, oranges, papayas, peaches, spinach, sweet red peppers, turnips, and yellow squash.

Lycopene protects against cell damage by acting as an antioxidant, and protects against cancers of the digestive tract (the colon, esophagus, mouth, rectum, stomach, and throat), as well as cancer of the bladder, cervix, lung, pancreas, and prostate. Food sources include, first and foremost, tomatoes. Heat treatment (cooking) tomatoes increases the absorption of lycopene as a nutrient. Lycopene is also found in apricots, cherries, guava, red and pink grapefruit, red pepper, strawberries, and watermelon.

Type: Xanthophylls

Xanthophylls are carotenoid compounds that contain hydroxyl groups, keto groups, or both.

Anthoxanthins act as antioxidants. Food sources include cabbage sprouts, cauliflower, and potatoes.

Beta-cryptoxanthin increases the activity of vitamin A and helps to protect against cervical cancer.

Canthaxanthin acts as an antioxidant, boosts immunity, slows the growth of cancer cells, and may help to prevent skin and breast cancers. Food sources include mushrooms, particularly reishi, maitake, and shiitake.

Zeaxanthin also protects against age-related macular degeneration. It improves the immune response and blocks the activity of peroxide free radicals. Food sources include beet greens, chicory leaf, collard, kale, kiwi, mangoes, mustard, okra, oranges, papayas, spinach, sweet red peppers, Swiss chard, turnip, and yellow squash.

Subclass: Monoterpenes

Monoterpenes act as antioxidants, limit cholesterol synthesis, and aid in the activity of protective enzymes that inhibit the actions of carcinogens. Some foods that monoterpenes are present in are basil, broccoli, cabbage, carrots, citrus fruits, cucumbers, eggplant, mint, parsley, peppers, and squash.

Type: Limonoids

Limonoids have been shown to protect lung tissue and guard against cancer. They induce protective enzymes, deactivate carcinogens, reduce cholesterol, protect against cataracts, and enhance immunity.

Limonene protects against cancer by stimulating anticancer enzymes and cancer-killing immune cells. Food sources include caraway, cardamom, celery, citrus fruits, fennel seed, and rosemary.

Perillyl alcohol may downgrade the malignancy of tumor cells. Food sources include apricots and cherries.

Type: Alpha-Pinene

Alpha-pinene is an aromatic monoterpene that acts as an antioxidant and anti-inflammatory. Food sources include allspice, anise, basil, bay leaves, bell peppers, caraway, cardamom, carrots, celery, cinnamon, coriander, cumin, fennel, ginger, grapefruit, lemons, limes, marjoram, oranges, oregano, parsley, peppermint, rosemary, sage, savory, spearmint, tangerines, tarragon, thyme, and turmeric.

Type: Capsaicin

Capsaicin acts as an antioxidant, lowers triglycerides and LDL cholesterol, reduces blood clotting, helps to prevent alcohol-induced stomach damage, protects against ulcers, speeds up the metabolism, and protects cell DNA from carcinogens. Capsaicin is also an effective painkiller and anti-inflammatory agent, and has been used effectively in the treatment of arthritis, cluster headaches, diabetic neuropathy, phantom limb pain after amputation, psoriasis, shingles, and trigeminal neuralgia. Food sources include chili peppers, cumin, and turmeric.

Subclass: Diterpenes

Diterpenes are one of the major constituents of plant resins and include compounds that act as sweeteners, fragrances, flavorings, and anticancer, antihypertensive, and anti-inflammatory agents. Diterpenes are found in most herbs, including oregano, rosemary, and stevia.

Type: Carnosol

Carnosol acts as an antioxidant, inhibits the development of tumors, and prevents fats in the body from oxidizing and damaging cells. The best food source is rosemary.

Type: Ginkgolides

Ginkgolides are bitter diterpenes found in the root, bark, and leaves of ginkgo biloba. Ginkgolides are antioxidants, anti-inflammatories, antiseptics, and anticoagulants. They are used in the treatment of asthma, tachycardia (rapid heartbeat), inflammation, and sepsis (blood poisoning).

Subclass: Phytosterols

Phytosterols protect against colon cancer by slowing down the reproduction of cells in the large intestine. They also enhance immunity, block the uptake of cholesterol in the intestines, and expedite the excretion of cholesterol from the body. They protect against heart disease, breast and prostate cancers, reduce inflammation, and alter tumor growth. The most common phytosterols are beta-sitosterol, stigmasterol, and campesterol. Food sources include vegetable oils, seeds, and nuts.

Subclass: Triterpenes/Triterpenoids

Triterpenoids may inhibit hormone-dependent steps in tumor formation. They also have antioxidant properties, help reduce cholesterol levels, and have been shown to inhibit breast cancer in laboratory tests. Food sources include cereal grains, cruciferous vegetables, citrus fruits, and licorice root.

Class: Phenols/Phenolic Compounds/ Polyphenols/Polyphenolic Compounds

This class of phytochemicals blocks the enzymes that cause inflammation, protects against inflammatory reactions caused by solar radiation, lowers the risk of heart disease and stroke, helps to prevent cell mutation, inhibits tumor formation and growth, and inhibits the production of prostaglandin, which causes blood clotting. These phytochemicals act as antioxidants, protect cells from structural damage, and reduce the risk of cancer by trapping carcinogens and assisting in their excretion from the body. They also form complexes with reactive metals, thus reducing their absorption. At least 8,000 phenolic compounds have been identified. Roughly half of them are flavonoids.

Subclass: Flavonoids

Flavonoids act as antioxidants, enhance the immune system, and inhibit enzymes responsible for metastasis (the spread of cancer cells throughout the body). They prevent cancer-promoting hormones from attaching to normal cells and guard against blood clots. They help to lower the risk of estrogen-related cancers, such as breast cancer, by blocking the enzymes that make estrogen. They also protect against heart disease and stroke, regulate the enzymes that control cell division, modify allergic reactions, reduce

capillary fragility, and enhance the function of vitamin C in the body.

Flavonoids are found in many foods, including apples, blueberries, citrus fruits, cranberries, chamomile tea, currants, flaxseed, lentils, onions, red wine, rice, soybeans, and both green and black tea.

Type: Tannins

Tannins occur in nearly every type of plant in the world. They protect plants from mold, fungi, bacteria, and foraging animals. They have an astringent quality that is readily noticeable in the taste of tea and wine. Tannins have antioxidant properties and are antimutagenic (they help to prevent cells from mutating), which makes them an important focus of cancer research. Tannins are generally categorized into two subgroups: hydrolyzable tannins, which include gallotannins, ellagitannins, and caffetannins; and condensed tannins, which are the oligomers and polymers of flavanols and include the proanthocyanidins.

Anthocyanidins and their precursors, *proanthocyanidins*, act as antioxidants, reduce the risk of macular degeneration by protecting the eyes from free radical damage, increase circulation, stabilize collagen structures (which hold tissues together), protect against heart disease and stroke by inhibiting the production of clot-promoting prostaglandins, and help the body to dispose of potential carcinogens. Food sources include beets, bilberries, blackberries, blueberries, cherries, citrus fruits, Concord grapes, cranberries, currants, eggplant, figs, green tea, persimmons, plums, pomegranates, radishes, raspberries, red cabbage, and strawberries.

Catechins act as antioxidants, protect the liver, boost fat metabolism, enhance immunity, lower cholesterol levels, and protect against respiratory and digestive infections. The catechins include epicatechin, epicatechin gallate, epigallocatechin, and epigallocatechin gallate. They are found in the highest amounts in green tea, black tea, and grapes, but are also found in berries, cherries, grapefruit, lemons, limes, oranges, and tangerines.

Ellagic acid acts as an antioxidant, decreases cell mutation, and inhibits damage to the cells' DNA from carcinogens. It also prevents the formation of cancer-causing substances called *nitrosamines* in the body. It slows tumor growth by blocking the production of enzymes used by cancer cells, inhibits lung and skin tumors, and is considered a vital nutrient in the fight against smoking-related lung cancer. Food sources include apples, blackberries, carrots, citrus fruits, cranberries, grapes, nuts, raspberries, strawberries, tomatoes, walnuts, and whole grains.

Ferulic acid prevents the formation of cancer-causing nitrosamines in the body. Food sources include apples, grapefruit, grapes, lemons, limes, oranges, red and white wines, red and yellow onions, shallots, and tangerines.

Caffeic acid triggers the production of enzymes that make carcinogens more water soluble, thereby making them easier to flush from the body. Food sources include many fruits and vegetables.

Chlorogenic acid, a conjugated form of caffeic acid, prevents the formation of cancer-causing nitrosamines in the body. Food sources include carrots, green peppers, pineapple, strawberries, and tomatoes.

Gallic acid is found in both green and black tea and has anticancer and antioxidant properties.

Resveratrol inhibits the formation and spread of cancerous tumors. It also modulates cholesterol metabolism and has chemical-detoxifying and anti-inflammatory properties. Food sources include grapes, mulberries, peanuts, and red wine.

Type: Curcuminoids

Curcuminoids are very powerful antioxidants, inhibit tumor growth, and protect DNA from damage by tobacco and other carcinogens. Studies have found that curcuminoids have the ability to break down amyloids—proteins that cause a plaque-like buildup that interferes with brain-cell communication and causes problems with memory recall. It also can reverse oxidative damage and inflammation, conditions that contribute to Alzheimer's disease. Curcuminoids increase the secretion of bile by stimulating the bile duct, protect the liver by detoxifying, stimulate and protect the gallbladder, help to protect against heart disease, help to inhibit platelet aggregation (thus improving circulation), inhibit enzymes that induce inflammatory prostaglandins, and help to break down fats and reduce LDL ("bad") cholesterol. Curcuminoids also soothe the stomach and prevent gas. Many curcuminoids have been discovered so far, including curcumin, tetrahydrocurcumin, demethoxycurcumin, and cassumunins A and B, among others. Food sources include curry, ginger, and turmeric.

Type: Flavones

Flavones have been found to stop the proliferation of human breast cancer cells and to act as monoamine oxidase inhibitors, which gives them the potential to be used as natural, safe antidepressants. This possibility is currently being studied.

Apigenin, a widely studied flavone, has been used in antiviral treatment for HIV and other infections, and in preparations for the treatment of inflammatory bowel disease and many skin conditions. The high concentration of apigenin in passionflower has led to its use in alternative medicine as an antispasmodic for Parkinson's disease and in easing asthma, reducing the pain associated with neuralgia, and treating shingles. Apigenin is an anticancer, anti-inflammatory, and antifungal agent. Food sources include apples, artichoke, barley, basil, broccoli, celery, chamomile, cherries, cilantro, cloves, endive, grapes, leeks, onions, oregano, parsley, tarragon, and tomatoes. It is also present in tea and wine.

Luteolin inhibits the growth of human leukemia cells and thyroid cancer cells; is an antioxidant, anti-inflammatory,

and anti-allergenic agent; and protects against atherosclerosis and autoimmunity. Food sources include artichokes, basil, celery, cruciferous vegetables, parsley, rosemary, and sweet red peppers.

Type: Flavonols

Flavonols are known for their antifungal, antibacterial, antioxidant, and anticancer properties, as well as their ability to protect against cardiovascular disease.

Rutin strengthens the walls of blood vessels and capillaries, including those in the eyes. It is used in the treatment of hemorrhoids, varicose veins, and poor circulation, and is helpful for those with arteriosclerosis and high blood pressure. Rutin also has a high level of superoxide anion scavenging ability, making it an important antioxidant. Rutin is found primarily in buckwheat.

Quercetin is one of the most abundant flavonoids and is readily available in many foods and beverages, including apples, berries, cruciferous vegetables, onions, red wine, tea, and many nuts and seeds. Quercetin provides cardiovascular protection, helps to prevent cataracts, and has anticancer, anti-inflammatory, anti-allergenic, antihistamine, and antiviral properties. In addition, it offers protection from ulcers. Quercetin has been shown to have activity against HIV, herpes simplex virus type 1, poliovirus type 1, respiratory syncytial virus, and parainfluenza virus type 3. Recent studies have shown that quercetin has activity against many different types of cancer cells, including gastric, endometrial, breast, leukemia, lung, colon, ovary, and squamous cell cancers. Quercetin has also been shown to be an important addition to nutritional supplementation for people with diabetes, as it protects against cataract and neurovascular problems.

Subclass: Isoflavones/Phytoestrogens

Isoflavones are a very important group of phytochemicals, also known as phytoestrogens. Phytoestrogens help to normalize estrogen levels in women. In men, they can block testosterone without causing feminine characteristics. They inhibit estrogen-related cancers; decrease postmenopausal symptoms; lower blood cholesterol levels; protect against breast cancer, prostate cancer, and osteoporosis; and decrease atherosclerosis. Isoflavones destroy enzymes that transform normal cells into cancer cells and prevent tumors from forming a blood supply, thus restricting their growth. Food sources include primarily soybeans and other soy products, such as soymilk and tofu. Isoflavones are also present in apples, beans, carrots, corn, flaxseeds, lentils, peanuts, peas, red clover, sesame seeds, sunflower seeds, and whole grains.

Type: Coumarin

Coumarin prevents abnormal blood clotting and stimulates anticancer enzymes. Food sources include cereal grains, citrus fruit, flaxseeds, licorice, parsley, strawberries, tomatoes, and vegetables.

Type: Daidzein

Daidzein is an estrogenlike compound that is formed from isoflavones. It helps to compensate for estrogen discharged from the body by the liver and the colon, lessening the effect of a decline in estrogen. It may help with bone formation and prevent and even reverse osteoporosis (bone thinning). Food sources include soy foods as well as alfalfa, beans, lentils, peanuts, peas, and sprouts.

Ipriflavones are synthesized from daidzein. They help to protect against osteoporosis by preventing bone reabsorption and by stimulating bone collagen synthesis. They are found in soybeans.

Type: Genistein

Genistein inhibits estrogen-related cancers and the growth of new blood vessels around cancer cells that are needed to feed growing tumors, decreases postmenopausal symptoms, lowers blood cholesterol levels, and reduces the risk of heart disease. It may aid in preventing both breast and prostate cancer. Genistein is found, like other isoflavones, in soy foods and in alfalfa, beans, lentils, peanuts, peas, and sprouts.

Type: Lignan

Lignan acts as an antioxidant, blocks body chemicals known as prostaglandins, and inhibits the production of estrogen by fatty tissues. Lignan helps lower cholesterol levels, protects against colon cancer, and helps to prevent the formation of gallstones. Food sources include barley, fatty fish, flaxseeds, legumes, millet, oats, plums, rice, soybeans, spelt, walnuts, and wheat.

Class: Thiols

Thiols are sulfur-containing phytochemicals. They are found in garlic, onions, and cruciferous vegetables. Thiols lower cholesterol levels, decrease blood clotting, and have antibacterial and antifungal properties.

Subclass: Allylic Sulfides

Allylic sulfides increases the production of enzymes that affect carcinogenic substances and help the body to get rid of them. These phytochemicals have anticancer, immune-enhancing, and memory-enhancing properties, along with antifungal, antiparasitic, and antiplatelet properties. They have also been reported to lower levels of LDLs while maintaining healthy levels of high-density lipoproteins (HDLs, or "good" cholesterol). Food sources include chives, garlic, leeks, onions, scallions, and shallots.

Type: Allicin

Allicin protects the stomach against the formation of ulcers and helps to treat intractable diarrhea resulting from infection with *Cryptosporidium parvum*. Allicin also has anticlot-

ting, antitumor, antibiotic, and antifungal properties. It lowers blood pressure, reduces the risk of heart disease and stroke, blocks the ability of carcinogens to mutate healthy cells into cancerous cells, boosts immunity, combats the fungal organism *Candida albicans,* and protects against damage from oxidizing agents and heavy metals. Allicin also reduces the production of cholesterol in the liver. Food sources include garlic, leeks, and onions.

Type: S-Allyl Cysteine

S-allyl cysteine may block the formation of harmful nitrosamines in the stomach, and may stimulate anticancer enzymes. Food sources include chives, garlic, and onions.

Subclass: Glucosinolates

Glucosinolates protect against breast cancer, stimulate anticancer enzymes, inhibit enzymes that cause cell mutation, and help rid the body of carcinogens contained in cigarette smoke. Food sources include cruciferous vegetables, garden sorrel, horseradish, mustard and turnip greens, rutabagas, radishes, and watercress.

Type: Dithiolthiones

Dithiolthiones suppress tumor growth and protect against DNA damage from carcinogens in tobacco smoke, helping to inhibit lung cancer. The best food source is broccoli.

Type: Isothiocyanates

Isothiocyanates protect against breast cancer, stimulate anticancer enzymes, inhibit enzymes that initiate cancer, and help rid the body of carcinogens contained in cigarette smoke. Food sources include cruciferous vegetables, garden sorrel, horseradish, mustard greens, radishes, rutabagas, turnips, and watercress.

Phenethyl isothiocyanate (PEITC) protects against breast cancer, activates the liver's production of enzymes that bind to carcinogens and transport them out of cells, inhibits enzymes that initiate cancer, and helps to rid the body of carcinogens contained in cigarette smoke. Food sources include cabbage and other cruciferous vegetables, garden sorrel, horseradish, kale, mustard greens, radishes, rutabagas, scallions, spinach, turnips, and watercress.

Sulfurophane protects against breast cancer, activates the liver to produce enzymes that bind to carcinogens and transport them out of cells, inhibits enzymes that contribute to cancer, and helps to rid the body of carcinogens contained in cigarette smoke. Food sources include cabbage and other cruciferous vegetables, garden sorrel, horseradish, kale, mustard greens, radishes, rutabagas, scallions, spinach, turnips, and watercress.

Subclass: Indoles

Indoles protect against breast and ovarian cancers by helping to prevent abnormal stimulation of estrogen. Indoles also inhibit enzymes that initiate cancer, and help to rid the body of carcinogens contained in cigarette smoke. Other benefits include improved immune response, retarded tumor growth, and assistance in the excretion of toxins from the body. Indoles also appear to combat cancer by sensitizing otherwise resistant cancer cells to cancer-fighting drugs. Food sources include cruciferous vegetables (particularly broccoli), garden sorrel, horseradish, mustard and turnip greens, radishes, rutabagas, and watercress.

Subclass: Tocopherols and Tocotrienols

The phytochemicals in this subclass act as antioxidants and protect against cancer, heart disease, and strokes. Tocopherols are used in the treatment of acne, alcohol-induced liver disease, allergies, anemia, arthritis, autoimmune disorders, cardiovascular diseases, cataracts, cervical dysplasia, diabetes, eczema, epilepsy, fibrocystic breast disease, gallstones, hepatitis, herpes, HIV/AIDS, immunodepression, infections, inflammation, lupus, macular degeneration, menopausal symptoms, menopause, multiple sclerosis, myopathy, neuralgia, neuromuscular degeneration, osteoarthritis, Parkinson's disease, peptic ulcers, periodontal disease, peripheral vascular disease, premenstrual syndrome, ulcerative colitis, Raynaud's disease, rheumatoid arthritis, scleroderma, seborrheic dermatitis, shingles, and skin ulcers. Food sources include asparagus, avocados, berries, green leafy vegetables, nuts and seeds, palm oil, tomatoes, and whole grains.

PART FOUR

PRESCRIPTION FOODS

INTRODUCTION

Food is such a powerful source of healing that we can, with conviction, say that "pharma-foods," including certain spices and herbs, are nature's safe prescriptions for health. Years of research have produced—and continue to produce—a real understanding of exactly how it is that food nurtures and heals and, more important, which disorders and conditions may be helped or cured by specific foods.

In Part Four, you will learn how to select and use the finest fruits, vegetables, sea vegetables, grains, flours, legumes, nuts, seeds, fish, and herbs and spices. Anyone who buys, eats, prepares, or stores food can use this section as a definitive reference. There is detailed information on how to select and store food to preserve freshness, flavor, and nutrition; how to ripen fruits and vegetables; how to prepare food for consumption; and what works best to eliminate wax and pesticides. For each type of food covered, you will learn about its medicinal value and healing properties; the key nutrients and phytochemicals it contains, and which plant parts to consume for their medicinal value. You will be introduced to the Magnificent 12—cruciferous vegetables that fight cancer, heart disease, and stroke—and a variety of nourishing sea vegetables, which are rich sources of protein, vitamins, minerals, essential fatty acids, and chlorophyll. You will also learn why fiber, nature's internal broom, is so important, and the best food sources of it; why eating fish is recommended by the nutritional community; which beverages are actually good for you, and how to make sure the water you drink is of good quality; the benefits of eating organic foods, including an explanation of new laws that regulate which foods can be labeled organic; and the importance of proper food combining—a complicated subject, made easy to understand, that can help you improve your digestion and maximize your nutritional intake.

Armed with the information in Part Four and an empty shopping cart, you can make decisions that will have a positive impact on your health from now on. This knowledge will help you to improve the quality and flavor of the food you eat, as well as expand your range of choices. It is an opportunity to nourish, regenerate, and heal your body as well as your appetite.

CHAPTER EIGHT

FABULOUS FRUITS . . .
AND BODACIOUS BERRIES

The Strawberry: Doubtless God could have made a better berry, but doubtless God never did.

—Dr. William Butler, *seventeenth-century English writer*

Fresh fruits and berries add color, variety, and powerful nutrition to any meal, snack, or dessert. The vitamins, minerals, and phytochemicals in fruit make it a food "superhero" and the ultimate brain fuel. Most fruits are 80 to 95 percent water (a composition much like the human body) and are naturally low in fat and calories. All fruits contain soluble fiber, which helps to lower blood cholesterol levels and regulate blood sugar; minerals such as potassium, iron, calcium, and magnesium; and many contain high amounts of vitamin C and beta-carotene. Fruits have low sodium levels and are cholesterol-free! Last, but not least, fruits do not have to be slaughtered to be eaten. In a natural cycle, humans and animals eat the fruits, then spread the seeds for propagation. Fruit is the ultimate environment-friendly food and takes little to no preparation to eat.

Fruits contain antioxidants that protect against cell damage, a proven source of disease and premature aging, plus bioflavonoids, which can prevent or slow tumor growth. Deep-colored fruits are particularly rich in antioxidants. Research shows that all kinds of berries (particularly bilberries, blueberries, huckleberries, and strawberries) have compounds that help to protect against cancer. (See Chapters 6 and 7.) In fact, berries are at the top of the list for the prevention of many physical disorders.

Although total fruit consumption in the United States has been increasing, the U.S. Department of Agriculture (USDA) states that on an average day, half of all Americans do not eat any fruit at all. Yet studies show that people who eat substantial amounts of fruits have a reduced rate of all cancer, heart disease, and most other illnesses.

SELECTING, STORING, AND RIPENING FRUIT

To gain the maximum benefit from the fruit you eat, there are a number of guidelines to keep in mind when purchasing and storing it. These include the following:

- Buy certified organic fruits whenever possible. These fruits are grown without synthetic pesticides and fertil-

izers, so there is little risk of exposure to residues of these chemicals. Studies suggest that organically grown fruit may be richer in some nutrients than comparable commercial products. The higher cost may seem prohibitive, but pound for pound, quality fruits and vegetables are still less expensive than most meat products. Do not expect organic produce to be as cosmetically *perfect* as fruits that have been protected from the occasional small pest bite by hazardous chemicals.

- Buy only as much fruit as you can use while it is fresh. The benefits of "live" fruit and fruit juices make a few extra shopping trips worthwhile.

- When selecting fruit, avoid any with large bruises, visible mold, or soft, mealy, mushy flesh. Watch for mold or mushiness around fruit stems, too. This is particularly important with melons.

- Most fruits should be firm and well colored. Fruit skins should be smooth, not bruised or shriveled. Do not buy fruit with broken flesh, cuts, or punctures. This can affect ripening and allows bacteria and other germs to enter.

- Berries should be high in color, plump, firm, and uniform in size.

- Keep on the lookout for deterioration. Even with the most modern handling methods, product quality can decline rapidly during display. Say no to any fruit with a sour smell.

- Fruits that are hard or tinged with green are usually unripe.

- Pick out any overripe fruits or berries before refrigeration or storage. Being stored with overripe or rotting fruit hastens the decay of other fruit.

- Once a piece of fruit is cut, exposure to oxygen and light starts to destroy vitamins (especially vitamin C). For optimum nutrition, cut fruits just before serving, preparing only enough for that day. Leftovers can be frozen for use later in baked goods or juices. Place berries on a baking sheet and separate them, then place the sheet in the freezer until the berries are frozen. You can then place them in a storage container. This way, they may be taken out as needed (per serving) with no large clumps.

- To ripen fruit quickly, place it in a paper bag. This traps ethylene gas produced by the fruit, which acts as a ripening agent.

WASHING FRUIT

Most fruit should be washed in cool water before refrigeration or room-temperature storage, even if you plan to peel it before eating. This is because the blade of the knife you use to peel or cut fruit can pick up pesticide residues, bacteria, or other undesirables from the rind and transfer it to the pulp. Sort out any stems, caps, twigs, or leaves while washing fruit or berries.

Pick out any overripe berries as soon as you get home so they do not hasten the decaying process of the other berries. Unlike most fruits, berries should not be washed immediately, as this promotes the growth of mold. Instead, place a paper towel around berries and put them in a container to keep moisture down. Rinse berries quickly in cool water and pick out any stems or leaves just prior to serving.

PESTICIDES AND WAX

Most of the fresh fruit available in grocery stores has been treated with pesticides while the fruit was growing. Residues of these chemicals pose a potentially substantial health risk. You should therefore wash all fruits well before eating them. Some types of fruit may even need to be peeled.

In addition to being treated with pesticides, many fruits are sprayed with a thin layer of wax to extend their shelf life and make them shiny and more "eye-appealing." Unfortunately, this wax coating also traps pesticide residue and prevents it from being washed away. You can often tell if a piece of fruit has been waxed by examining it (it will feel waxy), but if you are not sure, ask the produce manager at your supermarket which fruits have been waxed. If you must buy the waxed fruit, wash and peel them before eating.

FRUITS FROM A TO Z

There is an amazing variety of fruit on the market today, much of it available year-round. Following is a discussion of some of the many types of fruit, with explanations of the particular health benefits of each, the key nutrients and phytochemicals it contains, and, where applicable, special instructions for storing and preparing it.

Apples

One apple, eaten whole with the skin, has about 3.6 grams of fiber—nearly 17 percent of the recommended daily dietary fiber intake. This is enough to contribute substantially to colon health if eaten daily. Apples are good for anyone undergoing treatment for chronic enteritis, prostate problems, intestinal infections, inflammation of the colon, goiter, gout, diarrhea, arthritis, herpes, and acid stomach. Researchers at Cornell University say the phytochemical quercetin in apples has stronger anticancer properties than vitamin C. A strong anti-inflammatory, quercetin is known for its effectiveness in treating prostate problems. Apples help to detoxify metals in the body, protect against heart disease, clean the bladder, protect against the effects of radiation exposure, lower blood cholesterol and blood pressure, maintain circulatory and intestinal health, and stabilize blood sugar. Latest research shows that apples may help prevent lung disorders. The parts eaten include the skin, core, and flesh.

Key nutrients in apples include vitamin B_6, vitamin C, iron, potassium, sodium, phosphorus, calcium, sulfur, magnesium, boron, fiber, fructose, glucose, octacosanol, sucrose, zinc, copper, manganese, thiamine, riboflavin, niacin, pantothenic acid, folate, vitamin E, malic acid, and tartaric acid. Important phytochemicals include beta-carotene, quercetin, phytosterols, pectin, gallic acid, ellagic acid, ferulic acid, caffeic acid, tocopherol, chlorogenic acid, chlorophyll, catechin, P-coumaric acid, rutin, and sinapic acid.

Place apples in plastic bags and store them in the crisper compartment of the refrigerator. Apples purchased in good condition should keep for up to six weeks in the refrigerator.

Wash apples thoroughly before using them. Apples are on the list of produce with heavy pesticide residues. If the fruit has been waxed, peel the skin before consuming. To prevent the flesh from browning if it is not eaten immediately, rub the cut surfaces of the apple with a mixture of lemon juice and water.

Apricots

Apricots have been used to treat constipation, cancer, and bowel disorders. They also benefit the skin, heart, muscles, and nerve tissue. The parts eaten include the skin and the flesh.

Key nutrients in apricots include fiber, vitamin C, calcium, magnesium, vitamin B_3 (niacin), pantothenic acid, vitamin B_2 (riboflavin), vitamin B_1 (thiamine), phosphorus, folate, sodium, copper, fructose, glucose, sucrose, manganese, iron, and potassium. Important phytochemicals include beta-carotene, chlorogenic acid, isoquercitrin, limonene, lycopene, and tannin. Laetrile (also known as vitamin B_{17} and amygdalin) is a substance derived from the pit of the apricot that has been used to treat numerous disorders, including cancer. Though popular at one time, it has not been proven as a cancer preventive or cure. Laetrile contains enough cyanide to be fatal when eaten in large amounts. It is best not to eat the pit.

Choose fruit with a uniform golden-orange color. A pink blush on the fruit is a sign of sweetness. Ripe apricots will yield to gentle pressure on the skin and emit a perfumelike aroma.

Apricots should be stored in a paper bag at room temperature until fully ripened. Keep the bag away from heat or direct sunlight. Store fully ripened apricots in a plastic bag in the refrigerator, and they will keep for one to two days. Do not wash the fruit prior to storing.

When preparing apricots, if you are removing the skin, blanch them in boiling water for fifteen to twenty seconds, and then run them under cold water. The skin should slip off easily with the aid of a sharp knife.

Avocados

Avocados are good for the nerves, fatigue, hypoglycemia, and urinary tract infections, and they aid in convalescence after surgery. They are a good source of monounsaturated fats. A single avocado contains nearly 4 grams of protein—more than any other fruit.

Key nutrients in avocado include vitamin B_1 (thiamine), vitamin B_2 (riboflavin), vitamin D, calcium, sodium, folate, iron, phosphorus, vitamin B_3 (niacin), pantothenic acid, copper, manganese, magnesium, vitamin C, vitamin E, vitamin B_6, fructose, glucose, sucrose, zinc, potassium, fiber, amino acids, and small amounts of coenzyme Q_{10}. Important phytochemicals include alpha-carotene, beta-carotene, caffeic acid, chlorogenic acid, beta cryptoxanthin, P-coumaric acid, tocopherols, and tocotrienols. The flesh is the part eaten.

Choose a heavy fruit with an unblemished, unbroken skin. The fruit should yield to gentle pressure without denting. If it dents, it is overripe. Leave unripe avocados on the kitchen counter for a few days at room temperature to soften them.

Ripe avocados will keep for four to five days in the refrigerator. Unripe avocados stored in the refrigerator will never ripen.

To prepare avocados, wash the fruit well and run a sharp knife around the fruit lengthwise, then twist the two halves to separate them. Strike the pit of the fruit with the blade of the knife, and twist the knife blade in a clockwise motion to loosen the pit. Remove the pit and discard it. Peel the skin off the avocado halves with a paring knife, and scoop the flesh out with a spoon or melon baller (or you can slice the peeled halves). To prevent the flesh from discoloring, sprinkle it with a little lemon or lime juice as soon as it is cut.

Bananas

Bananas can provide nutrients vital to people with alcoholism, hypertension, hemorrhoids, heart disorders, high cholesterol, ulcers, diarrhea, potassium deficiency, high blood pressure, edema, and intestinal disturbances. Bananas are good for the nerves, muscles, liver, and kidneys, and they feed the good bacteria in the colon. They also help to lessen pain, aid sleep, and enhance immune function. Bananas are an excellent food for children and people who are recovering from illness. The flesh is the part eaten.

Key nutrients in bananas include potassium, folate, vitamin C, vitamin B_6, vitamin B_1 (thiamine), vitamin B_2 (riboflavin), biotin, pantothenic acid, vitamin B_3 (niacin), vitamin D, vitamin E, sodium, chlorine, calcium, iron, phosphorus, manganese, magnesium, fructose, glucose, sucrose, zinc, copper, fiber, and small amounts of lipids and amino acids. With the exception of avocados (which contain more fat) and dates (which have 60 percent more calories), bananas contain more potassium by weight than any other fruit. Important phytochemicals include beta-carotene, kaempferol, quercetin, rutin, stigmasterol, pectin, and phytosterols.

Select bananas that are free of bruises or obvious injury and that have intact stem ends and skins. The best eating quality is when the skin is solid yellow and newly speckled with brown spots.

Ripe bananas can be stored at room temperature for two to three days, or in the refrigerator for up to two weeks. The skins will darken in the refrigerator, but the flesh will be perfectly edible. Overripe bananas can be peeled, covered in plastic wrap, and frozen, to be used later in baking.

After peeling the banana, wash your hands with soap and water before eating it. Bananas from some countries are heavily sprayed. Dip the flesh in orange, lemon, or lime juice to prevent browning after peeling.

Blackberries

Blackberries are useful in the treatment of leukorrhea, enteritis, appendicitis, constipation, diarrhea, and anemia. The ellagic acid in blackberries is believed to help prevent cancer. The entire fruit is eaten. The leaves of the blackberry plant are used to make medicinal herbal teas.

Key nutrients in blackberries include fiber, vitamin C, magnesium, phosphorus, zinc, copper, manganese, vitamin B_1 (thiamine), vitamin B_2 (riboflavin), vitamin B_3 (niacin), pantothenic acid, vitamin B_6, fructose, glucose, sucrose, folate, vitamin E, iron, potassium, calcium, and small amounts of lipids. Important phytochemicals include beta-carotene, anthocyanins, chlorogenic acid, pectin, catechins, ellagic acid, ferulic acid, tocopherols, and tocotrienols.

When you purchase blackberries, open the container of berries immediately and remove any that are overripe—they will hasten the decaying process of the other berries. Blackberries should be used within two days after purchasing. Do not wash them until you are ready to eat them. They can be frozen and kept for up to twelve months.

Blueberries

Blueberries are at the top of the list of antioxidant-rich foods. They can be beneficial in the treatment of hypoglycemia, tinnitus, intestinal upsets, eye disorders, and urinary tract infections. Phytochemicals in blueberries help to strengthen blood vessels and are useful in treating varicose veins and spider veins. They promote heart health and aid the lymphatic system. The manganese in blueberries aids in keeping bones strong, and the high amount of vitamin C makes blueberries a powerful antioxidant and supporter of the immune system. The entire fruit is eaten. The pigment released from the blueberry's skin may be the most valuable nutrient in the berry, as it contains potent antioxidants called anthocyanins. The herb bilberry, also called the European blueberry, has the same health benefits as blueberries and is available in health food stores in liquid extract, capsule, and pill form.

Key nutrients in blueberries include fiber, vitamin C, folate, iron, manganese, potassium, calcium, magnesium, phosphorus, sodium, zinc, copper, fructose, glucose, sucrose, vitamin B_1 (thiamine), vitamin B_2 (riboflavin), vitamin B_3 (niacin), pantothenic acid, vitamin B_6, vitamin E, silicon, and small amounts of lipids and amino acids. Important phytochemicals include anthocyanins, alpha-carotene, beta-carotene, caryophyllene, chlorogenic acid, eugenol, limonene, myristicin, thymol, pectin, catechins, ellagic acid, tocopherols, and tocotrienols.

Select blueberries with a uniform dark bluish-gray color with a silvery bloom. Blueberries should be plump, firm, uniform in size, dry, and free from stems, caps, and leaves. Avoid moldy, bruised, or green berries. If you cannot find fresh blueberries, buy frozen ones—they are just as nutritious. Wild blueberries have more skin than flesh; however, both the wild and the cultivated variety contain powerful antioxidants that have the same health benefits.

Blueberries can be stored for longer than most other berries: up to ten days in the refrigerator for fresh, sound blueberries; or ten to twelve months when frozen. Do not clean blueberries until you are ready to use them.

To clean blueberries, place them in a basin of cold water. Any twigs, leaves, or unripe berries will float to the surface and can be skimmed off. Do this quickly, so berries do not become waterlogged if left in the water for too long.

Cantaloupe

Cantaloupes, also known as muskmelon, can help to lower blood cholesterol levels and high blood pressure. They help to lower the risk of heart disease and cancer, boost the immune system, protect against macular degeneration, and aid liver health. Cantaloupes have antitumor and anti-inflammatory properties. The part eaten is the flesh.

Key nutrients in cantaloupe include folate, fiber, vitamin C, potassium, calcium, iron, magnesium, phosphorus, sodium, fructose, glucose, sucrose, zinc, copper, manganese, vitamin B_1 (thiamine), vitamin B_2 (riboflavin), vitamin B_3 (niacin), pantothenic acid, vitamin B_6, vitamin E, and small amounts of lipids. Cantaloupes contain more beta-carotene than any other type of melon. Important phytochemicals include alpha-carotene, beta-carotene, beta-ionone, pectin, tocopherols, cucurbitacin B and E, myristic acid, flavonoids, and phytosterols.

Choose cantaloupes with a thick, coarse, corky surface, with veins standing out over a slightly golden colored rind. They should have a fruity aroma and round shape. A good cantaloupe will not have a stem, and it will yield slightly to thumb pressure on the nonstem end. Avoid cantaloupes with a pronounced yellow or green rind color, irregular shape, softening over the entire rind, and mold growth—especially in the stem scar.

Store cantaloupes at room temperature for up to four days, then refrigerate for up to five days. Refrigerate cut up melon in a covered container for up to three days.

Wash the cantaloupe under cool water before cutting to cleanse it of any mold or bacteria, which can be carried on the knife from the skin into the fruit. Cut the melon open and remove the seeds and strings.

Cherries, Sweet

Cherries have shown to be helpful in the treatment of gout, lumbago, rheumatism, paralysis, arthritis, stunted growth, and obesity. Black cherry juice is excellent for gout, and prevents tooth decay by stopping plaque formation. Cherries benefit the glandular system, remove toxic waste from tissues, and aid the functions of the gallbladder and liver. The ellagic acid content has cancer-preventing properties. The parts eaten are the skin and the flesh.

Key nutrients in cherries include vitamin C, potassium, calcium, iron, magnesium, phosphorus, fructose, glucose, sucrose, zinc, copper, manganese, vitamin B_1 (thiamine), vitamin B_2 (riboflavin), vitamin B_3 (niacin), pantothenic acid, vitamin B_6, folate, vitamin E, fiber, and small amounts of lipids. Important phytochemicals include beta-carotene, anthocyanins, ellagic acid, phytosterols, and perillyl alcohol.

Choose cherries that have been kept cool and moist. The flavor and texture of cherries suffer at warm temperatures. Select cherries that have a very deep maroon, mahogany, red, or black color. The surfaces should be bright, glossy, and plump-looking. Stems should look fresh and green. Avoid fruit that is shriveled or has dried stems. Pass on any cherries that have soft leaking flesh, brown discolorations, obvious signs of mold growth, or a dull appearance.

Cherries should be stored dry in the refrigerator loosely packed in plastic bags. Fresh cherries will keep for approximately one week in the refrigerator. Cherries can be frozen and kept for up to twelve months.

Wash cherries under cold water. You can pit cherries by cutting them in half and removing the pit with the tip of a knife.

Maraschino cherries are made by bleaching the fruit in sulfur dioxide brine and then toughening it with calcium salt or lime. The cherries are then dyed bright red, sweetened, flavored and packed in containers. Avoid this type of cherry.

Cranberries

Cranberries are good for the kidneys, bladder, and skin. They are useful in the treatment of asthma, cystitis, kidney stones, and bladder stones. They also are a good intestinal antiseptic. Natural compounds in cranberries keep bacteria, such as *Escherichia coli* (*E. coli*) from adhering to bladder cells. This activity allows the *E. coli* to be suspended in the bladder and then eventually flushed from the body, thus preventing bladder infections. The ellagic acid and anthocyanins in cranberries have an anticancer effect. Anthocyanins also promote formation of visual purple, a pigment present in the eyes that is instrumental in color and night vision. The entire fruit is eaten. Canned cranberry sauce contains up to 86 percent less vitamin C than an equal amount of fresh cranberries.

Key nutrients in cranberries include vitamin C, fiber, citric acid, malic acid, calcium, iron, magnesium, phosphorus, potassium, sodium, zinc, copper, manganese, fructose, glucose, sucrose, vitamin B_1 (thiamine), vitamin B_2 (riboflavin), vitamin B_3 (niacin), pantothenic acid, vitamin B_6, folate, vitamin E, and small amounts of lipids. Important phytochemicals include beta-carotene, ellagic acid, chlorogenic acid, eugenol, ferulic acid, quercetin, anthocyanins, and tocopherols.

Cranberries are usually sold packaged in plastic bags. Select a bag containing firm, bright-red berries. Avoid bags that contain pale berries and debris. At their peak, cranberries will bounce if dropped. There are many types of cranberries, but the most popular varieties are Searls, Early Black, Howes, and McFarlin.

Cranberries will keep for up to one month in their original packaging, stored in the refrigerator. Cranberries also can be frozen, in their original packaging, for up to one year.

Sort the berries before serving, and discard any berries that have "turned bad." To clean cranberries, place them in a basin of cold water. Any twigs, leaves, or unripe berries will float to the surface and can be skimmed off. Do this quickly, so that the berries do not become waterlogged. Do not wash the berries until you are ready to eat them.

Currants

Currants have been used to treat diarrhea, multiple sclerosis, and sore throat. They help to slow the aging process. The anthocyanins in currants have antibacterial and anti-inflammatory properties. Other flavonoids in currants inhibit cancer growth. The entire fruit is eaten. The dried currants that are commonly available in supermarkets are actually made from Black Corinth grapes, and are therefore a type of raisin.

Key nutrients in currants include fiber, vitamin C, potassium, calcium, iron, magnesium, phosphorus, sodium, fructose, glucose, sucrose, zinc, copper, manganese, vitamin B_1 (thiamine), vitamin B_2 (riboflavin), vitamin B_3 (niacin), pantothenic acid, vitamin B_6, folate, vitamin E, and small amounts of lipids. Important phytochemicals include beta-carotene, anthocyanins, pectin, and tocopherols.

Fresh currants are berries that grow on vines in clusters similar to grapes. They are very tart. They should be plump, firm, uniform in size, dry, and firmly attached to their branchlike stems. Avoid currants that are withered or crushed.

Remove from the container any currants that are overripe to prevent them from hastening the decaying process of the other currants. Store fresh currants in the refrigerator and use them within twenty-four hours.

Sort currants before serving, and discard any that have "turned bad." Wash the currants quickly under cold water. Do not wash the berries until you are ready to eat them.

Dates

Dates have a laxative effect and are linked to lower rates of certain cancers, especially pancreatic cancer. The parts eaten include the skin and the flesh.

Key nutrients in dates include potassium, vitamin C, vitamin B_1 (thiamine), vitamin B_2 (riboflavin), vitamin B_3 (niacin), boron, fiber, iron, calcium, fructose, glucose, sucrose, vitamin B_6, magnesium, phosphorus, sodium, zinc, copper, manganese, pantothenic acid, folate, vitamin E, and small amounts of lipids and amino acids. Important phytochemicals include beta-carotene.

Select fresh dates that are smooth-skinned, glossy, and plump. Avoid dates that are broken, cracked, dry, or shriveled, or that smell sour. Date sugar can be purchased in health food stores and substituted in equal measure for regular sugar. Though high in natural sugar, dates are fat-free.

Fresh dates can be stored for up to eight months in the refrigerator or for one to two months at room temperature. Fresh dates should always be stored in airtight containers to preserve freshness and to protect them from other food odors, which they readily absorb.

Slit each date open with a knife and push out the pit. If slicing the dates, place them in the freezer for one hour to firm them. The sweetness of dates makes them an excellent replacement for sugar in recipes. Chopped, they can be added to many baked items.

People who take monoamine oxidase inhibitor (MAOI) drugs, which are sometimes prescribed for depression, should avoid eating dates. Dates contain the amino acid tyramine, which can interact with these drugs and produce a life-threatening rise in blood pressure. Tyramine can also trigger migraine headaches in some people.

Figs

Figs kill bacteria and roundworms in the body, and they are useful for aiding digestion, treating hemorrhoids and chronic constipation, and lowering blood cholesterol. Figs are good for the thymus gland and the immune system, and they are useful in the treatment of coughs, hoarseness, respiratory and lung disorders, and uterine fibroids. With their high amounts of calcium and phosphorus, figs help build strong bones and ward off osteoporosis. Just three or four figs supply nearly 100 milligrams of calcium. The ancient Romans believed that they gave the elderly strength and kept them young. The entire fruit is eaten.

Key nutrients in figs include magnesium, potassium, calcium, iron, fiber, sulfur, vitamin B_6, folate, copper, phosphorus, zinc, vitamin B_2 (riboflavin), vitamin B_3 (niacin), vitamin B_1 (thiamine), fructose, glucose, sucrose, niacin, sodium, manganese, vitamin C, pantothenic acid, vitamin E, and small amounts of lipids and amino acids. Important phytochemicals include beta-carotene, anthocyanins, myristic acid, pectin, psoralen, and phytosterols.

Select fresh figs with a rich color, unbruised and unbroken skins, and a mild fragrance. Fresh figs should be soft to the touch, but not mushy. Slightly shriveled skins indicate sweetness. Avoid figs that smell sour. Black Mission figs are the most popular variety, but greenish-yellow skinned Kadota and Calimyrna are available also.

Ripe fresh figs should be stored in the refrigerator in a shallow dish lined with a paper towel and covered with plastic wrap. Fresh figs will keep for two to three days. Unripe figs can be placed on a plate and kept at room temperature, away from sunlight, until fully ripened. Turn them frequently as they ripen.

Wash figs under cold water and remove the hard portion of the stem end. Peel them if they have a thick skin.

Gooseberries

Gooseberries have been used to treat liver disorders, intestinal disorders, urinary tract infections, menstrual irregularities, and inflammatory disorders. The entire fruit is eaten. There are approximately 50 different species and more than 700 varieties of gooseberries.

Key nutrients in gooseberries include vitamin C, calcium, sodium, sulfur, vitamin B_1 (thiamine), potassium, iron, fructose, glucose, sucrose, magnesium, phosphorus, sodium, zinc, copper, manganese, vitamin B_2 (riboflavin), vitamin B_3 (niacin), pantothenic acid, vitamin B_6, folate, vitamin E, fiber, and small amounts of lipids. Important phytochemicals include beta-carotene, catechins, chlorogenic acid, ferulic acid, P-coumaric acid, pectin, tannin, and tocopherols.

Gooseberries should be plump, firm, uniform in size, dry, and free from stems and leaves. Gooseberries should *not* have stems or caps attached.

Once home, immediately remove any berries that are overripe, as these will hasten the decaying process of the other berries. Gooseberries should be used within two days after purchasing.

Sort the berries before serving, and discard any berries that have "turned bad." Wash the berries quickly under cold water. Do not wash the berries until you are ready to eat them.

Grapefruit

Grapefruit is good for the cardiovascular system because its chemicals and nutrients work to protect the arteries; the pectin content lowers blood cholesterol and high blood pressure. Grapefruit can reduce the risk of cancer, aid digestion, speed the breakdown of fat, feed the good bacteria in the intestines, and boost the immune system. As an anti-inflammatory, grapefruits also are useful for people with chest congestion, rheumatoid arthritis, lupus, and other inflammatory disorders. Grapefruit may help dissolve gallstones, cleanse the liver and gallbladder, and may be effective in the prevention and treatment of esophageal cancer. The part eaten is the flesh.

Key nutrients in grapefruits include potassium, folate, fiber, iron, fructose, glucose, sucrose, vitamin C, magnesium, phosphorus, sodium, zinc, copper, manganese, vitamin B_1 (thiamine), vitamin B_2 (riboflavin), vitamin B_3 (niacin), pantothenic acid, vitamin B_6, calcium, and small amounts of lipids and amino acids. Important phytochemicals include alpha-carotene, beta-carotene, flavonoids, beta-sitosterol, anthocyanins, lycopene, ellagic acid, ferulic acid, caffeic acid, pectin, phenethyl isothiocyanate (PEITC), limonoids, saponins, triterpenoids, quercetin, catechins, coumarin, beta-cryptoxanthin, esculetin, hesperetin, hesperidin, kaempferol, naringenin, P-coumaric acid, phloroglucinol, scopoletin, sinapic acid, stigmasterol, umbelliferone, rutin, terpenes, tocopherols, and monoterpenes. The pink, white, and red varieties also contain beta-carotene and lycopene.

Select smooth, glossy, round, firm, thin-skinned fruits that are heavy for their size, and have slightly flattened ends. Skin defects such as scars and discolorations do not affect the quality of the fruit. Avoid grapefruits that are coarse-skinned, soft, puffy, or pointed at one end.

Grapefruits can be stored at room temperature for up to a week, or in the refrigerator for six to eight weeks. Grapefruits are juiciest when slightly warm rather than when chilled.

If grapefruits are chilled, leave them at room temperature for at least thirty minutes before you juice or eat them. Wash grapefruits under cool water before cutting to rid them of any mold or bacteria, which can be carried on the knife from the skin into the fruit.

Grapefruit juice can interact with or boost the strength of certain medications. If you are in the habit of taking medications with grapefruit juice, consult your health-care provider concerning any possible complications. Grapefruit also can increase the risk of developing kidney stones.

Grapefruit seeds yield a natural antibiotic that is a good alternative to pharmaceutical antibiotics. Grapefruit seed extract, produced by grinding the seeds, fights bacteria and fungi, including candida, as well as viruses and parasites. You can either add liquid extract to fresh juice or take it in capsule form with a full glass of liquid. Never drink the liquid form without diluting it, as it is very strong and can burn the mouth, throat, or stomach that way. Some people experience minor side effects, principally mild stomach irritation and flatulence, but in general, it works quickly and is quite safe.

Grapes

Grapes help combat toxins in the body, stimulate the liver, increase energy, regulate blood cholesterol levels, reduce the action of platelets, lower the risk of cardiovascular disease, including heart attacks, and improve circulation. They have a cleansing effect on all tissues and glands. Grapes are useful in the treatment of fever, constipation, cancer, low blood pressure, low blood sugar, edema, and palpitations of the heart. They are good for the skin, and they strengthen the bladder and kidneys. The mineral content, including boron, makes grapes a preventive for osteoporosis (bone loss). Grapes contain salicylates, the same compounds used to make aspirin. Researchers believe that these compounds may discourage blood clots. The entire fruit is eaten.

Key nutrients in grapes include iron, potassium, phosphorus, calcium, magnesium, sulfur, sodium, fructose, glucose, sucrose, vitamin C, salicylates, fiber, zinc, copper, manganese, boron, vitamin B_1 (thiamine), vitamin B_2 (riboflavin), vitamin B_3 (niacin), pantothenic acid, vitamin B_6, vitamin E, vitamin K, folate, and small amounts of lipids and amino acids. Important phytochemicals include anthocyanins, pectin, lycopene, ellagic acid, ferulic acid, caffeic acid, chlorogenic acid, catechins, beta-cryptoxanthin, gallic acid, coumarin, P-coumaric acid, resveratrol, alpha-carotene, beta-carotene, quercetin, tocopherols, beta-ionone, beta-sitosterol, and myristic acid.

Select well-colored, plump grapes that are firmly attached to moist, flexible stems. Avoid soft or wrinkled grapes and grapes with lighter areas around the stem end.

Remove any spoiled fruit, and place unwashed grapes in a plastic bag in the refrigerator. Fresh grapes can be stored for up to one week in the refrigerator.

Wash grapes under cold water and remove any damaged fruit. Do not wash the grapes until you are ready to eat them.

Honeydew Melon

Honeydew melons can help to protect the body from esophageal cancer, as well as help to control high blood pressure. The potassium content, combined with high amounts of the antioxidants vitamin C and beta-carotene,

aids in preventing strokes. When ripe, the honeydew is the sweetest of all the melon varieties. The part eaten is the flesh.

Key nutrients in honeydew melons include vitamin C, potassium, fiber, calcium, iron, magnesium, phosphorus, sodium, fructose, glucose, sucrose, zinc, copper, manganese, vitamin B_1 (thiamine), vitamin B_2 (riboflavin), vitamin B_3 (niacin), pantothenic acid, vitamin B_6, folate, vitamin E, and small amounts of lipids. Important phytochemicals include pectin, lutein, chlorophylls, alpha-carotene, and beta-carotene.

Choose honeydews with a soft, velvety feel. There should be a slight softening at the blossom end of the fruit, and the rind should be a pale, creamy yellow or a light salmon color. Tiny freckles on the skin are a sign of sweetness. Avoid melons that are a flat white or greenish-white color. Pass on fruits that have large bruised areas or surface cuts.

Store honeydews at room temperature for up to four days, then refrigerate for up to five days. Refrigerate cut-up melon in a covered container for up to three days.

Wash the honeydew under cool water before cutting it to rid it of any mold or bacteria, which can be carried on the knife from the skin into the fruit. Cut the melon open and remove the seeds and strings before eating. Keeping the seeds intact helps to keep the fruit moist until you are ready to eat it.

Kiwi

Kiwi is slightly tart, tasting like a cross between strawberries and green grapes, and is known in China as the Chinese gooseberry. It contains pectin, a soluble fiber, which helps to control blood cholesterol levels. Kiwi is also useful in controlling high blood pressure. One large kiwi has only 46 calories and supplies more than twice the recommended dietary allowance (RDA) of vitamin C—that's more vitamin C than one medium-sized orange, half a grapefruit, or a cup of strawberries—as well as vitamin K and potassium. This fruit is a powerhouse of nutrients for its size! The entire fruit is eaten, including the skin if the fuzz has been rubbed off.

Chinese researchers used kiwi in an experiment for esophageal cancer. They found high levels of nitrites in their cancer patients and those who ate kiwi fruit were found to have a dramatic decrease in their nitrite readings.

Key nutrients in kiwi include vitamin A, vitamin B_6, vitamin C, vitamin K, calcium, phosphorus, sodium, folate, vitamin B_1 (thiamine), vitamin B_2 (riboflavin), vitamin B_3 (niacin), fructose, glucose, sucrose, potassium, magnesium, fiber, and small amounts of lipids. Important phytochemicals include beta-carotene, beta-cryptoxanthin, pectin, lutein, zeaxanthin, tannin, and tocopherols.

Select kiwi that is plump, fragrant, and yields to gentle pressure. Avoid ones that are shriveled, pulpy, bruised, or have wet spots.

Ripe kiwi will keep for two to three weeks and can be stored at room temperature or in the refrigerator. Do not store kiwi with other fruits because the ethylene gas emitted by other fruits will cause the kiwi to become overripe. However, if you want to hasten ripening, place kiwis in a paper bag with an apple or banana for a few days.

Wash kiwi under cold water before cutting to rid it of any mold or bacteria, which can be carried on the knife from the skin into the fruit. Kiwi can be peeled and sliced, or the flesh scooped out with a spoon after cutting it in half. When the fuzz is rubbed off, the entire fruit can be eaten. Because of its high vitamin C content, the kiwi does not discolor when it is cut and makes a good garnish.

Kiwi contains actinidin, an enzyme that inhibits gelling, so kiwi must be lightly cooked before adding to recipes that contain gelatin. Similarly, fresh kiwi should not be added to fruit gelatin (Jell-O) recipes, as the gelatin will not thicken.

Lemons

Lemons cleanse the bloodstream and liver, aid digestion, boost the immune system, prevent heart disease and cancer, lower blood cholesterol levels, lower high blood pressure, stimulate the liver, soothe insect bites and migraines, and reduce inflammation. Lemons are a solvent for uric acid and other toxins. They are useful in the treatment of influenza, common cold, sore throat, bronchitis, asthma, heartburn, gout, neuritis, diabetes, scurvy, fevers, and rheumatism. Lemon juice has been proven effective in protecting blood vessels from hardening. Lemons may help to dissolve gallstones, and may be effective in the prevention and treatment of esophageal cancer. The parts eaten include the flesh and the zest (shavings from the outermost part of the rind). The white part of the lemon peel can be rubbed against the gums to prevent bleeding. Another good use for lemons is to place freshly squeezed lemon juice in ice cube trays, freeze, and store the cubes in plastic bags in the freezer. The lemon juice cubes can then be added to herbal teas or defrosted to use whenever you need fresh lemon juice.

Key nutrients in lemons include vitamin C, fiber, fructose, glucose, sucrose, calcium, iron, magnesium, phosphorus, potassium, citron, citric acid, sodium, zinc, copper, vitamin B_1 (thiamine), vitamin B_2 (riboflavin), vitamin B_3 (niacin), pantothenic acid, vitamin B_6, and small amounts of lipids. Important phytochemicals include limonene, anthocyanins, pectin, psoralen, caffeic acid, ellagic acid, ferulic acid, hesperidin, monoterpenes, saponins, triterpenoids, quercetin, catechins, P-coumaric acid, sinapic acid, thymol, umbelliferone, rutin, coumarin, phenethyl isothiocyanate (PEITC), beta-carotene, and phytosterols.

Select firm and heavy fruit with a rich yellow color. The skin should be smooth, with a slight gloss. Avoid lemons that are dark yellow or dull in color, have hardened or shriveled skins, contain soft spots, or have a moldy surface.

Fruits with Super Nutrient Values

Researchers at Rutgers University in New Jersey analyzed twenty-five common fruits for their comparative nutrient values, then ranked the fruit according to nutrient density. The winner? Kiwi was first, with papaya and mango coming in second and third. Kiwi, along with papaya and apricots, also beat out bananas and oranges as the top potassium-rich fruits.

Lemons can be stored at room temperature for two weeks, or in a plastic bag, in the crisper compartment of the refrigerator, for up to six weeks. They can also be stored in a tightly sealed jar of water in the refrigerator.

If lemons are chilled, leave them at room temperature for at least thirty minutes before juicing or eating them. Wash lemons under cool water before slicing or peeling them to rid them of any mold or bacteria, which can be carried on the knife from the skin into the fruit. For easier juicing, roll lemons back and forth across the countertop for a few moments. Even better, submerge them in hot water for fifteen minutes—they will yield nearly twice as much juice. Lemons (and limes) are good in marinades for tenderizing meats.

People who have or are prone to urinary tract infections should avoid citrus fruits, as they produce alkaline urine, which encourages bacterial growth.

Limes

The phytochemicals in limes boost the immune system, prevent heart disease and cancer, lower blood cholesterol levels, and lower high blood pressure. Limes may help to dissolve gallstones, protect against scurvy, and may be effective in the prevention and treatment of esophageal cancer. The parts eaten are the flesh and the zest.

Key nutrients in limes include vitamin C, fiber, calcium, iron, fructose, glucose, sucrose, magnesium, phosphorus, potassium, citron, sodium, zinc, copper, manganese, vitamin B_1 (thiamine), vitamin B_2 (riboflavin), vitamin B_3 (niacin), pantothenic acid, vitamin B_6, folate, vitamin E, and small amounts of lipids and amino acids. Important phytochemicals include psoralen, anthocyanins, monoterpenes, pectin, saponins, triterpenoids, quercetin, catechins, rutin, limonene, caffeic acid, chlorogenic acid, eugenol, hesperidin, isoquercitrin, P-coumaric acid, tannin, tocopherols, ferulic acid, ellagic acid, coumarin, phenethyl isothiocyanate (PEITC), and beta-carotene.

Select limes with a glossy skin and a heavy weight for their size. Limes should be dark green, without any yellow areas. Avoid limes with a dull, dry skin, soft spots, or mold.

Purplish or brownish mottling does not indicate damage in early stages. Limes will turn a yellowish color as they ripen, but the best flavored are dark green.

Limes should be stored in the refrigerator, in a plastic bag, for up to six weeks. If limes are chilled, you will get twice the amount of juice from them if you leave them at room temperature for at least thirty minutes or drop them in hot water for a few minutes before you juice or eat them. For better juicing, roll them back and forth across the counter for a few moments to soften them. Wash limes under cool water before slicing or peeling them to rid them of any mold or bacteria, which can be carried on the knife from the skin into the fruit.

Limes contain the phytochemical psoralen, which can make the skin more sensitive to the sun. People who have or are prone to urinary tract infections should avoid citrus fruits, as they produce alkaline urine, which encourages bacterial growth.

Mangoes

Mangoes aid poor circulation. Mango juice combined with papaya juice helps to ease inflammation, digestive problems, fever, and pain. In parts of Asia, mango juice is used to relieve dehydration. Mangoes are one of the top fruit sources of beta-carotene, in addition to having a high vitamin C content. The tender flesh, which is the part eaten, also contains insoluble fiber.

Key nutrients in mangoes include vitamin C, vitamin E, potassium, fructose, glucose, sucrose, iron, fiber, calcium, magnesium, phosphorus, sodium, zinc, copper, manganese, vitamin B_1 (thiamine), vitamin B_2 (riboflavin), vitamin B_3 (niacin), pantothenic acid, vitamin B_6, folate, and small amounts of lipids and amino acids. Important phytochemicals include beta-carotene, pectin, gallic acid, limonene, myristic acid, tannin, lutein, zeaxanthin, and beta-cryptoxanthin.

Select mangoes that yield slightly when gently pressed, and have a flowery fragrance. The skin should be a deep or grass green, and have a "blush" of either red or orange-yellow. Avoid mangoes with a profusion of large black spots, or loose or shriveled skin. Their form resembles a very large California avocado.

Mangoes should be juicy when ripe. Ripe mangoes should be stored in the refrigerator, where they will keep for up to one week.

Wash mangoes under cool water before consuming or slicing them. Mangoes are good in sauces and chutneys; baked in custards, pies, breads, and muffins; or stewed with other fruits and used as toppings. Or simply peel the skin as you would a banana and enjoy after chilling.

Nectarines

Nectarines can help protect against cancer, control blood cholesterol levels, and prevent constipation. Nectarines have powerful antioxidant powers because of their high levels of potassium, beta-carotene, and vitamin C—twice that of peaches! The skin and the flesh are the parts eaten. Avoid eating nectarine pits. They contain amygdalin, a compound that is converted into cyanide in the stomach.

Key nutrients in nectarines include potassium, vitamin C, fiber, calcium, iron, magnesium, phosphorus, sodium, zinc, copper, fructose, glucose, sucrose, manganese, vitamin B_1 (thiamine), vitamin B_2 (riboflavin), vitamin B_3 (niacin), pantothenic acid, vitamin B_6, folate, vitamin E, and small amounts of lipids. Important phytochemicals include beta-carotene, lutein, zeaxanthin, beta-cryptoxanthin, and pectin.

Nectarines, first cousin to the peach, are thought of as "peaches without fuzz." Select ones that have a rich color and a sweet fragrance. They should be plump and soft along the seam. The coloration should be deep yellow under a red blush. Avoid nectarines that are hard, dull in color, have shriveled or cracked skins, or are overly soft.

Ripe nectarines should be stored in the crisper compartment of the refrigerator, and will keep for three to five days.

Wash nectarines under cold water before eating them. They will taste best if allowed to warm to room temperature.

Oranges

Adding oranges to the diet can help to cleanse the body, boost the immune system, prevent heart disease, lower blood cholesterol levels, combat acidosis, lower acid urine, prevent scurvy, combat fevers, dissolve gallstones, and lower high blood pressure. Oranges and orange juice have been used in the treatment of leukemia and other cancers, as well as diabetes. The high calcium level in oranges promotes the formation of strong bones and teeth. Studies have shown that the oil in the peel has terpenes, found to lower the incidence of chemically induced cancers. D-limonene, also found in oranges, is a natural cholesterol-lowering substance, has anticancer qualities, and may reduce tumors. The parts eaten are the flesh and the zest.

Key nutrients in oranges include vitamin C, folate, vitamin B_1 (thiamine), fiber, potassium, sodium, citric acid, fructose, glucose, sucrose, zinc, copper, iron, manganese, pantothenic acid, vitamin B_6, vitamin E, phosphorus, magnesium, sulfur, calcium, vitamin B_2 (riboflavin), vitamin B_3 (niacin), and small amounts of lipids and amino acids. Important phytochemicals include alpha-carotene, beta-carotene, beta-sitosterol, anthocyanins, pectin, ellagic acid, ferulic acid, caryophyllene, caffeic acid, naringenin, P-coumaric acid, sinapic acid, stigmasterol, rutin, hesperidin, limonene, monoterpenes, saponins, triterpenoids, quercetin, catechins, phenethyl isothiocyanate (PEITC), beta-cryptoxanthin, lutein, zeaxanthin, tocopherols, and coumarin.

Organically grown oranges are best. They should be firm and heavy, with a fresh, bright, smooth skin. Avoid oranges that are lightweight; have a rough skin texture or dull, dry skin; have a spongy texture; have spots and discolorations on the surface of the skin; have been dyed and/or waxed; and/or appear to be too "perfect" or look like a wax imitation.

If picked green, oranges may cause arthritic-like joint pains because the citric acid in green oranges has not had time to be converted into fructose (fruit sugar). Green oranges also have lower vitamin C levels than properly ripened oranges. Some oranges are colored orange with a red dye to appear ripe and then waxed to prolong shelf life. Many times, such oranges have been sprayed with a fungicide to retard rotting as well.

Oranges can be stored in the refrigerator, or at room temperature, for up to two weeks.

If oranges are chilled, leave them at room temperature for at least thirty minutes before you juice or eat them. Wash oranges under cool water before slicing or peeling them to rid them of any mold or bacteria, which can be carried on the knife from the skin into the fruit.

Papaya

Papaya assists digestion, protects mucous membranes from infection, constricts stomach ulcers, helps to ease inflammation, relieves acidosis, combats diarrhea and constipation, and helps rid the body of intestinal worms. Two important antioxidants in papayas, vitamins C and A, reduce the risk of cancer, heart disease, and cataracts. Papaya breaks down unwanted substances, including uric acid and other toxic acids in the body. It is good to add to infant formula to aid digestion. The parts eaten include the skin, flesh, and seeds.

Key nutrients in papaya include vitamin C, vitamin A, potassium, silicon, vitamin B_1 (thiamine), fiber, sodium, calcium, phosphorus, copper, iron, manganese, sulfur, magnesium, fructose, glucose, sucrose, zinc, vitamin B_2 (riboflavin), vitamin B_3 (niacin), pantothenic acid, vitamin B_6, folate, vitamin E, and small amounts of lipids and amino acids. Important phytochemicals include beta-carotene, beta-cryptoxanthin, papain, caryophyllene, lycopene, myristic acid, lutein, zeaxanthin, and pectin.

Select papayas that are yellow to orange-yellow in color. They should give slightly under gentle pressure, but they should not be soft or mushy at the stem end. The skin should be smooth, not bruised or shriveled. An uncut papaya should not give off any odor.

Ripe papayas should be stored in the refrigerator, in a plastic bag. They will keep for up to one week.

Wash papayas under cool water before cutting them to rid them of any mold or bacteria, which can be carried on the knife from the skin into the fruit. Papaya seeds can be cleaned, dried, and ground like peppercorns. Their peppery flavor makes them a good substitute for pepper.

Sprinkle ground seeds over foods to add important digestive enzymes.

Peaches

Adding peaches to the diet can aid the bladder, relieve cystitis, prevent edema, assist elimination, improve digestion, decrease gastritis, relieve constipation, and treat obesity. Peaches are good for those suffering from cancer, heart disease, and most types of illness because they are easily digested. Peaches contain salicylates, the same compounds used to make aspirin. Researchers believe these compounds may discourage unwanted blood clots from forming. The skin and the flesh are the parts eaten.

Key nutrients in peaches include vitamin C, potassium, fiber, magnesium, phosphorus, iron, calcium, sodium, manganese, silicon, fructose, glucose, sucrose, zinc, selenium, vitamin B_1 (thiamine), copper, vitamin B_2 (riboflavin), vitamin B_3 (niacin), pantothenic acid, vitamin B_6, vitamin K, folate, vitamin E, and small amounts of lipids and amino acids. Important phytochemicals include beta-carotene, pectin, chlorogenic acid, lycopene, quercetin, tannin, lutein, zeaxanthin, beta-cryptoxanthin, phytosterols, and tocopherols.

Choose mildly fragrant peaches that are firm or just a bit soft. The skin color between the red areas of the fruit should be yellow or creamy, and the skins should be unwrinkled. Avoid hard fruit and peaches with green coloring. Also avoid very soft fruit with large bruises or any sign of decay.

Peaches ripen quickly if placed in a cardboard box and covered with newspaper.

Ripe peaches should be stored in the crisper compartment of the refrigerator, and will keep for three to five days. Eat them as soon as they are ripe—they do not store well.

Wash peaches under cool water. Peaches can be consumed chilled or at room temperature.

Pears

Pears can be useful in treating inflammation of mucous membranes, colitis, chronic gallbladder disorders, arthritis, and gout. Pears can also be beneficial in lowering high blood pressure, controlling blood cholesterol levels, and increasing urine acidity. They are good for the lungs and the stomach. Most of the fiber is insoluble, making pears a good laxative. The gritty fiber content may cut down on the number of cancerous colon polyps. The skin and the flesh are the parts eaten. Most of the vitamin C, as well as the dietary fiber, are contained within the skin of the fruit.

Key nutrients in pears include vitamin C, folate, potassium, iron, fiber, vitamin B_1 (thiamine), vitamin B_2 (riboflavin), vitamin B_3 (niacin), calcium, magnesium, phosphorus, zinc, copper, manganese, fructose, glucose, sucrose, pantothenic acid, vitamin B_6, vitamin E, and small amounts of lipids and amino acids. Important phytochemicals include beta-carotene, caffeic acid, quercetin, pectin, and tocopherols.

Choose pears that are well-colored for their variety, and have few if any blemishes. Ripe pears will yield to gentle pressure at the stem end. Avoid pears that are soft at the blossom end of the fruit, shriveled at the stem end, or those with surface cuts or dark, soft spots.

Pears should be ripened at room temperature, and then placed in the refrigerator. Ripe pears will keep in the refrigerator for one to two days. Do not store pears in plastic bags, as this will cause the fruit to brown at the core.

Pears should be washed under cold water and eaten with their skins intact.

Pineapples

Pineapple works to cleanse the body, aid digestion, purify and thin the blood, prevent blood clots, increase circulation, aid menses, and regulate the glands. It is useful in the treatment of goiter, obesity, cancer, inflammation, influenza, common cold, sore throat, edema, allergies, bronchitis, pain, diabetes, rheumatic disorders, tendonitis, respiratory ailments, heart disease, high blood pressure, muscle disorders, arthritis, and liver and kidney ailments. The flesh is the part eaten. Fresh pineapple contains bromelain, an enzyme that reduces inflammation in the body. Bromelain is also available in pill and powdered forms.

Key nutrients in pineapple include vitamin C, vitamin B_6, folate, vitamin B_1 (thiamine), iron, magnesium, fiber, glucose, sodium, calcium, phosphorus, potassium, fructose, glucose, sucrose, zinc, copper, vitamin B_2 (riboflavin), vitamin B_3 (niacin), pantothenic acid, vitamin E, manganese, and small amounts of lipids and amino acids. Important phytochemicals include beta-carotene, bromelain, chlorogenic acid, pectin, P-coumaric acid, and tocopherols.

Choose pineapples with a bright, dark-green color. Ripe pineapples have a fragrant pineapple aroma, and are firm, plump, and heavy when mature. Avoid fruit with a dull yellowish-green color, dried appearance, and soft spots. Do not buy pineapples that smell sour or fermented.

Ripe pineapple can be stored in the refrigerator in a plastic bag. It will keep for three to five days. Cut-up pineapple can be stored in the refrigerator in an airtight container and will keep for up to one week.

Wash the pineapple under cool water, and remove the leafy crown. Cut the pineapple in quarters, and then remove the flesh from the skin.

Plums

Plums help to lower blood cholesterol levels, relieve constipation, and eliminate parasites from the body. They contain benzoic acid, which is useful in the treatment of liver disease, blood poisoning, and kidney disorders. Plums also contain salicylates, the same compounds used to make aspirin. Researchers believe these compounds may discourage the formation of unwanted blood clots. The skin and the flesh are the parts eaten. Avoid eating plum pits. They contain amygdalin, a compound that is converted into cyanide in the stomach.

Key nutrients in plums include vitamin C, vitamin B_2 (riboflavin), vitamin B_3 (niacin), potassium, fiber, vitamin B_6, vitamin E, vitamin K, calcium, iron, magnesium, phosphorus, fructose, glucose, sucrose, zinc, copper, manganese, vitamin B_1 (thiamine), pantothenic acid, folate, and small amounts of lipids and amino acids. Important phytochemicals include anthocyanins, beta-carotene, chlorogenic acid, ferulic acid, lutein, zeaxanthin, P-coumaric acid, beta-cryptoxanthin, pectin, and tocopherols.

Choose plums that are fairly firm to soft, plump, and well colored for their variety. Ripe plums are slightly soft at the stem and tip. Avoid plums with shriveled skins, mushy spots, breaks in the skin, or brownish discolorations. Also avoid plums that are overly hard.

Ripe plums stored in the refrigerator in a plastic bag will keep for up to three days. Wash plums under cool water before eating.

Pomegranates

Pomegranates have been used to treat halitosis, sore throats, hemorrhoids, intestinal worms, diarrhea, excessive perspiration, fevers, and leukorrhea. The peel contains about 30 percent tannin, which is an active astringent substance. The parts eaten are the juice and pulp. Pomegranate seeds also are edible and are high in fiber.

Key nutrients in pomegranates include calcium, phosphorus, iron, sodium, potassium, vitamin C, magnesium, fiber, fructose, glucose, sucrose, zinc, copper, vitamin B_1 (thiamine), vitamin B_2 (riboflavin), vitamin B_3 (niacin), pantothenic acid, vitamin B_6, folate, vitamin E, and small amounts of lipids. Important phytochemicals include beta-carotene, chlorogenic acid, anthocyanins, phytosterols, gallic acid, ellagic acid, pectin, and tannin.

Choose pomegranates that feel heavy for their size, with a bright color and blemish-free skin.

Ripe pomegranates should be stored in the refrigerator, and will keep for up to one month. The seeds, when packed tightly into an airtight container in the freezer, will keep for up to three months.

Wash pomegranates under cool water before cutting them to rid them of any mold or bacteria, which can be carried on the knife from the skin into the fruit. Cut the fruit in half and pry out the seeds, removing any of the light-colored membrane that may adhere to them.

Raspberries

Raspberries are good for the liver, muscles, blood, and kidneys, and they protect against viruses, cancer, and damage to DNA, the genetic material that governs cellular reproduction. They balance the nervous and vascular systems. Raspberries have been used to treat diarrhea, frequent urination, nervousness, depression, and impotence. The entire fruit is eaten.

Key nutrients in raspberries include calcium, folate, phosphorus, iron, manganese, selenium, potassium, sodium, silicon, fructose, glucose, sucrose, zinc, vitamin C, vitamin E, fiber, magnesium, copper, vitamin B_1 (thiamine), vitamin B_2 (riboflavin), vitamin B_3 (niacin), pantothenic acid, vitamin B_6, and small amounts of lipids. Important phytochemicals include alpha-carotene, beta-carotene, pectin, catechins, caffeic acid, ferulic acid, ellagic acid, anthocyanins, tannin, tocopherols, and tocotrienols.

Select raspberries with a uniform color. They should be plump and tender—avoid ones that are mushy or bruised. Raspberries should not have stems or caps attached. Pass on berries that are leaky or moldy, or are wet or have stained spots on the container.

Once home, immediately remove any overripe berries, as these will hasten the decaying process of the other berries. Raspberries should be used within two days after purchasing. Frozen, they will keep for up to twelve months.

Sort the berries before serving, and discard any that have "turned bad." Wash them quickly under cold water. Do not wash berries until you are ready to eat them. They are very fragile and should be handled with care.

Strawberries

Strawberries can help prevent night sweats, lower blood cholesterol levels, help prevent heart disease and strokes, dissolve tartar deposits on teeth, protect against viruses and cancer, protect against DNA damage, and protect against skin disorders. Strawberries have been used in the treatment of strep infections, gonorrhea, cancers, scurvy, anemia, eczema, dysentery, diarrhea, herpes simplex virus, and acne. Strawberries contain salicylates, the same compounds used to make aspirin. Researchers believe these compounds may discourage the formation of unwanted blood clots. The entire fruit is eaten.

Key nutrients in strawberries include vitamin C, folate, potassium, vitamin B_2 (riboflavin), vitamin B_3 (niacin), iron, fiber, calcium, magnesium, phosphorus, sodium, fructose, glucose, sucrose, zinc, copper, manganese, vitamin B_1 (thiamine), pantothenic acid, vitamin B_6, vitamin E, and small amounts of lipids and amino acids. Important phytochemicals include anthocyanins, pectin, catechins, caffeic acid, ellagic acid, gallic acid, ferulic acid, P-coumaric acid, beta-carotene, chlorogenic acid, tocopherols, and tocotrienols.

Choose clean and dry berries with a full red color, bright luster, firm flesh, and a cap stem still attached. Avoid berries with large colorless or seedy areas or a dull, shrunken appearance, or that are overly soft or have mold.

Always open a container of berries upon bringing them home, and remove any berries that are overripe. Berries that are overripe will hasten the decaying process of the other berries. Strawberries should be used within two days after purchasing. They can be frozen and kept for up to twelve months.

Wash strawberries thoroughly—they are at the top of the list of foods with pesticide residues. Sort the berries before serving, and discard any that have turned bad. Wash the berries quickly under cold water, and remove the caps and stems. Do not wash berries until you are ready to eat them.

Strawberries contain oxalic acid, which can aggravate kidney and bladder stones in some people. Oxalic acid may interfere with the body's ability to absorb iron and calcium. If you take supplements of these minerals, do not take them at the same time you eat strawberries.

Tangerines

Tangerines can help cleanse the body, boost the immune system, prevent heart disease and cancer, lower blood cholesterol levels, combat acidosis, prevent scurvy, combat fevers, dissolve gallstones, and lower high blood pressure. They contain more beta-carotene than any other type of citrus fruit. The flesh is the part eaten.

Key nutrients in tangerines include vitamin C, folate, vitamin B_1 (thiamine), potassium, phosphorus, magnesium, sulfur, calcium, iron, fiber, sodium, fructose, glucose, sucrose, zinc, copper, manganese, pantothenic acid, vitamin B_6, vitamin E, vitamin B_2 (riboflavin), vitamin B_3 (niacin), and small amounts of lipids and amino acids. Important phytochemicals include alpha-carotene, beta-carotene, caryophyllene, rutin, hesperidin, pectin, limonene, ellagic acid, ferulic acid, limonene, myristic acid, coumarin, beta-cryptoxanthin, monoterpenes, saponins, sesquiphellandrene, thymol, tocopherols, triterpenoids, quercetin, catechins, and phenethyl isothiocyanate (PEITC).

Select tangerines that have a deep orange color and feel heavy for their size. Skins should be loose but not shriveled. Avoid pale yellow or greenish fruits; however, small green areas on deeply colored fruit will not affect quality. Pass on fruit with cuts or punctures.

Tangerines should be kept in the refrigerator, and will keep for three to five days. Wash tangerines under cool water, peel off the skin, and separate the fruit into segments when you are ready to eat them.

People who have or are prone to urinary tract infections should avoid citrus fruits, as they produce alkaline urine, which encourages bacterial growth.

Watermelon

Watermelon is a natural diuretic, which makes it useful for weight loss, and is a blood purifier. It helps to cleanse tissues and combat canker sores. Watermelons are a good source of lycopene, an anticancer substance. Watermelon can help protect the body from esophageal cancer and help control high blood pressure. The flesh is the part eaten.

Key nutrients in watermelon include fiber, calcium, iron, magnesium, phosphorus, potassium, sodium, fructose, glucose, sucrose, zinc, copper, manganese, vitamin C, vitamin B_1 (thiamine), vitamin B_2 (riboflavin), vitamin B_3 (niacin), pantothenic acid, vitamin B_6, folate, vitamin E, and small amounts of lipids and amino acids. Important phytochemicals include lycopene, alpha-carotene, beta-carotene, lutein, zeaxanthin, cucurbitacin E, pectin, and phytosterols.

Select watermelons that are symmetrically shaped and are free of cracks, soft spots, or dark bruises. Choose a watermelon whose rind is neither very dull nor very shiny. The underside of the melon should be yellowish in color. The stem (if attached) should be dry and brown in appearance.

Uncut watermelon can be kept at room temperature and will keep for up to one week. Cut watermelon should be packaged in airtight containers. Refrigerated, it will keep for up to four days.

Wash watermelons under cool water before slicing to cleanse them of any mold or bacteria, which can be carried on the knife from the skin into the fruit.

A TASTE OF THE EXOTIC

The multicultural population of the United States has made it possible to find a variety of delicious, nutrient-rich foods from all over the planet in many supermarkets and farmer's markets. Every time you make a new fruit, vegetable, or herb a part of your diet, it expands the adventure that creative eating should be and allows you to access a larger range of powerful dietary healing.

For a different taste experience, look for some of the following more exotic fruits among the more familiar ones in your local market.

Breadfruit

This staple food of the tropics is an excellent source of vitamin C, supplying 50 percent of the recommended dietary allowance (RDA) in just 3½ ounces. It can be used at various stages of ripeness depending on the flavor desired. Fully ripe, it is fruity and sweet—and quite starchy. Edible only when cooked, breadfruit usually is prepared like potatoes or added to soup, stew, breads, and puddings. The seeds are edible and can be eaten boiled or roasted.

Key nutrients in breadfruit include vitamin A, vitamin C, vitamin E, vitamin B_6, calcium, potassium, folate, fiber, magnesium, manganese, phosphorus, vitamin B_1 (thiamine), vitamin B_2 (riboflavin), vitamin B_3 (niacin), and pantothenic acid. Important phytochemicals include beta-carotene.

Cactus Pear

Available July through March, this fruit tastes like watermelon. It can be peeled, seeded, and puréed into a topping for frozen yogurt. One cactus pear contains 42 calories and supplies 22 milligrams of potassium.

Camu-Camu

The Amazon rainforest produces a fruit that has more vitamin C than any other known plant in the world. Ounce for ounce, camu-camu has *thirty times* more vitamin C than an orange. This fruit is slightly bigger than a cherry and has a very sour taste. It grows wild in the swampy or flooded areas of the rainforest and is harvested from canoes. Some rainforest groups are investigating ways to cultivate camu-camu as a food crop. In Peru, it is made into drinks and ice cream. In addition to its high vitamin C content, camu-camu also has high amounts of calcium, fiber, phosphorus, and beta-carotene.

Carambola

This fruit is about the size of an avocado. If you slice a carambola crosswise, it is a perfect five-pointed star—which is why it's nicknamed "star fruit." It is golden when ripe, with four to six deep ribs edged in brown. The flesh is translucent, with a slight tartness; its flavor mixes hints of apple, plum, and citrus. Carambola originated in Asia and is now grown in South Florida. Carambola is a good source of potassium and vitamin C, contains no fat, and a single fruit contains only about 40 calories. Eden Winery in southwest Florida produces a fine table wine made entirely from carambola.

Key nutrients in carambola include calcium, vitamin A, vitamin B_6, vitamin C, vitamin E, fiber, folate, magnesium, phosphorus, potassium, and vitamin B_3 (niacin). Important phytochemicals include beta-carotene, beta-ionone, lutein, P-coumaric acid, and sinapic acid.

Chayote

This fruit tastes of cucumber and apple, and can be sautéed, boiled, or steamed. Three-quarters cup of chayote chunks contains 24 calories and supplies 150 milligrams of potassium and 18 percent of the recommended dietary allowance (RDA) of vitamin C.

Cherimoya

Also known as a custard apple, the cherimoya has a delicate, creamy flesh with large black seeds. It tastes like a blend of pineapple, banana, mango, and vanilla. When fully ripe, the flesh has the texture of firm custard.

Key nutrients in cherimoya include vitamin C, vitamin A, calcium, fiber, vitamin B_1 (thiamine), vitamin B_2 (riboflavin), vitamin B_3 (niacin), iron, phosphorus, magnesium, manganese, potassium, and zinc. Important phytochemicals include beta-carotene, beta-sitosterol, phytosterols, and stigmasterol.

Serve cherimoya well chilled. Cut it in half, remove the seeds, and spoon the fruit from the skin.

Guava

This sweet, fragrant large berry has an edible skin five times higher in vitamin C than an orange, which can be either white, yellow, pink, or green, depending on the variety. Similarly, the flesh may be white, yellow, or pink, and taste of different flavors, including pineapple, pear, and strawberry. It can be eaten fresh, used in fruit salads and desserts, and cooked and puréed as a condiment.

Key nutrients in guava include calcium, vitamin C, vitamin B_6, vitamin A, vitamin E, folate, fiber, iron, magnesium, manganese, phosphorus, potassium, vitamin B_1 (thiamine), vitamin B_2 (riboflavin), vitamin B_3 (niacin), pantothenic acid, and zinc. Important phytochemicals include limonene, beta-carotene, beta-ionone, ellagic acid, gallic acid, and myristic acid.

Horned Melon

This melon tastes like a combination of lime, cucumber, and banana. It can be cut into wedges or eaten straight from the rind.

Kumquat

At just one and one half inches in diameter, kumquats are the smallest of the citrus fruits. They are grown in China, Japan, and the United States. The name means "golden orange" in Cantonese. The entire fruit is edible; the rind is sweet, the flesh juicy and tart. They can be eaten whole or in fruit salads, sauces, and preserves.

Key nutrients in kumquats include calcium, fiber, vitamin C, vitamin B_6, vitamin A, vitamin E, iron, magnesium, manganese, phosphorus, potassium, zinc, vitamin B_1 (thiamine), vitamin B_2 (riboflavin), vitamin B_3 (niacin), and folate.

Lychee

The lychee originated in China some 2,000 years ago. The skin is tough and bumpy. Its milky-white flesh surrounds a single inedible seed. The flesh is juicy and sweet, with a perfumed aroma and a flavor similar to that of grapes. It is an excellent source of vitamin C and potassium.

Key nutrients in lychee include vitamin C, potassium, phosphorus, iron, and fiber.

Mesquite Pod

Mesquite grows in pods, much like that of the carob, in Argentina. The flavor of this fruit is sweet and spicy; the pods can be made into mesquite honey or brewed into tea. They are rich in compounds that may help control blood sugar.

Noni Fruit

Noni fruit, also known as Indian mulberry, is an evergreen tree that originated in India and grows in Tahiti, Hawaii, and Southeast Asia. Parts used are the bark, leaves, flowers, fruit, and seeds. It has been used medicinally as an analgesic, is reported to be antimalarial and anticancerous and is effective against fungus and parasites. Ripe noni fruit contains anthraquinones, phytochemicals that possess purgative activity, accounting for the cleansing effect described by users. Noni is not available fresh except in countries where it is grown, but it can be purchased freeze-dried, in capsules, as a liquid drink, and as powdered extract.

Passion Fruit

Native to Brazil, passion fruit has a tropical, perfumy fragrance. Its skin is tough and uneven in shades of red, lavender, purple, or yellow. When ripe, the skin is wrinkled and deep purple. The flesh has a sweet-tart flavor and contains tiny, edible seeds, which are rich in fiber. You can eat the fruit fresh and use it to make jams, sauces, and desserts. Three passion fruits contain 54 calories and supply 189 milligrams of potassium and 27 percent of the recommended dietary allowance (RDA) of vitamin C.

Key nutrients in passion fruit include calcium, vitamin C, vitamin B_6, vitamin A, vitamin E, fiber, magnesium, phosphorus, potassium, iron, zinc, vitamin B_2 (riboflavin), and vitamin B_3 (niacin). Important phytochemicals include beta-carotene, flavonoids, and xanthophylls.

Persimmon

Hachiya and Fuyu are the two main varieties of this native Japanese fruit that is now cultivated commercially in the United States. The shiny skins are red-orange. The creamy flesh is tangy and sweet, with hints of plum and pumpkin flavors. The Fuyu variety is high in vitamin C. Persimmons must be fully ripe before you eat them; otherwise, they will have a bitter taste. The Fuyu variety is crisp and can be eaten like an apple; the Hachiya's flesh is soft and is best spooned from the skin.

Key nutrients in persimmons include calcium, vitamin C, phosphorus, potassium, and iron. Important phytochemicals include beta-carotene.

Plantain

Plantain looks like a banana but is very different. Though a fruit, it is too starchy to be eaten raw and is used more like a vegetable—it is generally served fried, baked, mashed, sautéed, or stuffed. It can be used at each stage of ripeness, and has distinct flavors—and skin colors—as it matures. The skin of fully ripe plantain is entirely black. For a tasty side dish, slice plantain and sauté it in garlic oil. Before serving, add a dash of cinnamon, ginger, Herbamare seasoning, or sea salt. Plantain is also good sliced on top of fish before cooking.

Key nutrients in plantain include calcium, magnesium, phosphorus, potassium, vitamin C, vitamin A, folate, and fiber. Important phytochemicals include beta-carotene and phytosterols.

Prickly Pear

Literally hundreds of these medicinal plants grow in Mexico and the Southwestern United States where its sweet red fruit is called *tunas* in Spanish. Because it grows in clusters on certain varieties of desert cactus, the prickly pear is technically a berry. The fruit is oval and has spiny thorns, which should be removed before handling. The skin and flesh have several hues—orange, red, and purple. The firm flesh tastes something like watermelon and contains edible seeds. The Aztecs used prickly pears to mitigate fevers and soothe irritated livers. The Pima Native Americans apply prickly pear pads to the breasts of nursing mothers to increase milk flow. The pads are also used to ease pain of bites and burns, to treat type 2 diabetes, and to heal festering wounds. People with diabetes cut up the inner part and soak it in water and drink the liquid. Peel and slice the fruit for use in salads, sauces, desserts, and jams. It can also be grilled or broiled or juiced in a blender.

Key nutrients in prickly pear include calcium, fiber, vitamin C, vitamin B_6, vitamin A, phosphorus, potassium, magnesium, iron, zinc, vitamin B_1 (thiamine), vitamin B_2 (riboflavin), vitamin B_3 (niacin), and folate.

Pummelo

The largest citrus fruit, pummelo is also known as Chinese grapefruit. It originated in Southeast Asia and is the ancestor of the familiar grapefruit grown in the United States. It comes in a variety of colors, sizes, and shapes. Like grapefruit, it has a thick skin and membranes between the inner segments. Pummelo flesh is either pink or white and less acidic than grapefruit. It can be used just like grapefruit.

Key nutrients in pummelo include calcium, fiber, magnesium, phosphorus, potassium, iron, zinc, vitamin C, vitamin B_6, vitamin B_1 (thiamine), vitamin B_2 (riboflavin), and vitamin B_3 (niacin).

Quince

Quince is a bumpy yellow or green fruit, similar to an apple in shape and size. The fruit should be hard when purchased. Fresh quince is hard and bitter, making it inedible raw. Cooking alters this fruit into a food of the gods. It is similar to a baked apple when cooked, only it tastes even better. The flavor is tart, yet sweet, firm but still pliant, and very juicy. It is free of fat, high in vitamin C, and contains minerals and B vitamins. Quince is used primarily to make

jelly and preserves. Traditionally, quince jelly was used to settle the stomach, help digestion, and ease constipation.

Key nutrients in quince include calcium, magnesium, phosphorus, potassium, vitamin C, vitamin A, vitamin E, folate, and fiber. Important phytochemicals include amygdalin, beta-carotene, chlorogenic acid, ferulic acid, myristic acid, P-coumaric acid, pectin, and tannin.

Red Banana

Grown in Central and South America and Mexico, the red banana is smaller than the yellow variety and can be very sweet. When ripe, the skin has a maroon to dark-purple hue. Its flesh is creamy white, sometimes with a pink tinge. It can be used in fruit salads or cooked for dessert. It is especially good in bread. One red banana has 118 calories and supplies 22 percent of the recommended dietary allowance (RDA) of vitamin C and 10 percent of the RDA of vitamin A.

Key nutrients in red banana include vitamin C, calcium, folate, fiber, iron, magnesium, manganese, pantothenic acid, phosphorus, potassium, vitamin B_2 (riboflavin), vitamin B_3 (niacin), vitamin B_1 (thiamine), and zinc. Important phytochemicals include beta-carotene, beta-sitosterol, kaempferol, myristic acid, pectin, phytosterols, quercetin, rutin, stigmasterol, and tocopherols.

Tamarind

Tamarind is an evergreen tree native to Asia and Northern Africa and is grown extensively in India. It also grows in South Florida. The tree produces large pods containing seeds and a pulp that is high in both acid and sugar. The pulp has a flavor that is like a combination of dates and apricots. Tamarind pulp can be puréed and added to chutneys and curries, and it is a main ingredient in Worcestershire sauce. Tamarind's flavor is something like a combination of dates and apricots. Traditionally, it is used as a mild laxative.

One-half cup of tamarind pulp has 144 calories and supplies 377 milligrams of potassium and 17 percent of the recommended dietary allowance (RDA) of vitamin B_1 (thiamine). Other key nutrients in tamarind include calcium, iron, magnesium, phosphorus, potassium, vitamin C, vitamin A, vitamin E, vitamin B_3 (niacin), folate, and fiber. Important phytochemicals include limonene, myristic acid, pectin, and tannin.

Ugli Fruit

Marketed under the trademark name Ugli, this tangelo has its origins in Jamaica, where it once grew wild. It was developed into a commercial variety as a hybrid of the tangerine, grapefruit, and Seville orange. Also known as unique fruit, it is unusual in appearance, with skin that is thick, wrinkled, and yellow-green. The Ugli fruit's flesh, however, is sweet and juicy, with few seeds. You can eat and prepare it in much the same way as other citrus fruits.

Key nutrients in Ugli fruit include vitamin C.

FRUIT RECIPES

HONEY FRUIT BOAT

This is great for that special luncheon—and it's fast to prepare.

2 cantaloupes or honeydew melons
2 red sweet grapefruits
1 cup honey
1 cup finely grated coconut
3 tablespoons lemon juice
1 pint fresh strawberries
2 bananas, sliced
1 small bunch seedless grapes
1 pint fresh blueberries (optional)
1 cup creamy yogurt
1 cup chopped nuts (optional)

1. Cut the melons in half and remove the seeds.
2. Peel the grapefruits and pull them apart by segments. Coat the segments with honey, roll in finely grated coconut, and set aside.
3. Mix the lemon juice and the remaining honey and coconut together.
4. Halve the strawberries and slice the bananas. Stir them, together with the grapes and blueberries (if desired), into the lemon juice mixture.
5. Spoon the coated fruit (except for the grapefruit) into the melon halves. Top each with ½ cup yogurt and arrange the coated grapefruit pieces on top. Sprinkle with nuts, if desired. If you like, you can serve the stuffed melon in a bowl with lettuce leaves arranged around it.

Variation: If you are on a sugar-free diet, omit the honey and substitute rice or barley malt syrup. Add more yogurt if desired.

QUICK PEACH CRISP

This dessert is easy to make and nutritious!

1 5-ounce can unsweetened sliced peaches, drained
3 tablespoons fructose *or* raw sugar *or* 1 teaspoon barley malt sweetener
2 tablespoons flour *or* 3 tablespoons tapioca *or* arrowroot powder
2 tablespoons quick-cooking oats
½ teaspoon cinnamon
1 dash nutmeg
1 dash ginger
1 tablespoon expeller-pressed vegetable oil or margarine

1. Preheat the oven to 350°F.
2. Pour the peaches into a small baking dish.

3. Mix together the fructose, flour, oats, cinnamon, nutmeg, and ginger. Top the peaches with this mixture. Brush the top of the mixture with the oil.
4. Bake for twenty-five to thirty minutes.

Variations: If you prefer, you can substitute an equal amount of any other fruit for the peaches. If you are in a hurry, simply top the peaches with crumbled cookies, apple-cinnamon granola, or other granola of your choice, brush with oil, and bake as above. If desired, serve the dessert topped with honey, ice cream, yogurt, or chopped nuts.

APPLE RAISIN CRISP

This dessert is a healthy classic.

5 cups cored, sliced apples
1 teaspoon cinnamon
1 cup pure maple syrup or honey
1 cup quick cooking oats
½ cup expeller-pressed vegetable oil
½ cup raisins
1 cup chopped nuts

1. Preheat the oven to 350°F.
2. Lightly oil a shallow baking pan. Place sliced apples over bottom and sprinkle with cinnamon.
3. Mix together the remaining ingredients, except for the nuts. Spread the mixture over the apples. Top with the nuts.
4. Bake for thirty to thirty-five minutes. Serve warm.

Variation: Instead of the oat topping, crumble oatmeal cookies on top and bake as above.

FROZEN BANANA SUPREME

This is quick, easy, and delicious. Kids love it!

1 cup carob pieces
2 tablespoons expeller-pressed vegetable oil
3 peeled bananas, cut in half crosswise and frozen
1 cup finely chopped nuts

1. Melt the carob pieces and vegetable oil together in a double boiler. Pour the melted carob into a tall glass.
2. Dip each banana half in carob coating, then roll in the nuts. Return coated bananas to the freezer until the carob has hardened. Keep them frozen until ready to serve.

NO-COOK FRUIT PUDDING

This healthy dessert provides protein along with the fruit.

2 cups tofu
2 cups any fresh fruit or mashed bananas
¼ cup expeller-pressed vegetable oil

1 teaspoon powdered barley malt sweetener or ½ cup
   honey (omit sweetener if using bananas).
1 tablespoon lemon juice
1 teaspoon vanilla
1 baked pie shell
½–1 cup sliced fresh strawberries

1. Blend all the ingredients in a blender or food
    processor until smooth.
2. Pour into the pie shell and chill for two hours.
3. Top with enough sliced fresh strawberries to cover the
    top before serving.

Variations: If you prefer, substitute any other fruit of your
choice for the strawberries. If desired, you can use crumbled
cookies or graham crackers as a crust in place of the pie
shell, or simply chill the pudding without crust in pudding
cups. For a chocolate flavor, add 1 tablespoon carob or
cocoa powder (or to taste) to the blender with the other
ingredients. Check the taste for sweetness before pouring
the mixture into the pie shell.

COOL FRUIT SALAD

This fruit salad is great for relieving digestive disorders.

1 fresh pineapple
1 cup melon balls
1 cup diced papaya or fresh peaches
3 cups yogurt
3 tablespoons honey or other sweetener of your
   choice
2 cups sliced strawberries
4 whole strawberries (optional)
4 springs fresh mint (optional)

1. Cut the whole pineapple in quarters and remove the
    core. Cut the pineapple away from the shell and cube
    the flesh. Refrigerate the shells until serving time.
2. Stir together 1 cup of cubed pineapple with the
    melon balls and papaya. Chill for at least two hours.
3. Mix the yogurt and honey together and spoon ⅓ cup
    onto each pineapple-shell quarter and cover with
    sliced strawberries.
4. Spoon a layer of the remaining honey-sweetened
    yogurt on top. If desired, garnish each dessert with a
    whole strawberry and a sprig of mint before serving.

CHAPTER NINE

MOM WAS RIGHT!
EAT YOUR VEGETABLES

I do not like broccoli. And I haven't liked it since I was a little kid and my mother made me eat it. And I'm President of the United States, and I'm not going to eat any more broccoli.

—*George H. W. Bush, U.S. President*

Vegetables provide a wealth of nutrients that are critical for optimal health. They contain necessary essential fatty acids, vitamins, minerals, and trace minerals the body needs, as well as many unidentified nutrients. They are virtually fat-free, cholesterol-free, and a superior source of fiber. If weight control is a concern for you, you should be aware that vegetables offer the maximum amount of nutrition for the minimum amount of calories. In addition, the energy in most vegetables comes in the form of complex carbohydrates, which do not cause blood sugar highs and lows. Because of their healing properties, raw vegetables and juices made from them are used around the world as curatives for many illnesses.

Nutrition research shows that eating a diet rich in vegetables reduces the risk of many chronic diseases. Harvard University researchers found that eating five servings per day of fruits and vegetables (particularly cruciferous vegetables such as broccoli, bok choy, cauliflower, and Brussels sprouts) is associated with a 30 percent lower risk of ischemic strokes, the third largest cause of death in the United States. The lower incidence of cancer that exists in some countries, such as Japan, has been linked to a diet that consists mostly of vegetables, rice, and soy products. The likelihood of getting eye disorders, such as cataracts and macular degeneration, is known to be lower in people who eat diets high in beta-carotene, which is found in leafy greens, carrots, and numerous other vegetables. Ongoing research into the thousands of phytochemicals and antioxidants found in vegetables has shown they have the ability to neutralize the kind of free radical damage that is linked to aging and virtually every kind of degenerative disease. (See Part 3.)

In the traditional American diet, vegetables have been served as side dishes, but more and more people are turning to a vegetarian diet and have eliminated or restricted their consumption of meat, poultry, fish, and dairy products. Once considered radical, a proper vegetarian diet is acknowledged by the U.S. Food and Drug Administration (FDA) as healthy and able to meet the recommended dietary allowances of those vitamins and minerals for which standards have been established. (See Chapter 35.)

SELECTING VEGETABLES

Whenever possible, it is best to purchase organically grown vegetables. Commercial farmers' routine use of pesticides, herbicides, and fungicides can leave toxic residues in vegetables. Choosing organic vegetables, when available, eliminates the potential risk posed by these chemicals. (See Chapter 18.) If this is not possible, try to eat a variety of vegetables to help prevent repeated exposure to any one pesticide. Eating produce during its peak growing season also minimizes exposure. Since vegetables in season usually do not have to be shipped long distances to local markets, they are less likely to be treated with irradiation or the chemicals or waxes necessary to retard spoilage. Waxes may seal in pesticide residues. If it is not possible to tell whether a vegetable has been waxed, ask your supermarket's produce manager or the person selling the produce.

Always wash vegetables thoroughly with a stiff vegetable brush and a vegetable wash. Most health food stores sell nontoxic vegetable washes that remove up to 97 percent of the water-insoluble residues left on produce from pesticides, fungicides, and herbicides. VegiWash from Consumer Health Research, Inc., and Allens Biodegradable Fruit and Veggie Wash are two that work well.

TYPES OF VEGETABLES

Most vegetables fall into one of several categories: leafy vegetables (or leafy greens); seeds and pods; roots, bulbs, and tubers; "fruit" vegetables; and flowers, buds, and stalks. There is some overlap among categories—for example, kale is classified as a cruciferous vegetable but also may be considered a leafy green; rutabaga and turnips, two other cruciferous vegetables, are also root vegetables. Still, the potential benefits of a vegetables depend, to some extent, on the types of vegetable they are.

The nutritional content of vegetables varies, depending on the species and the climate and other variables in growing conditions. Preparation methods also affect the nutrient content of the vegetables you eat. In all the sections that follow, the information concerning phytochemical and nutrient content are derived from raw vegetables.

Green and Leafy Vegetables

Green and leafy vegetables, such as collards, dandelion, kale, spinach, endive, chicory, watercress, lettuces, and other salad greens, are highly nutritious. They are a rich source of beta-carotene, iron, chlorophyll, and dietary fiber. All leafy vegetables can be eaten in salads. The darker colored greens are more nutritious and have higher amounts of beta-carotene. Try adding small amounts of "cooking greens" to salads. Blanch strong greens, such as collards and kale, in broth and add to soups and stews. Leafy greens have the added advantage of being excellent sources of vitamins, minerals, proteins, and fiber while being very low in calories, and reducing overall calorie consumption is one thing that has been clearly associated with a longer life span.

Seeds and Pods

Seeds and pods are the parts of plants that store energy. Examples include snow peas, green beans, okra, and corn. These kinds of vegetables contain more protein than other vegetables. They tend to be high in carbohydrates, which turn to starch when they are ripe.

Roots, Bulbs, and Tubers

Roots, bulbs, and tubers are the parts of a plant that store nutrients. Potatoes, rutabaga, turnips, beets, and carrots are among the most popular. More exotic tubers and root vegetables, such as celeriac, malanga, and oca, are also commonly available. Vegetables from this group are not generally as low in calories as other vegetables, but they are mineral-rich and very filling. Roots, bulbs, and tubers are a good source of fiber and can be used as low-calorie alternatives to other starches, such as rice or pasta.

"Fruit" Vegetables

"Fruit" vegetables, such as tomatoes, avocados, squashes, and peppers, contain the ripened ovaries (seeds) of pollinated flowers. The fleshy pulp surrounding the seed is the part to eat. With the exception of avocado, these "fruits" are usually low in calories and provide a wide range of tex-

ture and flavor to work with in the kitchen. They are often used in salsa, relishes, and other condiments.

Flowers, Buds, and Stalks

Flowers, buds, and stalks include celery, rhubarb, asparagus, cauliflower, and broccoli. These plants tend to be rich in vitamin C and dietary fiber. Try some of the less traditional edible flowers, such as peppery-flavored nasturtiums or borage flowers in a salad; rose petals are delicately sweet-tasting and dress up any cake or fruit salad.

COOKING AND PREPARING VEGETABLES

Ideally, vegetables should be consumed either raw or lightly cooked. Cooking vegetables destroys their enzymes and many of the phytochemicals and vitamins. Some of the water-soluble vitamins will bind to various chemicals during the cooking process and pass through the body unabsorbed. Researchers are finding, however, that certain phytochemicals (particularly the lycopene in tomatoes) are not only heat-stable, but their compounds are actually released by heat and become more available when cooked.

One of the best ways to prepare vegetables is to steam them. Steamers are inexpensive and using them is simple. Cooking times vary depending upon the type of vegetable. Most vegetables are still crunchy when properly cooked. Another cooking method that minimizes the loss of nutrients is to cook thoroughly washed vegetables for just a short time in a small amount of water. The water remaining from cooking is nutritious and good to use in gravies and stock.

Vitamin C begins to break down upon exposure to air. Once a vegetable containing vitamin C is cut, it is best to consume (or cook) it immediately. Minimize the number of cuts so that less surface area is exposed to the air. It's best to tear leafy vegetables by hand rather than use a knife to cut them to minimize nutrient loss.

FRESH VEGETABLES VERSUS FROZEN OR CANNED

Canned vegetables are the least desirable form of produce. The heating that is a part of the canning process destroys many vitamins. Furthermore, sodium is usually added during processing. The flavor is not "true to nature" and canned vegetables lack texture.

If you must purchase canned vegetables, select ones labeled "reduced sodium" or "low sodium." Also read labels to make sure that there is no sugar or monosodium glutamate (MSG) added. Store the cans in a cool, dry place since high temperatures can destroy the remaining vitamins. Don't discard the juice—instead, drink it or use it to make vegetable stock.

Vegetables that are "flash frozen" soon after harvesting retain most of their nutrients. Properly prepared, frozen vegetables are a good alternative if fresh produce is not available or if you do not have enough time to prepare fresh vegetables. Some phytochemicals in vegetables are preserved by freezing, so frozen vegetables may actually be more nutritious than fresh ones that have been sitting in the refrigerator too long.

Buy frozen vegetables in plastic bags rather than in cardboard containers so that you can feel the shape of the individual vegetables through the bag. Do not purchase bags that are frozen in a solid clump. Remember, frozen vegetables prepared in cream sauce, butter, or seasonings can be calorie and fat laden. When storing frozen vegetables, be sure the freezer remains at zero degrees Fahrenheit since temperatures above zero can destroy nutrients.

CRUCIFEROUS VEGETABLES: THE MAGNIFICENT TWELVE

Eating more vegetables can dramatically reduce and prevent disease. The twelve vegetables known as the cruciferous vegetables are particularly powerful protectors against cancer, heart disease, and strokes—the top three killers in the United States. The cruciferous vegetables all have flowers with four petals that botanists described as resembling a cross—crux in Latin; hence the name cruciferous. Botanically, these vegetables all belong to the Cruciferae family, which includes plants of the genus Brassica. The magnificent twelve are broccoli, Brussels sprouts, cabbage, cauliflower, collards, kale, kohlrabi, mustard greens, horseradish, rutabaga, turnips, and watercress.

Consume three one-cup servings from this list each day. Eat one cup raw and two cups slightly steamed, except for horseradish. Use horseradish grated fresh in sauces and spreads. To ensure a variety of nutrients necessary for optimal health, alternate vegetables daily. Over time, most monotonous diets become nutritionally deficient (as well as boring) from lack of variety, which, in turn, leads to problems in certain areas of the body. Cruciferous vegetables are also thought to depress thyroid function because of certain substances they contain, but researchers have concluded that cooking neutralizes the thyroid-depressing substances. It is believed that green vegetables, along with dark-orange vegetables, act as antidotes to cancer-forming processes that can go on for years after exposure to carcinogens.

If consuming cruciferous vegetables causes an upset stomach, bloating, or gas, a lack of alpha-galactosidase, an enzyme that breaks down certain complex sugars, may be to blame. To avoid this, add increasing amounts of these vegetables gradually so that your digestive system learns to tolerate them. Start by adding one-half cup twice a week and gradually increase from there. Beano, or BeSure by Wakunaga, products that provides the missing enzyme, may also help and can be found in health food stores and many pharmacies.

Broccoli

Broccoli is best known for its ability to prevent cancer by protecting cells from free-radical damage and carcinogens.

It lowers the risk primarily of cancer of the rectum, colon, esophagus, larynx, lung, prostate, oral cavity, pharynx, and stomach. Experiments in the 1950s discovered that broccoli helped to protect guinea pigs from lethal doses of radiation. Cabbage also worked, but broccoli was more effective. It also protects against heart disease, cataracts, constipation and hemorrhoids, diabetes, arthritis, and allergies; helps to normalize body fluid levels; controls high blood pressure; and promotes bowel health. Further, women who consume more broccoli are less prone to cervical cancer. Broccoli is one of the best vegetable sources of calcium, and just one-half cup daily exceeds the recommended dietary allowance (RDA) of vitamins C and E.

Research has found that broccoli sprouts contain the powerful cancer-fighting compound sulforaphane in far higher concentrations than those found in mature broccoli. Sulforaphane is the most powerful natural chemical for stopping the growth of tumors. Reported in the May 2002 issue of Proceedings of the National Academy of Science, sulforaphane killed Helicobacter pylori (H. pylori), which is the bacteria that causes stomach ulcers and stomach cancers. The sulforaphane even worked when H. pylori was resistant to often used antibiotics. Although long-term studies will be needed to determine exactly how much sulforaphane must be consumed to gain full protection, one of the researchers, Jed W. Fahey of the Johns Hopkins University School of Medicine, has stated that the levels that were tested could be achieved by eating broccoli or broccoli sprouts. Broccoli blocks cell mutations that foreshadow cancer, possibly due to the abundance of chlorophyll. The parts eaten are the immature flower head (or florets) and the stalks.

Key nutrients in broccoli include calcium, iron, magnesium, phosphorus, potassium, sodium, zinc, chromium, copper, manganese, fiber, vitamin C, vitamin B_6, vitamin K, vitamin B_2 (riboflavin), vitamin B_3 (niacin), vitamin B_1 (thiamine), folate, pantothenic acid, and small amounts of amino acids and lipids. Phytochemicals include alpha-lipoic acid, beta-carotene, beta-sitosterol, caffeic acid, chlorogenic acid, chlorophyll, ferulic acid, kaempferol, P-coumaric acid, phytic acid, quercetin, quercitrin, rutin, sinapic acid, squalene, stigmasterol, lutein, sulforaphane, indoles, tocopherols, isothiocyanates, monoterpenes, triterpenoids, glucosinolates, chlorophyll, and dithiolthione.

The florets should be compact and uniformly green. Varieties with a purple or bluish-green cast are higher in beta-carotene than the green. Bright color is an indication of nutritional quality. Yellowing spots are a signal that the broccoli is not fresh. Fresh broccoli has a clean smell. It should also have a strong cabbagelike odor. The florets and stalks should be free of soft or slippery spots. Select broccoli that has been kept cold. Otherwise, its sugar will convert to lignin, a type of fiber that will not soften during cooking.

Unwashed broccoli stored in an open plastic bag in the crisper compartment of the refrigerator will keep for three

---

Baby Broccoli Arrives

A hybrid developed by Sakata Seed Corporation in Japan has produced a "new" vegetable dubbed *broccolini*. Basically a baby broccoli, it is a cross between conventional broccoli and gai lan, or Chinese broccoli. Broccolini's stems are thin, like spears, and grow only to six inches long. Its head is a loose cluster of florets. Use it like regular broccoli; it does have a milder taste and lasts longer—up to twenty-one days in the refrigerator. Broccolini is available in some grocery stores.

---

to five days. Cooked broccoli can be stored in an airtight container for two to three days.

Wash broccoli under cold running water. Remove the leaves, if any, and add them to fresh salads. You also can peel and slice the stalks and add them to stir-fry dishes and vegetable dips.

Broccoli should be cooked quickly in small amounts of water, steamed, or stir-fried. Overcooking releases foul-smelling sulfur compounds, which can turn broccoli brown by interacting with the chlorophyll it contains. Broccoli should be served crisp and bright green. It needs less time to cook than most vegetables, so prepare it last.

Brussels Sprouts

Researchers have found specific substances (chlorophyll, dithiolthiones, carotenoids, indoles, and glucosinolates) in Brussels sprouts that retard cancer. Countries where Brussels sprouts are consumed frequently have a low incidence of gastrointestinal cancer. Brussels sprouts may also help protect against estrogen-related cancers such as breast, uterine, and endometrial cancer. Brussels sprouts may inhibit the formation of polyps, precancerous growths that can progress to colon cancer. In research trials, the glucosinolates found in Brussels sprouts detoxified aflatoxin, a potent carcinogen from mold that is linked to high rates of cancer, particularly of the liver. Aflatoxin often contaminates peanuts, corn, and rice, and is a serious threat in developing countries. A juice made of Brussels sprouts, string beans, lettuce, and carrots provides the needed elements to regenerate and improve the insulin-producing capacity of the pancreas. A diet rich in Brussels sprouts and cabbage may improve the functioning of the metabolic system, further aiding in cancer prevention. The part eaten is the immature flower bud.

Key nutrients in Brussels sprouts include calcium, fiber, iron, magnesium, phosphorus, potassium, sodium, zinc, copper, manganese, vitamin C, vitamin B_6, vitamin A, vitamin E, vitamin K, vitamin B_1 (thiamine), vitamin B_2 (riboflavin), vitamin B_3 (niacin), pantothenic acid, folate, and small amounts of lipids and amino acids. Phyto-chemicals include alpha-lipoic acid, beta-carotene, caffeic acid, ferulic acid, lutein, P-coumaric acid, quercetin, rutin, sinapic acid, glucosinolates, indoles, isothiocyanates, sulforaphane, dithiolthiones, triterpenoids, tocopherols, and chlorophyll.

Brussels sprouts should be firm with compact, bright green heads. Yellowed or wilted leaves indicate aging. Check around the stems for tiny wormholes or black smudges. This may be a sign that there are aphids on the inside. The stems should be white.

Store unwashed, untrimmed sprouts in a perforated plastic bag for up to five days in the crisper compartment of the refrigerator. If purchased in a pint or quart tub with cellophane covering, remove the sprouts and inspect them for yellowed leaves, holes, or smudges. Remove any wilted or yellowed leaves before storing.

Soak sprouts in a basin of warm water for ten minutes, then rinse with cool water. Remove the coarse outer leaves. Trim the ends, leaving a small nub intact. To ensure even cooking, cut a small x into the bottom of the stem. Cook the sprouts just until tender. Overcooking will produce an overpowering sulfur smell.

Cabbage

Cabbage stimulates the immune system, and kills bacteria and viruses. It helps to inhibit the growth of cancerous cells; protects against tumors; controls hormone levels; affects sex drive, fertility, cardiovascular disease, and menopause symptoms; and curbs the formation of cancer-causing substances. Cabbage can speed up the metabolism of estrogen, which reduces the risk of breast cancer and inhibits the growth of polyps, an early sign of colon cancer. Eating cabbage once each week may reduce the chances of colon cancer by as much as 60 percent. It is therapeutically effective in conditions of scurvy, diseases of the eyes, gout, rheumatism, pyorrhea, asthma, tuberculosis, cancer, and gangrene. It is excellent as a revitalizing agent and blood purifier. The chlorophyll in raw cabbage also helps to prevent anemia.

Cabbage is a good source of fiber, another protective measure against colon cancer. A study in Japan discovered that people who consumed the most cabbage had the lowest death rate from all cancers. This puts cabbage in the same category as yogurt and olive oil as potential life extenders. The high levels of vitamin A aid in tissue rejuvenation, and the sulfur content helps fight infection and protects the skin from eczema and other rashes.

In its raw form and especially as a juice, cabbage contains ascorbigen, formerly called cabbagen or vitamin U, which heals and protects against stomach ulcers. To heal ulcers, drink one quart a day of a mixture composed of equal parts of quality water, cabbage juice, and celery juice. Celery juice also contains an antiulcer factor. Spring and summer cabbage are more effective than fall or winter. If you like, you can add pineapple or apple juice to the mixture for extra flavor. When juicing cabbage, drink it immediately, as ascorbigen is quickly destroyed. Excessive consumption of cabbage and cabbage juice can cause goiter, a thyroid condition.

The part of cabbage that is eaten is the head.

Key nutrients in cabbage include calcium, fiber, iron, magnesium, phosphorus, potassium, sodium, zinc, copper, manganese, vitamin C, vitamin B_6, vitamin K, vitamin E, vitamin B_1 (thiamine), vitamin B_2 (riboflavin), vitamin B_3 (niacin), pantothenic acid, folate, and small amounts of lipids and amino acids. Phytochemicals include beta-carotene, beta-sitosterol, caffeic acid, chlorogenic acid, ferulic acid, dithiolthiones, kaempferol, P-coumaric acid, phenolic acids, quercetin, sinapic acid, indoles, isothiocyanates, phenethyl isothiocyanate (PEITC), sulforaphane, monoterpenes, triterpenoids, glucosinolate, and tocopherols.

Of the many varieties of cabbage, the most familiar are green, red, Savoy, napa, and bok choy. Cabbage heads should be free of brown spots or wilted leaves. Green and red cabbages should have firm, compact heads with smooth leaves. The head should feel heavy for its size. Napa and Savoy cabbage will have crinkled leaves that are not as compact. Bok choy should have smooth, white stalks topped with leafy greens free of yellow spots.

Red and green cabbage can be stored unwashed and uncut for up to twenty days. If kept cold, it will retain its vitamin C content. Once the surface is cut, it should be tightly wrapped with plastic wrap and the remainder used within three or four days. Savoy, napa, and bok choy do not store as well and should be consumed within three to five days of purchase.

Wash heads of green or red cabbage under cold running water, then cut into quarters, leaving the stem intact to hold the leaves together. As each quarter is used, remove the stem. Rinse cabbage after shredding, slicing, or chopping. Napa and Savoy cabbage can be torn or shredded by hand in much the same way as lettuce. Wash torn pieces in a colander under cool, running water. The white stems of bok choy can be used like celery. Remove the leafy green portion and chop stalks in pieces. The leaves can be added to soups or stir-fry dishes.

Cauliflower

Cauliflower helps to protect against stomach, rectum, prostate, colon, and bladder cancer. It contains compounds (such as indoles) that stimulate the body's detoxification system to neutralize carcinogens, preventing them from attacking healthy cells; slows tumor growth; lowers circulating estrogen levels in the body, which reduces the risk of breast and uterine cancers; and minimizes the risk of lung cancer. It is not as high in chlorophyll and carotenes as some of the brassicas, so it is less likely to inhibit lung and other smoking-related cancers. It is better than cabbage for people with diabetes. The parts eaten are the undeveloped flower buds, or florets.

Broccoflower

Broccoflower is a cross between broccoli and cauliflower. Except for a green head, it looks like cauliflower. Broccoflower cooks more quickly and has a milder taste than cauliflower, plus it contains some types of beta-carotene not found in cauliflower.

Key nutrients in cauliflower include calcium, iron, magnesium, fiber, phosphorus, potassium, sodium, zinc, copper, manganese, vitamin C, vitamin B_6, vitamin K, vitamin E, vitamin B_1 (thiamine), vitamin B_2 (riboflavin), vitamin B_3 (niacin), pantothenic acid, folate, and small amounts of lipids and amino acids. Phytochemicals include beta-carotene, sulforaphane, flavonoids, indoles, glucosinolates, triterpenoids, isothiocyanates, anthoxanthins, tocopherols, kaempferol, P-coumaric acid, quercetin, and sinapic acid.

Look for cauliflower heads that are firm, with compact florets. The heads should be a creamy white with no bruises or discoloration. Any leaves on the head should be crisp and green.

Cauliflower will keep in the crisper compartment of the refrigerator for up to five days. It should be stored unwashed in an open or perforated plastic bag.

To prepare cauliflower, remove any green leaves from the head. Break the florets from the head using your hands or a sharp knife. Trim off any brown or discolored spots. Slice large florets in half lengthwise. To cook the whole head, remove the bottom of the core to ensure even cooking. Rinse cauliflower under cool running water prior to cooking.

If you have Crohn's disease, it is wise to eat this vegetable in moderation, as cauliflower has been linked to flare-ups of symptoms in persons with Crohn's disease.

Collards

Collards improve the function of the glands and the nervous, respiratory, skeletal, and urinary systems. They protect against estrogen-related cancers, retard tumor growth, and minimize the effects of cigarette smoke. They stimulate anticancer enzymes and retard the growth of carcinogens related to cigarette smoke; improve immune response; protect against lung, colon, esophageal, and prostate cancers; and reduce the risk of age-related macular degeneration. Collards may not only reduce the risk of certain cancers, but may also prevent the metastasis of breast cancers. They can protect against osteoporosis and strokes as well as minimize the neurological damage resulting from a stroke. The parts eaten are the leafy greens and, sometimes, the tender stems.

Key nutrients in collard greens include calcium, iron, magnesium, phosphorus, potassium, sodium, zinc, copper, manganese, vitamin C, vitamin B_6, vitamin E, vitamin B_1 (thiamine), vitamin B_2 (riboflavin), vitamin B_3 (niacin), pantothenic acid, fiber, folate, and small amounts of lipids and amino acids. Phytochemicals include beta-carotene, indoles, lutein, myristic acid, zeaxanthin, glucosinolates, isothiocyanates, sulforaphane, chlorophyll, and triterpenoids.

Look for large, smooth leaves that are dark green to bluish-green in color. The leaves should be stiff and attached to a long stalk with no spots or discoloration around the edges.

Store unwashed greens in an open plastic bag in the crisper compartment of the refrigerator for up to five days.

To prepare collards, tear the leafy green portion away from the stalks. If the veins extending into the leaf are tough and raised, remove them as well. Gently agitate greens in a basin filled with cool water. Drain water and repeat the process until greens are clean.

A cooking suggestion for collards: Blanch them for eight to twelve minutes, then drain and chop them. Sauté one large onion, chopped, and two cloves of garlic, minced, in a little olive oil until tender. (You can adjust the amount of onion and garlic to suit your taste.) Add the collards and heat through. Season them with lemon juice and sprinkle with toasted almonds.

Collard greens contain a high amount of oxalates—compounds that can combine with calcium and form stones in susceptible individuals. If you have a history of kidney stones, it is wise to minimize your consumption of collard greens and other oxalate-containing foods, including beet greens, leeks, rhubarb, rutabaga, spinach, and Swiss chard.

Kale

Kale is one of the best known cancer-fighting vegetables on the planet. It is the richest of all leafy greens in carotenoids and contains an abundance of lutein, a phytochemical that scientists think may be more protective against cancer than beta-carotene. Kale helps regulate estrogen and wards off many forms of cancer, including breast, bowel, bladder, prostate, and lung cancers; protects against heart disease; and regulates blood pressure. The calcium in kale is more absorbable by the body than the calcium in milk. Also, ounce for ounce, kale contains more calcium than milk. Kale's calcium is easily assimilated, making it a wonder food to protect against osteoporosis, arthritis, and bone loss. Heat destroys some of the carotenoids, but the resulting balance is more available to the body, and the chlorophyll content does not seem to be affected. It is wise to consume kale in both raw and cooked forms. The part of the plant that is eaten is the leaves.

Key nutrients in kale include calcium, iron, magnesium, phosphorus, potassium, sodium, zinc, copper, manganese, vitamin C, vitamin B_6, vitamin E, vitamin K, vitamin B_1 (thiamine), vitamin B_2 (riboflavin), vitamin B_3 (niacin),

pantothenic acid, fiber, folate, and small amounts of lipids and amino acids. Phytochemicals include alpha-carotene, beta-carotene, canthaxanthin, kaempferol, myristic acid, quercetin, lutein, sulforaphane, indoles, zeaxanthin, glucosinolates, isothiocyanates, tocopherols, tocotrienols, chlorophyll, and triterpenoids.

If not kept chilled, kale will wilt and become bitter, so look for it in a refrigerated case or on ice. Kale greens should be crisp and dark green with ruffled edges. Smaller leaves are more tender and mild.

Store unwashed kale leaves wrapped in paper in a plastic bag for up to five days in the crisper compartment of your refrigerator.

To prepare kale, tear the leafy green portion away from the stalk. If the veins extending into the leaf are tough and raised, remove them as well. Gently agitate the greens in a basin filled with cool water. Drain the water and repeat the process until the greens are clean. Kale has a strong flavor, so it is best steamed or added to soups.

A cooking suggestion for kale: Blanch one bunch for eight to twelve minutes, drain, and chop. Sauté two cloves of garlic, minced, and a pinch of crushed red pepper flakes in 2 tablespoons of olive oil. (You can adjust the seasonings to suite your taste.) Add the kale, one 15-ounce can of cannelloni beans, and enough reserved blanching water (or low-sodium chicken or vegetable broth) to moisten the mixture. Heat it through while mashing the beans. Season with lemon juice.

Kohlrabi

A cross between a turnip and a cabbage, kohlrabi reduces the incidence of hormone-dependent cancers such as breast, uterine, and endometrial cancers, and helps to reduce the carcinogenic effects of cigarette smoke. It is good for treating indigestion, jaundice, diabetes, the lymphatic system, and alcoholism. An excellent source of vitamin C, kohlrabi can help the body to ward off infection. It contains ample quantities of vitamin E, which helps to prevent plaque buildup in the arteries, thus minimizing the risk for heart disease. Its high potassium content helps the body maintain a proper fluid balance. In China, the fresh juice is used to stop nosebleeds, and the seed powder is used to improve eyesight and help urination after childbirth. The part eaten is the bulb.

Key nutrients in kohlrabi include calcium, iron, magnesium, phosphorus, potassium, sodium, zinc, copper, manganese, vitamin C, vitamin B_6, vitamin E, vitamin B_1 (thiamine), vitamin B_2 (riboflavin), vitamin B_3 (niacin), pantothenic acid, fiber, folate, and small amounts of lipids and amino acids. Phytochemicals include beta-carotene, indoles, isothiocyanates, glucosinolates, dithiolthiones, flavonoids, sulforaphane, triterpenoids, myristic acid, and quercetin.

Kohlrabi bulbs should be firm and pale green without scars or blemishes. Younger bulbs are more tender and do not need to be peeled. The bulbs can be stored for up to two weeks in a plastic bag in the refrigerator.

Wash kohlrabi with a vegetable brush under cool running water. Cut into uniform-sized chunks and add them to soups, or serve them steamed or roasted as a side dish. Raw kohlrabi can be shredded and added to salads.

Mustard Greens

Mustard greens help to inhibit tumor growth; protect against cancer and heart disease; and help strengthen the immune system. Their high iron and calcium content helps to prevent anemia and build strong bones and teeth. Mustard greens are superior to spinach. The calcium benefit is not lost because of the lower oxalic acid content. The part eaten is the leaves. In Russia, many people use mustard seed oil in place of olive oil.

Key nutrients in mustard greens include calcium, iron, magnesium, phosphorus, potassium, sodium, zinc, copper, manganese, vitamin C, vitamin B, vitamin K, vitamin E, vitamin B_1 (thiamine), vitamin B_2 (riboflavin), vitamin B_3 (niacin), pantothenic acid, fiber, folate, and small amounts of lipids and amino acids. Phytochemicals include beta-carotene, indoles, lutein, zeaxanthin, glucosinolates, isothiocyanates, sulforaphane, chlorophyll, tocopherols, and tocotrienols.

Mustard greens are more tender than collards or kale, and are a lighter, grass-green color. They should be crisp, with no spots or signs of wilting. Those with seeds attached are overmature. Store them in a plastic bag in the crisper compartment of the refrigerator.

To prepare mustard greens, separate the leafy portion from stems and gently swirl them in a basin of cold water. Empty and refill the basin and repeat this procedure until the greens are free of dirt or grit.

A cooking suggestion for mustard greens: Blanch one bunch of mustard greens for six to eight minutes, then drain and chop them. Sauté one large onion, chopped, and two cloves of garlic, minced, in a little vegetable oil until tender. Add the mustard greens, one 15-ounce can of black-eyed peas, and enough reserved blanching water (or low-sodium chicken or vegetable broth) to moisten the mixture. Toss it lightly, and do not overcook. Season with apple cider vinegar and hot pepper sauce or any other seasoning you like—you can always adjust seasonings to suit your personal preference.

Radishes

Radishes stimulate the appetite; relieve respiratory infections; cleanse the gallbladder and liver; ease cold and flu symptoms; and are a natural diuretic. In Chinese medicine, radishes are used to promote digestion, break down mucus, soothe headaches, and heal laryngitis. The juice is mixed with ginger juice to cure laryngitis. For sinusitis, drink the juice of six radishes, one cucumber, and one apple. This is also a very beneficial drink for the liver and the gallbladder. Radishes contain salicylates, the same compounds used to make aspirin. Researchers believe these compounds may help to discourage the formation of unwanted blood clots. The part of the plant eaten is the root.

Though not supernutritious, radishes are low in calories and a good source of vitamin C. Radishes are used in salads to add zest and crunch. Varieties such as the daikon radish, also called the Japanese or oriental radish, have a richer taste and can be used to flavor soups and stews. Black radishes have such a pungent flavor that they usually are not eaten alone, but are grated or shredded to spice up salads and slaws.

Horseradish, a relative of the radish, belongs to the mustard family. It benefits asthma, bronchitis, and lung disorders, lymphatic congestion, and is a digestive stimulant. Its strong bite comes from the mustard oils released when it is cut. Fresh horseradish left in contact with the skin will cause blistering. You should avoid contact with the eyes and wash your hands after handling horseradish. Horseradish can be grated and used raw as a condiment, and adds zing to tartar sauce.

Key nutrients in radishes include calcium, iron, magnesium, phosphorus, potassium, sodium, zinc, copper, manganese, vitamin C, vitamin B_6, vitamin A, vitamin E, vitamin B_1 (thiamine), vitamin B_2 (riboflavin), vitamin B_3 (niacin), pantothenic acid, fiber, folate, and small amounts of lipids and amino acids. Phytochemicals include anthocyanins, beta-carotene, caffeic acid, ferulic acid, myristic acid, P-coumaric acid, sinapic acid, glucosinolates, indoles, isothiocyanates, and sulforaphane.

The familiar red globe variety should be bright red and small- to medium-sized—larger radishes tend to be pithy. Black radishes should have a smooth, glossy appearance and feel heavy for their size. The carrot-shaped daikon radish should be well formed and free of any rootlets. All radishes should be free of cracks or blemishes. If the greens are attached, they should be crisp and green with no signs of wilting. The roots should be smooth and firm.

Remove the tops before storing and radishes will keep better. Red globe and daikon radishes will keep for one to two weeks in sealed plastic bags in the refrigerator. If kept dry, black radishes can keep for up to one month. Store them in a perforated plastic bag on the refrigerator shelf.

To prepare radishes, remove the root and tops of radishes with a knife and scrub them with a brush under cool running water. The oils that give radishes their peppery taste are in the skin, so peel them to tone down their pungent flavor.

Rutabaga

Rutabaga, a cross between a turnip and cabbage, is loaded with cancer-fighting compounds. Slightly more nutritious than its distant cousin, the common white turnip, rutabaga is a good source of complex carbohydrates that supply energy to the body. Its high fiber content helps control blood cholesterol levels, thus potentially reducing the risk of heart disease, stroke, and diabetes. Rutabagas can help clear up mucus and congestion and have an alkalizing effect on the body. Their high fiber content can help reduce the risk of colon or rectal cancer. Rutabagas should not be consumed by anyone who has kidney problems, as they contain mustard oil and may cause gas. The part eaten is the root.

Key nutrients in rutabagas include calcium, iron, fiber, magnesium, phosphorus, potassium, sodium, zinc, copper, manganese, vitamin C, vitamin B_6, vitamin E, vitamin B_1 (thiamine), vitamin B_2 (riboflavin), vitamin B_3 (niacin), pantothenic acid, and small amounts of lipids and amino acids. Phytochemicals include beta-carotene, lycopene, glucosinolates, indoles, isothiocyanates, and sulforaphane.

Rutabagas can be distinguished from turnips by their round, slightly lumpy shape, purple top and yellowish base. They are usually waxed to prevent moisture loss, with the stems and rootlets removed. The root should be hard, with no soft spots or scars. Smaller rutabagas have the best flavor.

Like all root vegetables, rutabaga stores well. At room temperature, an unwashed root will keep for a week to ten days; in the refrigerator, it will keep for up to three weeks.

Always peel rutabagas to get rid of the waxed skin. Remove the crown by cutting a thin slice off the top. Using a large chef's knife, cut the rutabaga into quarters. Peel each quarter using a paring knife, then cut into chunks, dice, or slice julienne strips. Rutabagas are a hearty, flavorful addition to vegetable broth.

Turnips

Turnips balance the calcium in the body, reduce mucus, help ease asthma and bronchitis, and relieve sore throats. Turnip root helps protect against heart disease, cancer, and viral infection, and can be helpful in controlling blood cholesterol levels. Eaten raw, the root helps lower the amount of circulating estrogen in the body, which reduces the risk of estrogen-related cancers. Turnips contain high amounts of vitamin C. The greens contain significant amounts of beta-carotene, a phytochemical that protects against various forms of cancer. The parts eaten are the roots and leafy greens.

Key nutrients in turnips include calcium, iron, magnesium, phosphorus, potassium, sodium, zinc, copper, manganese, vitamin C, vitamin B_6, vitamin E, vitamin K (turnip greens), vitamin B_1 (thiamine), vitamin B_2 (riboflavin), vitamin B_3 (niacin), pantothenic acid, fiber, folate, and small amounts of lipids and amino acids. Phytochemicals in turnip root include beta-carotene, lycopene, indoles, sulforaphane, isothiocyanates, phenethyl isothiocyanate (PEITC), tocopherols, and tocotrienols. Turnip greens also contain beta-carotene, glucosinolates, and lutein.

Freshly harvested turnips are frequently sold in bunches with their leaves. Turnips with their greens removed are either packaged in plastic bags or sold loose. The leaves should be crisp and green, with no signs of wilting or discoloration. Turnip roots should be smooth and heavy for their size.

Remove the greens from the root prior to storing them. Store the greens in a plastic bag for two to three days. The root will keep for up to a week in the crisper compartment of the refrigerator.

To prepare turnip greens, place them in a basin of water and gently swirl them around to remove any dirt. Remove the greens from the basin, empty, refill, and repeat the procedure as necessary. To prepare the turnips themselves, remove the crown of the root with a sharp knife. Using a vegetable peeler, remove a thin layer of skin from the root. The root can be sliced, cut into large chunks, or diced. The slighly peppery flavor of turnips adds spice to stir-fry dishes. Or you can steam, braise, boil, or roast turnips and serve them with black pepper and lemon juice. Small turnips can be cooked whole.

If you have thyroid disease, it is wise to limit your consumption of turnips. Turnips contain substances that can promote growth of a goiter in people with thyroid disease.

Watercress

A member of the mustard family, watercress is rich in vitamin C and beta-carotene, potent antioxidants that help to fight cancer. Watercress is also a wonderful food for treating anemia, calcium deficiencies, blood purification, catarrhal conditions, liver and pancreatic problems, appetite stimulation, thyroid problems, and arthritis. In research trials on the phytochemical phenethyl isothiocyanate (PEITC), smokers were served watercress three times a day for three days. After just three days, they excreted "detoxified" carcinogens in their urine. Watercress may help protect against the development of lung cancer in smokers and in people exposed to secondhand smoke. Chewing a few stalks of watercress daily can help improve most illnesses. The leaves and stems are the parts eaten.

Key nutrients in watercress include calcium, iron, magnesium, phosphorus, potassium, sodium, zinc, copper, manganese, vitamin C, vitamin E, vitamin K, vitamin B_1 (thiamine), vitamin B_2 (riboflavin), vitamin B_3 (niacin), pantothenic acid, fiber, folate, and small amounts of lipids and amino acids. Phytochemicals include beta-carotene, glucosinolates, indoles, lutein, isothiocyanates, phenethyl isothiocyanate (PEITC), sulforaphane, chlorophyll, tocopherols, and tocotrienols.

Watercress is sold in bunches. The small round leaves should be dark green, not wilted or spotted. The stems should be firm and crisp. To store watercress, wrap the roots in a moist paper towel and place in a closed plastic bag. They should keep for four to five days.

Precautions for Heart Patients

Vegetables rich in vitamin K, such as broccoli, cabbage, and Brussels sprouts, may lower the effectiveness of the blood thinner medication warfarin (Coumadin), a drug frequently prescribed for people with a history of cardiovascular problems and/or surgery to prevent clots from forming in blood vessels. Since vitamin K aids blood clotting, too much of it can counteract the blood-thinning actions of warfarin. Eating small amounts of vitamin K-rich foods daily should not be harmful. However, if you do not normally eat these vegetables, but overindulge—for instance, having a meal with lots of greens in a Chinese restaurant—there could theoretically be some health risk. If you take a blood-thinning medication, you may want to discuss this with your health-care provider.

To prepare watercress, remove the roots. Hold the bunch by the stems and swirl them in a basin of cool water. Empty the basin and repeat until the leaves and stems are free of grit. Watercress can be added to soups and other cooked dishes, but it is most often used in salads. Its mustardlike flavor complements sandwiches as well as bean, grain, and pasta dishes.

Watercress grows readily in streambeds; however, because streams often harbor bacteria and parasites, and because it is not easy to distinguish watercress from potentially harmful plants, it is not a good idea to pick it in the wild.

GREEN AND LEAFY VEGETABLES

Green is a powerful healing color, and one of the most plentiful on the planet. Looking at a landscape or forest is calming and releases stress. Green has the same peaceful effect *inside* the body.

Green and leafy vegetables should be an important part of your daily diet. Leafy greens with the darkest, most intense colors contain the highest levels of nutrients. Greens contain the vitamins, minerals, calcium, and beta-carotene necessary to maintain the immune system. They also help ward off diseases such as cancer. Leafy greens are excellent for the gallbladder, spleen, heart, and blood, and they are a good brain food.

Greens can be cooked in many ways, used in fresh juices, and added raw to salads. Because greens contain ample sodium, you should not add additional salt when preparing them. The sodium content varies from 22 milligrams per cup in cooked mustard greens to 316 milligrams in a cup of Swiss chard. This is a natural form of sodium that is needed by the body in a correct balance with

potassium. All greens are good in soups, stews, and casseroles. They are also good simply steamed and seasoned before serving.

Include all these marvelous raw greens in power juices, too. The wide range of nutrients in greens makes them essential for health and healing.

Arugula

Arugula, also known as roquette, helps to normalize body acids with its high alkalinity and can be used to treat acidosis. Its mild peppery flavor is a perfect accent to pasta salads, and it blends well with oranges and berries. Toss it with milder greens in a salad and serve with robust vinaigrette.

Key nutrients in arugula include fiber, calcium, iron, magnesium, phosphorus, potassium, sodium, zinc, copper, manganese, vitamin C, vitamin B_1 (thiamine), vitamin B_2 (riboflavin), vitamin B_3 (niacin), pantothenic acid, vitamin B_6, fiber, folate, vitamin E, and lipids. Phytochemicals include beta-carotene.

Arugula is sold in small bunches. Avoid limp, wilted, or yellowed leaves. Look for those that are smooth, dark green, and free of brown spots.

The leafy greens should be stored in sealed plastic bags in the coldest part of the refrigerator. Do not store washed arugula; instead, prepare small amounts just before consumption. Trim any roots from the stems, then separate the leaves. Place the leaves in a large basin of cool water. Gently agitate the water. Remove the leaves, then allow the dirt to settle. Empty the basin and repeat the process until the leaves are clean.

Beet Greens

Best used in juices, the leafy green tops of beets are a rich source of carotenes and minerals. The folate in beet greens helps to protect against birth defects and fights lung cancer and heart disease. Beet greens increase the body's alkalinity and may help to reduce nicotine cravings. They are a must in juices for treating blood disorders, to improve liver function, and to help correct problems related to the flow of bile.

Key nutrients in beet greens include calcium, iron, magnesium, phosphorus, potassium, sodium, vitamin C, vitamin E, vitamin B_6, vitamin B_1 (thiamine), vitamin B_2 (riboflavin), vitamin B_3 (niacin), pantothenic acid, fiber, folate, small amounts of zinc, copper, and manganese. Phytochemicals include beta-carotene, beta-sitosterol, caffeic acid, chlorogenic acid, ferulic acid, lutein, zeaxanthin, and tocopherols.

The leafy tops should be crisp and dark green in color. Smaller leaves are preferable to large one, which may be bitter. The greens are delicate and should be consumed within two to three days. Store them in a closed plastic bag in the crisper compartment of the refrigerator.

Before using the greens, gently agitate them in a basin filled with cool water. Drain the water and repeat the process until greens are clean.

Chicory

Chicory can aid liver function and blood disorders. It contains high amounts of magnesium, which promotes uptake of other minerals and plays an important role in protecting against heart disease. It helps build and mend bones, and is useful in treating osteoporosis. Chicory also can be used to reduce the swelling and discomfort of tendinitis.

Key nutrients in chicory include calcium, iodine, iron, magnesium, phosphorus, potassium, sodium, zinc, copper, manganese, vitamin C, vitamin B_6, vitamin E, vitamin B_1 (thiamine), vitamin B_2 (riboflavin), vitamin B_3 (niacin), pantothenic acid, fiber, folate, and small amounts of lipids and amino acids. Phytochemicals include beta-carotene, myristic acid, caffeic acid, zeaxanthin, and chlorophyll.

Look for crisp greens that are free of yellow spots and signs of wilting. Store unwashed chicory in a plastic bag in the crisper compartment of the refrigerator for up to one week.

To prepare chicory, twist off the core and separate the leaves. Thoroughly rinse the leaves under cold running water. Chicory is a bitter salad green related to endive and escarole. The outer leaves have the strongest flavor and can be added in small amounts to other salad greens for a robust, peppery flavor. Roasted chicory root is ground and used to flavor coffee or even as a coffee substitute.

Dandelion Greens

Dandelion greens help fight cancer; boost immunity; thwart the aging process; build bones, teeth, and blood; and protect against heart disease. Ancient herbalists relied on dandelion greens as a liver tonic to treat liver maladies. Modern research has shown that due to their choline content, dandelion greens stimulate production of bile, enabling the liver to do its job more efficiently. They also cleanse the gallbladder. Dandelion greens seem to have a general tonic effect on the body. The parts generally eaten are the leaves and tender stems. The blossoms and roots are also edible.

Key nutrients in dandelion greens include calcium, iron, magnesium, phosphorus, potassium, sodium, zinc, copper, manganese, vitamin C, vitamin B_6, vitamin E, vitamin B_1 (thiamine), vitamin B_2 (riboflavin), vitamin B_3 (niacin), pantothenic acid, fiber, folate, and small amounts of lipids and amino acids. Phytochemicals include beta-carotene, chlorophyll, tocopherols, and tocotrienols.

Dandelion greens should be purchased with the roots intact. Ideally, they should be gathered just before the plants flower. The leaves have jagged edges, and should be moist and crisp with no signs of wilting or yellowing. The "weed" with saw-toothed leaves and yellow flowers that pops up in springtime on lawns and in gardens is essentially the same dandelion cultivated for sale in markets today. However, the cultivated variety has longer, more tender leaves than the wild variety. If you decide to forage for your own wild greens, here are a few precautions: Do not pick wild greens from an area that has been treated with pesticides, and do not collect greens from roadsides, since the soil there is almost certainly contaminated with lead from exhaust fumes (even though lead is no longer permitted in gasoline). Avoid pastures or areas that are popular with dog walkers, as the soil may contain parasites or worms. Most important, be absolutely certain that you identify correct species of plant. Many plants have look-alikes that may not be edible. As an alternative, many seed companies now sell dandelion seeds and you can grow your own in pots in the backyard or even on your windowsill.

To store dandelion greens, encase the greens, unwashed, in moist paper towels and place them in a plastic bag in the refrigerator. Greens will keep for three days, but try to consume them within one day of purchase to ensure optimum nutritional value.

To prepare them, remove the roots and separate stems. Trim any tough or thick stems. Swirl the greens in a basin of cool water. Remove the greens from the water and allow the dirt to settle to the bottom. Empty the basin, refill, and repeat until greens are free of grit or dirt.

Endive

Endive, also known as Belgian endive, is related to chicory and escarole and has similar healing properties and nutrient content. It is purposely grown to prevent the development of chlorophyll. This process produces creamy white leaves with a yellowish-green tinge. It has a crunchy, velvety texture and a slightly bitter taste.

Key nutrients in endive include calcium, iron, magnesium, phosphorus, potassium, sodium, zinc, copper, manganese, vitamin C, vitamin B_6, vitamin K, vitamin E, vitamin B_1 (thiamine), vitamin B_2 (riboflavin), vitamin B_3 (niacin), pantothenic acid, fiber, folate, and small amounts of lipids and amino acids. Phytochemicals include beta-carotene, caffeic acid, kaempferol, lutein, myristic acid, quercetin, tocopherols, and tocotrienols.

Choose small, compact heads of long, delicate yellow and white leaves with pale green tips. Store them in the original container or wrapping for three to four days.

To prepare endive, remove the core and rinse the outer leaves under cold running water. Tear into bite-sized pieces for salad or use an entire leaf on sandwiches or as a cosmetic "dish" for salads. Belgian endive is delicious served with Roquefort or goat cheese and combines well with fruits such as apples and pears. It is good in salads dressed with raspberry vinaigrette.

Lettuce, Butterhead (Boston and Bibb Type)

Butterhead lettuces have a soft velvety texture and a sweeter flavor than other lettuces. They help to regulate bowel function and may help to prevent colon and rectal cancer and protect against heart disease, stroke, and diabetes. One cup of Boston lettuce supplies 10 percent of the recommended dietary allowance (RDA) of vitamin A and folate.

Key nutrients in butterhead lettuce include calcium, iron, magnesium, phosphorus, potassium, sodium, zinc, copper, manganese, vitamin C, vitamin B_6, vitamin E, vitamin K, vitamin B_1 (thiamine), vitamin B_2 (riboflavin), vitamin B_3 (niacin), pantothenic acid, fiber, folate, and small amounts of lipids and amino acids. Phytochemicals include beta-carotene, tocopherols, tocotrienols, and psoralen.

Bibb lettuce is small and cup-shaped, with crisp grass-green leaves. Boston lettuce is a larger, loose head with bright yellowish-green leaves. Both should be free of any sign of wilting or yellowing or slimy spots. Both types will keep for up to five days in a tightly closed plastic bag in the crisper compartment of the refrigerator.

To prepare butterhead lettuce, twist off the core, separate the leaves, then swirl them in a basin of cool water. Remove the leaves and allow any dirt to settle to the bottom. Empty and refill the basin and repeat as necessary. If you do not plan to use an entire head, simply remove as many leaves as needed and wash them under cold running water. These lettuces are delicious mixed with peppery greens such as arugula or watercress and served with raspberry vinaigrette.

Lettuce, Looseleaf

These are good all-purpose varieties of lettuce containing antioxidants known to inhibit cancer. Their high fiber content helps to regulate bowel function and may prevent colon and rectal cancer.

Key nutrients in looseleaf lettuce include calcium, iron, magnesium, phosphorus, potassium, sodium, zinc, copper, manganese, vitamin C, vitamin B_6, vitamin E, vitamin B_1 (thiamine), vitamin B_2 (riboflavin), vitamin B_3 (niacin), pantothenic acid, fiber, folate, and small amounts of lipids and amino acids. Phytochemicals include beta-carotene, lutein, and psoralen.

Look for a large, loose head with ruffled leaves that are crisp. The leaves may be light green or tipped in red. There should be no visible signs of wilting or yellow spots. Looseleaf lettuce will keep for up to four days in a plastic bag in the crisper compartment of the refrigerator.

To prepare it, twist off the core and separate the leaves, then swirl them in a basin of cool water. Remove the leaves and allow any dirt to settle to bottom. Repeat this procedure as necessary, using clean water each time. If you are not using the entire head, simply remove as many leaves as needed and wash them under cold running water.

Lettuce, Romaine

Romaine lettuce, also known as cos lettuce, is a good source of fiber and has a higher nutrient content than any other type of lettuce. Two cups of romaine supply more than 50 percent of the recommended dietary allowance (RDA) of vitamin A.

Key nutrients in romaine include calcium, iron, magnesium, phosphorus, potassium, sodium, zinc, copper, manganese, vitamin A, vitamin C, vitamin B_6, vitamin E, vitamin B_1 (thiamine), vitamin B_2 (riboflavin), vitamin B_3 (niacin), pantothenic acid, fiber, folate, and small amounts of lipids and amino acids. Phytochemicals include beta-carotene, chlorophyll, lutein, zeaxanthin, and psoralen.

A head of romaine should be elongated, with crisp, dark-green, oval-shaped outer leaves and paler leaves in the interior. There should be no signs of wilting, yellow spots, or brown edges. Try to buy smaller heads, as the larger ones may be bitter and tough. Romaine lettuce will keep for up to four days in a plastic bag in the crisper compartment of the refrigerator.

To prepare romaine, twist off the core and separate the leaves, then swirl them in a basin of cool water. Remove the leaves and allow any dirt to settle to the bottom. Repeat this procedure as necessary using clean water each time. Traditionally used for Caesar salad and salad Nicoise, this versatile green combines well with most dressings and strong flavors.

Sorrel

Sorrel is a powerful antioxidant with the same healing properties as kale.

Key nutrients in sorrel include calcium, vitamin C, fiber, iron, magnesium, manganese, vitamin B_3 (niacin), phosphorus, potassium, vitamin B_2 (riboflavin), vitamin B_1 (thiamine), and zinc. Phytochemicals include beta-carotene, indoles, isothiocyanates, quercetin, rutin, tannin, and sulforaphane.

Choose sorrel with smaller leaves, which will be tender. Paler leaves indicate a milder flavor. It is best bought fresh, without wilting or discoloration. Wrap unwashed sorrel in damp paper towels, place in a plastic bag, then store in the crisper compartment of the refrigerator. Sorrel is a delicate green, so use it within two to three days.

To prepare sorrel, remove the stems, as they are tough. Swirl the leaves in a basin of cool water until they are free of any dirt. Sorrel has a pleasantly tart and slightly lemon flavor. Try it in salads, or as a seasoning in soups, casseroles, and omelets.

Spinach

Spinach is a nutritional bonanza. Multiple studies have validated its ability to protect against cancer. It prevents the body's cells from undergoing mutation, reduces the risk of lung cancer, and blocks the formation of nitrosamines, which are potent carcinogens. One Harvard University study showed that women with diets high in carotenoids had a 39 percent lower risk of developing cataracts. Another study found that the phytochemicals zeaxanthin and lutein, which are abundant in spinach, form the yellow pigment in the macula of the eye and that persons with a diet rich in these two compounds had a 43 percent lower risk of developing macular degeneration. Spinach contains alpha-lipoic acid, whose potent antioxidant activity, researchers believe, protects nerve cells; it has been used in Germany to treat nerve damage in people with diabetes. It is also a good source of vitamin B_2 (riboflavin), which is proven to lessen the risk of cancer and helps the body to cope with stress. As a rich source of manganese, it is beneficial for persons with juvenile onset diabetes. The folate content helps prevent birth defects, certain cancers, and heart disease. Its calcium and magnesium content help to build strong bones and teeth and to lower blood pressure.

Key nutrients in spinach include calcium, iron, magnesium, phosphorus, potassium, sodium, zinc, copper, manganese, vitamin C, vitamin B_6, vitamin E, vitamin K, vitamin B_1 (thiamine), vitamin B_2 (riboflavin), vitamin B_3 (niacin), pantothenic acid, fiber, folate, and small amounts of lipids and amino acids. Phytochemicals include alpha-lipoic acid, beta-carotene, ferulic acid, kaempferol, myristic acid, P-coumaric acid, quercetin, rutin, lutein, zeaxanthin, tocopherols, tocotrienols, and chlorophyll.

If possible, buy loose spinach so that you can examine the leaves carefully. Choose small leaves that are dark green in color, with no signs of wilting or yellow spots. Fresh spinach leaves have a slightly rubbery texture. If you purchase spinach packaged in a plastic or cellophane bag, squeeze the bag to see if the leaves seem springy.

Loosely pack unwashed spinach in a plastic bag and store it in the crisper compartment of the refrigerator for up to a week.

To prepare spinach, separate the leaves, removing any stems that are fibrous and tough, then swirl them in a basin of cold water. Remove the leaves and allow any dirt to settle to the bottom. Repeat this procedure until the leaves are dirt-free. It may take some time to make sure all the grit is gone.

Spinach contains oxalic acid, a compound that interferes with the body's ability to absorb calcium and other minerals. Serving spinach with orange slices or a squeeze of fresh lemon juice will increase the absorption of the many minerals found in spinach. It is most beneficial served raw.

A cooking suggestion for spinach: Cut up a bunch of spinach into large pieces, leaving small leaves whole (keep in mind that spinach cooks down to about one-fourth of the amount and size you start with). Lightly stir-fry with 1 teaspoon of minced fresh ginger, two cloves of garlic, minced, in 2 tablespoons of olive oil until fragrant. Add the spinach, toss, and heat a few minutes more, just until

A Baker's Dozen: Top Nutritious Vegetables

The thirteen vegetables listed below are particularly nutritious. They have high amounts of vitamins A and C, calcium, fiber, beta-carotene, folate, iron, potassium, and copper.

- All dark-green leafy vegetables
- Sweet potato
- Carrot
- Spinach
- Collards
- Bell pepper, red
- Kale
- Dandelion greens
- Broccoli
- Brussels sprouts
- Peas
- Winter squash
- Swiss chard

wilted. Do not overcook. Season with 1 teaspoon tamari sauce and 3 tablespoons rice or balsamic vinegar. Sprinkle with toasted sesame seeds.

OTHER VEGETABLES

Cruciferous and leafy green vegetables are powerhouses of nutrition and should be a part of your everyday diet. There are also many other vegetables that are important components of a well-rounded diet. Some are available only during certain seasons, but you should eat them when you can get them. Others are available most of the time and the nutrition they provide is a valuable complement to the cruciferous and leafy green vegetables. Alternating among a wide variety of vegetables in the diet helps to alleviate culinary boredom and ensures superior nutrition.

Artichokes

Artichokes have diuretic properties and are useful in treating water retention. They have a stabilizing effect on the metabolism and help to lower blood cholesterol and blood sugar. The chemical compound cynarin, found originally in artichokes, is now duplicated synthetically and marketed as a pharmaceutical drug to lower blood cholesterol. Artichokes are also known to protect the liver and stimulate bile flow. The parts eaten are the outer leaves, inner petals, and the choke, or bottom.

Key nutrients in artichokes include fiber, calcium, iron, magnesium, phosphorus, potassium, sodium, zinc, copper, manganese, vitamin C, vitamin B_1 (thiamine), vitamin B_2 (riboflavin), vitamin B_3 (niacin), pantothenic acid, vitamin B_6, folate, and small amounts of lipids and amino acids. Phytochemicals include beta-carotene, beta-sitosterol, caffeic acid, myristic acid, stigmasterol, chlorophyll, polyphenols, and cynarin.

Look for artichokes that are compact, with thick, fleshy leaves. Check the stems for small holes, which may be a sign of worm damage. Artichokes will keep for up to five days in the refrigerator in a plastic bag. To prevent them from drying out, sprinkle a few drops of water into the bag. Do not wash or trim them prior to storing.

To prepare an artichoke, hold it by the stem and swish it around in a bowl of cold water. Cut one inch off the top of the bud. Trim the outer leaves using kitchen shears. Remove any coarse leaves from the bottom and trim the stem so that it is flush with the bottom. If you want to prepare the bottom (or heart), cut the artichoke in half lengthwise to make removal easier. Drop the prepared artichoke into a bowl of water to which you have added a tablespoon of lemon juice to prevent the cut parts from darkening.

Artichokes (which are the flower of the plant) may provoke an allergic reaction in people who are sensitive to ragweed.

Asparagus

Asparagus has potent diuretic properties and helps to regulate glandular disorders and kidney dysfunction. It neutralizes excess ammonia in the body, a condition that causes lethargy and sexual dysfunction; aids in the health of the prostate gland; inhibits the development of cataracts; eliminates toxins from the liver; and is good for people with kidney disorders. The high amounts of carotene, vitamin C, and selenium make this vegetable excellent for cancer treatment. Fresh asparagus contains high amounts of histones, folic acid, and nucleic acid, which simulate immune function. It is a good source of folate, a B vitamin that plays an important role in cell division and may help to prevent birth defects and protect against heart disease and cervical cancer. The parts eaten are the tips and entire spear (when tender).

Key nutrients in asparagus include fiber, calcium, iron, magnesium, phosphorus, potassium, sodium, zinc, copper, manganese, vitamin C, vitamin B_1 (thiamine), vitamin B_2 (riboflavin), vitamin B_3 (niacin), pantothenic acid, vitamin B_6, vitamin E, vitamin K, folate, and lipids and amino acids. Phytochemicals include beta-carotene, chlorophyll, tocopherols, and tocotrienols.

Look for bright-green spears that are firm and straight with a uniform diameter (so that they will all cook in the same amount of time). The tips should be compact and have a slightly purplish color.

Asparagus deteriorates quickly unless it is kept cold. To store it, trim a ¼ inch off the lower end of the stalks, and wrap the stalks in a moist paper towel and store in the crisper compartment of the refrigerator. Or stand the trimmed, wrapped stalks in an inch of water—they will keep for up to three days.

To prepare asparagus, wash the spears under cool running water. If there is any sand in the tips, dunk them in and out of water until they are clean. You can then steam the spears. To use the tips only, snap them off at the point where they break easily; this is the "choice" part of asparagus. You can then peel the lower, woody stems with a vegetable peeler and add them to soups or stir-fry.

If you have a history of gout, consume asparagus in moderation only. It contains purines, compounds that can trigger gout attacks in susceptible individuals.

Beans, Edible-Podded

A rich source of iron, edible-podded beans are a valuable addition to the diet for treating anemia. This category includes wax, green, and snap beans. They can help to minimize the effects of declining estrogen levels and regulate bowel function. They are a rare source of the nutrient inositol, and have been found to promote the normal function of the liver and pancreas. The entire pod (with the ends trimmed) is eaten. Edible-podded beans have most of the same qualities as shelled beans. They are not as high in fiber and some other nutrients, but they do contain high amounts of beta-carotene and vitamin C.

Key nutrients in edible-podded beans include fiber, calcium, iron, magnesium, phosphorus, sodium, zinc, copper, manganese, vitamin C, vitamin B_1 (thiamine), vitamin B_2 (riboflavin), vitamin B_3 (niacin), pantothenic acid, vitamin B_6, vitamin E, vitamin K (in green beans), folate, and small amounts of lipids and fatty acids. Phytochemicals include alpha-carotene, beta-carotene, and daidzein.

Buy edible-podded beans in loose form so that you can select pods of uniform size to ensure even cooking. The pods should be straight and firm, and free of spots. If the beans show through the pods, they are too mature and will be tough.

Store unwashed, unsnapped beans in resealable plastic bags in the crisper compartment of the refrigerator. Beans will keep for up to five days. To prepare them, wash the beans in cool water and snap both ends of each bean, removing any strings. Cut into two-inch lengths or leave them whole.

Beans, Shelled

Shelled beans, including lima, pinto, and fava beans as well as black-eyed peas and garbanzos, are high in fiber and protein and have little fat. The regular consumption of beans can lower cholesterol and help lower blood pressure, two major contributing factors to heart disease. Beans help to inhibit estrogen-related cancers; prevent the conversion of normal cells to malignant ones; and protect against cancerous tumors and prevent new capillary growth in tumors. They also help to prevent diabetes and, in people who already have diabetes, to keep it under control. Their abundant supply of manganese helps keeps bones strong. In a research study at the University of Texas, women with osteoporosis were found to have about one-third less manganese in their blood than do unaffected women. The fiber in beans regulates bowel function, combats constipation and hemorrhoids, and lowers the risk of colon cancer. Shelled beans, such as navy and red beans, absorb stomach acid and can control ulcer attacks. The parts eaten are the mature fresh seeds.

Key nutrients in shelled beans include fiber, calcium, iron, magnesium, phosphorus, sodium, zinc, copper, manganese, vitamin C, vitamin B_1 (thiamine), vitamin B_2 (riboflavin), vitamin B_3 (niacin), pantothenic acid, vitamin B_6, vitamin E, folate, and small amounts of lipids and amino acids. Phytochemicals include beta-carotene, daidzein, and genistein.

Fresh shelled beans should be firm and uniform in size. The color will differ according to variety, but it should be clear and bright. The seeds should protrude through the pod and feel firm. The pods should be free of blemishes. They can be stored for three to four days in their pods in sealed plastic bags in the refrigerator. Once shelled, the seeds can be stored for one or two days in the refrigerator in sealed plastic bags.

To prepared shelled beans, rinse them in cool water. Remove the seeds by splitting the pod with your thumb. The seeds (now beans) should be rinsed and any membranes removed. Mature fava beans are tough, and the seed needs to be peeled before (or after) cooking. Split the skin with a sharp paring knife and remove the skins. Cooked fava beans are easier to peel.

Fava beans can raise blood pressure. They should be avoided by anyone taking monoamine oxidase inhibitor (MAOIs), a type of drug sometimes prescribed for depression. Also, fava beans contain vicine, a substance that can be toxic but that most people's bodies break down easily. However, Mediterranean people in particular seem to lack the necessary digestive enzyme to break down vicine. This can result in anemia.

Beets

Beets have been used for medicinal purposes since ancient times. They have a cleansing effect on the liver and can be used to treat liver maladies, kidney stones, and disorders of the gallbladder, stomach, and intestines. Beets aid digestion and the lymphatic system. They also help flush out uric acid and table salt. They can combat anemia, debility, and general weakness. Beets tone the blood and build red blood cells.

Key nutrients in beets include calcium, iron, magnesium, phosphorous, potassium, sodium, zinc, copper, man-

ganese, vitamin C, vitamin B_1 (thiamine), vitamin B_2 (riboflavin), vitamin B_3 (niacin), pantothenic acid, vitamin B_6, folate, and small amounts of lipids and amino acids. (For information about the nutritional content on the leafy green beet tops, see page 83.) Phytochemicals include beta-carotene, lutein, and zeaxanthin.

Beets should be smooth and hard, with a deep red color. They should be round, with a slender extended taproot and free of blemishes or soft spots. Small to medium beets are best since the larger ones may be tough. The leafy tops should be crisp and dark green in color. Smaller leaves are preferable to large leaves, which may be bitter. Since the greens perish quickly, wilted tops are not always a sign that beet bulbs are bad. If the greens are wilted, be sure to check the bulb.

Removing the greens from the bulb helps to prevent moisture from being lost. Leave at least one inch of the red stalks. Placed in a plastic bag, the unwashed bulbs will keep for up to three weeks in the refrigerator.

Remove the greens from the bulb and use them as directed earlier in this chapter. Gently wash the bulbs, taking care not to break the skin. Once the skin is broken, the pigment will bleed out, leaving a dull-brown beet. Peel beets after cooking and serve them whole or sliced. Adding vinegar or lemon juice will help the beets to retain their brilliant magenta color. Beets can be baked, boiled, or steamed, or shredded raw and added to slaws or salads.

The pigment betacyanin found in beets may make your urine or stool red. This is not cause for alarm. In fact, this pigment is also extracted and used as a natural food dye. Although cooking beets concentrates their minerals, they lose most of their vitamin A, vitamin C, and B-complex vitamins when cooked, so in addition to eating cooked beets, use them raw to add flavor, color, and nutrients to salads and juiced mixtures.

Burdock

Burdock is an excellent blood purifier and can help the body eliminate toxins, making it a useful treatment for arthritis and rheumatic pains. It is also helpful in treating kidney and urinary tract infections and eliminating excess water weight. The root is the part that is eaten.

Key nutrients in burdock include calcium, iron, fiber, magnesium, phosphorus, potassium, sodium, zinc, copper, manganese, vitamin C, vitamin B_6, vitamin A, vitamin E, vitamin B_1 (thiamine), vitamin B_2 (riboflavin), vitamin B_3 (niacin), pantothenic acid, folate, and small amounts of lipids and amino acids. Phytochemicals include beta-carotene, caffeic acid, chlorogenic acid, lignin, myristic acid, and stigmasterol.

Fresh burdock root should be slender (up to one inch in diameter), firm and brown with a spongy, fibrous center that is white. It should be free of blemishes or soft spots.

The fresh root can be stored "as is" for up to one month in the crisper compartment of the refrigerator. If it begins to shrivel, trim the ends and soak it in cool water for one-half hour and then store it in a plastic bag in the crisper compartment.

To prepare burdock root, thoroughly wash it with a vegetable brush. Fresh burdock root is often muddy or dirty. Once it is clean, cut it into chunks for soups or shred or slice it and add it to stir-fry or grain dishes.

Pregnant woman should not consume burdock root, as it may stimulate the uterus.

Carrots

Carrots are one of the best dietary sources of beta-carotene, which boosts the immune system and reduces the risk of many cancers, including, breast, rectal, larynx, and lung cancer. Almost all epidemiological studies on the subject have concluded that the regular consumption of beta-carotene might reduce the risk of developing cancer by 40 to 70 percent. Carrots also contain lutein, another anti-cancer carotenoid. Research suggests that it is the synergy of all the compounds in carrots that makes them such an important deterrent in the development of cancer. Eating just one medium-sized raw carrot four times a week can reduce the odds of developing lung cancer. Carrots stimulate production of T-helper cells, immune cells that protect the body from all types of infection; guard against cardiovascular disease; reduce inflammation; and slow the aging process. They build healthy skin, tissue, and teeth; improve eyesight; prevent eye and mucous membrane infection; stimulate the appetite; and prevent dehydration. They are excellent for treating infantile diarrhea and acute colitis. Adults with acute enterocolitis, diarrhea, or colon disorders can benefit from carrot soup or juice. The fiber content in whole carrots helps suppress the low-density (LDL, or "bad") cholesterol and raise the high-density (HDL, or "good" cholesterol), an important precautionary measure against heart disease. Research has also established that eating a beta-carotene-rich food at least once a day significantly reduces the risk of macular degeneration. Carrots contain an estrogenlike compound that stimulates libido. They are excellent used in raw juices, but you should never eat or juice the tops, as they are very bitter. The root is the part of the plant eaten.

Key nutrients in carrots include fiber, calcium, iron, magnesium, phosphorus, potassium, sodium, zinc, copper, manganese, vitamin C, vitamin B_6, vitamin K, vitamin E, vitamin B_1 (thiamine), vitamin B_2 (riboflavin), vitamin B_3 (niacin), pantothenic acid, folate, and small amounts of lipids and amino acids. Phytochemicals include alpha-carotene, beta-carotene, lutein, tocopherols, apigenin, beta-ionone, beta-sitosterol, caffeic acid, caryophyllene, chlorogenic acid, chlorophyll, coumarin, eugenol, ferulic acid, kaempferol, limonene, lycopene, myrcetin, myristic acid, myristicin, P-coumaric acid, pectin, psoralen, quercetin, quercitrin, scopoletin, and stigmasterol.

Look for carrots that are reddish-orange. The deeper the color, the higher the beta-carotene content. Carrots should be medium to slender in size, since larger carrots tend to be more fibrous. Avoid buying carrots with "rootlets," as this is a sign of immaturity. A pale-green rim at the top portion of the carrot is a sign that the carrot is beginning to age. Avoid carrots that have dark-green or black rims at the top.

Carrots store well. They will keep in their original packaging for up to four weeks. Loose carrots should be stored unwashed in a closed plastic bag.

Celeriac

Available August through May, also known as celeriac, celery root is a knobby and often muddy root. It comes from a celerylike plant of which only the root is edible. It tastes of celery and walnut, and adds a very mellow flavor to soups and stews. Celeriac contains water-soluble fiber that lowers cholesterol and may reduce the risk of heart attack. One celery root (about ⅓ cup sliced) contains 39 calories, 300 milligrams of potassium, and no fat. It is high in phosphorus, and is beneficial to the nervous, lymphatic, and urinary systems.

Key nutrients in celeriac include calcium, iron, fiber, magnesium, phosphorus, potassium, sodium, zinc, copper, manganese, vitamin C, vitamin B_6, vitamin E, vitamin B_1 (thiamine), vitamin B_2 (riboflavin), vitamin B_3 (niacin), pantothenic acid, and folate. Phytochemicals include beta-carotene.

Celeriac should be round with tough outer skin that has small "knobs." Look for small, hard roots with a smooth skin. It can be stored for up to one month in the refrigerator. Store unwashed root in open or perforated plastic bags.

To prepare celeriac, scrub the root thoroughly, then peel the outer skin. The flesh should be white with a celerylike smell. Celeriac can be shredded, sliced, or cut into cubes. To prevent discoloration, place celeriac in a bowl of cool water with lemon juice. Soak for three to five minutes, then drain. To eat it raw, peel and cut it into julienne strips, and coat with vinaigrette dressing. Celeriac can be used in much the same way as celery. Add raw celeriac to salads, purée it for soups and stews, or add it to stir-fry dishes.

Celery

Celery may protect against certain cancers, especially stomach cancer. Eating two to four celery stalks daily can lower blood pressure, particularly if high blood pressure is related to stress. Celery has mild diuretic properties and aids in digestion and weight loss. It is helpful in diseases of chemical imbalance and has detoxifying effects. It helps to regulate the nervous system and controls dizziness and headaches. Celery also aids kidney and liver function and stimulates the sex drive. It balances acidity in the body and helps to clear up skin problems. Celery is also good for people with diabetes and is an excellent addition to raw vegetable juices.

Key nutrients in celery include calcium, iron, magnesium, phosphorus, potassium, sodium, zinc, copper, manganese, vitamin C, vitamin B_6, vitamin K, vitamin E, vitamin B_1 (thiamine), vitamin B_2 (riboflavin), vitamin B_3 (niacin), pantothenic acid, fiber, folate, and small amounts of lipids and amino acids. Phytochemicals include beta-carotene, phytosterols, phthalides, polyacetylenes, psoralen, tocopherols, coumarin, eugenol, myristic acid, myristicin, and P-coumaric acid.

Look for stalks that are pale green and smooth. Avoid bunches that have cracks or dark spots. Darker green stalks tend to be tough and stringy. The leaves should be crisp and dark green. Unwashed celery stored in an open plastic bag in the crisper compartment of the refrigerator will keep up to two weeks.

To prepare celery, peel outer ribs with a vegetable peeler to remove strings that make it tougher. It is not necessary to peel the inner stalks or "celery hearts." Trim about one-quarter inch from the base of the stalk and remove the outer leaves. Thoroughly rinse the stalks in cold running water. Prepared ahead of time, celery stalks can "stand" in ice water for up to an hour. Similarly, if celery becomes limp, you can revive it by soaking it in ice water. The leafy green tops can be chopped finely and added to salads or dried and added to soups and stews.

Chard

A member of the beet family, chard (also known as Swiss chard) is a good source of folate, the B vitamin that helps fight lung cancer and prevent neural-tube birth defects. Folate deficiency is linked to mental decline and heart disease in the elderly. Eating chard can improve digestion, boost energy levels, and correct calcium deficiency. It is also a diuretic and a laxative, and when mixed with carrot juice, it helps to control urinary tract infections, hemorrhoids, and skin disease.

Key nutrients in chard include calcium, iron, magnesium, phosphorus, potassium, sodium, zinc, copper, manganese, vitamin C, vitamin B_6, vitamin E, folate, and small amounts of lipids and amino acids. Phytochemicals include alpha-carotene, beta-carotene, kaempferol, lutein, P-coumaric acid, quercetin, zeaxanthin, and chlorophyll.

Look for broad, dark-green leaves with either a white or red stalk. The leaves should be crisp and free of any spots or discoloration. Unwashed greens can be stored in damp paper towels wrapped in plastic. Chard will keep for three to four days in the crisper compartment of the refrigerator.

To prepare chard, trim the ends, then swirl in a basin of cool water. Remove the leaves and allow the dirt to settle to the bottom. Refill the basin and repeat until all grit and sand are removed. Chard can be added raw to salads or cooked. When cooking greens, remove the stems and cook them for a few minutes before adding the leaves. Two pounds of raw greens will yield approximately 1 cup of cooked greens.

A cooking suggestion for chard: Wilt the chard by boiling or sautéing it briefly, then drain and chop. Sauté slivered onion, red bell pepper, and minced garlic in a little vegetable oil until tender. Add chard and toss until heated. Season with balsamic vinegar. (Note: Chard stems require a longer cooking time than the leaves. Boil or steam chopped stems separately until tender, about five minutes, then mix into cooked greens.)

Corn

Corn is a good source of dietary fiber and is useful in treating irritable bowel syndrome and regulating bowel function. It is a bone and muscle builder and is good for weight gain. Corn is hard to digest and must be thoroughly chewed. Corn's high potassium content may help to regulate blood pressure and heart function, thereby reducing the risk of stroke and heart attack. Corn protects against cancer and viral infection, and may lower cholesterol and help prevent hardening of the arteries. It is a brain food, and is also good for the nervous system. The parts eaten are kernels of the immature plant. Yellow corn contains the most nutrients, and cornmeal enriched with lysine is a complete protein. People who have digestive disorders or who are on a weight-loss program should avoid corn.

Key nutrients in corn include calcium, iron, magnesium, phosphorus, potassium, sodium, zinc, copper, manganese, vitamin C, vitamin B_6, vitamin E, vitamin B_1 (thiamine), vitamin B_2 (riboflavin), vitamin B_3 (niacin), pantothenic acid, fiber, folate, and small amounts of lipids and amino acids. Phytochemicals include beta-carotene, alpha-carotene, beta-cryptoxanthin, eugenol, ferulic acid, gallic acid, indoles, myristic acid, P-coumaric acid, squalene, stigmasterol, thymol, monoterpenes, and phytoestrogens.

When buying corn in the husk, look for green husks that are "tight" and moist. Never buy corn in the husk that is yellowed and dry. The kernels should be plump and in close rows. When punctured, a kernel should spurt a milky liquid. The silk should be soft and pale yellow, never brown or wiry. Corn should not be piled in unrefrigerated bins at the supermarket.

Corn must be kept refrigerated to prevent its sugar from turning into starch. Store for two to three days in the crisper compartment of the refrigerator. If corn cannot be consumed within that time, parboil it and store it in plastic bags in the refrigerator.

To prepare corn, remove the husks and snap off the ends. Remove the silk using a stiff, dry vegetable brush. Rinse the corn under cool running water. Corn can be boiled, grilled in the husk, or baked in the oven. To cut the kernels off the cob, hold the ear vertically, then slice downward with a sharp knife. Do not press too hard, as part of the cob may be removed.

If you suspect you may have food allergies, pay close attention to how you feel after eating corn. Corn, and cereals and sweeteners made from corn, are among the most common causes of food allergies or sensitivities.

Cucumber

Cucumbers are approximately 95 percent water and are not quite as high in vitamins as most other vegetables. Nevertheless, they help to normalize heart rhythm, regulate blood pressure, ensure proper function of nerves and muscles, and maintain the body's fluid balance. They are low in calories, a good source of fiber, and lend lots of flavor and crunchy texture to recipes. Their sterol content may help prevent heart disease by lowering cholesterol. The highest concentration of sterol is in the skin. The skin also contains vitamin A, so if possible, buy unwaxed cucumbers and eat the skin after scrubbing. Applying cucumber juice or puréed cucumber to insect stings, poison ivy, or sunburn is cooling and helps to reduce itching and inflammation. A slice of cucumber placed over the eyelid and surrounding area helps to reduce puffiness.

Key nutrients in cucumbers include calcium, iron, magnesium, phosphorus, potassium, sodium, zinc, copper, manganese, vitamin C, vitamin B_6, vitamin K, vitamin E, vitamin B_1 (thiamine), vitamin B_2 (riboflavin), vitamin B_3 (niacin), pantothenic acid, fiber, folate, and small amounts of lipids and amino acids. Phytochemicals include beta-carotene, monoterpenes, sterols, tocopherols, beta-sitosterol, caffeic acid, chlorogenic acid, cucurbitacin B and E, ferulic acid, myristic acid, and squalene.

Select firm cucumbers with rounded tips. The skin should be a dark green with no yellowing. Typically, smaller cucumbers have fewer and smaller seeds. Pickling cucumbers are smaller in size, lighter in color, and have small bumps. Cucumbers must be refrigerated to remain fresh.

Waxed cucumbers will keep for about a week in the crisper compartment of the refrigerator. Unwaxed cucumbers (which are preferable) will keep for three to four days. Once cut, a cucumber should be wrapped in plastic and stored in the crisper compartment. Unwaxed cucumbers can be washed with a vegetable brush, the ends removed, and served in slices or quarters. The skin of waxed cucumbers should always be peeled away before serving.

Eggplant

Eggplant can enhance immunity, help to lower cholesterol, and fight heart disease. It boosts tumor-fighting activity and inhibits the production of cancer-causing nitrosamines. Eggplant is diuretic and antibacterial, and may counteract the effects of fatty foods. It binds cholesterol in the intestinal tract so that fat is not absorbed into the bloodstream. It works best when eaten with foods containing essential fatty acids and cholesterol. Some of the phytonutrients in eggplant help to prevent convulsions. The Chinese use eggplant to aid the function of the large intestines, spleen, and stomach. The entire fruit is eaten.

Key nutrients in eggplant include calcium, iron, magnesium, phosphorus, potassium, sodium, zinc, copper, manganese, vitamin C, vitamin B_6, vitamin E, vitamin B_1 (thiamine), vitamin B_2 (riboflavin), vitamin B_3 (niacin), pantothenic acid, fiber, folate, and small amounts of lipids and amino acids. Phytochemicals include beta-carotene, caffeic acid, chlorogenic acid, lycopene, pectin, scopoletin, tannin, phytosterols, monoterpenes, phenolic acids, and anthocyanins.

Several types of eggplant are available. The most common is the purple-black, oval-shaped variety. The slender, elongated variety often referred to as Japanese eggplant is slightly sweeter and not as likely to be bitter. Italian, or "baby," eggplants are more rounded and have thinner skin and fewer seeds. All eggplants come in a variety of colors, ranging from white to dark purple. Regardless of the variety, eggplants should be firm, weighty, and free of scars or cuts. The skin should be smooth and free of wrinkles. When you press an eggplant with your thumb, any indentation should quickly fill back out.

Unwashed, uncut eggplant will store for up to three days in the crisper compartment of the refrigerator. To prepare it, gently wash the eggplant under cool running water. Remove the stem and cap with a sharp knife. Eggplant may be cooked with or without skin, as a matter of personal preference. To avoid bitterness, slice or dice the eggplant, lightly sprinkle it with salt, then place it in a colander to drain the natural juices for a half-hour. Rinse the eggplant and pat dry with a paper towel before cooking. You should never fry eggplant. It soaks up oil more than any other vegetable, almost like a sponge. Instead, try grilling, roasting, oven-baking, or sautéing it with a small amount of canola oil. If you have arthritis, see the cautions pertaining to eggplant in the section on nightshade vegetables on page 98.

Fennel, Sweet

Sweet fennel, also known as anise, is a vegetable related to the celery family. It has a firm, crisp white bulb and green fronds. The fronds are similar to those of the dill plant. The lower part of the plant is a large white bulb that is much larger than a bunch of celery. The flavor is sweet, pleasant, and licoricelike. Fennel is high in vitamins A and C. Fennel seeds are edible and help to rid the intestinal tract of mucus and aid in relieving flatulence.

Throughout history, fennel has been used as a healing food. The ancient Greek physician Hippocrates prescribed fennel tea to stimulate milk production in nursing mothers; the medieval English herbalist Nicholas Culpeper treated kidney stones, liver, and lung ailments, and gout with fennel. Chewing fennel seeds is an age-old remedy for hunger pangs. Nutritionists today agree that fennel aids digestion, and it may prevent certain cancers. Fennel has been a popular ingredient in French cuisine for many years. It is easy to grow and forms a tall, lovely plant. Fennel makes a pungent, licorice-flavored tea.

Key nutrients in fennel include calcium, iron, magnesium, phosphorus, potassium, sodium, zinc, copper, manganese, vitamin C, vitamin B_6, vitamin A, vitamin B_1 (thiamine), vitamin B_2 (riboflavin), vitamin B_3 (niacin), pantothenic acid, fiber, folate, and small amounts of lipids and amino acids. Phytochemicals include beta-carotene, psoralen, beta-sitosterol, caffeic acid, limonene, ferulic acid, isoquercitrin, myristicin, P-coumaric acid, pectin, quercetin, rutin, scopoletin, sinapic acid, stigmasterol, tocopherols, and umbelliferone.

The bulbs should be firm and moist with no signs of splitting or brown spots. If the stalks are intact, they should be straight and firm. If the stalks have been cut, the ends should not be dry. The feathery leaves should be bright green with no signs of wilting or yellowing.

To store fennel, remove stalks from the bulb and wrap them separately in plastic. They can be stored in the crisper compartment of the refrigerator for up to three days. Use the stalks first as they do not keep as well as the bulbs.

The leaves can be used like an herb to season fish, eggs, and pork. Trim the base from the bulb and wash under cold running water. The bulb can be diced or cut into chunks, or individual layers can be removed and cut into small strips or squares. If you are slicing the bulb, leave the core intact so that the layers will hold together. The stalks can be used in much the same way as celery although the flavor is delicately sweet and similar to licorice.

Try eating fennel raw, in salads, or with a dip. Or sauté it in vegetable oil until tender, but crisp, then cover with ½ inch of water and simmer for twenty minutes. Another method of cooking fennel is to slice the bulb in half and boil it for about fifteen minutes.

Jerusalem Artichoke

Jerusalem artichokes, also know as sunchokes, help to build the blood, stimulate the growth of beneficial intestinal bacteria that reduce constipation, and lower blood pressure and cholesterol. Three-fourths of a cup of sliced artichoke has 76 calories and supplies 19 percent of the recommended dietary allowance (RDA) of iron and 13 percent of the RDA of vitamin B_1.

A natural source of insulin, Jerusalem artichokes are a good food choice for people with diabetes and gluten allergies. Jerusalem artichokes are an excellent source of iron and a nonstarchy substitute for potatoes. The tuber is the part eaten.

Key nutrients in Jerusalem artichokes include calcium, iron, magnesium, phosphorus, potassium, sodium, zinc, copper, manganese, vitamin C, vitamin B_6, vitamin E, vitamin B_1 (thiamine), vitamin B_2 (riboflavin), vitamin B_3 (niacin), pantothenic acid, fiber, folate, fructooligosaccharides, and small amounts of lipids and amino acids. Phytochemicals include beta-carotene.

Select tubers that are clean and firm and free of blemishes. The skin should be glossy and tan to brown in color, with no sign of green. Choose tubers that have the least amount of "knobs" and show no signs of sprouting.

Jerusalem artichokes can be stored in a plastic bag for up to two weeks in the crisper compartment of the refrigerator, or in a cool, dry place away from light. Available from October through June, this tuber can be scrubbed, sliced, and stir-fried. It is a wonderful substitute for potatoes and has less starch. There is no need to peel it. To prepare them, scrub with a stiff vegetable brush. Like potatoes, most of the nutrients are just beneath the skin. If peeling is needed, use a vegetable peeler. Cut them into chunks for soups, use slices like potatoes or turnips, or bake them whole and serve like a potato. Raw shredded Jerusalem artichoke can be added to salads or slaw. They are delicious pickled or marinated and served as a condiment.

Okra

Okra helps inhibit cellular mutations associated with cancer and may also reduce the likelihood of stroke or heart attack by inhibiting plaque formation in the arteries. It also helps to prevent constipation, which protects against colon and rectal cancer, and lowers blood cholesterol levels. Okra is an excellent demulcent and helps to relieve intestinal disorders including colitis, inflammation of the colon and spastic colon, diverticulitis, and stomach ulcers. The pods are the parts eaten. Okra is a very prolific plant. When one pod is picked, another grows.

Key nutrients in okra include calcium, iron, magnesium, phosphorus, potassium, sodium, zinc, copper, manganese, vitamin C, vitamin B_6, vitamin E, vitamin B_1 (thiamine), vitamin B_2 (riboflavin), vitamin B_3 (niacin), pantothenic acid, fiber, folate, and small amounts of lipids and amino acids. Phytochemicals include alpha-carotene, beta-carotene, myristic acid, pectin, and zeaxanthin.

Fresh okra pods are tender and moist, with a downy covering similar to "peach fuzz." They should have a bright green color. Choose smaller pods (up to 3½ inches) since larger pods tend to become tough and fibrous.

Okra can be stored for three to four days in a closed plastic bag in the crisper compartment of the refrigerator.

To prepare okra, wash the pods under cool running water. With a knife, remove the cap and the end, and cut into slices for stir-frying or sautéing. When cooking the whole pod, prevent the juices from being released from the inner capsule by removing only a tiny part of the cap. This also will reduce its gelatinous consistency. Okra is also less gelatinous when prepared with an acidic vegetable, such as tomato.

Onions

Onions have been used throughout the ages as a food and a medicine. The Egyptians regarded the onion as a symbol of the universe because of its sheaths (the layers that encircle the bulb). The daily consumption of onions (¼ to 1 cup diced) has been shown to lower cholesterol, inhibit cancerous tumor growth, and help manage diabetes. Onions are a blood tonic and have anticoagulant properties that may reduce the risk of heart attack and aid in high blood pressure. The anti-inflammatory properties of onions may provide relief for people with asthma, hay fever, and allergies, and they are also useful for helping to relieve croup and lung infections. Onions help to inhibit carcinogens, bacteria, and tumor growth. They are also useful in treating intestinal problems. Syrup made from the juice of one onion mixed with honey is an age-old remedy for the common cold, asthma, sore throat, and bronchitis. Onions also can be used as a digestive aid, expectorant, antiseptic, and antifungal. Adding onions to fatty foods may minimize the clot-promoting abilities of these foods. The part eaten is the bulb.

Key nutrients in onions include calcium, iron, magnesium, phosphorus, potassium, sodium, zinc, copper, manganese, vitamin C, vitamin B_6, vitamin E, vitamin K, vitamin B_1 (thiamine), vitamin B_2 (riboflavin), vitamin B_3 (niacin), pantothenic acid, fiber, folate, and small amounts of lipids and amino acids. Phytochemicals include beta-carotene, quercetin, allylic sulfides, allicin, allyl cysteine, tocopherols, isothiocyanates, beta-sitosterol, caffeic acid, ferulic acid, kaempferol, myristic acid, P-coumaric acid, pectin, phloroglucinol, phytosterols, rutin, sinapic acid, and stigmasterol.

Onions are available in several varieties, with flavors ranging from pungent to mild. When purchasing onions, consider whether they will be used to flavor cooked dishes or will be used raw in salads or sandwiches. Globe onions should be dry and firm with no soft spots or discoloration. The skins should be shiny and the tops should be closed with no green sprouts. Shallots, a type of onion with a mild, savory flavor, should be firm and dry with no soft spots or sprouts. Scallions, or green onions, should have crisp, grass green tops and white bottoms. Leeks resemble large scallions but should have firm, straight root ends that are free of splits. A bulbous root end is indicative of over-maturity. The tops should be fresh and green, with no signs of yellowing or wilting.

Leeks and scallions should be stored in plastic bags in the crisper compartment of the refrigerator. Scallions should be used within three or four days of purchase, while leeks will keep for a week. Globe type onions and shallots do not have to be stored in a refrigerator. They can be stored in baskets or spread out in a single layer in a dry, cool place away from light. They can be stored unwrapped in the crisper compartment of the refrigerator for up to a month. Onions should not be stored with potatoes since potatoes release a gas that can hasten the onions' ripening process. Once cut, an onion tightly wrapped in plastic can be kept in the refrigerator for two to three days.

Trim the tops and bottoms from the onion. Peel the skin and the first layer of membrane underneath, which is often sticky. Once peeled, onions can be sliced, chopped, diced, or grated depending upon your intended use. Prepare a scallion by trimming the rootlet using a sharp knife. Peel away any sticky membrane. The green tops can be chopped and added to salads, omelets, or stews for a mild chivelike flavor. Pearl onions can be served as a side dish. Larger globe onions can be cored, stuffed, and baked as an entree. To reduce the fiery flavor of onions, pour boiling water over thin slices and allow them to stand for five minutes. After cutting onions, rinse your hands with lemon juice to remove the tear-provoking odor.

Parsnip

Parsnips are in the same botanical family as carrots, celeriac, and celery. They have a surprisingly sweet flavor that complements bitter or smoky foods. The National Cancer Institute is investigating their ability to inhibit the formation and growth of cancerous cells. They have anti-inflammatory properties and are a good source of dietary fiber. They are good for colon disorders, constipation, and high blood pressure. Parsnips can help boost immunity. The part eaten is the root.

Key nutrients in parsnips include calcium, iron, magnesium, phosphorus, potassium, sodium, zinc, copper, manganese, vitamin C, vitamin B_6, vitamin E, vitamin B_1 (thiamine), vitamin B_2 (riboflavin), vitamin B_3 (niacin), pantothenic acid, fiber, folate, and small amounts of lipids and amino acids. Phytochemicals include beta-carotene, flavonoids, limonene, myristic acid, myristicin, quercetin, psoralen, polyacetylenes, and phenolic acids.

A parsnip looks like a pale version of a carrot, with color ranging from yellow to off-white. They should be firm and sturdy with no pitting, discoloration, cracks, or soft surface areas. If the tops are still attached, they should be fresh and green. Parsnips are a winter vegetable and their flavor is best after exposure to cold weather.

Remove the green tops (if any) to prevent moisture loss. Store in a plastic bag in the refrigerator for up to one month.

Parsnips are fairly tough and are not usually eaten raw. Trim any rootlets or knobs and scrub the parsnips with a stiff vegetable brush. Peel with a vegetable peeler or sharp paring knife. Parsnips can be cut into slices, diced, halved, or quartered for baking or steaming. To purée parsnips, peel them after cooking. Parsnips make a hearty, flavorful addition to soups and stews, and can be served as a side dish similar to potatoes.

Peas, Green

Green peas are a storehouse of vitamins and nutrients. A ½-cup serving provides more than 20 percent of the recommended dietary allowance (RDA) of vitamin C, which bolsters the immune system. Peas help to normalize the fluid levels of the body and maintain cell function. They are also a good source of soluble fiber that helps to lower cholesterol levels and control blood sugar. Research has shown that peas aid in preventing prostate cancer. Studies in Wales and England have found a connection between pea consumption and low rates of acute appendicitis. Puréed peas can be used as a treatment for ulcers. They also contain an antifertility compound, m-xylohydroquinone, so it may be wise to avoid them if you are trying to become pregnant. The unripe seeds are the parts eaten.

Key nutrients in green peas include calcium, iron, magnesium, phosphorus, potassium, sodium, zinc, copper, manganese, vitamin C, vitamin B_6, vitamin E, vitamin K, vitamin B_1 (thiamine), vitamin B_2 (riboflavin), vitamin B_3 (niacin), pantothenic acid, fiber, folate, pectin, and small amounts of lipids and amino acids. Phytochemicals include alpha-lipoic acid, beta-carotene, daidzein, and chlorophyll.

Look for medium-sized pods with a firm texture. The pod surface should be bright green, smooth, and slightly bulging. Store unshelled peas in a perforated plastic bag in the refrigerator for two to three days.

To prepare fresh peas, rinse the pods in cool water. Snap off the stems and pull the strings downward. Using your thumb, pop peas out of the pod into a colander, then rinse to remove any membranes.

Peppers, Chili

This category of pepper includes cascabel, cayenne, habanero, jalapeño, and serrano (the hottest), and Anaheim, ancho, cherry poblano, and Hungarian wax (moderately hot). Capsaicin, the compound that gives chili peppers their fiery flavor, is largely responsible for their healing qualities as well. Chili peppers can help improve circulation, prevent bronchitis, clear the sinuses, soothe the bronchial passages and the lungs, aid in asthma and hypersensitive airways, reduce swelling of the tracheal and bronchial cells caused by cigarette smoke and other irritants, act as expectorant and decongestant, and boost metabolism. They have been thought to irritate the stomach lining and promote ulcers, but in fact chili peppers prevent ulcers and improve digestion. Regular consumption of chili peppers has a beneficial effect on blood cholesterol, lowering the bad cholesterol and triglycerides. Chili peppers also help to protect against cancer, heart attack, and stroke and are higher in vitamin C than citrus fruits. Capsaicin has also been shown to block the substance that transmits pain signals to the central nervous system. The fleshy fruit is the part eaten.

Key nutrients in chili peppers include calcium, iron, magnesium, phosphorus, potassium, sodium, zinc, copper, manganese, vitamin C, vitamin B_6, vitamin A, vitamin E, vitamin B_1 (thiamine), vitamin B_2 (riboflavin), vitamin B_3 (niacin), pantothenic acid, folate, and small amounts of lipids and amino acids. Phytochemicals include capsaicin, flavonoids, and phenolic acids.

Peppers have different shapes and colors, depending on the variety. They should have a firm, glossy skin free of soft spots, discoloration, or wrinkles. Dried hot peppers should be shiny, with unbroken skins. Some varieties wrinkle when dried.

Unwashed peppers will keep for seven to ten days in a closed plastic bag in the refrigerator. Dried chili peppers can be stored in an airtight container at room temperature for three months.

To prepare chili peppers, wash them, then cut them in half lengthwise. Scraping out the seeds and membranes, and rinsing peppers under cold running water will remove much of the heat. Place chilies cut side up on a cutting board and cut them into strips. You can then chop or dice them to add to salsas, sauces, and stir-fry dishes. The uncut halves can be roasted or grilled. The capsaicin in chili peppers can cause blistering of the skin and irritation to the eyes and nasal passages. Wearing gloves can minimize the risk of irritation. Be sure to thoroughly wash your hands, cutting board, and utensils with hot soapy water after handling chilies. The burning sensation from eating hot peppers can be neutralized by eating plain, low-fat yogurt.

Researchers from institutions in Mexico and the National Cancer Institute in the United States compared patients who had gastric cancer with cancer-free volunteers. They found that the highest risk of gastric cancer occurred in patients who consumed the most capsaicin—the equivalent of nine to twenty-five jalapeño peppers per day. Gastric cancer rates have fallen dramatically in most countries, but not in Mexico, which was what prompted the study.

Peppers, Sweet

Sweet peppers, including bell, banana, and pimento, are low in calories and high in vitamin C, which helps to fight infections, heart disease, and cancer. When allowed to ripen on the vine to a deep red color, the lobe-shaped bell pepper will contain twice as much beta-carotene and vitamin C as the immature green fruit. The fully mature red pepper helps to protect against certain types of cancer, particularly bladder, ovarian, and pancreatic cancer. Since cancer and most degenerative diseases thrive in an acidic environment, sweet peppers are a good alternative to citrus fruits. The fleshy fruit is the part eaten.

Key nutrients in sweet peppers include calcium, iron, magnesium, phosphorus, potassium, sodium, zinc, copper, manganese, vitamin C, vitamin B_6, vitamin A, vitamin K, vitamin E, vitamin B_1 (thiamine), vitamin B_2 (riboflavin), vitamin B_3 (niacin), pantothenic acid, fiber, folate, and small amounts of lipids and amino acids. Phytochemicals include alpha-carotene, beta-carotene, phenolic acids, flavonoids, caffeic acid, capsaicin, caryophyllene, cryptoxanthin, eugenol, limonene, myristic acid, scopoletin, stigmasterol, hesperidin, chlorogenic acid, chlorophyll, P-coumaric acid, lutein, tocopherols, and zeaxanthin.

Sweet peppers should have glossy skin that is free of blemishes or soft spots. The four-lobed bell varieties should feel heavy for their size. Store unwashed peppers for up to six days in a sealed plastic bag in the crisper compartment of the refrigerator.

To prepare sweet peppers, cut around the stalk and core, then twist and pull it off in one piece. Cut the pepper in half, and scrape out the seeds and the fleshy white membranes.

Bell peppers are frequently waxed to preserve freshness and color. Waxed peppers should be peeled before you use them.

Potatoes

Potatoes are a satisfying food and a wise choice for healthy eaters and dieters alike. Their rich stores of potassium (more than bananas) help to maintain fluid balance and regulate blood pressure and heart function. Raw potato juice is an excellent source of potassium and is good for helping to treat all heart disorders. The ample supply of vitamin B_6 in potatoes helps to bolster immunity. The fiber content of potatotes supports proper bowel function. Potatoes help to fight infection and protect against cancer and heart disease. They also contain anticancer substances and balance alkalinity and acidity in the body. Potatoes can be detrimental for people with diabetes, however, as they raise insulin and blood sugar levels quickly. People with arthritis also should eat potatoes in moderation only, if at all. The tuber is the part eaten.

Key nutrients in potatoes include calcium, iron, magnesium, phosphorus, potassium, sodium, zinc, copper, manganese, vitamin C, vitamin B_6, vitamin K, vitamin E, vitamin B_1 (thiamine), vitamin B_2 (riboflavin), vitamin B_3 (niacin), pantothenic acid, fiber, folate, and small amounts of lipids and amino acids. Phytochemicals include alpha-lipoic acid, beta-carotene, anthoxanthins, tocopherols, caffeic acid, chlorogenic acid, ferulic acid, myristic acid, P-coumaric acid, pectin, rutin, scopoletin, sinapic acid, and umbelliferone.

Though there are hundreds of varieties of potatoes, there are four main types that are grown commercially: russet, long white, round white, and round red. Some of the newer varieties available today, such as Yukon Gold, Yellow Finn, and purple, have all the same nutritional qualities as the traditional potatoes but have richer, sweeter flavors. Regardless of variety, the basic guidelines for selection are the same. Look for clean, firm tubers with no eyes or sprouts. Sprouts contain solanine, a toxic substance. Avoid potatoes with a green tint to the skin since this also indicates the presence of solanine. A purplish tint to the skin or to the peeled potato may also indicate the presence of toxins.

Refrigerating potatoes causes their starch content to convert into sugar. Potatoes will keep for one to two months in a cool, dark place stored in a perforated plastic bag or an open brown paper bag. Check them periodically and remove any soft or shriveled potatoes or potatoes that have sprouted. Potatoes that have sprouted contain elevated levels of solanine. They should not be stored for more than two months since naturally occurring toxins called glycoalkaloids build up as potatoes mature.

Scrub potatoes with a vegetable brush under cold running water. Most of a potato's mineral content is found just underneath the skin, while its vitamins and starch content are in the center of the potato. The skin is also a good source of fiber. However, unless you are buying organic potatoes, you may want to peel them. Steam potatoes instead of boiling to avoid losing the potassium. To enjoy the taste of fried potatoes without the calories of the fat, preheat your oven to 400°F, thinly slice a potato, *lightly* coat a cookie tray with a small amount of oil, arrange potatoes in a thin layer, and bake them for thirty minutes, turning them once during cooking.

Pumpkin

Pumpkin helps to prevent cancers, cataracts, and arteriosclerosis. It helps the body to fight infection and maintain fluid balance; protects against heart disease and cancer; and regulates blood pressure. The seeds are high in protein and contain a significant amount of vitamin E, iron, and vitamin B_6. The flesh is the part most commonly eaten, but the seeds and flowers are edible also.

Key nutrients in pumpkin include calcium, iron, magnesium, phosphorus, potassium, sodium, zinc, copper, manganese, vitamin C, vitamin B_6, vitamin E, vitamin B_1 (thiamine), vitamin B_2 (riboflavin), vitamin B_3 (niacin), pantothenic acid, fiber, folate, and small amounts of lipids and amino acids. Phytochemicals include beta-carotene, alpha-carotene, lutein, monoterpenes, tocopherols, cryptoxanthin, ferulic acid, myristic acid, and phytic acid.

Look for pumpkins with a rich orange color that are free of blemishes or soft spots. The surface should be smooth and dull—a shiny rind indicates immaturity. The more mature a pumpkin is, the sweeter the meat. Pumpkins can be stored in a cool, dry place for up to one month. Refrigerating pumpkin hastens the ripening process and promotes deterioration.

To prepare fresh pumpkin, first rinse the outer shell to remove any mold and debris. Pierce the rind all the way through. Cut the pumpkin in half, then scoop out the seeds and any stringy fibers. Cut into smaller chunks and remove the rind from each chunk, then steam, boil, or purée. Or you can bake an entire pumpkin in the rind by cutting out a "lid" and, with a spoon, scooping out the seeds and fibrous membrane. Bake it at 350°F until tender. Also, wash the seeds to remove any trace of pulp or fiber. Allow them to dry thoroughly and bake them on a lightly oiled cookie sheet at 250°F for one hour.

Snow Peas and Sugar Snap Peas

Snow peas and sugar snap peas are harvested immaturely, so they do not have as high a protein content as green peas, but they contain twice as much vitamin C. They are a good source of iron, and because they are eaten in the pod, they provide a lot of insoluble fiber, which helps to prevent constipation. The entire pod is eaten.

Key nutrients in snow peas include calcium, iron, magnesium, phosphorus, potassium, sodium, zinc, copper, manganese, vitamin C, vitamin B_6, vitamin E, vitamin B_1 (thiamine), vitamin B_2 (riboflavin), vitamin B_3 (niacin), pantothenic acid, folate, pectin, and small amounts of lipids and amino acids. Phytochemicals include alpha-carotene, beta-carotene, daidzein, and chlorophyll.

Pods should be flat and glossy, with very slight protrusions where the peas are. They should be firm and bright green, with no signs of wilting or yellowing. Sugar snap peas are somewhat plumper than snow peas. Both varieties should be consumed within a day or two. Store them in perforated bags in the crisper compartment of the refrigerator.

To prepare the peas, wash them under cold running water. Sugar snap peas have a string that needs to be removed prior to cooking. Snap one end, then pull the string downward, snap the other end, then pull the string back up the other side. Cooking pod peas quickly preserves their flavor and crunchy texture. Use them in stir-fry dishes or steam them and serve as a side dish.

If you have a history of gout, you may want to limit your consumption of snow peas and sugar snap peas. Both contain purines, a compound that can cause a person with gout to suffer a flare-up.

Squash, Summer

Researchers at the National Institutes of Health have discovered compounds in the pulp and seeds of summer squash that can inhibit development of viruses and carcinogens in the intestinal tract, minimizing the risk of stomach cancer. Summer squash also strengthens immunity; helps prevent birth defects; fights depression; and cuts the risk of lung cancer. The parts eaten are the skin, meat, and seeds of the edible gourd.

The nutritional content of summer squash varies among the different species and depends on growing conditions, but in general, summer squash contains calcium, iron, magnesium, phosphorus, potassium, sodium, zinc, copper, manganese, vitamin C, vitamin B_6, vitamin B_1 (thiamine), vitamin B_2 (riboflavin), vitamin B_3 (niacin), pantothenic acid, fiber, folate, and small amounts of amino acids. Phytochemicals include beta-carotene, myristic acid, pectin, monoterpenes, and lutein.

Some varieties to choose from include zucchini, crookneck, yellow straightneck, chayote, and pattypan (also called cymling, sunburst, or scallop). Look for small, well-formed squash with a uniform, bright color. The surface should be free of nicks or blemishes and have a shiny appearance. Squash can grow quite large, but when it is allowed to do so, the skin is tough, the flesh stringy, and the seeds large and tough.

Summer squash can be stored for up to one week in sealed plastic bags in the crisper compartment of the refrigerator. Pattypan and chayote, which have a tougher skin, may keep a little longer.

The word *squash* is derived from several Native American words that, roughly translated, mean "something eaten raw." Raw squash is a tasty addition to salads, crudités platters, and slaw (grated). First wash squash with a vegetable brush and trim the ends. If the skin is tough, peel the squash using a vegetable peeler; however, the beta-carotene content is in the skin. Small squash can be steamed whole and served as a side dish. Its delicate, unassuming flavor makes it an ideal addition to casseroles and vegetable medley dishes. When cooking squash in other dishes, minimize water loss by lightly salting the squash prior to cooking, then allowing it to stand on paper towels for ten minutes before adding it to your recipe. Larger squash can be halved lengthwise and baked. Top them with brown sugar, herbs, or soymilk cheese. The meat can be scooped and mixed with grains then placed back in the hull.

Squash blossoms are edible and have a flavor similar to that of the squash. Most commonly, zucchini and yellow crookneck blossoms are eaten. The blossoms contain beta-carotene, potassium, and vitamin C. The raw blossoms are a stunning addition to salads or vegetable platters. You can also gently steam them or sautée them in a small amount of oil.

Squash, Winter

The deep-orange flesh of winter squash is loaded with beta-carotene—it is one of the best plant food sources of this nutrient, which is converted into vitamin A in the body. Winter squash may also minimize the risk of cataracts and help to preserve normal eyesight. Smokers and people who are regularly exposed to secondhand smoke may minimize their risk of lung cancer by including winter squash in their diet a couple of times a week. Winter squash can help ward off infections; protect against cancer, stroke, and heart disease; and maintain a proper fluid and electrolyte balance in the body. The part eaten is the meat of the edible gourd.

Key nutrients in winter squash include calcium, iron, magnesium, phosphorous, potassium, sodium, zinc, copper, manganese, vitamin C, vitamin B_6, vitamin B_1 (thiamine), vitamin B_2 (riboflavin), vitamin B_3 (niacin), pantothenic acid, and small amounts of lipids and amino acids. Phytochemicals include alpha-carotene, beta-carotene, and lutein.

Winter squash can grow quite large. Unlike summer squash, the longer it remains on the vine, the sweeter it becomes. Winter squash should be heavy, with smooth, dull rinds that are free of cuts or blemishes. It comes in an array of shapes and colors, with each variety offering a different flavor and texture.

It is unnecessary to refrigerate winter squash. It can keep for up to three months in a cool, dry place. The beta-carotene content increases while the squash is stored. Cut squash can be tightly wrapped and stored for a week in the refrigerator.

To prepare winter squash, rinse the squash under cool running water. Since winter squash has thick rinds and can be difficult to cut, use a meat cleaver or large chef's knife, depending on the size and variety. Squash can be cut into chunks, then peeled with a knife. It is not advisable to boil squash, but it can be steamed or baked. The chunks can be mashed like potatoes. Some varieties have very tough rinds and are easy to peel after cooking. Varieties such as banana and butternut can be cut into halves, the seeds and pulp removed, then baked and served in the rind. Butternut and acorn squash can also be stuffed with a grain or with seasoned bread crumbs prior to baking. Winter squash can also be substituted for pumpkin in pie, bread, or soup recipes. Spaghetti squash can be cooked whole, or cut in half lengthwise and steamed, cut side up. After cooking, remove the seeds and pulp and, using a fork, scrape the sides. The flesh will separate into strands that are similar to pasta. Serve it with a tomato sauce or toss them with other vegetables, fresh herbs, and vinaigrette dressing.

Sweet Potatoes

Sweet potatoes are a "power food" with many therapeutic properties, including high fiber. They are lower in carbohydrates than white potatoes. They contribute to healthy gums and strong connective tissue, and help to promote rapid healing of wounds. They reduce the risk of cancer and osteoporosis, promote bone and tooth development, and help the body release energy from nutrients ingested. They also help to lower cholesterol levels and protect against heart disease and disease-producing viruses. Some research has indicated that sweet potatoes may increase the likelihood of having twins. Sweet potatoes contain high levels of hormonelike agents that stimulate the production of a follicle-stimulating hormone (FSH). FSH stimulates the ovaries to produce more than one ovum (egg), thereby increasing the likelihood of a double conception. Sweet potatoes are high in carbohydrates that initiate production of the brain chemical serotonin. Serotonin helps fight depression. Sweet potatoes and yams are not the same vegetable—in fact, in botanical terms, they are not even distantly related. The part eaten is the tuber.

Key nutrients in sweet potatoes include calcium, magnesium, phosphorus, potassium, sodium, zinc, copper, manganese, vitamin C, vitamin B_6, vitamin E, vitamin B_1 (thiamine), vitamin B_2 (riboflavin), vitamin B_3 (niacin), pantothenic acid, fiber, folate, and small amounts of lipids and amino acids. Phytochemicals include beta-carotene,

caffeic acid, chlorogenic acid, isoquercitrin, pectin, polyphenols, protease inhibitors, quercetin, squalene, and tocopherols.

Choose firm, smooth, unblemished sweet potatoes. Avoid any that have shriveled or have soft spots. Store them in a cool, dry, well-ventilated place for up to three weeks. If refrigerated, they lose their taste.

To prepare a sweet potato, thoroughly scrub it with a vegetable brush. Prick the potato in several spots with a knife and bake on a cookie sheet. Try seasoning sweet potatoes with apple or orange juice, cinnamon, nutmeg, or honey rather than with butter. Sweet potatoes can be used in any recipe that calls for a white potato.

Tomatoes

Tomatoes help the body to resist infection and fight cancer. Lycopene, a phytochemical in tomatoes, has potent anti-cancer properties. It is plentiful in raw tomatoes, but not all of it is available to the body unless the tomatoes have been cooked. Heat breaks down the tomato's cell walls, releasing the lycopene. Cooked tomato products such as tomato sauce, pasta sauce, and ketchup are good sources of lycopene. Lycopene is absent, however, in green and yellow tomatoes. Tomatoes also can help to lower blood pressure, aid in cleansing toxins, and benefit the kidneys. Studies have also shown that tomatoes can offer protection against acute appendicitis and digestive disorders. The part eaten is the fruit. Sun-dried tomatoes have excellent flavor but are not as nutritious as fresh tomatoes.

Key nutrients in tomatoes include calcium, magnesium, phosphorus, potassium, sodium, zinc, iron, copper, manganese, vitamin C, vitamin B_6, vitamin K, vitamin E, vitamin B_1 (thiamine), vitamin B_2 (riboflavin), vitamin B_3 (niacin), pantothenic acid, fiber, folate, and small amounts of lipids and amino acids. Phytochemicals include alpha-lipoic acid, beta-carotene, beta-sitosterol, caffeic acid, chlorophyll, eugenol, ferulic acid, lycopene, P-coumaric acid, curcumin, kaempferol, myristic acid, naringenin, pectin, ferulic acid, ellagic acid, tocopherols, tocotrienols, phenol, quercetin, quercitrin, rutin, squalene, stigmasterol, and chlorogenic acid.

Tomatoes are one of the most consumed vegetables in the United States. Due to the incredible demand for tomatoes, modern agribusiness farmers have developed tomatoes with thicker skins that can be picked green and then ripened by external application of ethylene gas. Ethylene gas is formed internally in many fruits and vegetables when they are allowed to ripen naturally. External application of this gas doesn't necessarily destroy its nutritional value, but it does affect the texture and flavor. When purchasing tomatoes, choose plump ones that are free of bruises or soft spots. Tomatoes should be firm with taut, shiny skins and free of cracks. Fresh tomatoes, even unripe green ones, will have a distinct fragrance. Tomatoes that have been gassed to ripen will never have an odor, except when they begin to rot. Never buy tomatoes from a refrigerated case. Exposure to lower temperatures (below 55°F) prevent tomatoes from ever being able to ripen. Sun-dried tomatoes, which are dehydrated, are often sold packed in oil that can add unnecessary fat and calories to your diet. Look for sun-dried tomatoes in the dehydrated form and reconstitute them yourself by soaking in boiling water.

If tomatoes are not quite ripe, hasten the ripening process by placing them in a brown paper bag. Adding a banana will accelerate the process even more, since the banana will emit ethylene gas. Placing tomatoes in a sunny window will cause uneven ripening. A ripe tomato will keep at room temperature for two to three days. Once ripe, tomatoes can be stored in the refrigerator for another day or two. For maximum flavor, allow tomatoes that have been refrigerated to come to room temperature before serving them.

To prepare tomatoes, wash them in cool water. When slicing a tomato for a sandwich or salad, place it upright and cut from top to bottom—the slices will keep their juice better than ones cut from side to side. Tomatoes can be baked, broiled, stewed, or sautéed. If you plan to cook tomatoes and do not want to include the skins in your recipe, freeze the whole tomatoes first. The skins will slip off easily when the tomatoes are defrosted.

Consider growing your own tomatoes. They are one of the easiest vegetables to cultivate at home. With thousands of varieties to choose from, even the novice gardener can grow tomatoes. At the very least, tomatoes can be grown in a container in a sunny window. If you have arthritis, you should eat tomatoes in moderation or eliminate them from your diet.

NIGHTSHADE VEGETABLES: TOMATOES, POTATOES, EGGPLANT, AND PEPPERS

One class of vegetables that deserves a bit of special attention is the nightshade vegetables. Originally cultivated in South America, the nightshade vegetables were discovered by Spanish explorers and brought to Europe and Asia as seeds gathered in Mexico and Columbia. Their name supposedly comes from the fact that they grow at night, unlike mushrooms or other fungi that grow in the shade. These vegetables belong to the *Solanaceae* family, which comprises 92 genera with more than 2,000 species. Members of this family include tobacco, henbane, mandrake, and belladonna, a deadly nightshade. Edible nightshades include tomatoes, potatoes, eggplant, aubergines, and a majority of popular peppers (green, red, chili, paprika, cayenne, hot, and sweet), with the exceptions of black and white pepper.

Nightshade vegetables contain high levels of glycoalkaloids—specifically, solanine in potatoes and eggplants, and tomatine in tomatoes. These levels seem to decline as the vegetable ripens; however, a noticeable amount remains. Some edible nightshades have even been found with consistent amounts of nicotine, depending on how ripe they

are. Solanine levels can increase dramatically if a potato is stored improperly (subjected to too much light and heat). At certain levels, glycoalkaloids can be toxic and cause gastrointestinal inflammation, nausea, diarrhea, dizziness, and other symptoms severe enough to require hospitalization.

Arthritis and Nightshades

A less ominous yet farther-reaching effect of these glycoalkaloids is that they apparently can disrupt the metabolization of calcium in the body. Ironically, nightshade vegetables are quite often consumed with high-calcium foods such as cream or cheese—as in eggplant parmigiana, potatoes and sour cream, or tomatoes and cheeses of all kinds. They may block valuable calcium from assimilating and therefore deplete already low calcium levels in people with arthritis. If you eat a low-fat diet or do not consume dairy foods, it is a good idea to limit your consumption of nightshade vegetables.

Norman F. Childers, a former professor of horticulture at Rutgers University in New Jersey, had arthritis and noticed increased joint pain and stiffness after consuming any type of tomatoes. He was already aware of the potential toxicity of nightshade plants. After observing livestock eating weeds containing solanine and consequently kneeling, apparently due to joint pain, Dr. Childers decided to test nightshade vegetables one at a time. Months later, after he had eliminated all nightshade vegetables from his diet, he reported that his arthritis pain had subsided. Dr. Childers eventually concluded that people sensitive to nightshade vegetables could cure arthritic aches and pains simply by avoiding nightshades. Childers, who has worked with solanaceous plants all his life, concluded, "Regular consumption of tomatoes, potatoes and eggplants is a primary cause of arthritis."

Green Spots on Potatoes

In *Unsafe at Any Meal* (McGraw-Hill, 2002), Dr. Earl Mindell speaks about the issue of solanine content of potatoes, especially potatoes with green patches or sprouting eyes. Although the green referred to is probably harmless chlorophyll, it denotes the youth, or lack of ripening, of the potato and hence, high solanine levels. Mindell writes, "Solanine, present in and around these green patches and in the eyes which have sprouted, can interfere with the transmission of nerve impulses, and can cause jaundice, abdominal pain, vomiting, and diarrhea."

Good News about Nightshades

The glycoalkaloids found in nightshade vegetables have a prohibitive effect on the assimilation of milk products. Cow's milk, for example, can have as much as four times the amount of calcium as human mother's milk. This can wreak havoc on the digestive system. When nightshades are consumed with calcium-rich diets, they can keep calcium from being deposited in the wrong places. The Agricultural Service of the U.S. Department of Agriculture (USDA) is currently working on a new method of testing glycoalkaloid levels in nightshade vegetables, and is also testing a method that drastically lowers solanine levels in potatoes.

FOR A DIFFERENT TASTE . . .

In addition to all the familiar vegetables discussed above, many "new" vegetables are becoming available in specialty food stores and many supermarkets. Try sampling some of these unique vegetables.

Chayote

An important food in tropical regions, chayote is a variety of summer squash with pale-green skin and deep ridges. It contains a single edible seed and can vary in size from several ounces up to 2 pounds. Chayote takes longer to cook than other squashes, and it can be served fried, boiled, baked, mashed, pickled, or steamed. Its flavor has hints of cucumber and apple.

Key nutrients in chayote include calcium, magnesium, phosphorus, potassium, zinc, copper, manganese, vitamin C, vitamin A, folate, and fiber. Phytochemicals include beta-carotene.

Hearts of Palm

A dieter's dream, hearts of palm contain only 21 calories per cup. What other food can compare? Hearts of palm are very rich in vitamin A. With their delicate flavor, they can be added to countless dishes, seafood, soups, gumbos, and salads.

In the United States, this delicate vegetable comes from palmetto trees grown in Florida. Some species of South American palms also produce edible hearts. As they are rarely sold fresh (they perish very quickly), it is more likely you may find canned hearts of palm in stores. The canned hearts are ivory-colored cylinders of smooth layered flesh. Rinse them after opening the can, then slice them and add them to salads.

Key nutrients in hearts of palm include calcium, iron, magnesium, phosphorus, potassium, zinc, copper, manganese, selenium, vitamin C, vitamin B$_3$ (niacin), folate, and fiber.

Jicama

Also known as Mexican potato, jicama (HEE-kah-mah) is a large root vegetable resembling a turnip. It has a thin brown skin and white flesh that is similar to the radish. Three-quarters of a cup of sliced jicama has 41 calories and supplies 175 milligrams of potassium and meets 33 percent of the recommended dietary allowance (RDA) of vitamin C. Jicama has anticoagulant properties that were first reported as a result of the substitution of *sar quort* (another name for jicama) for water chestnuts in a Chinese recipe.

Jicama should be peeled and sliced; it has a sweet, nutty, crunchy flavor and can be eaten raw or cooked. Try it in stir-fry dishes. Or you can use it in place of potatoes—it is less starchy and has fewer calories. Its texture is similar to that of water chestnut.

Key nutrients in jicama include calcium, iron, magnesium, phosphorus, potassium, zinc, copper, manganese, selenium, vitamin C, vitamin A, vitamin E, folate, and fiber.

North American Indian Groundnut

This is a tuber that has three times the protein of potatoes and is thought to contain anticancer agents. It is edible when cooked. It can also be made into flour and used in bread or fried into hash browns.

Nuna

Nuna is also called pop beans because it puffs and bursts in half when heated. It is higher in protein and fiber than popcorn. Nuna is grown in the Andes of Peru and Bolivia, and, unfortunately, is not easy to find in the United States at the present time, but this may change in coming years.

Plantain

Plantains look like bananas but are very different. Though a fruit, plaintain is too starchy to be eaten raw and is used more like a vegetable—it is generally served fried, baked, mashed, sautéed, or stuffed. Plantains have higher amounts of vitamin A and potassium than bananas, but are similar in their low-fat and sodium content. They are also high in fiber.

Plantains can be used at each stage of ripeness, and have distinct flavors—and skin colors—as they mature. The skin of fully ripe plantain is entirely black. For a tasty side dish, slice plantain and sauté it in garlic oil. Before serving, add a dash of cinnamon, ginger, Herbamare seasoning, or sea salt. Plantain is also good sliced on top of fish before cooking.

Key nutrients in plantain include calcium, magnesium, phosphorus, potassium, vitamin C, vitamin A, folate, and fiber. Important phytochemicals include beta-carotene and phytosterols.

Taro Root

Taro is a starchy tropical tuber with a stringy skin and off-white or light-purple flesh. It is most familiar as the main ingredient in poi, a native Hawaiian dish that consists of cooked taro root that has been pounded to a paste and mixed with water. Raw taro has a bitter taste; however, cooking gives it a nutty flavor. It tastes like a combination of potato and water chestnut. One cup has 107 calories and supplies 591 milligrams of potassium. Taro is very easy to digest and can be boiled, baked, or steamed. It can also be used to thicken stews and soups.

Key nutrients in taro include calcium, magnesium, phosphorus, potassium, vitamin C, folate, and fiber. Phytochemicals include phytosterols and saponin.

Tepary Beans

These North American beans are white and golden brown. They are only about half the size of navy beans, although they are much higher in fiber and protein, and are thought to contain a substance that controls blood sugar. Tepary beans make a delicious, rich, nutty-flavored soup.

Winged Beans

This tropical legume from Southeast Asia is unique in that it is entirely edible—and its shoots, flowers, seeds, green pods, leaves, and tuberous roots are high in protein, fiber, and vitamins. The pods grow up to ten-inches long. The seeds also produce edible oil. The immature pods can be eaten raw in salads or cooked like green beans. The roots are nutty-tasting tubers that can be peeled and eaten like potatoes—and contain four times the protein. The leaves of this plant are spinachlike, the pods are similar to green beans, and the tendrils resemble lacy asparagus. The unripe seeds can be eaten like peas. The seeds contain up to 42 percent protein, and their vitamin A content is one of the highest recorded. Look for winged beans in specialty produce markets (some supermarkets carry them also). Winged beans are also known as goa beans.

Key nutrients in the raw mature beans include calcium, iron, magnesium, phosphorus, potassium, zinc, copper, manganese, vitamin B_1 (thiamine), vitamin B_2 (riboflavin), vitamin B_3 (niacin), pantothenic acid, vitamin B_6, and folate. Phytochemicals include beta-carotene and myristic acid.

WAYS TO EAT SIX SERVINGS OF VEGETABLES AND FRUITS A DAY

People often look at the recommendation to eat at least six servings of vegetables and fruits each day and wonder how to do it. Following are some creative serving suggestions that may help you increase the amount of fruits and vegetables in your, and your family's, daily diet:

- Serve soup. Use vegetables and legumes as a base for soups or as additional ingredients.

- Thicken sauces without using fat. Substitute cooked and puréed vegetables for cream or whole milk.

Preserving Living Vegetables

Vegetables are living, breathing organisms. Once harvested, a vegetable draws from its nutrient content to continue to "breathe." The special plastic that precut vegetables are packaged in can slow down a vegetable's "respiration rate." This slower respiration rate results in a higher retention of nutrients.

When you purchase whole, unprocessed vegetables, you can use Evert-Fresh produce storage bags to extend the life of fresh produce and significantly reduce nutrient loss. These bags are made with a natural mineral that absorbs the ethylene that fruits and vegetables emit as they ripen, and that in turn hastens ripening.

- Be creative. Pasta and stir-fry dishes are ideal ways to incorporate lots of different vegetables into your meals while using small portions of meat.

- Enhance old standbys. Add fruit to hot or cold breakfast cereals. Also, add fruit or raw, grated vegetables such as carrots or zucchini to muffin and cookie recipes.

- Try different types of lettuce. Choose a wider variety of greens, including arugula, chicory, collards, dandelion greens, kale, mustard greens, spinach, and watercress.

- Steam vegetables and serve them over rice to create a beautiful, healthy meal. Most vegetables taste better and are much more nutritious when steamed.

GREEN POWER FOOD

Wheatgrass, barley grass, and spirulina, often referred to as *green foods*, are excellent sources of beta-carotene, chlorophyll, and minerals. They are good for helping to treat all colon disorders, HIV/AIDS, cancer, and virtually every other type of illnesses. Wheatgrass is best when juiced fresh and combined with other vegetables. Barley grass is available in a powdered form that can be added to quality water. Spirulina is high in protein, beta-carotene, gamma-linolenic acid (GLA), and nutrients essential for the formation of hormones. It is good for vegetarians because it is one of the few available vegetable sources of vitamin B_{12}, which is lacking in most vegetarians' diets. It is also rich in calcium, iron, RNA, DNA, and trace minerals.

A Japanese study detailed the effects of adding spirulina to the diet of rats with serum cholesterol problems induced by a high-fructose diet, which increases the level of cholesterol and triglycerides in the blood. When spirulina was added to the diet, levels of both cholesterol and triglycerides were consistently reduced. Kazuko Iwata and colleagues at the Kagawa Nutrition College in Japan found that including spirulina in the diet increased the activity of the enzyme lipoprotein lipase, which is involved in fat metabolism.

Wheatgrass, barley grass, and spirulina will be vital foods of the future. They contain everything that is currently known to build a healthy immune system. All are available in powdered and tablet forms *now*!

VEGETABLE RECIPES

APPLE YAM DELIGHT

16 ounces yams or sweet potatoes
¾ cup instant rolled oats
¾ cup date raw sugar or other sweetener of choice
⅓ cup Hain's Soft Safflower Oil Margarine or other margarine of your choice
2 apples
½ cup barley malt powder or other powdered sweetener of your choice
1 teaspoon cinnamon
16 ounces chunky applesauce

1. Preheat the oven to 350°F.
2. Cut the sweet potatoes into bite-sized pieces.
3. Process the oats in blender to make oat flour. Combine oat flour and sugar, and cut in the margarine until crumbly.
4. Slice the apples and arrange half of the apple slices in an oiled 10-inch by 6-inch baking dish. Mix the cinnamon and barley malt and sprinkle half of it over the apple slices.
5. Add the sweet potatoes and applesauce in layers and sprinkle with the remaining cinnamon-sugar mixture. Top with the oat, sugar, and margarine mixture.
6. Bake for forty-five minutes. Serve warm.

Variation: Omit the barley malt and cinnamon and substitute ¼ to ½ cup pure maple syrup. Top with chopped nuts.

SPINACH OR BROCCOLI BAKE

2 cups mashed tofu or low-fat cottage cheese or ricotta cheese
2 green peppers, chopped
1 cup cooked brown rice
1 1-pound package spinach, raw or fresh-steamed and patted dry, and/or raw broccoli
1½ teaspoons sea salt
½ teaspoon granulated or powdered garlic
1 dash cayenne pepper
½ cup chopped raw almonds
2 cups grated cheese of your choice

1. Preheat the oven to 350°F.
2. Combine the first seven ingredients, mix well, and place them in a medium baking dish. Top with the almonds and cheese.
3. Bake for thirty to forty-five minutes. Serve hot.

Variation: If you wish to add meat to this dish, add ½ to 1 pound broiled boneless chicken chunks to the ingredients in step 2.

ALMOND CREAM GREEN BEANS

1 pound fresh, frozen, or home-jarred green beans
½ teaspoon sea salt
½ cup almonds, slivered or in large pieces
3 tablespoons expeller-pressed vegetable oil
2 teaspoons oat or whole-wheat flour
½ plain yogurt, sour cream, or mashed tofu
1 dash cayenne pepper

1. Clean the beans and place them in a saucepan with just enough water to cover. Add the sea salt. Bring the pot to simmering temperature, and allow the beans to simmer for fifteen minutes. Drain.
2. Sauté the almonds in 1 tablespoon of the oil until they are lightly browned, and remove them from the pan.
3. Add the rest of the oil to pan, add the flour, and cook over medium heat, stirring constantly, until thickened and well blended. Add the yogurt, mix until smooth, and continue cooking until the mixture is thickened.
4. Add the drained beans and half of the almonds, season with cayenne pepper, and allow to cook briefly to make sure the beans are heated through. Top with the rest of the almonds. Serve warm.

Variation: If you prefer, you can substitute onions for the almonds.

24-HOUR CABBAGE SLAW

½ medium cabbage
1 small halved sweet or red onion
½ medium green pepper
2 carrots
½ teaspoon Italian seasoning
⅔ cup apple cider vinegar
⅓ cup vegetable oil
1 dash barley malt sweetener
½ teaspoon sea salt (optional)

1. Slice the cabbage into wedges, finely chop the onion and pepper, and place them in a large mixing bowl.
2. Shred the carrots and add to the cabbage mixture.
3. Mix the remaining ingredients together and stir them into the cabbage mixture.
4. Refrigerate for at least eight hours before serving. (This can be made a day or two in advance.) At serving time, stir thoroughly and drain off excess liquid.

TOMATO SALSA

   3 medium vine-ripened tomatoes
   1 large clove garlic
   2 scallions
   ½ cup parsley
   ½ teaspoon sea salt (optional)

1. Dice or chop the tomatoes into small pieces and place in a medium mixing bowl.
2. Finely mince the garlic and chop the scallions and parsley into small pieces and add them to the tomatoes.
3. If desired, season with sea salt.
4. Mix all the ingredients together. Serve as a side dish; spoon over rice or pasta; or use as a dip with tortilla chips or as a dressing for salads.

TOFU AND BROCCOLI IN GARLIC SAUCE

   2 pounds tofu
   ½ cup tamari or soy sauce
   2 cups water
   2 cubes vegetable bouillon or 1 tablespoon miso
   4 tablespoons olive oil
   ½ cup chopped onions
   ½ pound fresh sliced mushrooms
   3 cloves garlic, crushed
   1 tablespoon prepared mustard
   3 tablespoons honey
   ½ sweet red pepper, chopped
   ¼ teaspoon ginger or 1 teaspoon fresh ginger, peeled and grated
   1 pound broccoli florets

1. Cube the tofu and marinate it in the tamari sauce for two hours or overnight, turning occasionally.
2. Boil the water, add the bouillon, and set aside.
3. Drain the tofu, reserving the marinade. Over medium heat, brown both sides of the tofu in 3 tablespoons of olive oil. Remove from the pan.
4. Sauté onions and mushrooms in 1 tablespoon olive oil until soft. Stir together the garlic, bouillon-water mixture, mustard, honey, red pepper, and ginger. Add to the sautéed vegetables.
5. Add the tofu and the reserved marinade. Simmer over medium heat for one minute.
6. Add the broccoli and simmer for three more minutes. Remove from heat and let sit for five minutes before serving. Serve over brown rice or noodles.

CUCUMBER-TOMATO SALAD

   4 cups sliced cucumber
   3 cups sliced tomato
   1 cup sliced celery
   ½ large onion, sliced
   ½ cup chopped parsley or 1 tablespoon dried parsley

   ½ pound drained tofu, mashed
   3 tablespoon lime juice or lemon juice
   2 tablespoons olive oil
   1 teaspoon barley malt sweetener or sweetener of your choice
   1 clove minced garlic
   1 dash of sea salt (optional)
   ¼ teaspoon cayenne pepper (optional)

1. Mix together the cucumber, tomato, celery, onion, and parsley in a large mixing bowl.
2. In a separate bowl, mix together the mashed tofu, lime juice, olive oil, barley malt, garlic, and, if desired, sea salt and cayenne pepper. Blend the dressing together until smooth.
3. Add the dressing to the vegetables and toss to blend flavors. Serve chilled over lettuce leaves.

CAULIFLOWER CASSEROLE

   3 scallions, with tops, chopped
   2 cloves garlic, minced, or 1 teaspoon garlic powder
   1 teaspoon expeller-pressed vegetable oil
   1 cup soymilk or other milk of your choice
   ½ cup plain yogurt or sour cream
   1 package dry cheese soup mix of your choice
   2 tablespoons chopped or dried parsley (optional)
   1 teaspoon sea salt (optional)
   1 dash cayenne pepper (optional)
   1 cup shredded soy cheese or other cheese of your choice
   1 large head cauliflower, broken into large florets
   ¾ cup crackers or bread crumbs

1. Preheat the oven to 350°F.
2. Sauté the scallions and garlic in the oil over high heat, just until scallions are tender.
3. Add the milk, yogurt, and soup mix, stirring constantly. Add the parsley, sea salt, and cayenne pepper, if desired. Add the cheese. Stir until the cheese melts, then remove from heat.
4. Place the cauliflower in well-oiled casserole dish. Pour the sauce over the cauliflower and top with crackers or bread crumbs. Cover the dish and bake for twenty minutes.
5. Uncover and bake until golden brown, about ten minutes more. Serve hot.

Variation: If desired, spread tomato slices over the top of the casserole before topping with the crackers or bread crumbs.

ANTICANCER ROOT SALAD

   2 small beets, washed
   3 radishes, diced
   2 turnips, diced
   1 parsnip, diced

1 cup shredded cabbage
1 onion, minced
2 cloves garlic, minced
2 tablespoons apple cider vinegar
1 tablespoon olive oil
2 tablespoons fresh thyme
½–1 teaspoon grated fresh horseradish
1 dash cayenne pepper (optional)
¼ cup minced fresh parsley

1. Place the beets in a pan with enough water to cover and bring to a boil over high heat. Reduce heat and cook for thirty minutes. Remove from heat, drain, and allow to cool. Peel and dice the beets after they have cooled down.

2. While the beets are cooking, steam or boil the radishes, turnips, parsnip, and cabbage in another pan until tender.

3. When all the vegetables are cooked and cooled, mix them together in a large mixing bowl.

4. Mix together the onion, garlic, vinegar, oil, thyme, horseradish, and cayenne pepper, if desired. Whisk into a creamy dressing.

5. Add the dressing to the vegetable salad and toss together. Top with parsley and serve.

CHAPTER TEN

SEA VEGETABLES: POWER-PACKED OCEAN FOODS

Some algae are a delicacy for the most honoured guests, even for the King himself.

—*Sze Teu, Chinese writer (c. 600)*

The world's oceans are a rich source of many nourishing sea vegetables that are high in essential minerals, trace minerals, chlorophyll, iodine, protein, essential fatty acids, calcium, and vitamins. More than 160 species of sea vegetables, commonly known as seaweed, are consumed throughout the world, particularly in Japan and China, where they have been a staple food for thousands of years. Dulse, edible seaweed, has supplemented diets in Scotland and Ireland for centuries. When we add the ocean's bounty to meals, we are tapping into nature's restorative source of all life.

Seaweed is the common term used for large marine algae growing in the shallow waters along ocean shores. They are plants, though less complex ones than land plants. Without roots or intricate tissues, seaweed must absorb nutrients from the water. To survive, they form rootlike parts in order to attach themselves to rocks or other stable items. Seaweeds are grouped into three types according to their characteristic color: brown, red, or green. Brown algae thrive in cooler water at depths of nearly 50 feet. This group includes kelp, whose length can be as much as 1,500 feet. Red algae, such as dulse, have compounds with the ability to gel foods. Green algae are the bridge between land and sea plants, as evidenced by their ability to store food as starch the same as land plants. Of the green algae, nori is the most popular. Brown and red algae grow almost exclusively in seawater, whereas green algae also thrive in freshwater ponds and lakes.

The most commonly consumed seaweeds, which grow in both the Atlantic and Pacific oceans, are alaria, arame, hijiki, nori, dulse, and several kinds of kelp.

SEAWEED NUTRITION

Seaweed is a remarkable dietary staple for many reasons. No other type of food is as rich a source of the minerals essential to maintaining and improving one's health as sea-

weed. Collectively, seaweeds have all fifty-six minerals and trace minerals deemed necessary for the human body. One-half cup of cooked hijiki has as much calcium as one cup of milk and more iron than two eggs. Seaweed is high in protein and dietary fiber, low in calories, and naturally fat-free. Additionally, it has significant amounts of calcium, iron, potassium, phosphorus, magnesium, zinc, iodine, and the vitamins A, C, E, and K, and the B-complex vitamins, including vitamin B_{12}, which is rare in plant foods. Seaweed has natural sugars, such as mannitol, and natural glutamic acid, which enhances flavor. Important phytochemicals in seaweed include carotenoids.

MEDICINAL USES OF SEA VEGETABLES

Through traditional use in Oriental medicine and in research studies, seaweed is known to strengthen immune function; reduce cholesterol; have antiviral and antibacterial actions; lower blood pressure; have anticoagulant properties; and improve metabolism and digestion.

The darker sea vegetables, such as arame, wakame, hijiki, and varieties of kelp, contain sodium alginate, which converts heavy metals in the body into a harmless salt that is easily excreted. Research at Canada's McGill University found that the dark sea vegetables also can remove radioactive strontium from the body.

The *Canadian Medical Association Journal* reported the importance of different marine algae in preventing the body's absorption of radioactive products, and in their use as possible natural decontaminates. Additional studies show that seaweed's natural iodine can lower the amount of radioactive iodine absorbed by the thyroid by as much as 80 percent.

Seaweed contains calcium phosphate, which helps to stave off osteoporosis by nourishing the bones. Calcium, as well as iodine and sodium alginate, in seaweed also serve as buffers against cancer. Seaweed may be an important

Iodine in the Diet

The overuse of commercial iodized table salt can lead to excess iodine in the system. High iodine intake may actually impair thyroid function. Early symptoms of excess iodine include rough skin, hyperactivity, mental and emotional imbalances, and poor concentration.

Unlike iodized salt, the natural iodine in sea vegetables is balanced with many other nutrients, which most Americans need, plus the vitamin B_{12} vegetarians need.

Be aware that there is a difference between eating sea vegetables and taking iodine supplements. While sea vegetables can be eaten as frequently as desired, supplement intake should be carefully monitored.

factor in the low rates of certain cancers in Japan. Japanese scientists found several varieties of kelp to be effective in the treatment of tumors. Researchers at Harvard University Medical Center reported that eating a diet consisting of 5 percent kelp significantly delayed the onset of breast cancer in animals. Other laboratory studies in which sea vegetables were used in the treatment regimen for leukemia have shown great promise. Extracts from two red algae have been found to inhibit the herpes simplex virus. (These have not been tested on humans, however.) Statistically, according to Canadian researcher Zoltan Rona, M.D., supplementing with sea vegetables may be a very effective form of breast cancer prevention. An association has been made between low thyroid function and breast cancer; as a source of iodine and other trace minerals, sea vegetables provide optimal nutrition for the thyroid gland.

The high content of potassium in seaweed is good for the heart and kidneys. The iodine in seaweed aids in weight loss also. Seaweed nourishes membranes, making it good for nervous disorders, skin conditions, colds, and constipation. It is high in chromium, which helps to control blood sugar levels.

COOKING WITH SEA VEGETABLES

The balanced combination of minerals in sea vegetables rounds out the flavor of foods. They lend a saltiness without the high sodium of table salt, and have a range of tastes from mild to a deep-sea pungency. Experiment with different varieties and start with small amounts in foods until you get used to the taste. Seaweed can be used in dried form as a condiment, eaten as a snack, or added to soup, salads, stews, and grain dishes—even desserts. To make beans more digestible and less "gassy," add seaweed during cooking.

To rehydrate dried seaweed, immerse it in water for a few minutes until soft. Remember that most seaweed varieties expand to many times their original volume in liquid, so small amounts go a long way.

Seaweed is available in health food stores in dried, powder, flake, and granule forms. Organic seaweed products are available also from companies such as Maine Coast Sea Vegetables, who also make Sea Pickles from fresh, undried kelp.

SEAWEED VARIETIES

Each sea spawns its own diverse vegetables that vary in taste, nutritional content, and healing properties from those found or grown elsewhere. Try a small amount of each of the following varieties until you find one that pleases your palate or fills a specific dietary need.

Alaria

Alaria, harvested in North America, is nearly identical to the Japanese seaweed wakame, though it has a more delicate taste. It also requires a longer cooking time—at least twenty minutes in soups or stews. After a brief soaking, alaria can be eaten uncooked in salads. It is rich in vitamin A, the B vitamins, and calcium.

Arame

A dark, nearly black seaweed with a stringy texture, arame has a mild taste and aroma. Before it is ready to be sold, arame must be cooked for seven hours, then dried in the sun. It can be served as a side dish or tossed with pasta, salads, and stir-fry dishes. When cooking arame, soak it for ten minutes, then simmer until tender. It has high amounts of calcium, potassium, iron, and vitamin A and B vitamins.

Dulse

Dulse is a native sea vegetable harvested in the North Atlantic and Pacific Northwest. It is little known in Asia. Dulse has a strong, distinctive flavor and chewy texture. It can be eaten as a snack directly from the bag. Use dulse in a variety of ways: in soups, stews, casseroles, salads, and sandwiches. You also can pan-fry it on medium heat or roast in the oven at 250°F until crisp, then crumble it over pastas, pizza, soups, and salads. Dulse is rich in protein, potassium, iron, and vitamin K, which is necessary for blood clotting.

Hijiki

A brown alga harvested primarily in Japan, hijiki has a slight licorice flavor. When dried, it is black and brittle. It cooks to a firm texture and expands five to six times its original size. Use it as any other vegetable in soups, casseroles, and stews. Hijiki has the highest amount of calcium of all the sea vegetables—1,400 milligrams per 3.5-ounce serving. Its potassium content is remarkably high, too, at 14,700 milligrams for each 3.5 ounces. It is a mineral-rich, high-fiber seaweed, high in vitamin A and carotenes.

Kelp

Kelp is the generic name for edible species of flat, leaflike brown algae belonging to the *Laminariaceae* family. These various species of kelp are known by different names: *kombu* (also *konbu*) and *wakame* in Japan; *haidai* and *qundai-cai* in China; and simply *kelp* in the United States.

Kelp contains vitamins A, D, E, and K, is a main source of vitamin C, and is very rich in minerals. Algin, agar, and carrageenan are kelp gels that revitalize gastrointestinal health and aid digestion. It is a demulcent and can help ease herpes outbreaks.

Kombu (*Laminaria*) has been cultivated in Japanese waters since 1730 and is considered to have great nutritional healing value. It is cooked with fish and meat dishes, served as a vegetable with rice and used as the basis of dashi, a flavorful soup stock. It is a meaty, high-protein food. Kombu has ample amounts of calcium, iron, potassium, and vitamins A and K. Kombu is also a decongestant for excess mucus, helps to lower blood pressure, and contains a powerful skin-healing nutrient, germanium.

Wakame (*Undaria*) is used in soups and simmered dishes, toasted and crumbled as a condiment, and served with rice. It is nearly as high in calcium as hijiki and is rich in protein, iron, potassium, and vitamin K. Wakame boosts calcium uptake from the digestive tract and supports bone formation.

Edible kelp (*Laminaria longicruris*) native to Eastern United States coasts is similar to Japanese kombu in looks and taste, but unlike kombu, it is more tender, cooks quickly, and easily dissolves when cooked longer than twenty minutes in dishes such as soups, beans, and stew.

All kelp contains glutamic acid, which acts as a tenderizer when cooked with beans. Roast bite-sized pieces of kelp in light oil until they are crisp and greenish for delicious "chips." Or dry-roast it for flakes that can be sprinkled on a variety of dishes. Granulated or powdered kelp can be used as a condiment or a flavoring. Kelp's natural saltiness makes it an excellent substitute for table salt. It can also be eaten raw. To tenderize or pickle kelp, marinate it in vinegar or tamari sauce. The white powder on the surface of kelp is a flavor component, not mold, and should not be wiped or washed off.

For its many health benefits, I recommend using kelp daily in small amounts in the diet. If you do not like the flavor of kelp, you can purchase it in tablet or liquid form at a health food store. Kelp is a chief source of iodine, which is essential for thyroid function. It has been used to treat arthritis and rheumatism, to aid digestion, and to stimulate the immune system.

Kelp also helps to reduce side effects from radiation and chemotherapy. When traveling by plane, take kelp beforehand to lessen the effects of radiation exposure that are inevitable with air travel. Kelp liquid, available from World Organics, is tasteless when a few drops are added to water.

Key nutrients in kelp include calcium, phosphorus, potassium, iodine, silicon, zinc, chromium, selenium, barium, B vitamins, and vitamins A, D, E, and K.

Nori

Nori is one of the most familiar sea vegetables because of its use in sushi as a wrap for rice balls and seafood. Nori ranges in color from dark green and purple to black. It comes in paper-thin sheets that can be lightly toasted and flaked to use as a garnish or seasoning on a wide assortment of dishes. It has a sweet, meaty taste when dried, and is higher in assimilable protein than any other sea plant.

Nori is exceptionally high in protein and vitamin A, and a rich source of B vitamins, vitamin C, vitamin E, vitamin K, iodine, and potassium.

Laver, another variety of nori (not sold in sheets), can be mixed with oats and fried into a flatbread. Laver bread is a traditional dish in Great Britain.

SEAWEED FOOD ADDITIVES

Seaweed-based food additives are used so often in fast food and processed food that if you live in North America or Europe you probably eat some every day. They are found in hamburgers, yogurt, and even strawberry ice cream. The following commonly used additives account for over $600 million of the $5 billion seaweed market.

Agar-Agar

Also called agar, kanten, and Japanese gelatin, this tasteless gelatin is extracted from several species of red seaweed. Agar-agar is used commercially and in the home as a thickener and setting agent. It can replace gelatin derived from animal protein. Because agar-agar does not need to boil to thicken, more nutrients are preserved. Agar-agar can be used in fruit pies, flavored gelatin, jellies, jams, and soups. It comes in flake, bar, and granulated forms. Use 2 tablespoons of flakes, 1 tablespoon of granulates, or seven inches of bar to 3 cups of liquid. Always soak the agar-agar in one cup of liquid for five minutes before adding the rest of the liquid. If it is not as thick as you like, remember that it thickens when it cools. Agar-agar adds fiber to the diet and helps to cleanse the digestive tract.

Alginic acid

Also called algin, alginic acid is a thick jellylike substance derived from several types of brown algae. It can absorb as much as 300 times its own weight in water. Alginic acid is used as a stabilizer and thickener in many processed foods, including ice creams, puddings, fruit drinks, salad dressings, and cheeses. It has the ability to draw harmful pollutants, such as lead, from the body.

Carrageenan

A gum extracted from certain species of red algae, carrageenan (also known as Irish moss) has thickening, gelling, and binding properties. It is used to stabilize emulsions in dairy products; to improve the quality of foods such as soups, salad dressings, sauces, and fruit drinks; and to give a creamy thick texture to milk products.

ON THE HORIZON

Sea-based products in medicine are rare, but some experts say the world's oceans and waterways may harbor the next generation of drugs, biologics, and even a few medical devices. Dozens of promising products, including a cancer therapy made from algae and a painkiller extracted from sea snails, are in development at research laboratories. Other products, such as an anti-inflammatory drug extracted from an organism called the Caribbean sea whip, are under review by the U.S. Food and Drug Administration (FDA). Researchers have identified nearly 4,000 compounds from sea plants and animals that have anti-inflammatory, antitumor, and antileukemia potential.

CHAPTER ELEVEN

GRAINS AND FLOURS: WHOLE-FOODS GOODNESS

Plant a kernel of wheat and you reap a pint; plant a pint and you reap a bushel. Always the law works to give you back more than you give.

—*Anthony Norvell, twentieth-century thinker and author*

Grains have been the staple food of many cultures for thousands of years for a good reason. Grains are loaded with protein, fiber, vitamins, and minerals. They are extremely versatile, relatively inexpensive, and easy to cook. Use them in soups, salads, side dishes, main dishes, and even desserts. Their nutty flavor and hearty texture make them a perfect base for breakfast cereals, pasta, and baked goods. Grains should be whole, and flours should be made from whole grains. The risk of diabetes, heart disease, stroke, and cancer can be reduced through the simple act of substituting whole grains for refined grains. Refined foods such as white flour and white rice are stripped of the fiber and nutrients that whole grains still possess. The first word on the label must be *whole*—don't be fooled by artificial brown or caramel coloring.

An array of uniquely different and interesting grain varieties, such as amaranth, quinoa, and spelt, have joined the familiar wheat, corn, and oats in health food store bins.

GRAIN GOODNESS

Grains are not all in the same botanical family. True grains, which include wheat, rice, oats, rye, millet, corn, triticale, and barley, belong to the grass family. Amaranth, quinoa, buckwheat, and others are in different families; however, all grain kernels have a similar makeup. The kernel consists of three parts:

- Bran. Bran enfolds and protects the kernel's inner layers. It is high in fiber, B vitamins, and zinc and other minerals. It is the top source of fiber.

- Endosperm. The endosperm is the largest part of each seed kernel, about 83 percent, and is made up mostly of starchy complex carbohydrates and protein. It nourishes the sprouted seed.

- Germ. Located at the kernel's base, the germ sprouts during germination, when the kernel is sown. Highly

nutritious, it is full of enzymes, protein, vitamins, minerals, and polyunsaturated fats. Wheat germ oil is rich in vitamin E. The germ is the only part that contains fat. The kernels of some grains are covered by an inedible protective covering called the hull, or husk.

Another thing grains have in common is the types of nutrients they supply; chief among them are fiber and complex carbohydrates.

Fiber

Whole grains provide both soluble and insoluble fiber. Insoluble fiber, concentrated in the bran, is typically removed in the milling process. Soluble fiber, in all grains, lowers blood cholesterol and is thought to reduce heart disease risk. Insoluble fiber prevents constipation and protects against certain cancers. It can aid in weight loss by giving the dieter a sense of being full with less food. (See Chapter 16.)

Carbohydrates

Grains are an excellent source of complex carbohydrates, which help curb the appetite. Carbohydrates are fuel for the body's vital energy needs. They provide energy in a time-release fashion to ensure a steady blood sugar level. Endurance athletes and bodybuilders often "stoke up" on complex carbohydrates—to fill up without filling out. High-carbohydrate foods are not fattening. Carbohydrates have less than half the calories found in fat. Research shows that women who eat carbohydrates recover more quickly from symptoms of premenstrual syndrome (PMS) than those who do not, and that carbohydrates, due to complex chemical reactions in the brain, act as a tranquilizer and are beneficial for people with seasonal adaptive disorder and depression.

Other Important Nutrients

In addition to fiber, carbohydrates, and high concentrations of protein, whole grains contain essential vitamins and minerals, including B vitamins (thiamine, riboflavin, and niacin), vitamin E, folate, calcium, selenium, iron, magnesium, and zinc. Grains also contain phytochemicals, the nonnutritive biochemistry to help to prevent disease. (See Chapter 7.) The main phytochemicals in whole grains are beta-glucans, lignin, tocotrienols, phytoestrogens, and phytic acid. They help to lower cholesterol and prevent cancer and heart disease.

Combined with legumes and vegetables, whole grains provide complete nourishment.

REFINED GRAINS

Since they were first cultivated, grains have been milled (refined) to make them easier to cook and digest. Milling is a mechanical process in which grinders and rollers remove the hull, bran, and germ, leaving only the endosperm. At this stage, the endosperm may be crushed into meal or flour, or cracked into small pieces for faster cooking. Refined grain products include flours, breads, and breakfast cereals.

Though refined grains remain fresh longer than unrefined ones, they also lose twenty-two essential nutrients in the process. For instance, white flour retains only 20 percent of the vitamins and minerals and 25 percent of the fiber contained in the whole-wheat kernel. For an illustration, of the effects of refining grain on the nutritive value of foods, see Table 11.1 below.

Today, most refined grain products are "enriched." That means they must meet standards set by the FDA for adding back the lost nutrients in amounts at or near the levels found in the original kernel.

TABLE 11.1 EFFECTS OF REFINING ON THE NUTRIENT CONTENT OF BREAD

The table below compares the nutrition offered by a slice of whole-wheat bread with that offered by a slice of white bread. It illustrates clearly that refining grains has a detrimental effect on nutrient levels.

NUTRIENT	WHOLE-WHEAT BREAD (1 SLICE)	WHITE BREAD (1 SLICE)
Calories	69	67
Dietary fiber	2 grams	0.6 grams
Vitamin B_2 (riboflavin)	0.06 milligrams	0.08 milligrams
Vitamin B_3 (niacin)	1.8 milligrams	1 milligram
Iron	0.9 milligrams	0.7 milligrams
Magnesium	24 milligrams	6 milligrams
Potassium	71 milligrams	30 milligrams

FLOUR

Typically, flour, a soft dry powder, is milled from grain; however, it can be made from seeds, fruits, and even vegetables and fish. Because milling removes moisture, flour generally has a higher concentration of calories than the raw material used to produce it. For instance, a pound of raw potatoes has 350 calories; a pound of potato flour has a whopping 1,600 calories. Virtually all wheat flour is refined (white) flour, which is made solely from the wheat kernel endosperm. Whole-wheat flour retains all three parts of the kernel, which are recombined after milling. White flour is available in many types, including the following:

- All-purpose flour. This is a blend of hard and soft wheat that is used mostly for breads, cakes, and pastries.

- Bleached flour. This is flour that has been treated with chemicals such as benzoyl peroxide or acetone peroxide to bleach it white.

- Bread flour. This is made from hard wheat only.

- Bromated flour. This is flour to which a maturing agent has been added to help make dough-kneading easier and to develop the gluten, a protein substance required to make bread and other baked goods rise.

- Cake flour. This is made from soft wheat only. It is finer textured than all-purpose flour.

- Durum flour. This is the highest in protein of any wheat flour. It is often used to make pasta.

- Graham flour. This is made from winter wheat. The kernel is ground to the consistency of refined flour, while the bran is left coarse and flaky. It is good for all baked goods. It was named after Sylvester Graham, a physician who rebelled against white bread, which he called, "even less than useless." Graham crackers also were named after him.

- High-gluten flour. This is flour from which the starch has been removed, leaving twice as much gluten as regular bread flour. Used as a strengthener in other flours that are low in gluten, it is high in protein.

- Semolina flour. This flour is refined from hard durum wheat. It is used especially in commercial pasta products.

- Self-rising flour. This type of flour is made from soft wheat. Salt, leavening, and an acid-releaser are added.

BUYING AND STORING GRAINS

Grains are available already boxed, in cellophane bags, or in bulk from bins. When buying prepackaged grains, make sure the package is tightly sealed. Check the freshness date also. When buying bulk grains, it is a good idea to shop at stores that have a high turnover to ensure the freshest supply. Rather than stocking up, buy small amounts often. It is important, too, that the bins be emptied before new stock is added. Grains should be dry, clean of debris and chaff, and fresh smelling. It is best to buy grains that have been refrigerated.

Though they have a comparatively long shelf life, whole grains can spoil. Their natural oils become rancid. Insects and mold can attack them also. Keep them in containers that can be closed tightly. If stored in a cool, dry place, they will keep for about a month. Grains stored in the refrigerator in moisture-proof containers have a longer life—up to five months. Most grains that are frozen will keep almost forever. Two exceptions, however, are oats and oat bran, whose high fat content makes them more apt to turn rancid after two or three months.

BUYING AND STORING FLOURS

Flour production is not standardized, so the same kind of flour from two different manufacturers may be made from different blends of wheat. This makes for varying results in the kitchen. The flours sold in the southern United States, for example, tend to contain more soft wheat, which is needed to produce the light biscuits favored there.

Most nonwheat flours can be found in health food or specialty stores. Because they contain little or no gluten, nonwheat flours have to be mixed with wheat flours to ensure that baked goods will rise. Some are sold premixed by the manufacturer. Or you can prepare a mixed flour at home by adding one part of nonwheat flour to four parts of wheat flour.

Flour that is not stored properly or kept too long may develop an unpleasant flavor as well as absorbing moisture. Also, whole-grain flours can turn rancid within weeks because of the fat in the germ. As with grains, flours should be stored in containers with tight-fitting lids and/or in the freezer to extend shelf lives.

When reading the labels on flours or products made from them, keep the following in mind:

- Ingredients are listed in order of quantity. Thus, there is more of the first item in the product than of those that come after.

- If wheat flour is listed first in the ingredients, it still may be mostly white flour, since the terms are used synonymously.

- When bread is labeled "white bread," it is made from refined flour.

- To qualify for the "whole-wheat" label, a product must be made from 100 percent whole-wheat flour, which contains the same proportion as in the original kernel.

- The FDA has not set regulations for use of the term "natural." However, many manufacturers use it to mean that preservatives were not used in the product.

- The term *unbleached* means the flour or grain was not chemically whitened.

Stone-ground grains are best. Because this process does not use heat, it leaves all the nutrients intact. Purchase only flours that meet this criteria, and buy them from a store that keeps grains refrigerated or in a freezer. Keep all whole-grain flours in the refrigerator.

Information about sources of uncommon kinds of grains and flours can be found in the Resources section.

TYPES OF GRAINS AND FLOURS

Many grains, although staples in other cultures, are not commonly used in the United States. Some of these grains are nutritionally equal and even superior to the everyday varieties Americans are accustomed to. The cost of introducing a new grain into your daily menus is relatively low, and you may even find that you prefer the taste.

Amaranth

Amaranth, also known as kiwicha, is high in protein, particularly the amino acid lysine, which is normally not found in plants. The seed resembles millet and is higher in nutrition than most other grains. It is frequently popped like popcorn and glued together with honey to create a bar that is eaten like a granola bar. This food is native to Central and South America.

A staple of the ancient Aztec culture, amaranth flour is milled from the seed of the amaranth plant. Though not technically a grain, flour made from this cereal-like herb can be used just like wheat flour: for cereals, in baking mixes, as a side dish, and for making crackers and flatbreads. It can also be added to soups, tabbouleh, and pilafs. It has a distinctive taste, so start with a small amount initially—⅓ cup of amaranth flour to 1 cup of whole wheat. To make a highly nutritious breakfast, stir ⅓ cup of amaranth flour into 1 cup of boiling water and cook for two to three minutes.

Key nutrients in amaranth include protein, calcium, fiber, lysine, B vitamins, methionine, magnesium, zinc, copper, and iron.

Barley

Barley has been used as far back as the Stone Age for everything from a type of currency to an ingredient in medicines. Add it to vegetable soups and stews, or use it in cereals and breads. Whole hulled barley, with only the outer husk removed, is the most nutritious.

Barley stimulates the liver and lymphatic system, enhancing the body's discharge of toxic waste. It helps suppress cholesterol in the liver. Beta-glucans in barley work with other soluble fibers to help prevent intestinal absorption of dietary fats and cholesterol. Containing both soluble and insoluble fiber, this grain aids bowel regularity. Barley broth is excellent for the ill and convalescing, as well as for those with heart problems. Potassium is abundant in unrefined barley. Mugi, a seasoning paste (miso) made from soy and a specific type of barley has been shown to reduce tumors and body fat. Barley is best purchased as "whole hulled," rather than pearled.

Key nutrients in barley include fiber, magnesium, manganese, vitamin E, the B-complex vitamins, zinc, copper, iron, calcium, protein, potassium, sulfur, and phosphorus. Phytochemicals include tocotrienols, lignin, and beta-glucans.

Buckwheat

Not really part of the wheat family, buckwheat is made from the seeds of a plant related to rhubarb. Kasha, or hulled, toasted buckwheat, has a nutty flavor and is popular as either whole groats or cracked. Used extensively in Slavic cooking, buckwheat can be enjoyed in pilafs, as a cereal side dish, or as fillings and hot porridge—or in the familiar pancake mix.

Its high rutin content makes buckwheat good for people with arteriosclerosis and for strengthening capillaries and reducing the risk of hemorrhage. (Rutin can also be purchased in pill form.) Buckwheat is a good blood builder and neutralizes acidic wastes. It is beneficial for the kidneys, helps to lower blood pressure, and reduces serum cholesterol.

Buckwheat is an excellent source of protein (missing in most grains except millet), fiber, B vitamins, potassium, lysine, phosphorus, vitamin E, calcium, and iron. Phytochemicals include rutin.

Bulgur Wheat

A staple throughout the Middle East, bulgur is produced by steaming, drying, and then cracking whole-wheat kernels. There is also a newer processing method, whirling, which removes the bran but retains essential nutrients. Precooked by steaming, bulgur can be soaked for thirty minutes and is ready to use in salads, pilafs, and sandwich fillings such as tabbouleh. It is also used in cereals, stews, soups, baked goods, and desserts.

Key nutrients in bulgur wheat include fiber, potassium, choline, B vitamins, iron, and calcium.

Corn

A Northern Hemisphere original and high in carbohydrates, corn has been a nourishing mainstay for thousands of years. Though usually thought of as a vegetable, the corn plant is in fact a grass, and the kernels are the grain. Cornmeal flour is the basis for traditional Southern breads, such as cornbread and corn pone. It can also be used as breading for baked fish and chicken. In the United States, corn (in the form of corn syrup) is used extensively as a sweetener, especially by beverage manufacturers.

Corn germ makes a great breading for chicken or fish. It is also good added to cereals and toppings. Nutrient-rich, it contains ten times more zinc than wheat germ and it has a longer shelf life.

Corn grits, or hominy, are another form of corn. The term *grits* refers to a processing method in which grains, particularly barley, buckwheat, brown rice, soy, wheat, and corn, are hulled and coarsely ground. Hominy is corn kernels hulled by a caustic solution, then washed. Grits are good as a cereal or side dish. They can be added to breads and also can be used to bread fish and chicken.

Though high in protein, corn itself is not an adequate protein source. It lacks two essential amino acids required to be a complete protein, which is why some food manufacturers fortify corn products with lysine and tryptophan. Replace these missing nutrients by eating corn with legumes or rice.

Key nutrients in corn include protein, fiber, vitamin A, B vitamins, vitamin C, calcium, folate, magnesium, phosphorus, potassium, and iron. Phytochemicals include alpha-carotene, phytosterols, phytic acid, and phytoestrogens.

Jerusalem Artichoke

Known also as the sunchoke, the Jerusalem artichoke is a tuberous vegetable of the sunflower family. Its underground stem, which resembles ginger root or a small knobby potato, can be dehydrated and ground into flour. Popular in pasta, Jerusalem artichoke flour has a slightly sweet and nutty flavor. It can be used in all baked goods (mix one part to nine parts of any other kind of flour), sprinkled over cereals and yogurt, or blended with fruit and vegetable juices. It adds low-calorie bulk that aids healthy digestion.

Jerusalem artichoke tubers contain the highest known *natural* level of fructooligosaccharides (FOS). (FOS can be made synthetically from sugar.) FOS, which cannot be digested by the human body, move to the colon where they feed beneficial bacteria. In turn, these "friendly" bacteria promote health by inhibiting the growth of toxic bacteria in the colon that have been linked with high blood pressure, elevated cholesterol levels, and even carcinogens. Jerusalem artichoke flour is also available in tablet form as a dietary supplement from several manufacturers, including Zumbro, Inc., whose tablets are made from organically grown whole Jerusalem artichoke tubers.

Key nutrients in Jerusalem artichoke flour include protein, fiber, calcium, vitamin A, vitamin C, vitamin B_3 (niacin), folate, iron, magnesium, potassium, and phosphorus.

Kamut

A relative of durum wheat, Kamut (pronounced ka-MOOT) is a reincarnation—and registered brand name—of an ancient Egyptian grain. Though it does contain gluten, clinical studies have shown that many people with wheat allergies are able to tolerate Kamut, which has 40 percent more protein than modern hybridized wheat. It has a higher nutrititive value and delivers more energy than other wheat products. Its protein is complete, as it contains all eight essential amino acids. Kamut's flavor is rich and buttery. Various Kamut products are available in health food stores, including cereal, pasta, flour, breads, and snacks. It also is used to make wheatgrass juice.

Key nutrients in Kamut include protein, fiber, calcium, iron, magnesium, phosphorus, potassium, B vitamins, vitamin E, and folate.

Millet

Except for quinoa and amaranth, millet has the most complete protein of any grain. It is a staple in China, India, and Africa, but in the United States it is used mainly as birdseed. The whole grain makes a good-tasting cereal. It can be added to breads and homemade granola, or ground into a flour or meal.

Less allergenic than wheat, millet is also naturally alkaline, which is beneficial to the spleen, pancreas, and stomach. It is good for people with acidosis, colitis, ulcers, and urinary disorders. Its significant amounts of iron, lecithin, and choline help keep cholesterol in check and stop the formation of certain types of gallstones.

Key nutrients in millet include protein, fiber, iron, magnesium, potassium, B vitamins, manganese, iron, phosphorus, and copper. Phytochemicals include lignin.

Oats

A great source of complex carbohydrates, oats are high in protein as well, containing twice as much as brown rice and one and a half times as much as bulgur wheat. Oats, the only grain almost always eaten in its whole form, contain the highest amount of fat of all grains, which warms the body and gives it stamina. Oats and oat flour are capable of normalizing blood glucose, a benefit to people with diabetes, and are good for those with a sluggish thyroid. Oat bran and oatmeal lower cholesterol and are high in fiber.

The different forms in which oats are available include steel-cut, rolled, bran, groats, flakes, flour, and instant. Oats retain more of their food value through processing than does wheat. Use oat flour in baking; it adds exceptional flavor to any bread recipe. Rolled or flaked oats require longer cooking time—around twenty to thirty minutes. Steel-cut oats, which are sliced, have the most nutrients left in the grain.

All types of oats are enjoyable as a hot breakfast cereal or as a cold cereal in granola and muesli. To make a good thickener in stews, soups, stuffing, and pancakes, cook 1 cup of steel-cut oats in 2 cups of water for thirty minutes.

Oat Milk from Nordic Farmers is a product available at many health food stores. A nondairy, vanilla-flavored drink, it is made from organic Swedish oats and can be used as a milk substitute.

Key nutrients in oats include protein, fiber, iron, manganese, phosphorus, calcium, B vitamins, and vitamin E. Phytochemicals include tocotrienols, beta-glucans, saponins, lignin, ferulic acid, and caffeic acid.

Potato

Potatoes are not a grain, but flour can be made from steamed and dried potatoes. One pound of potato flour equals five pounds of whole potatoes. Potato flour is used in baking and as a thickener and flavoring for soups. It is good in gravies, sauces, stews, muffins, and breads. For instant mashed potatoes, try the flour in flake form.

Key nutrients in potatoes include protein, fiber, vitamin B_6, vitamin C, potassium, copper, iron, magnesium, manganese, and vitamin B_3 (niacin).

Quinoa

Though an herb rather than a true grain, quinoa (pronounced either key-NOH-wah or KEEN-wah) has gained a reputation as a "super-grain" because of its high nutritional value. It provides all of the essential amino acids, including lysine, a scarce amino acid in vegetables, plus methionine and cystine in an almost perfect profile. These are especially important for vegetarians because most plant sources have inadequate amounts of these amino acids. Compared with other grains, it is not only high in protein but also in iron, vitamin B_3 (niacin), vitamin B_6 and phosphorus.

Quinoa was the principal fare of the ancient Incas, who referred to it as the Mother Grain and revered it as sacred. Today, most quinoa sold in the United States is imported from South America. Grown in thousands of varieties, its color can range from beige to black. Because it contains all essential amino acids, quinoa is considered a complete protein. With its light, delicate taste, quinoa works well as a substitute for most other grains. People who are allergic to various cereal grains usually can tolerate quinoa because it is gluten-free. A modern, highly nutritious convenient food, it is quick and easy to prepare as a side dish or hot cereal, or to use in pilafs, soups, salads, stews, and chili. It can also be made into flour that lends a nutty flavor to baked goods. For an unusual breakfast cereal or dessert, sweeten cooked quinoa with juice, fresh fruit, maple syrup, or sweet spices.

Each quinoa kernel is coated with saponin, a bitter compound that repels harmful insects and birds. Saponin is removed during processing. To make basic quinoa, cook it as you would rice.

Key nutrients in quinoa include protein, fiber, vitamin B_6, copper, folate, iron, magnesium, manganese, vitamin B_3 (niacin), phosphorus, potassium, vitamin B_2 (riboflavin), vitamin B_1 (thiamine), and zinc. Phytochemicals include saponins (when unwashed).

Rice

Rice is rich in complex carbohydrates yet low in fat and calories. Its protein is good quality, as it contains fairly high levels of the amino acid lysine. Like grain, when rice is milled, it loses important nutrients. In the United States, most white rice has been refined and then enriched with vitamin B$_1$ (thiamine), vitamin B$_3$ (niacin), and iron. In fact, all rice starts out brown; the milling process makes it white. Truly versatile, rice can be used as a side dish, as hot and cold breakfast cereal, and in salads, soups, and stews. Rice bran is a good bulking agent for baked foods.

Rice aids digestion and helps to reinstate normal bowel function after a bout with diarrhea. It also helps regulate glucose metabolism in people with diabetes. Rice bran helps to lower cholesterol, and some studies have shown it may help prevent bowel cancer. According to the *American Journal of Clinical Nutrition*, a study of women in southern China, where they eat a rice-based diet, found they had a lower risk for diabetes, obesity, high cholesterol, and heart disease than women in northern China where wheat is the dietary staple. Many children with health and behavior problems caused by food sensitivities have found relief after switching to a rice-based diet.

There are a number of different types of rice that are more or less commonly available. These include the following:

- Brown rice. This is rice from which only the inedible husk has been removed. More nutritious than any other type of rice, it is the only form that contains vitamin E. It has a nutty flavor and chewy texture. Cooking time is longer than for white rice, as the bran layer is intact.

- Black rice. Imported from Thailand, this is a whole-grain rice with a glutinous texture. It is good in dishes where cohesiveness rather than fluffiness is desired, such as paella, risotto, or rice-based desserts.

- White rice. The most popular type of rice, it is available enriched or parboiled. Enriched rice has had nutrients replaced after milling. Because they are applied in a solution to the outside of the grain, rinsing enriched rice before cooking washes away the added nutrients. Parboiled (or converted) rice has been steamed and dried before milling to force nutrients from the bran and germ into the center of the grain. Neither enriched nor parboiled rice is a good fiber source. White rice has more calories than brown or wild rice.

- Instant rice. This can be white or brown. It is rice that has been milled, cooked, then dehydrated. It reduces cooking time to about five minutes.

- Wild rice. This is not actually a type of rice, but an aquatic grass seed native to North America. Though expensive, it contains more protein than other rice and is richer in the amino acid lysine. It has a woodsy, earthy flavor.

Grain size and shape dictate the texture rice will have when cooked. Short-grain rice, which is oval, is sticky; medium-grain is moist and tender; long-grain is dry and the grains tend to stay separate. Brown rice comes in short or long grain. Short grain is best in recipes that need to hold together as it is stickier. Long grain stays separate better and is best as a side dish, in fried rice, or with vegetables. Both are good in salads.

Key nutrients in brown rice include protein, fiber, calcium, magnesium, manganese, phosphorus, potassium, iron, B vitamins, and vitamin E. Nutrients in enriched white rice include protein, calcium, magnesium, phosphorus, potassium, folate, iron, vitamin B$_3$ (niacin), vitamin B$_1$ (thiamine), and manganese. Phytochemicals include lignin and phytic acid. Table 11.2, below, illustrates the nutrient content of brown rice.

For a different taste experience, or to prepare ethnic dishes, look for specialty rices in health food and gourmet shops. Aromatic varieties are especially intriguing. They have a nutty flavor and delicate fragrance. Some available specialty rices include the following:

- Arborio rice. This is a creamy white rice grown in Italy used for the classic rice dish risotto. It is also good in paella and rice pudding.

- Basmati rice. Highly fragrant, from India and Pakistan, basmati almost doubles in length when cooked. It is available in both brown or white, and can be substituted for regular rice in most recipes.

- Black japonica rice. The black bran of this kind of rice liquefies when cooked, turning the water dark purple. It has an earthy flavor and is usually blended with other varieties. It works well in stuffing and pilaf.

- Jasmine rice. Originally from Thailand but now grown in the United States, jasmine rice is similar to basmati in flavor but has a more flowerlike aroma. It is good in Southeast Asian dishes.

- Mochi rice. Sweet rice, a sticky type of short-grain rice, is the basis for mochi, a traditional Japanese food. Once steamed, the rice is pounded or ground to break open

TABLE 11.2 NUTRIENT CONTENT OF BROWN RICE

The table below illustrates the nutrient content of ½ cup of cooked brown rice.

CALORIES	340
Protein	7.31 grams
Fat	2.68 grams
Fiber	3.22 milligrams
Vitamin B$_6$	0.46 milligrams
Calcium	21 milligrams
Magnesium	131 milligrams
Iron	1.36 milligrams
Copper	0.26 milligrams
Zinc	1.86 milligrams

the grains until they stick together, then formed into a thin block and dried. Usually sold in 12-ounce blocks, mochi must be cut and cooked before being eaten. Grated and chopped, it can be used in soups, stews, and sauces; cut and baked, it can be used to make waffles, breadsticks, or biscuits.

- Red yeast rice is a popular Chinese spice that is the end result of Went yeast fermented on rice. The Chinese have used it to promote healthy heart function for centuries. Current research believes it is promising as a tool to lower LDL cholesterol as it contains compounds that inhibit cholesterol synthesis in the liver.

- Texmati rice. Developed in the United States as a cross between basmati and Texas long-grain rice, this rice is also called popcorn rice because of its aroma.

- Valencia rice. Grown in the Spanish province of the same name, this rice is used to make paella. It easily absorbs other flavors.

- Wehani rice. This is a type of rice that was developed and is grown at California's Lundberg Family Farms. It has a rust-colored bran that turns mahogany when cooked. The flavor is buttery and nutty.

Rye

Rye has been cultivated for nearly 2,000 years. It thrives in Eastern Europe and Scandinavia where climates are too wet and cold for other grains. Low in gluten, rye needs to be supplemented with other high-gluten flours. It is used in breads and crackers. Whole rye, which can be cooked as a cereal, comes cracked and in flakes and berries. Because of its strong flavor, it is more palatable when cooked with milder-tasting grains.

Rye boosts the glandular system. It is also good for a weight-loss diet, because its low gluten content makes it dense and more filling.

Key nutrients in rye include protein, fiber, vitamin B_6, vitamin E, calcium, copper, folate, iron, magnesium, manganese, phosphorus, potassium, vitamin B_3 (niacin), vitamin B_2 (riboflavin), vitamin B_1 (thiamine), and zinc.

Soy

Roasted soybeans are ground into a fine powder to make high-protein flour that is more nutritious than grain flour. Soy flour comes in two types: natural, which contains all of the soybean's oils; and defatted, which has the oils removed during processing. Of the two, defatted has more concentrated protein. Soy flour can be used as it is, or toasted in a dry skillet over moderate heat to bring out its nutty flavor. To use soy flour in baking, substitute it for one-quarter of the recipe's primary flour. Soy flour can be added to almost any recipe for hot cereals, soups, stews, breads, and pancakes. To reduce cholesterol in baking

recipes, replace eggs with 1 tablespoon of soy flour and 2 tablespoons of water per egg.

Key nutrients in soy flour include protein, B vitamins, vitamin E, lecithin, phosphorus, potassium, calcium, iron, and zinc.

Spelt

More than 5,000 years old, spelt is once again resuming a prominent place among preferred grains. Its sweet, nutty taste works well in salads, soups, and stews. It tops wheat in amino acids, protein, some minerals, and B vitamins. Spelt also is used to make a variety of pastas and can be substituted in most recipes calling for wheat or rice.

Gluten-sensitive people tolerate spelt better than any other grain. High in carbohydrates, it contains more crude fiber and protein than wheat. Spelt also has all eight essential amino acids necessary in the daily diet to ensure proper cell maintenance. Spelt has special carbohydrates called mucopolysaccharides, which play a decisive role in blood clotting and stimulate the immune system. Spelt's other immune-stimulating properties are in its cyanogenic glucosides, which support the body's cancer-fighting abilities.

Key nutrients in spelt include protein, fiber, B vitamins, iron, copper, manganese, vitamin A, calcium, and potassium. Phytochemicals include lignin.

Sunflower

This seed of the sunflower plant can be used to make a flour that can add a lot of nutrients to baked goods and is especially good in cookies. Use it to replace a portion of the flour in your favorite recipe. If you grind your own sunflower seed flour at home, make sure the seeds are fresh. Select packages that contain few off-color or dark seeds. For best results, grind the seeds just before using them, as they can become rancid once exposed to air.

Key nutrients in sunflower seed flour include protein, fiber, potassium, calcium, iron, vitamin B_1 (thiamine), vitamin B_3 (niacin), vitamin B_6, folic acid, phosphorus, magnesium, zinc, and copper.

Tapioca

The dried starch of the cassava root, a tropical tuber, is milled into flour. Like cornstarch or arrowroot, tapioca is used primarily as a thickener in puddings, fruit pies, and soups.

Key nutrients in tapioca include protein, fiber, calcium, magnesium, phosphorus, potassium, vitamin A, vitamin C, and folate.

Triticale

Scottish botanist A. Stephen Wilson developed triticale (pronounced tri-ti-CAY-lee) in the late 1800s. A wheat and rye hybrid with higher protein content than either, it is available as whole berries, flakes, flour, and meal. A robust grain with a nutty flavor, triticale works well in baked goods, pilafs, or casseroles, or as porridge.

Key nutrients in triticale include protein, fiber, copper, iron, manganese, vitamin B_1 (thiamine), calcium, magnesium, phosphorus, and zinc.

Teff

At a mere 1/32 inch in diameter, teff certainly qualifies as the world's smallest grain. A mainstay of Ethiopian cooking, teff flour is used to make a pancake-type bread called injera. Due to its small size, the bran and germ layers make up a larger portion of the kernel than other grains. These nutrient-rich layers remain intact after milling. Teff has a mild, nutty flavor, with a slightly molasseslike sweetness. It can be used in flat breads, muffins, waffles, breakfast cereal, and cookies. Add it to soups, stews, and gravies as a thickener. Teff is now being grown in Idaho and is available in some health food stores.

Key nutrients in teff include protein, fiber, calcium, iron, and vitamin B_1 (thiamine).

Wheat

One of the oldest cultivated grains, wheat is the world's most important cereal crop. Nearly 2 billion people regularly use wheat in their diets. Whole wheat, in which the bran and germ remain intact, is a nutritional powerhouse. Wheat bran, for instance, is packed with 12 grams of fiber per ounce. And it is mostly insoluble fiber, which helps to protect against colon cancer. Wheat germ, though fairly high in polyunsaturated fat, delivers 9 grams of protein per ounce.

In the United States, wheat is consumed mostly in the form of refined flour used in breads, cakes, cereals, and numerous other baked goods. Wheat is high in gluten, which strengthens dough and makes bread rise. However, many people are unable to tolerate gluten, which is a tough protein substance. Celiac disease, an intestinal disorder caused by gluten intolerance, is a condition in which this intolerance leads to irritation and damage of the intestinal lining, which in turn causes poor absorption of nutrients and water. Wheat causes allergic reactions in some people, too, resulting in a range of physical and emotional problems. Wheat products should be eaten in moderation, or not at all if intestinal disorders are a problem.

The thousands of varieties of wheat are known by planting season, grain hardness, and kernel color. The most common categories are hard red winter, hard red spring, soft red winter, hard white, soft white, and durum. Soft and hard white wheat are milled into flour used mainly for baking. Soft wheat flour is higher in carbohydrates and is good for making pastries, crackers, and cookies. Flour made from hard wheat is higher in protein and is good for breads because of its higher gluten content. Cracked wheat, made from wheat berries, is good for hot cereals and can be sprouted. Rolled wheat, similar to rolled oats,

can be used in granola and cookies. Durum, the hardest type of wheat, is primarily processed into semolina flour to make pasta.

Key nutrients in whole wheat include protein, fiber, B vitamins, vitamin E, iron, folate, magnesium, and manganese. Phytochemicals in whole wheat include tocotrienols, ferulic acid, phytic acid, beta-glucans, lignin, and ellagic acid.

COOKING GRAINS

There are a few basic rules and steps to follow when cooking grains:

1. Bring liquid to a boil.
2. Add the grain and boil for five minutes.
3. Cover the pot with a tight-fitting lid and turn the heat down very low (the lowest setting) and allow it to simmer for the designated amount of time. Do not lift the lid until the recommended time has passed.

Table 11.3 below gives a general guide to the amounts of grain, liquid, and cooking time for different grains.

The goal is to steam the grain. Heating for longer than the time listed in Table 11.3 will not hurt, as long as the heat is sufficiently low. The heat may also be turned off without lifting the lid so the steam will not escape, allowing the grain to sit for a while.

An easy way to make whole-grain cereal is to place grain and boiling water in a thermos the night before, and the cereal will be ready to eat in the morning, with all the nutrients intact.

TYPE 11.3 BASIC COOKING GUIDE FOR GRAINS

Use the table below to calculate how much grain and how much liquid you need to produce the amount of cooked grain you would like—and how much time it will take to cook it.

GRAIN	AMOUNT OF GRAIN	AMOUNT OF WATER, MILK, OR BROTH	COOKING TIME IN MINUTES	YIELD (APPROXIMATE)
Barley, flaked	1 cup	3 cups	15	3 cups
Barley, pearled	1 cup	1 cup	30–40	1¼ cups
Buckwheat groats	1 cup	2 cups	20	3 cups
Bulgur	1 cup	2 cups	15	2½ cups
Cornmeal	1 cup	3½ cups	30	3 cups
Millet	1 cup	3 cups	30	4 cups
Oat groats	1 cup	3 cups	40–50	2½ cups
Oats, quick	1 cup	2 cups	1	2 cups
Oats, rolled	1 cup	2–3 cups	15–20	4 cups
Quinoa	1 cup	2 cups	15	2¾ cups
Rice, brown	1 cup	2 cups	35–40	2½ cups
Rye flakes	1 cup	3 cups	20	3 cups
Wheat groats	1 cup	2½ cups	35	3 cups
Rye berries	1 cup	3 cups	35	3 cups

GRAIN RECIPES

QUINOA PILAF

Use as a side dish similar to rice. Good with any meal.

2 tablespoons canola or olive oil
1 small red onion, chopped
3 ounces quinoa
1 pint quality water
½ teaspoon sea salt (optional)

1. Place oil in medium deep skillet. Add the onion and quinoa, stirring until slightly brown.
2. Add the water and salt, if desired, and place a lid on the skillet. Cook until soft, about 15 minutes. Serve hot.

RICE SALAD

What a refreshing way to serve rice! This dish supplies all the nutrients needed for a "complete" meal.

2 cups cooked brown rice
1 cup shredded carrots
1 cup Good Things House Dressing (see page 182)
1 package frozen green peas or fresh peas, slightly steamed
½ cup chopped celery
½ cup fresh chopped parsley
½ cup chopped onion
½ cup shredded red cabbage
1 cup Cherry tomatoes, cut up
1 dash garlic powder

1. Place the cooked rice in a bowl.
2. Add the remaining ingredients and toss to mix. Chill before serving.

SUMMER RICE SALAD

Another nutrient-packed salad that is good for everyone—a "healing" dish.

½ cup sliced mushrooms (try reishi or shiitake)
½ cup chopped celery
1 green pepper, diced
2 tablespoons garlic oil
1 cup chopped fresh raw or lightly steamed pea pods
4 cups cooked brown rice
3 tablespoons chopped fresh or 1½ tablespoons dried parsley
1 tablespoon dill weed
1 dash cayenne pepper
¾ cup cold-pressed safflower or eggless mayonnaise
2 tablespoons apple cider vinegar
1 teaspoon barley malt concentrated sweetener or honey
2 cups cherry tomatoes cut in half or large tomatoes, diced (optional)
2 teaspoons sea salt (optional)

1. In a skillet, sauté mushrooms, celery, and green pepper in garlic oil until tender.
2. Add pea pods, cooked rice, and seasonings. Cook for two to four minutes, then allow the mixture to cool.
3. Combine the mayonnaise, vinegar, and sweetener. Pour it over the rice mixture.
4. Add the tomatoes and sea salt, if desired. Toss to mix. Serve on a bed of lettuce or stuffed in an avocado or tomato. Serve warm or chill before serving.

Variations: If desired, substitute a mixture of ½ cup Good Things House Dressing (see page 182) and ½ cup eggless mayonnaise for the dressing above. Or add ½ cup lightly steamed broccoli or cauliflower.

FRUIT OATMEAL COOKIES

This recipe makes a big batch of delicious cookies that are good frozen and keep well! DELICIOUS!

8 cups oats
6 cups whole-wheat flour
2½ cups date sugar or other dry sweetener or fructose
1½ teaspoons ginger
1 teaspoon baking powder
1 teaspoon cinnamon
4 eggs or egg replacement
3 cups honey or maple syrup
2 cups expeller-pressed vegetable oil (such as Canola)
1½ cup frozen apple juice concentrate
2 teaspoons pure vanilla extract
1 cup chopped dried fruit of choice—apples and/or apricots are good (optional)
2 cups chopped nuts of choice (optional)

1. Preheat the oven to 350°F.
2. In a large mixing bowl, combine the dry ingredients.
3. In a separate bowl, mix together the wet ingredients.
4. Fold the dry mixture into the wet. Fold in fruit and nuts, if desired.
5. Drop by full tablespoons on an oiled cookie sheet and press down slightly with the bottom of a drinking glass. Bake for twelve to eighteen minutes.

Variations: Apple cider spiced juice from a health food store is good to use in place of the apple juice concentrate. Or substitute any favorite fruit juice. This recipe is fun to play with. Add nuts, nut butters, carob chips, peanut butter chips, seeds or any kind of dried chopped fruit. Try different combinations. Here's a good idea for holiday treats: divide the dough in half or thirds and mix in different ingredients, such as carob chips, chopped dried apples, and raisins, to make an assortment of cookies.

QUINOA STIR-FRY

Quinoa's unusually high-quality protein has nearly ideal amino acid balance, which is difficult to obtain in the plant kingdom. It is also a good source of fiber, complex carbohydrates, calcium, phosphorous, iron, and vitamins B and E.

1 cup chopped broccoli
1 cup sliced mushrooms
½ cup chopped celery
1 onion, sliced
1 red pepper, chopped
½ cup sliced carrots
½ cup cauliflower pieces
3 cloves garlic, minced
½ cup sliced almonds
¼ cup sunflower seeds
2 tablespoons sesame oil
2 tablespoons teriyaki sauce
1 teaspoon Vegit seasoning or seasoning of choice
2 cups cooked quinoa

1. Sauté the vegetables, garlic, almonds, and sunflower seeds in sesame oil until vegetables are crisp, not soft.
2. Add the teriyaki sauce, seasoning, and quinoa. Stir until mixed and warmed through. Serve immediately.

RICE BREAD

This bread is wheat-free and yeast-free. It's good for people with candidiasis.

3 cups brown rice flour
1 cup soy flour or oat flour
4 tablespoons aluminum-free baking powder (Rumfords aluminum-free baking powder can be found in health food stores)
½ teaspoon sea salt
2 eggs, separated
1 cup soymilk or milk of your choice
½ cup rice syrup, honey, or barley malt syrup
½ cup yogurt
4 tablespoons expeller-pressed safflower oil

1. Preheat the oven to 350°F.
2. In a large mixing bowl, combine all the dry ingredients.
3. Whip egg whites until stiff but not dry. Beat the yolks until creamy.
4. Add the milk, syrup, yogurt, and oil to dry ingredients and mix well. Add the yolks and mix well. Fold in the egg whites.
5. Bake for approximately one hour in a well-oiled standard loaf pan.

CHAPTER TWELVE

BOUNTIFUL BEANS AND LEGUMES: THE NEAR-PERFECT FOOD

You don't have to cook fancy or complicated masterpieces—just good food from fresh ingredients.

—Julia Child, American chef and author

Worldwide, legumes are grown in thousands of varieties—some are plants, others are vines, trees, and shrubs. Their shared characteristic is the production of edible seeds inside of pods. Beans, dried peas, and lentils are all considered legumes. Peanuts, clover, alfalfa, and fenugreek are legumes also, though usually not classified as such. Among the oldest agricultural crop, beans, peas, and lentils may even predate grain cultivation. Legumes are important in crop rotation programs, as they replenish the soil with nitrogen, a vital nutrient that grain crops deplete.

Since they readily absorb the flavors of other foods, herbs, and spices, legumes work well in a range of dishes, from casseroles and soups to stews, salads, vegetables, and pasta. They also make nutritious, filling side dishes.

LEGUME NUTRITION

Legumes have more protein than any other plant-derived food. Their protein is not considered "complete," as they are missing one or more of the essential amino acids. The deficiency can be corrected by serving legumes with rice, grains, or nuts, which provides the amino acids necessary for complete protein. The soybean, higher in protein than any other legume, is the exception— its protein is complete.

Legumes are loaded with energizing complex carbohydrates, calcium, iron, folic acid, B vitamins, zinc, potassium, and magnesium. They contain large amounts of both soluble and insoluble dietary fiber, more than any plant source except wheat. Soluble fiber helps to reduce blood cholesterol levels and normalizes blood sugar. Insoluble fiber helps regulate bowel function, eases some digestive problems, and may possibly help to prevent colon cancer. Ample amounts of legumes can help people with diabetes to keep blood sugar levels under control. Legumes are digested slowly and provide a gradual, steady supply of glucose, rather than a quick surge like most simple carbohydrates. Studies show that foods high in fiber, such as

legumes, can help lower blood pressure. Legumes also contain certain phytochemicals that have potential health benefits, including the following:

- *Protease inhibitors*, which slow tumor growth.

- *Phytosterols*, which protect against colon cancer.

- *Isoflavones*, which lower the risk of breast and ovarian cancer.

- *Saponins*, which stop cancer cells from multiplying.

Dried legumes are naturally low in fat (except for soybeans and peanuts), calories, and sodium, and are cholesterol-free. A true nutritional bargain, legumes are an inexpensive protein source and have a long shelf life.

Though legumes are high in iron, it is not the type the body absorbs well. This can be remedied by eating vitamin C–rich foods with legumes, which will boost iron absorption.

BUYING AND STORING LEGUMES

Select legumes that are uniform in size and color and not broken or cracked. Look for small marks, which could indicate insect infestation. If stored in a cool, dry place in tightly sealed containers to keep out moisture and humidity (both increase the cooking time), legumes will keep for as long as a year. If using clear storage containers, be sure to keep them out of direct sunlight to prevent loss of color, which can alter the taste of legumes. Mixing new legumes with stored legumes will cause them to cook unevenly. Refrigerate cooked leftovers in sealed containers and they will keep several days.

COOKING AND "UN-GASSING"

Beans, lentils, and peas contain certain compounds, such as lectins, tannins, and enzyme inhibitors, which potentially can be toxic if not cooked thoroughly. These substances interfere with the action and absorption of some vitamins and minerals. However, proper preparation of dried legumes—soaking and cooking—makes them harmless.

Beans are infamous for causing intestinal distress (bloating) and flatulence (gas). When sugars, starches, and fiber reach the large intestine without being digested or absorbed, friendly bacteria in the bowel consume them. Gas is a byproduct of this bacterial action. Bloating and gas are more likely if beans are not eaten regularly. Build up a tolerance for beans by eating small amounts at first, then gradually increase intake, which gives the body time to adjust. Rinse beans thoroughly before cooking. Adding ½ cup of uncooked brown rice or 1 teaspoon of fennel seeds to beans while cooking will help reduce gas and bloating. Adding sea vegetables during cooking is another remedy. Products like Beano, Say Yes to Beans from Nature's Plus, or Be Sure from Wakunaga of America, also help to prevent gas and bloating. They must be taken with the first bite of beans. These products can also be effective in preventing the gas and bloating caused by eating certain vegetables, such as cauliflower or cabbage.

TYPES OF LEGUMES

The inexpensive cost and wide variety of legumes make them perfect foods to introduce into your diet. We all recognize the standard, pinto, lima, navy, and red beans that Mom served, but there is a new generation of legumes, such as cranberry, fava, and mung beans, that offer variety as well as a complete protein.

Adzuki Beans

Also called azuki or aduki, these small tender red beans, native to the Orient, are often added to brown rice dishes. Their delicate, sweet flavor goes well with soups (they are delicious in barley soup), casseroles, salads, stir-fry dishes, bean cakes, and pasta dishes. The adzuki bean is a popular staple in the macrobiotic diet. In traditional Japanese medicine, it is used to treat kidney ailments.

Key nutrients in adzuki beans include protein, fiber, calcium, iron, magnesium, phosphorus, potassium, zinc, copper, manganese, B vitamins, folate, beta-carotene, and small amounts of lipids and amino acids.

Anasazi Beans

Originally cultivated by the Anasazi Indians in Colorado, anasazi beans are grown in the Southwest. Similar to the pinto bean, the anasazi has a full flavor and is generally sweeter and meatier than other types of beans. Use in chili, stews, succotash, and a variety of Mexican dishes, such as refried beans, burritos, and bean dips.

Key nutrients in anasazi beans include protein, fiber, iron, phosphorus, and vitamin B_1 (thiamine).

Black Beans

A favorite in Latin American, Caribbean, and Oriental cooking, black beans (also called turtle beans and frijoles negros) are deep black, with an earthy flavor. Their soft, mealy texture makes them easy to purée for black bean soup, refried beans, and bean dips. They go well with rice and other grains, for a complete protein, as well as with tomatoes and corn.

Key nutrients in black beans include protein, fiber, calcium, iron, magnesium, phosphorus, potassium, zinc, copper, manganese, vitamin B_1 (thiamine), vitamin B_3 (niacin), pantothenic acid, folate, and small amounts of amino acids and lipids. Phytochemicals include beta-carotene.

Black-Eyed Peas

Distinguished by a dark spot along their ridge, black-eyed peas are creamy white, medium-sized beans whose taste is similar to peas. They are also sometimes called black-eyed beans, black-eyed Suzies, and cowpeas. Add them to stews, soups, and salads.

Key nutrients in black-eyed peas include protein, fiber, calcium, potassium, folate, magnesium, phosphorus, iron, copper, zinc, and selenium.

Chickpeas

Small and compact, chickpeas resemble hazelnuts or acorns. A favorite in Indian, Latin, and Middle Eastern dishes, these chewy, nutty beans can be cooked with grains, added to salads and vegetable burgers, mixed with pasta, and roasted. Hummus, a Middle Eastern dip, is made from mashed chickpeas mixed with oil and tahini, a sesame seed paste. Falafel is made from mashed chickpeas, which are formed into balls, then deep-fried. Also called garbanzo beans and ceci beans, chickpeas take longer to cook than most beans.

Key nutrients in chickpeas include protein, fiber, calcium, iron, magnesium, phosphorus, potassium, zinc, copper, manganese, vitamin C, vitamin B_3 (niacin), vitamin B_1 (thiamine), pantothenic acid, vitamin B_6, folate, and small amounts of lipids and amino acids. Phytochemicals include beta-carotene.

Cranberry Beans

The speckled, cranberry-colored skin of cranberry beans turns pink when cooked. A small oval bean, their flavor is somewhat nutty and similar to pinto beans. Use them in chili, salads, soups, stews, and casseroles.

Key nutrients in cranberry beans include protein, fiber, calcium, iron, magnesium, phosphorus, potassium, zinc, copper, manganese, vitamin B_1 (thiamine), vitamin B_3 (niacin), vitamin B_2 (riboflavin), folate, pantothenic acid, vitamin B_6, and small amounts of lipids and amino acids. Phytochemicals include beta-carotene.

Fava Beans

These large, lima-shaped beans have a granular texture and robust, slightly bitter flavor. Also called broad beans, they have tough skins and need to be peeled before eating. They go well with zesty herbs and other pungent ingredients. Use in soups, stews, or casseroles.

Key nutrients in fava beans include protein, fiber, calcium, phosphorus, potassium, magnesium, zinc, copper, manganese, vitamin C, vitamin B_3 (niacin), folate, and small amounts of lipids and amino acids. Phytochemicals include beta-carotene.

Great Northern Beans

Great Northern beans are the largest, and most popular, of the white beans. They have a mild flavor, which makes them a versatile substitute in most any bean dish. Use them as the basis for baked beans, or in casseroles, soups, stews, and vegetable chowders.

Key nutrients in Great Northern beans include protein, fiber, calcium, potassium, phosphorus, magnesium, iron, zinc, copper, manganese, vitamin C, vitamin B_1 (thiamine), vitamin B_3 (niacin), pantothenic acid, folate, and small amounts of lipids and amino acids. Phytochemicals include beta-carotene.

Kidney Beans

So called because of their shape, kidney beans are most familiar as the large red type, but they are grown in a variety of colors, shapes, and sizes. Great Northern, black beans, and navy beans all belong to the kidney bean family. Red kidney beans are popular in chili, soups, and salads, and such dishes as red beans and rice, and jambalaya.

Key nutrients in kidney beans include protein, fiber, potassium, phosphorus, calcium, magnesium, iron, zinc, manganese, copper, vitamin C, vitamin B_3 (niacin), pantothenic acid, vitamin B_6, folate, and small amounts of lipids and amino acids. Phytochemicals include beta-carotene.

Lentils

The lentil belongs to the pea family. This tiny, disk-shaped legume comes in a rainbow of colors, though red, brown, and green lentils are the most common in the United States. A principal food during Biblical times and a favorite in Middle Eastern, Indian, and North African cooking, lentils have a delicate flavor and creamy texture. They do not need presoaking and cook quickly. Because they become quite soft after cooking, they make excellent bases for purées and soups. Also use them cold in salads or cook them with other vegetables. Lentils are a wonderful crunchy addition to salads when sprouted.

Key nutrients in lentils include protein, fiber, potassium, folate, phosphorus, magnesium, manganese, vitamin B_3 (niacin), iron, copper, vitamin A, vitamin B_6, calcium, and phosphorus.

Lima Beans

These flat beans are grown in two sizes: baby limas and large limas. Both are white and creamy-textured; baby limas are smaller and milder. Fordhooks, also a lima bean, are large and light green. The starchy, meaty texture of the lima adds substance to soups, casseroles, chowders, salads, and succotash.

Key nutrients in lima beans include protein, fiber, potassium, phosphorus, magnesium, calcium, iron, manganese, zinc, vitamin C, folate, vitamin B_6, and small amounts of lipids and amino acids. Phytochemicals include beta-carotene.

Lupine Beans

Though grown in limited amounts in the United States, the lupine bean is used in numerous dishes in other parts of the world, particularly the Mediterranean area and South America. A remote cousin of Texas bluebonnets, the lupine bean grows wild there in the spring. Researchers at North Dakota State University in Fargo have found that flour made from lupine beans combined with semolina flour makes a low-calorie pasta more nutritious than conventional pastas.

Key nutrients in lupine beans include protein, fiber, potassium, and calcium. Phytochemicals include beta-carotene.

Mung Beans

Fresh sprouts are probably the most familiar form of this legume, though the dried beans are used as well. Native to India, mung beans have a sweet flavor and are popular in curries. They are small, olive-colored, and fast cooking. They are found in natural food stores and Asian markets.

Key nutrients in mung beans include protein, fiber, potassium, phosphorus, magnesium, calcium, iron, zinc, copper, manganese, vitamin C, vitamin B_6, folate, vitamin B_3 (niacin), vitamin B_2 (riboflavin), pantothenic acid, and small amounts of lipids and amino acids. Phytochemicals include beta-carotene.

Navy Beans

These small white beans are another version of Great Northern beans. So named because of their extensive use in the U.S. Navy's dietary program, navy beans can be used in any recipe calling for white beans. Oblong and cream-colored, they work especially well in soups, stews, or as a main course with corn bread. Navy beans commonly are the base for Boston baked beans.

Key nutrients in navy beans include protein, fiber, potassium, magnesium, phosphorus, calcium, iron, zinc, copper, manganese, vitamin C, vitamin B_1 (thiamine), vitamin B_3 (niacin), pantothenic acid, vitamin B_6, folate, and small amounts of lipids and amino acids. Phytochemicals include beta-carotene.

Pinto Beans

In Spanish, *pinto* means "painted." These reddish beans are splashed with pink and black speckles that fade during cooking. They are high in calories and are not a compete protein. Highest in fiber of the legumes, pinto beans are a favorite in Southern, Southwestern, Tex-Mex, and Mexican cooking. Use them in chili, soups, or as a main dish.

Key nutrients in pinto beans include protein, fiber, potassium, phosphorus, magnesium, calcium, iron, zinc, copper, manganese, vitamin C, vitamin B_1 (thiamine), vitamin B_3 (niacin), vitamin B_2 (riboflavin), pantothenic acid, vitamin B_6, folate, and small amounts of lipids.

Soybeans

The ordinary soybean, a staple in Asian cooking, is a major medicinal food. A substantial body of scientific evidence points to the health benefits of soybeans and soy-based products. The soybean's therapeutic agents are so numerous that an entire chapter of this book is devoted to this remarkable legume (see Chapter 24) and another to a single product of the soybean, tofu (see Chapter 25).

Split Peas

Fresh green and yellow peas split in half when they are dried and their skins are removed. Typically used to make a thick hearty soup with vegetables, split peas also can be puréed and can be used in place of lentils.

Key nutrients in split peas include protein, fiber, calcium, iron, phosphorus, magnesium, manganese, vitamin B_3 (niacin), phosphorus, vitamin B_1 (thiamine), folate, copper, vitamin B_6, and vitamin C. Photochemicals include beta-carotene.

COOKING BEANS

Beans are easy to cook, but there are a few general guidelines to keep in mind. First and foremost, always use quality water when cooking beans. And do not overcook beans or allow the water you are cooking them in to boil for more than ten minutes. Beans should be tender but firm. Simmering brings the best results. Although beans come in a wide variety of shapes and sizes, the same cooking directions apply to all of the beans listed in this chapter.

Use 5 cups of quality water for each 1 cup of beans you are cooking. In a good, heavy pot or saucepan, place the beans in the water, bring the water to a boil, then reduce the heat and allow them to simmer for two to three hours, until they are tender. The cooking time will vary depending on the size of the beans.

The only exception to these instructions concerns chickpeas, Great Northern beans, and soybeans, which must be simmered longer than three hours.

BEAN RECIPES

PROTEIN-RICH LENTIL BURGERS

2 cups washed lentils
1½ quarts quality water
1 green or red pepper, finely chopped
½ pound mushrooms, finely chopped
1 onion, finely chopped
Olive oil to coat the sauté pan
1 carrot, shredded
1 pinch sea salt or to taste
¼ cup oat bran or quick-cooking rolled oats or
    1 cup cooked sweet short-grain rice
¼ cup ketchup or tomato paste

1. Cook the lentils in the water over medium heat for one and a half to two hours. When the lentils are soft, remove them from the heat and drain.
2. Lightly sauté the pepper, mushrooms, and onion in olive oil. Add the carrot and season with sea salt.
3. Mash the lentils or process them in a blender at medium speed. Gradually add the sautéed vegetables to the mashed lentils until mixed but not mushy.
4. Add the bran, oats, or rice to the mixture, then add the catsup or tomato paste. Mix well. The mixture should be approximately the consistency of raw hamburger. If it is too soft, gradually add more of the grain until you achieve the proper consistency.
5. Form into patties and broil or sauté mixture until golden brown. Serve in a sandwich or place on top of vegetables and rice or pasta. Or pour Hain's or Mayacamas gravy mix over the patties and serve with mashed potatoes and a vegetable.

BEAN BURRITOS WITH SWEET POTATOES

1 large onion, finely chopped
1 tablespoon expeller-pressed olive or canola oil
4 cloves of garlic, finely minced
½ green pepper, chopped
6 cups cooked adzuki, kidney, or garbanzo beans
    (or a mixture)
2 cups of the bean liquid, drained and set aside
    after cooking the beans
2 tablespoons chili powder
2 teaspoons ground cumin
½ tablespoon prepared mustard

1 dash of cayenne pepper (optional)
2 to 3 tablespoons tamari sauce
8 large whole-wheat tortilla
3 cups cooked, mashed sweet potatoes
1 medium tomato, diced
1 tablespoon prepared salsa or to taste
1 cup plain yogurt
1 avocado, thinly sliced
½ cup chopped Romaine lettuce
1 tablespoon chopped scallion or to taste (optional)

1. Preheat the oven to 375°F.
2. Sauté the onion in the oil until almost transparent, then add garlic and green pepper. Mix in the beans, bean liquid, chili powder, cumin, mustard, and, if desired, cayenne pepper. Bring to a boil, then reduce the heat, cover, and simmer for twenty minutes.
3. Stir in the tamari. Using a potato masher, mash the drained beans in the cooking pot. Continue to simmer and cook uncovered, until excess liquid is gone and it is the consistency of mashed potatoes. Remove from heat.
4. Spread approximately ⅔ cup of the bean mixture down the middle of each tortilla and top with approximately ½ cup of the sweet potatoes. Roll the tortillas and place them seam side down in a casserole dish, keeping them close together. Bake for five to ten minutes.
5. While the burritos are in the oven, mix the tomato, salsa, and plain yogurt.
6. When the burritos are done, remove them from the oven and top them with the avocado slices, lettuce, and tomato mixture. Sprinkle with chopped scallions if desired.

Variation: Use cooked brown rice instead of sweet potatoes.

Lentil Stew with Pumpkin and Greens

Lentil stew is high in all needed nutrients. It is excellent for those with cancer or heart disorders, and is great for anyone in need of a highly nutritious meal.

2 tablespoons olive or canola oil
1 large onion, minced
1 tablespoon minced fresh ginger
1 tablespoon whole cumin seeds
¾ teaspoon ground cinnamon
½ teaspoon ground coriander
¼ teaspoon ground cardamom
4½ cups water
1¼ cups lentils, rinsed
2 pounds pumpkin, peeled and cut into
    1-inch cubes
½ cup golden raisins
1 cup diced apples
½ pound fresh cooking greens

1. Heat oil in a large saucepan. Sauté the onion and fresh ginger for about five minutes.
2. Stir in cumin seeds and other spices, 2½ cups of the water, and the lentils. Bring to a boil, cover, and reduce heat and simmer for thirty minutes.
3. Add the pumpkin, raisins, apples, and the remaining water. Cover and simmer over medium heat until the lentils are barely tender, about ten minutes.
4. Stir in the greens, cover, cook a few more minutes, until the lentils are tender. Serve with cooked brown rice.

Variation: If you wish, you can substitute an equal amount of sweet potatoes for the pumpkin.

Fiesta Bean Dip

1½ cups Taste Adventure Pinto Bean Flakes or
    cooked, mashed beans of your choice
½ cup plain yogurt or sour cream mixed with taco
    seasoning to taste
1 dash of cayenne pepper (optional)
½ cup chopped olives
¼ cup chopped green onions
½ cup guacamole or fresh, mashed avocado
½ cup grated soy cheese
½ cup fresh diced tomatoes
3 tablespoons salsa

On a plate, layer the ingredients in the order listed, beginning with the beans. Serve with corn chips.

Tasty Veggie Chili

This dish freezes well in individual dishes. Pop one in the oven or microwave for a tasty meal.

3 pounds red kidney beans
2 quarts chopped tomatoes
2 cans tomato purée or tomato sauce
3 large onions, chopped
3 stalks celery, chopped
1 garlic clove, finely chopped
3 green peppers, chopped
2½ tablespoons cumin
2 tablespoons tamari sauce
2 tablespoons chili powder
1 tablespoon sea salt
½ teaspoon onion powder
¼ teaspoon cayenne powder
¼ teaspoon garlic powder
2 tablespoons vegetable or chicken bouillon

1. Soak red kidney beans overnight, then cook until tender usually about 45 to 60 minutes. Do not overcook.
2. Add tomatoes and tomato purée or sauce.

3. In a large skillet, sauté the onions, celery, green peppers, and garlic in garlic oil or safflower oil until tender. Add sautéed vegetables to the cooked beans.
4. Mix cumin, tamari, chili powder, sea salt, onion powder, cayenne pepper, and garlic powder into the bean mixture.
5. Add vegetable or chicken bouillon. Simmer over very low heat for one to two hours. Serve over brown rice and top with grated cheese and fresh avocado slices.

Variations: If desired, add additional tomatoes when you add the bouillon. You can also add granulated soy protein to give the dish a meaty look and taste. Tomato or mixed-vegetable juice can be used to add flavor in place of tomatoes (or you can use half and half).

BARLEY BEAN SOUP

Adzuki and anasazi beans are highest in nutrients of all beans.

> ½ pound adzuki or anasazi beans
> ½ pound barley
> 2 carrots, diced
> 1 large onion, diced
> 2 stalks celery, chopped
> 2 tablespoons garlic oil or safflower oil
> 2½ quarts water
> 6 tablespoons vegetable broth or 2 tablespoons
>   miso mixed with 4 tablespoons water
> 1 dash sea salt
> 1 dash cayenne pepper (optional)
> ½ cup dried vegetables or 1 box Hain's dry
>   Vegetable Soup mix (optional)
> ¼ cup parsley, chopped or dried (optional)

1. In a large pot, bring the beans and barley to a boil in the water. Reduce the heat and cover. Simmer for 1½ hours.
2. When the beans and barley are done, in a large skillet, sauté the carrots, onions, and celery in oil, and add to the beans and barley along with broth or miso. Barley swells a lot, so you may need to add additional water. Stir in sea salt, cayenne pepper (if desired), dried vegetables, and parsley (if desired). Simmer for fifteen minutes and serve.

Variations: Substitute 1 quart of Knudsen Very Veggie juice or Very Veggie Chili Juice for 1 quart of water for a spicier flavor. Vegetarians should especially like the added flavor from these juices. If you prefer soup without beans, eliminate them and use another pound of barley instead.

BLACK BEAN SOUP

> 2 cups black beans
> 1 whole bay leaf
> 6 cups water

> 1 teaspoon celery seed
> ½ teaspoon sea salt
> 1 dash cayenne pepper
> ¼ teaspoon basil
> 2 tablespoons expeller-pressed oil
> 2 stalks celery, chopped
> 2 onions, chopped
> 1 large carrot, chopped
> Juice of one-half lemon
> 1 tablespoon tamari sauce

1. Soak the beans and bay leaf overnight in water in a pressure cooker. Leaving the beans in the water they soaked in, pressure-cook them for one and a half hours or cook them slowly in a regular pot or saucepan for two to three hours.
2. Remove the bay leaf. Purée beans in a blender and return them to the pot. Add the salt, cayenne pepper, and basil.
3. In a skillet, sautée the celery, onions, and carrot in the oil until tender. Add them to the pot.
4. Simmer for fifteen minutes more, then add the lemon juice and tamari sauce. Serve garnished with a dollop of plain yogurt or sour cream and chopped chives.

HEARTY LIMA BEAN SOUP

> 1½ quarts water
> 1 pound lima beans
> 2 tablespoons vegetable bouillon or miso
> 1 large onion, chopped
> 2 stalks celery (hearts and leaves), chopped
> 1 large carrot, chopped
> 3 tablespoons garlic oil or expeller-pressed
>   vegetable oil with 1 crushed clove garlic added
> 3 tablespoons chopped fresh parsley or 1 table-
>   spoon dried parsley
> 2 tablespoons tamari
> 1 whole bay leaf
> 1 dash sea salt
> 1 dash cayenne pepper
> 1 cup potato flakes or boiled mashed potatoes or
>   raw cubed potatoes (optional)

1. In a large pot, pour the water over the beans and allow to soak overnight.
2. Leaving the beans in the water they soaked in, bring to a boil, then turn down to a simmer and allow the beans to simmer until they are tender, about one and a half hours. Add the vegetable bouillon.
3. In a skillet, sauté the onion, celery, and carrot in hot oil. Add the sautéed vegetables and seasonings to the beans.
4. If desired, stir in potato flakes; they add to the flavor and the thickness. Continue to simmer until the beans have completely finished cooking. Serve hot.

Sweet Red Bean Salad

¼ cup tofu or eggless mayonnaise
¼ cup lowfat plain yogurt
1 tablespoon honey or touch of sweetener of
 choice
1 dash sea salt or seasoning of choice to taste
1 dash cayenne powder (optional)
4 cups cooked red kidney beans
1 cup diced tofu
½ cup chopped celery
½ cup chopped onions
½ cup honey pickle relish

1. In a small bowl, combine the tofu or mayonnaise, yogurt, honey or sweetener, and seasonings.

2. In a medium bowl, mix together the kidney beans, tofu, celery, onions, and pickle relish.

3. Pour the tofu or mayonnaise mixture over the beans and vegetables and toss to mix. Serve at room temperature or chilled.

Variations: Use a total of 4 cups of any three different kinds of beans in place of only kidney beans. You can also use Good Things House Dressing (see page 182) in place of the dressing described here.

CHAPTER THIRTEEN

NUTS AND SEEDS:
BENEFICIAL PLANT-DERIVED FATS

Every oak tree started out as a couple of nuts that decided to stand their ground.

—Unknown

Nuts and seeds house the embryo from which a plant propagates future generations. The seed itself is the ripened ovule of a flowering plant. Nuts are the single-seeded fruit of shrubs or trees that have a hard shell that protects the kernel.

Moderate use of nuts and seeds in the diet can add variety and nutrition and supply good plant-derived fats with no cholesterol. The fatty acids nuts contain are high in beneficial monounsaturated and polyunsaturated fats, which form part of the molecules that move cholesterol through the bloodstream. That means nuts can be very good for the heart. However, they should still be eaten in moderation due to their high caloric content. Butters made from nuts are very close in nutritive value and fat content to whole nuts, so you should use nut butters also in moderation. A comparison of the fat content of different types of nuts can be found in Table 13.1 below.

Nuts and seeds are often thought of as snack foods, to be eaten one handful at a time. It is easier to monitor the amount eaten (and the fat intake) if you use them instead

as a food and incorporate them into meals. You can eat nuts and seeds without thawing, cooking, or seasoning, and even, at times, without silverware! Some vegetarians say that adding nuts to a meal dramatically increases their satisfaction level, supplying crunch, chewiness, and a nice blast to the taste buds.

A recommended serving of nuts is ¼ cup. Nuts are an excellent source of protein, fiber, vitamin E, magnesium, zinc, copper, selenium, potassium, phosphorous, zinc, vitamin B$_2$ (riboflavin), biotin, and iron, as well as "good" fat and many phytochemicals. All nuts contain comparatively high levels of compounds called *protease inhibitors,* which are known to block cancer in tests on laboratory animals. Further, a six-year survey of 26,000 individuals conducted at Loma Linda University in California concluded that participants who ate nuts frequently (at least five times a week) had half the rate of heart attack and coronary death as those who rarely ate them. Although the benefits were greatest for frequent nut eaters, people who ate them even once a week had a 25 percent lower incidence of heart disease

TABLE 13.1 A COMPARISON OF THE FAT CONTENT OF DIFFERENT TYPES OF NUTS, NUT BUTTERS, AND SEEDS

NUT, NUT BUTTER, OR SEED	SERVING SIZE	FAT CONTENT	SATURATED FAT CONTENT	CHOLESTEROL CONTENT
Almonds	1 ounce	15 grams	1 gram	0 grams
Cashews, dry-roasted	1 ounce	13 grams	3 grams	0 grams
Chestnuts, roasted	1 ounce	0.6 grams	0.1 grams	0 grams
Hazelnuts	1 ounce	19 grams	1 gram	0 grams
Macadamia, roasted in oil	1 ounce	22 grams	3 grams	0 grams
Peanut butter	2 tablespoons	16 grams	3 grams	0 grams
Peanuts, roasted in oil	1 ounce	14 grams	2 grams	0 grams
Pecans	1 ounce	20 grams	2 grams	0 grams
Pistachios	1 ounce	15 grams	2 grams	0 grams
Sesame seeds	1 tablespoon	4 grams	0.6 grams	0 grams
Sunflower seeds	1 ounce	14 grams	2 grams	0 grams
Walnuts	1 ounce	16 grams	1 gram	0 grams

Caution: When to Say No to Nuts

In moderation, nuts are nutritious, but not all nuts should be eaten by everyone. Peanuts (especially those used for commercially prepared peanut butter) may be contaminated by a mold called *Aspergillus flavus*, which produces aflatoxin, a carcinogen.

Coconuts are high in saturated fat, which can raise blood cholesterol, so it should be eaten in limited amounts only.

Most nuts contain the amino acid arginine, high levels of which can lead to flare-ups of herpes, so if you are prone to herpes outbreaks, you should probably consume them sparingly. Also, you should not eat nuts if you have been diagnosed with colitis, Crohn's disease, or diverticulitis. Consult your physician for more information.

Never use roasted nuts or seeds, because the oils they contain turn rancid when exposed to heat. Use only raw nuts that have been in a tightly sealed container. Do not buy nuts that have been exposed to light and air, like those in bins and in heated showcases. The good oils in raw nuts rapidly become rancid in this type of environment, and rancid fats are a source of toxic free radicals. Consume only raw nuts or those tightly sealed in bags. Avoid nuts that are processed with added oil, sugar, or artificial flavors.

than those who ate no nuts at all. In addition, a report issued jointly by the American Institute for Cancer Research and the World Cancer Research Fund concluded that a diet high in nuts could prove to be protective against some cancers.

Seeds, which also add a concentrated burst of flavor to meals and breads, are making a comeback in trendy restaurants and on vegetarian menus. It is not unusual to see a sprinkling of sunflower, coriander, poppy, fennel, sesame, mustard, pumpkin, or cumin seeds on hot and cold salads, in baked goods, and in main dishes. The oils of the seeds can be used in sauces, salad dressing, and baked goods, and to season meat and fish, although heating alters the chemical structure and makes it harder for the body to use the nutrition. (See Chapter 28.) Raw seeds are most flavorful when simply toasted in a dry skillet over low heat until they color slightly. Many seeds can also be sprouted, and this live food is a superior form of nutrition. (See Chapter 23.)

TYPES OF NUTS AND SEEDS

With so many to choose from, everyone should be able to find some kinds of nuts and seeds to give a pleasing flavor and texture to just about any meal.

Almonds

Almonds are called the king of nuts because they are high in calcium, potassium, magnesium, phosphorus, folic acid, and protein. They are higher in calcium and fiber than any other nut. Almond oil is good for the skin and almond butter is nutritious.

At one time, cancer clinics around the world were using laetrile, a compound derived from the phytochemical amygdalin, found in apricot pits and raw bitter almonds to treat cancer. Laetrile was thought to be an anticancer agent, but research has never successfully proven its value, and bitter almonds are not generally available. However, phytochemicals in almonds have been shown to inhibit the growth of lung, prostate, and breast tumors. Many clinics

still recommend eating a handful of raw almonds daily, chewing them thoroughly until they are almost liquid.

Key nutrients in almonds include protein, fiber, calcium, iron, magnesium, phosphorus, potassium, sodium, zinc, copper, manganese, selenium, vitamin C, vitamin B_1 (thiamine), vitamin B_2 (riboflavin), vitamin B_3 (niacin), pantothenic acid, vitamin B_6, folate, and vitamin E. Almonds are high in monounsaturated fatty acids and contain essential amino acids. Phytochemicals include quercetin, kaempferol, alpha-tocopherol, gamma-tocopherol, glutamic acid, myristic acid, phytosterols, and serine.

Brazil Nuts

Gathered from trees in the Amazon basin of Brazil, this is the only variety of nut that is not cultivated. Brazil nuts are a good source of calcium, phosphorus, and vitamin B_1 (thiamine), and are among the richest sources of selenium, a vital mineral lacking in most U.S. soils and therefore in most food grown in this country. A one-ounce serving of Brazil nuts (six to eight kernels) contains over 800 milligrams—more than ten times the recommended dietary allowance (RDA) of selenium, which is 40 to 75 micrograms. These nuts also have antioxidant and anticancer action and protect against heart disease.

Key nutrients in Brazil nuts include protein, fiber, calcium, iron, magnesium, phosphorus, potassium, sodium, zinc, copper, manganese, selenium, vitamin C, vitamin B_1 (thiamine), vitamin B_2 (riboflavin), vitamin B_3 (niacin), pantothenic acid, vitamin B_6, folate, and vitamin E. They are high in monounsaturated and polyunsaturated fatty acids and contain essential and nonessential amino acids. Phytochemicals include alpha-linolenic acid, gamma-tocopherol, beta-carotene, and tocopherol.

Cashews

Grown primarily in India, cashews are high in iron, potassium, magnesium, vitamin A, and fat. The shell of this plant, a relative of sumac and poison ivy, contains a caustic, toxic resin that can blister human skin, so cashews are available in the consumer marketplace shelled. A one-ounce serving contains 7.7 grams of monounsaturated fatty acids, 2.2 grams of polyunsaturated fatty acids, and only 2.5 grams of saturated fat.

The distinctive flavor of the cashew is a robust addition to main dishes, vegetables, bread, and dessert recipes.

Key nutrients in cashews include protein, fiber, calcium, iron, magnesium, phosphorus, potassium, sodium, zinc, copper, manganese, selenium, vitamin B_1 (thiamine), vitamin B_2 (riboflavin), vitamin B_3 (niacin), pantothenic acid, vitamin B_6, folate, and vitamin E. They are high in monounsaturated fatty acids and contain essential amino acids. Phytochemicals include gamma-tocopherol, alpha-catechin, gallic acid, naringenin, and phytosterols.

Chestnuts

Good raw, boiled, or roasted, the European chestnut is lowest in fat content of any nut. Not to be confused with the Chinese water chestnut, which is a tuber of a marsh plant, chestnuts are a good source of vitamin B_6, vitamin C, and folate. They are a low-fat nut snack that can provide distinctive flavor and texture in cooking or salad preparation. Flour made from chestnuts is used to make bread in Italy.

Key nutrients in chestnuts include protein, fiber, calcium, iron, magnesium, phosphorus, potassium, sodium, zinc, copper, manganese, selenium, vitamin C, vitamin B_1 (thiamine), vitamin B_2 (riboflavin), vitamin B_3 (niacin), pantothenic acid, vitamin B_6, folate, vitamin B_{12}, vitamin A, vitamin E, essential amino acids, and the nonessential amino acids glutamic acid and serine.

Chia Seed

The often-ridiculed seed of the "instant pet," chia seeds have a history as a nutritious flavoring for soups and beverages. They were used by ancient mountain and desert-dwelling Native American civilizations. Aztec warriors used carbohydrate-rich chia seeds as an energy booster. The tiny black seeds are also high in protein and may be sprinkled on foods whole or ground in a blender.

The two varieties of chia, native to California and Mexico, respectively, add flavor and nutrients to cottage cheese, sandwiches, soups, and salads. Adding chia to protein or fiber drinks can help stimulate bowel function.

Key nutrients in chia seeds include protein, fiber, calcium, iron, magnesium, phosphorus, potassium, sodium, zinc, copper, manganese, selenium, vitamin C, vitamin B_1 (thiamine), vitamin B_2 (riboflavin), vitamin B_3 (niacin), pantothenic acid, vitamin B_6, folate, vitamin A, and vitamin E. They contain saturated, monounsaturated, and polyunsaturated fatty acids, as well as essential amino acids and the nonessential amino acids glutamic acid and serine. Phytochemicals include caffeic acid, ferulic acid, myristic acid, P-coumaric acid, and vanillic acid.

Hazelnuts (Filberts)

Hazelnuts originated in wild trees in Asia and Europe. People have been picking the nut in the wild since prehistoric times. Hazelnuts have also been known as Cob, and the cultivated varieties, which are bigger, are now called filberts. Filberts were developed from the species of hazelnuts from Southeast Europe. They are used often in sweet and savory dishes and stews. These nuts have also been ground and made into oil and hazelnut butter. The flavor of hazelnuts is sometimes added to coffee. Hazelnuts are lower in fat than most of the nut family. Nutritionally, 100 grams (about 3.5 ounces) of hazelnuts yields 7.6 grams protein, yet the nuts do not present a fat problem when used in salads, cookies, or cakes.

High in potassium, sulfur, and calcium, hazelnuts have a mild flavor and are good cooked with vegetables and grains.

Key nutrients in hazelnuts include protein, fiber, calcium, iron, magnesium, phosphorus, potassium, sodium, zinc, copper, manganese, selenium, vitamin C, vitamin B_1 (thiamine), vitamin B_2 (riboflavin), vitamin B_3 (niacin), pantothenic acid, vitamin B_6, folate, vitamin A, and vitamin E. They are high in monounsaturated fatty acids and contain essential amino acids. Phytochemicals include tocopherols, beta-carotene, myristic acid, and phytosterols.

Flaxseeds

These nutty-flavored seeds taste good sprinkled on cereal, yogurt, in soups, and salads. Flaxseed flour and ground flaxseed can be added to breads, muffins, cookies, and other baked goods. The oil of flaxseed is the richest source of omega-3 linolenic acid, the type of essential fatty acid most deficient in the American diet. (See Chapter 28.)

Flaxseeds are effective as a laxative and as a soothing agent in inflammatory respiratory problems. They can be brewed into a tea or applied as a poultice to treat abscesses, boils, and other skin swellings. Adding flaxseed oil to the diet can help to lower cholesterol and may protect against stroke, as well as slow the progression of rheumatoid arthritis and atherosclerosis.

Key nutrients in flaxseeds include protein, fiber, calcium, iron, magnesium, phosphorus, potassium, sodium, zinc, copper, manganese, selenium, vitamin C, vitamin B_1 (thiamine), vitamin B_2 (riboflavin), vitamin B_3 (niacin), pantothenic acid, vitamin B_6, folate, and vitamin E. They are one of the richest sources of polyunsaturated fatty acids, and also contain essential amino acids. Phytochemicals include apigenin, tocopherols, beta-sitosterol, chlorogenic acid, luteolin, myristic acid, pectin, squalene, stigmasterol, phytoestrogens, and lignins.

Peanuts

Peanuts, though technically a legume, are usually thought of as nuts. They are a complete protein, and have recently been found to contain resveratrol, the phytonutrient found in red wine that has been shown to help reduce heart disease.

Key nutrients in peanuts include protein, fiber, calcium, iron, magnesium, phosphorus, potassium, sodium, zinc, copper, manganese, selenium, vitamin C, vitamin B_1 (thiamine), vitamin B_2 (riboflavin), vitamin B_3 (niacin), pantothenic acid, vitamin B_6, folate, and vitamin E. They are high in monounsaturated and polyunsaturated fatty acids and contain essential amino acids and the nonessential amino acids glutamic acid and serine. Phytochemicals include alpha-tocopherol, caffeic acid, chlorogenic acid, delta-tocopherol, ferulic acid, gamma-tocopherol, glutamic acid, serine, sinapic acid, and myristic acid.

There are some concerns about peanuts as a part of the diet, however. They are often contaminated with aflatoxin, a known carcinogen that is produced by certain types of mold. Also, many people are allergic to peanuts, and peanut allergies can be quite severe, even life-threatening. Studies have shown that the incidence of peanut allergies and sensitivities is higher among people who were given peanut butter before the age of three. For that reason, it is probably wise to avoid giving any peanut products to a child younger than three.

Pecans

A native North American member of the hickory family, pecans are high in potassium and vitamin A. Rich in essential fats, pecans are good for baking and are a popular ingredient in candy.

Studies have shown that pecans can help to lower low-density lipoprotein (LDL, or "bad") cholesterol levels. This southern nut favorite is probably most well known for its contribution to the famous pies of the region. As with the similar hickory nut, pecans are also tasty additions to ice cream, cake, and the noted praline.

Key nutrients in pecans include protein, fiber, calcium, iron, magnesium, phosphorus, potassium, sodium, zinc, copper, manganese, selenium, vitamin C, vitamin B_1 (thiamine), vitamin B_2 (riboflavin), vitamin B_3 (niacin), pantothenic acid, vitamin B_6, folate, and vitamin E. They are high in monounsaturated fatty acids and contain essential amino acids. Phytochemicals include gamma-tocopherol and beta-carotene.

Pine Nuts (Pignolia)

Used extensively in Middle Eastern and Italian dishes, pine nuts are chewy and sweet, which makes them good in salads or combined with fruits. Their distinctive taste adds an interesting flavor to vegetable dishes and entrées.

Key nutrients in pine nuts include protein, fiber, calcium, iron, magnesium, phosphorus, potassium, sodium, zinc, copper, manganese, selenium, vitamin C, vitamin B_1 (thiamine), vitamin B_2 (riboflavin), vitamin B_3 (niacin), pantothenic acid, vitamin B_6, folate, vitamin A, and vita-

min E. They are high in monounsaturated and polyunsaturated fatty acids, and contain essential amino acids and the nonessential amino acids glutamic acid and serine. Phytochemicals include phytosterols.

Pistachios

Pistachios have a sweet, mild flavor. You may see holes in these nuts made by a tiny worm, which gives each nut its unique flavor. Foreign pistachios are often dyed red to make them more appealing and to hide imperfections created during the roasting process. Pistachios from the United States, introduced in 1976 and now primarily from California, are most often undyed and sold in their natural tan shell. One of the highest sources of potassium of all nuts, pistachios are a great snack and a welcome addition to ice cream and other desserts.

Key nutrients in pistachios include protein, fiber, calcium, iron, magnesium, phosphorus, potassium, sodium, zinc, copper, manganese, selenium, vitamin C, vitamin B_1 (thiamine), vitamin B_2 (riboflavin), vitamin B_3 (niacin), pantothenic acid, vitamin B_6, folate, vitamin A, and vitamin E. They are high in monounsaturated fatty acids and contain essential amino acids and the nonessential amino acids glutamic acid and serine. Phytochemicals include gamma-tocopherol, alpha-tocopherol, beta-carotene, beta-sitosterol, myristic acid, pectin, phytosterols, and stigmasterol.

Pumpkinseeds

Pumpkinseeds actually contain more iron than liver by weight. Pumpkinseeds are an excellent source of essential fatty acids that promote good prostaglandin production. A popular treatment for prostate problems, pumpkinseeds are a popular herbal remedy that can be used as a mild laxative with additional diuretic action.

Key nutrients in pumpkinseeds include protein, fiber, calcium, iron, magnesium, phosphorus, potassium, sodium, zinc, copper, manganese, selenium, vitamin C, vitamin B_1 (thiamine), vitamin B_2 (riboflavin), vitamin B_3 (niacin), pantothenic acid, vitamin B_6, folate, vitamin A, and vitamin E. They are high in polyunsaturated and monounsaturated fatty acids and both essential and nonessential amino acids. Phytochemicals include phytosterols.

Sesame Seeds

These tiny oval seeds, which grow on a tall annual plant, are basic to many of the world's cuisines, including those of Africa, China, and India. They can be purchased hulled or unhulled. The unhulled ones are darker in color, have the bran intact, and are a good source of calcium, iron, and phosphorus. Sesame seeds are often used on breads and buns. By weight, sesame seeds actually have a higher iron content than liver.

Key nutrients in sesame seeds include protein, fiber, calcium, iron, magnesium, phosphorus, potassium, sodium, zinc, copper, manganese, selenium, vitamin C, vitamin B_1 (thiamine), vitamin B_2 (riboflavin), vitamin B_3 (niacin), pantothenic acid, vitamin B_6, folate, vitamin A, and vitamin E. They are high in monounsaturated fatty acids, and contain both essential and nonessential amino acids. Phytochemicals include phytosterols.

Sunflower Seeds

Did George Washington and Benjamin Franklin snack on sunflower seeds? Could be. Historical references dating back to 1744—thirty-two years before the American Revolution—indicate that sunflower seeds had already been discovered as a tasty treat in Colonial times. Originally thought of as a delicacy for the wealthy, sunflower seeds today enjoy a universal appeal and are widely accepted as a delicious, nutritious snack food. The crisp, crunchy kernel brings an extra spark of interest to any dish and is a trendy addition to salads, breakfast cereals, and baked goods. Sunflower kernels have a unique flavor—somewhat nutty, yet subtle. Sunflower kernels are higher than any other nut or seed products in the antioxidant phytochemical tocopherol, which may help to protect against cardiovascular disease. Sunflower kernel oil is a healthy alternative for cooking oil or salad oil.

Key nutrients in sunflower seeds include protein, fiber, calcium, iron, magnesium, phosphorus, potassium, sodium, zinc, copper, manganese, selenium, vitamin C, vitamin B_1 (thiamine), vitamin B_2 (riboflavin), vitamin B_3 (niacin), pantothenic acid, vitamin B_6, folate, vitamin A, and vitamin E. They are high in polyunsaturated fatty acids, and contain essential and nonessential amino acids. Phytochemicals include tocopherol, choline, betaine, lignan, and phenolic acids.

Walnuts

Shelled walnuts are delicious in baked goods, sprinkled on salads, and as a topping on desserts. The oil from walnuts is high in polyunsaturated fatty acids and tends to lower blood cholesterol. Walnut oil is used in cooking and is high in potassium, phosphorous, magnesium, and vitamin A.

Key nutrients in walnuts include protein, fiber, calcium, iron, magnesium, phosphorus, potassium, sodium, zinc, copper, manganese, selenium, vitamin C, vitamin B_1 (thiamine), vitamin B_2 (riboflavin), vitamin B_3 (niacin), pantothenic acid, vitamin B_6, folate, vitamin A, and vitamin E. They are high in polyunsaturated fatty acids, and contain essential amino acids. Phytochemicals include alpha-linolenic acid, gamma-tocopherol, and beta-carotene.

NUT AND SEED RECIPES

Currant Nut Dessert

This dessert is high in the essential fatty acids found in walnuts and pecans.

1 cup yogurt
¼ cup currants or raisins
¼ cup chopped raw walnuts or pecans
1 pinch cinnamon
1 teaspoon vanilla
1 dash of barley malt sweetener (optional)

Mix ingredients together in a serving bowl and and chill.

Almond Milk

This is an excellent addition to children's and infant's diets. It's also good for adults as a milk substitute. Substitute almond milk for soymilk if you are allergic to soy.

1 cup almonds
3 cups water
½ fresh papaya (optional; good for babies)
1 teaspoon blackstrap molasses (optional; a good mineral source)
1 teaspoon pure vanilla extract (optional)
1 tablespoon brewer's yeast or wheat germ or both (optional)

1. In a grinder, food processor, or blender, grind the nuts into a powder. Gradually add the water and other ingredients while continuing to blend.
2. Store almond milk in the refrigerator and serve chilled.

Note: Using molasses and papaya makes this a complete milk for infants, especially for those who are allergic to cow's milk. If you plan to use this as a drink for adults, start by adding ½ teaspoon of brewer's yeast to the recipe and gradually increase to 1 tablespoon over a couple of weeks' time. Omit the wheat germ if you plan to use almond milk for cooking or on cereals.

Sesame Milk

This milk is sweet enough without additional sweetener. It is high in protein and essential fatty acids, and is an excellent drink for those with bowel problems.

1 cup sesame seeds
1 tablespoon flaxseed
1½ cups of water
4 pitted dates

1. In a blender or food processor, grind sesame seeds and flaxseed to a powder. Gradually add the water and dates while continuing to blend.
2. Store sesame milk in the refrigerator and serve chilled.

Variations: If constipation is a problem, substitute soaked prunes for the dates. Try adding different fruits and even fresh carrot juice to taste for a refreshing and nutritious breakfast. Substitute cashews or sunflower seeds for the sesame seeds to make cashew milk or sunflower milk.

CHAPTER FOURTEEN

THE FISH STORY:
SWIMMING IN FAVORABLE FATS

Fish-dinners will make a man spring like a flea . . .

—*Thomas Jordan, seventeenth-century English poet*

The Inuit people in Greenland, whose diets consist principally of fatty fish, have less arteriosclerosis and fewer deaths from heart disease than people in the United States. Japanese women, who consume more fish than their American counterparts, have a lower incidence of both heart disease and breast cancer. At the University of Leidi in Holland, researchers studied 852 men who ate 7 to 11 ounces of fish weekly. There was a 50 percent lower death rate from heart disease among those who ate fish compared with those who did not consume any fish. And *The Journal of the American Medical Association* reported on a study by Brigham and Women's Hospital that found that eating at least one meal of fish weekly can cut the risk of sudden cardiac death in men in half. Clearly, fish can make a vital contribution to dietary wellness.

The health benefits of the omega-3 fatty acids present in fish oil have been recognized since the early 1980s, when their cholesterol-lowering capabilities were first identified. Fish oils also reduce the likelihood of unwanted blood clots, lower blood pressure, and strengthen the walls of the heart, and may prevent stroke and the spread of existing cancers. The anti-inflammatory effect of fish oils is also well established. Additionally, studies now indicate a possible link to the prevention of mood swings from postpartum depression in new mothers and increased mental function in people with Alzheimer's disease. Laboratory experiments also indicate that fish oil fatty acids can inhibit the growth of several types of human cancer cells.

A University of Wyoming study showed that 40 percent of asthma sufferers who participated in the study experienced a significant improvement in breathing ability and a better resistance to asthma attacks while on a high fish oil diet. In addition, researchers at the University of Sydney in Australia reported that the regular consumption of oily fish is associated with a reduced risk of developing asthma during childhood.

TYPES OF FISH

There are many different types of fish, some with greater potential health benefits than others. The primary health effects are linked to the level of omega-3 essential fatty acids the fish contain. (For a comparison of the omega-3 content of selected popular species, see Table 14.1 below.) In general, fish are divided into two categories: saltwater (or marine) fish and freshwater fish. Recent years have seen the growth of what may be considered a third category, farm-raised fish.

TABLE 14.1 OMEGA-3 CONTENT OF SELECTED POPULAR FISH SPECIES

SPECIES	GRAMS OF OMEGA-3 ESSENTIAL FATTY ACIDS PER 3.5-OUNCE (100-GRAM) SERVING
Norway sardines	5.1
Atlantic mackerel	2.6
Atlantic herring	1.7
Albacore tuna	1.5
Atlantic sturgeon	1.5
Halibut	1.5
Sablefish	1.6
Atlantic salmon	1.4
Bluefish	1.2
Mullet	1.1
Striped bass	0.8
Silver hake	0.6
Florida pompano	0.6
Shark	0.5
Swordfish	0.2

Saltwater Fish

Saltwater fish are caught in marine environments, typically oceans. They are often divided into three categories, depending on fat content:

- Fatty fish include sardines, mackerel, salmon, smelt, anchovies, mullet, and herring.

- Medium-fat fish include halibut, ocean perch, red snapper, sole, sea trout, and albacore tuna.

- Low-fat saltwater fish include flounder, haddock, swordfish, cod, shellfish, and whiting.

All of the above fish above are among the best to consume, as they contain good fats.

Freshwater Fish

Freshwater fish are caught in lakes, rivers, and streams. They too are divided into groups according to fat content:

- Fatty fish include lake trout, mullet, smelt, catfish, and rainbow trout.

- Medium-fat fish include carp.

- Low-fat fish include bass, bream, pike, and lake perch.

One concern about freshwater fish is that they may be more subject to certain types of contamination, especially high levels of mercury, depending on where they are caught. If you consume freshwater fish, it is wise to know where it came from and to find out about any advisories concerning fish from that area. You can eliminate some of any mercury that may be present by broiling the fish on a rack so that it remains above the juices that run.

Farm-Raised Fish

The omega-3 essential fatty acids found in saltwater fish come from a diet of deep-water plankton and smaller fish. Farm-raised species of fish (especially Atlantic salmon transplanted to the Pacific Northwest for farming in pens in the Pacific Ocean) do not appear to have as high an omega-3 content as their wild-caught cousins. Farm-raised fish are fed grain feeds that do not produce as high a content of the omega-3 essential fatty acids docosahexaenoic acid (DHA) and eicosapentaenoic acid (EPA).

BUYING AND STORING FISH

Unless you live in a coastal area (or catch the fish yourself!), frozen fish is probably a better choice than fresh fish, because fresh fish at the market may be five to ten days old. Fish are normally frozen within four hours of being caught. Any fish you buy should not smell "fishy" or ammonialike, but should have an odor more like a fresh-grated cucumber. If a fish smells, that means that the fatty acids have started to break down and the fish is becoming rancid.

Identifying fresh seafood is not that difficult. There are a number of simple steps that can be taken to verify that the fish is fresh. The fish's eyes should be clear and bulge a little. Only a few fish, such as walleye, have naturally cloudy eyes. Whole fish and fillets should have firm and shiny flesh. Dull flesh may mean the fish is old. Fresh whole fish also should have bright red gills free from slime. If the flesh doesn't spring back when pressed, the fish isn't fresh. There should be no darkening around the edges of the fish or brown or yellowish discoloration.

Other tips for selecting fish, courtesy of the U.S. Food and Drug Administration (FDA), include the following:

- Buy only from reputable sources. Be wary, for example, of vendors selling fish out of the backs of pickup trucks.

- Buy only fresh seafood that is refrigerated or properly iced.

- Don't buy cooked seafood, such as shrimp, crabs, or smoked fish, if they are displayed in the same case as raw fish. Cross-contamination can occur.

- Don't buy frozen seafood if the packages are open, torn, or crushed on the edges. Avoid packages that are above the frost line in the store's freezer. If the package cover is transparent, look for signs of frost or ice crystals. This could mean that the fish has either been stored for a long time or thawed and refrozen.

- Put seafood on ice, in the refrigerator, or in the freezer, immediately after buying it.

- When eating fish caught recreationally, follow state and local government advisories about fishing areas and warnings about eating fish from certain areas.

The length of time raw fish can be stored safely depends on the type of fish. Lean fish, such as cod, flounder, and haddock, can be kept in the refrigerator for one to two days or frozen for up to six months. Fatty fish, such as blue perch and salmon, can also be kept in the refrigerator for one to two days but should be frozen for only two to three months.

FISH CONTAMINATION

In recent years, cases of hepatitis A, a viral infection that inflames the liver and causes gastroenteritis (a mild flulike illness), have been linked to consumption of raw clams and oysters. Also, some ocean fish are contaminated with parasites that can cause infection in humans. Cooking fish to at least 140°F or freezing it at a temperature below 0°F will kill these parasites. Therefore, unless fish used to prepare sushi has been frozen, it should be considered contaminated and dangerous. People with diabetes, liver disease, gastrointestinal disorders, or other diseases affecting the immune system should eat only thoroughly cooked fish and seafood.

A Consumer Reports team conducted a six-month investigation in urban and suburban New York City, Chicago, and the San Jose–Santa Cruz area of California. They went to grocery stores and specialty stores, sampling salmon, flounder, sole, catfish, swordfish, lake whitefish, and clams. They found that 40 percent of the fish were either contaminated or beginning to spoil and 30 percent were rated poor due to bacterial contamination, polychlorinated biphenyls (PCBs), or mercury. Fish requires storage temperatures between 30°F and 32°F, but some store display cases reach 45°F. Some unscrupulous markets defrost frozen fish and sell it as "fresh," letting it sit for days in their display cases. Some restaurants soak fish in milk to reduce the "fishy" taste and to make the meat whiter. If you are allergic to dairy products, be cautious when eating out.

FISH RECIPES

Nondairy Cheddar Salmon Loaf

2 teaspoons tamari
2 teaspoons miso (optional)
2 cups canned salmon (with the bones for extra calcium)
1½ cups soft bread crumbs or cracker crumbs
1 egg
1 cup cooked sweet or short-grain rice
½ cup finely diced celery
½ cup grated Tofutti soy cheese or Cheddar or other cheese of your choice
3 tablespoons oat flour or other flour of your choice
3 tablespoons water
2 tablespoons finely minced onion
1 tablespoon chopped or dried parsley
¼ teaspoon garlic granules or powder (not garlic salt)
2 teaspoons sea salt (optional)
1 dash cayenne (optional)
1–3 tablespoons water (optional, if needed to form a loaf)

1. Preheat the oven to 350°F.
2. In a large mixing bowl, combine the tamari and, if desired, the miso.
3. Add the rest of ingredients, mix well, and form into a loaf shape with your hands. If the mixture is too stiff, gradually add water until the desired consistency is reached.
4. Pack into an oiled loaf pan. Bake for forty-five to fifty-five minutes and serve.

Variations: Instead of using a loaf pan, form the mixture into patties before baking and eat like burgers. Or cook individual servings in a muffin pan. Serve the loaf or patties with the sauce of your choice. Or top with the grated cheese of your choice before serving.

Halibut à la Greco

4 fresh or frozen halibut steaks, ¾-inch thick
2 tablespoons virgin olive oil
2 teaspoons arrowroot powder or 1 egg white
½ cup soymilk or skim milk
1 cup crumbled feta cheese
⅛ teaspoon plus 1 dash cayenne pepper
1 large fresh tomato, chopped
¼ cup chopped pitted ripe olives
¼ cup toasted pine nuts or slivered almonds
Juice of 1 lemon
1 tablespoon snipped parsley
1 dash of sea salt (optional)

1. Thaw halibut in refrigerator if frozen.
2. Preheat the oven to 400°F.
3. In a large skillet, cook halibut in olive oil over medium-high heat for three minutes on each side. The fish will be only partially cooked.
4. Place halibut in a baking dish. In a small bowl, stir together the arrowroot or egg white and milk. Stir in cheese, ⅛ teaspoon cayenne pepper, and salt and spoon over halibut. Sprinkle with chopped tomato, olives, and nuts.
5. Bake, uncovered, for ten minutes. Sprinkle lemon juice, parsley, and dash of cayenne pepper on top and serve immediately. (Go easy on the cayenne; it is very hot, but it's good for those with circulatory and heart disorders.)

Salmon Steaks

4–6 thick salmon steaks
Sea salt to taste (optional)
1 dash of cayenne pepper
Juice of one lemon
2 tablespoons olive or other vegetable oil
2 tablespoons oat flour or whole-wheat flour
2 teaspoons dried dill
1 tablespoon eggless mayonnaise (Vegenaise) (optional)
2 teaspoons horseradish powder (optional)
1½ cups yogurt or Tofutti soy sour cream
2 large sweet onions, sliced
1 red pepper, sliced thin, or ½ cup canned pimentos

1. Preheat the oven to 400°F.
2. Place fish in casserole dish and season with sea salt, cayenne pepper, and lemon juice.
3. Put oil in a small saucepan and stir in the flour and the dill, mayonnaise, and horseradish powder, cooking over medium heat until well blended. Add the yogurt or sour cream and stir until just boiling. Remove from heat.
4. Arrange onion and pepper slices over the steaks. Pour the sauce on top and bake, covered for fifteen minutes. Uncover and bake another five to ten minutes. Do not

overcook. Check for doneness by using a fork; the fish should flake easily. Sprinkle with a bit of dried parsley, if desired, and serve.

EASY HALIBUT

4–5 pounds halibut steaks
Sea salt to taste
Juice of one lemon
1½ cups chopped celery
1 large onion, chopped
1 can tomato soup or 1 package Hain's dry soup
    mix plus ½ cup water
1 cup plain yogurt
1 dash cayenne pepper
Slice of thick tomato for each serving
1 tablespoon dried or fresh, chopped parsley
1 dash garlic powder for each serving

1. Preheat the oven to 350°F.
2. Season steaks with sea salt and lemon juice and place in a shallow baking dish.
3. Mix together the celery, onion, tomato soup mix, yogurt, and cayenne pepper, and pour over the fish. Top each steak with a slice of tomato, a sprinkle of parsley, and a dash of garlic powder.
4. Bake until the fish flakes easily when probed with a fork, approximately twenty-five to thirty-five minutes. Do not overcook or the fish will become tough. Serve immediately.

FLOUNDER FLORENTINE

¼ cup chopped onion
2 tablespoons expeller-pressed canola oil
10 ounces fresh spinach, chopped
1 tablespoon fresh lemon juice
1 tablespoon fresh dill or 1 teaspoon dried dill
1 dash sea salt (optional)
1 dash garlic powder (optional)
¼–½ cup sliced, slivered, or chopped almonds
2 pounds flounder fillets

1. Preheat the oven to 375°F.
2. Sauté the onion in oil until transparent. Add the spinach, cover, and cook until spinach is barely wilted. Remove from heat.
3. Add the lemon juice, seasonings, and almonds. Stir to blend and allow to cool.
4. Rinse the flounder. Place each fillet on a cutting board with the skin side down. Spoon equal amounts of filling onto each fillet and roll up. Use a toothpick to hold the roll together if it will not stay rolled up.
5. Place the rolls, seam side down, on an oiled baking dish and cover. Bake until the fish is tender and flaky, about twenty to twenty-five minutes. Serve immediately.

BREADED FISH

4–6 fish fillets of your choice (perch, haddock, and whitefish are good choices)
1 fresh lemon, cut in half
1 dash garlic powder for each serving
1 dash sea salt for each serving
1–1½ cups bread crumbs (make these by processing croutons, crackers, bread, or cornflakes of your choice in a blender or food processor until fine)
1 sprinkle dried parsley

1. Preheat the oven to 350°F.
2. Wash the fillets and pat dry. Place them on a platter, squeeze lemon over them, and sprinkle with garlic powder and sea salt. Allow to sit for a few minutes.
3. Pour bread crumbs into a large plastic bag. Shake the fillets one at a time in the bag until evenly coated.
4. Place the breaded fillet in a well-oiled baking dish and sprinkle with dried parsley. Bake for twenty-five to thirty-five minutes, just until the fish flakes easily and the fish looks solid white (all signs of translucency should disappear). Serve immediately as a main dish or in a sandwich.

EASY BROILED FISH

Any number of servings of the fish of your choice
1 dash garlic powder (not garlic salt) for each serving
1 dash sea salt for each serving
1 dash cayenne pepper for each serving
½ teaspoon olive or other vegetable oil for each serving
1 lemon, cut in half
1 tablespoon tamari for each serving
1 teaspoon fresh or ½ teaspoon dried parsley for each serving

1. Preheat the broiler.
2. Place the fish on an oiled baking dish. Season with garlic powder, sea salt, and cayenne pepper. Dot with the oil. Squeeze lemon juice over the fish and sprinkle the tamari on top.
3. Broil for ten minutes. Baste the fish with juices from the bottom of the baking dish. Broil another five minutes or until the fish is solid white, not translucent, and flakes easily with a fork. Baste once. Sprinkle with parsley and serve immediately. Broiled fish is excellent served over cooked brown rice with a lemon wedge on the side, and/or with steamed broccoli or any vegetable of your choice.

Variations: During the last few minutes, top with a plantain sliced lengthwise and/or slivered almonds for a more exotic dish. Or pour tomato soup with chopped onion, celery, and green peppers over the fish before baking.

CHAPTER FIFTEEN

COOL, CLEAR, AND CLEAN WATER

Water is the only drink for a wise man.

—*Henry David Thoreau, nineteenth-century American writer*

Humans can go without food for thirty to forty days, but without water, life would end in three to five days. Quality water is the best frontline treatment for every physical disorder of any living organism. With drinking water threatened by droughts, environmental pollution, and contaminants, it is important to consider where water comes from and its vital contribution to health.

The human body is composed of approximately 70 percent water, with content varying considerably from person to person and from one body part to another. The body's water supply is responsible for and involved in nearly every physical process, including digestion, absorption, circulation, and excretion.

A drop in the body's water content is reflected as a decline in blood volume. The lowering of the water content in the blood triggers the hypothalamus, the brain's thirst center, to send out the demand for water. This causes a slight rise in the concentration of sodium in the blood, which quickly triggers a sensation of thirst. People often consume only enough liquid to quench a dry or parched throat but not enough to cover normal water loss. Adults can become dehydrated quickly, as the percentage of water the body reserves drops with age. As we age, our sense of thirst dulls.

It is beneficial to always drink more water than the body craves or needs. You should try to make it a habit to drink water even when you are not feeling thirsty. It is, in fact, vital to health to drink eight or more glasses of quality water each and every day.

Drinking enough water could probably eliminate many bowel and bladder problems and even the common headache. Toxins build up in the system, which can cause headaches if not enough water is consumed to flush them out. The bladder also functions better with plenty of water. Drinking a full glass of water has been known to relieve anxiety attacks, food intolerance reactions, heartburn, acid stomach, muscle pain, colitis pain, hot flashes, and many other disorders. Flushing the system can relieve such symptoms more quickly than can using any herb, drug, or food. Quality water maintains, heals, rejuvenates, and rehabilitates the body.

Chronic fatigue syndrome (CFS), which is on the rise in this country, is just one of the disorders that can be helped by drinking at least eight glasses of water daily. Toxins and chemicals that cause symptoms of muscle aches, headaches, and extreme fatigue, which are very common complaints, can be flushed out by water. Without water, these metabolic waste products and toxins would poison the body.

The kidneys remove wastes like uric acid, urea, and lactic acid that must be dissolved in water. If not enough water is present, these substances are not removed effectively and may cause damage to the kidneys. Digestion and metabolism also rely on water for certain enzymatic and chemical reactions in the body. Water carries nutrients and oxygen to cells through the blood, and regulates body temperature through perspiration. Drinking plenty of water is especially important for athletic people and for those with arthritis or musculoskeletal problems, as it lubricates the joints. Water is essential for breathing—the lungs must be moistened by water to facilitate oxygen intake and carbon dioxide excretion. Approximately one pint of liquid is lost each day through exhaling. If not enough water is taken in for fluid balance, every body function could be impaired. The more you exercise, the more water you must consume to keep your body's water level in balance.

Excess body fat, poor muscle tone, digestive problems, organ malfunction, joint and muscle soreness, and water retention all may be related to not taking in enough fluids. In fact, in many cases, the way to eliminate fluid retention is to drink more water, as it is a natural diuretic. Proper water intake assists weight loss. If not enough water is consumed, the body cannot metabolize fat, which leads to water retention and weight gain.

Does all this seem too simple to be true? The simple things that God created are often the best medicine. Humankind has gotten away from the natural substances provided for healing. If the medical system could profit from charging a high price for water (and plant foods) as a prescription and an aid to healing, they would.

There are even more benefits from hydrating the body with water. Consuming water can slow down the aging process. Arthritis, kidney stones, constipation, arteriosclerosis, obesity, glaucoma, cataracts, diabetes, hypoglycemia, and many other diseases can be prevented and/or improved by consuming quality water. Drinking eight to ten glasses of water daily can make a noticeable difference in a person's health and quality of life.

TYPES OF DRINKING WATER

In the discussion above, you will notice that I do not just emphasize the importance of getting enough water, but of getting enough *quality* water. This is an important distinction. There is significant variation in the quality of drinking water available from different sources.

Bottled Water

Bottled water is water that is intended for human consumption and that is sealed in bottles or other containers with no added ingredients except for optional antimicrobial agents that must be identified on the label. The label may also contain other terms that it is important to understand.

Artesian water, or artesian well water, is water from a well where the water is brought to the surface by natural pressure or flow.

Ground water comes from water underground in the water table under pressure equal to or greater than atmospheric pressure that does not come in contact with surface water. Ground water must be pumped mechanically for bottling.

Mineral water is water containing not less than 250 parts per million (ppm) total dissolved solids (TDS), originating from a geologically and physically protected underground water source or spring that has been tapped at the spring opening or through a borehole. Mineral water is distinguished from other types of water by its constant level and relative proportions of minerals and trace elements at its source, allowing for variations in concentration due to seasonal differences. No minerals may be added to this water. If the TDS content of mineral water is below 500 ppm, the water may be labeled low mineral content. If it is greater than 1,500 ppm, the label *high mineral content* may be used.

Bottled water that has been produced by distillation, deionization, reverse osmosis, or other processes and meets the legal definition may be labeled *purified water* or *demineralized water.* Alternatively, the water may be called *deionized water* if the water has been processed by deioniza-tion, *distilled water* if it is produced by distillation, or *reverse osmosis water* if the water has been processed by reverse osmosis.

Water that contains the same amount of carbon dioxide that it had at emergence from the source may be labeled *sparkling bottled water.* An important note: soda water, seltzer water, and tonic water are not considered bottled waters. They are considered soft drinks, may contain sugar and calories, and are regulated separately.

Sparkling water is water that has been carbonated. It can be a healthy alternative to soda and alcoholic beverages, but if it's loaded with fructose and other sweeteners, it may be no better than soda pop. Read the label!

Understanding where the carbonation in sparkling water comes from isn't always easy. A "naturally sparkling water" drink must get its carbonation from the same source as the water. If water is "carbonated natural water," that means the carbonation came from a source other than the one that supplied the water. That doesn't mean the water is of poor quality. It can still be called "natural" because its mineral content is the same as when it came from the ground, even though it has been carbonated from a separate source. People suffering from intestinal disorders or ulcers should avoid carbonated water.

In addition, most states have no rules governing appropriate labeling, so a number of bottled water claims may be misleading or incorrect. The following is a guide to understanding what the most commonly used classifications of bottled water mean and how these varying waters may help or harm the body.

Spring water is water coming from an underground formation from which water flows naturally to the surface of the earth. Spring water must be collected only at the spring or through a borehole tapping the underground formation feeding the spring. To meet the definition of "spring," there must be natural force bringing the water to the surface opening. The location of the spring must be identified on the label of any water labeled spring water.

Well water comes from a hole bored, drilled, or otherwise constructed into the ground, which taps the water of an aquifer (an underground water source).

The phrase *from a community water system* or *from a municipal source* must appear on the label of water that comes from the same source as the water that flows through the pipes of a city or town. About 25 percent of bottled waters now sold come from the same water supply that flows into some household taps.

The regulations allow for the defined terms to be used with one another if the bottled water meets the various definitions, so it is possible for some water labels to include a number of the different terms.

Tap Water

Tap water is the water that comes out of your kitchen and bathroom faucets. Depending on where you live, where the water comes from, and what has been done to it, there is tremendous variability in the quality of tap water. The one constant is that, as a general rule, it is the *least* desirable source of drinking water.

Tap water almost always contains inorganic materials that enter the bloodstream when you drink it. Traces of these substances adhere to the artery walls. Cholesterol sticks to them causing the arteries to narrow and creating a potential risk of possible blockage. Other deposits of inorganic materials occur where blood flow is slowest, in such locations as:

- The joints, where they may contribute to arthritis.

- Small veins, where they may contribute to varicose veins.

- Small arteries, where they may contribute to hardening of the arteries.

- The inner ear, where they may contribute to hearing loss.

- The lens of the eye, where they may contribute to cataracts.

- The lungs, where they may contribute to emphysema.

Tap water is also full of harmful chemicals that the body cannot use. Approximately half of the tap water in the United States comes from lakes, rivers, or other surface sources. Underground aquifers or wells provide 35 percent, and the remaining 15 percent comes from private wells. Private wells are not government regulated, except at the local level, and it is up to the individual to determine what the quality of such water might be. It is known that such substances as residues of pharmaceutical drugs given to people and animals—including antibiotics, hormones, painkillers, tranquilizers, and chemotherapy drugs—and runoff from garden and agricultural chemicals such as fertilizers and pesticides are detectable in much ground water, surface water, and tap water. Bacteria and parasites, and the chlorine with which municipal water supplies are routinely treated, are other concerns. Because of increased concern over drinking water contaminated with microorganisms, the U.S. Centers for Disease Control and Prevention (CDC) and the EPA have issued suggestions that people with compromised immune systems boil tap water for at least one minute before using it, use an appropriate filtration system, or buy quality bottled drinking water.

More than 90 percent of the major water treatment plants in the United States use treatment methods that date from before World War I. These treatment systems do not take advantage of modern processes, like activated charcoal filtration or ozone treatment, for removal of chemical contaminants.

Interestingly, it is known that people who have Parkinson's disease are more likely than those without that disorder to have drunk well water and lived in rural areas, where agricultural runoff is significant. It therefore seems reasonable to suppose that the risk of Parkinson's disease may be linked to an overload of environmental toxins.

William Koller, M.D., a neurologist and researcher at the University of Kansas, has said that he believes toxins are the cause of this disease, but which specific toxins are unknown.

If you live in an agricultural area and use well water, you should have your water tested for nitrates, which can cause a serious blood disorder in infants and adults. Nitrates enter ground water when the nitrogen in chemical fertilizers and manure work down into the soil and eventually into the water that feeds the local wells.

Radon, a naturally occurring gas formed in the earth's crust, can migrate into water systems and may be implicated in lung cancer. The United States Environmental Protection Agency (EPA) estimates that 8 million Americans have high levels of radon in their water. This radon becomes airborne when the water runs in the home. Those most likely to have this problem are those who have private wells or get their water from other underground sources. Areas of the country known to have high concentrations of radon in the soil include parts of New Jersey, New York, Pennsylvania, North Carolina, New England, and Arizona, but it is not limited to these areas.

Government agencies and environmental organizations have reported that lead is another potential hazard and that some 42 million Americans are drinking water contaminated with high levels of lead. Water testing is advised especially if your household includes children under age six or if you are pregnant or likely to become pregnant. Small children and developing fetuses are particularly vulnerable to the brain-damaging effects of lead. Lead may also cause liver and kidney problems, and harm the cardiovascular, immune, and gastrointestinal systems.

More than one-third of all community water systems have been cited for failure to meet the EPA's water safety standards. Consumer activist Ralph Nader commissioned a study that identified more than 2,100 contaminants in tap water in the United States. The EPA monitors contaminants in seven categories: fluoride, volatile organics, coliform and surface water treatment, inorganics, organics, lead and copper, and other interim standards. The total number of contaminants currently monitored is only 79.

Waste and pollution create more problems than contamination of drinking water—they also affect our animal friends. *Pfiesteria*, a microorganism generated by human waste has reportedly killed billions of fish in the Chesapeake Bay and North Carolina areas, with other kill sites located from Mexico to Delaware. *Pfiesteria* thrives in unclean waters that are high in nitrogen and phosphorus. This is common near agricultural and industrial areas and it is perfect for *Pfiesteria*, but deadly for fish. Pfiesteria also affects humans who are continually exposed to contaminated waters, causing symptoms such as lesions, inability to concentrate, disorientation, and memory loss.

The United Nations Environmental Program says that there is a global water crisis, and that this is the most immediate and serious human health problem facing the planet. Three million people die every year from diarrheal diseases, such as cholera and dysentery, caused by contaminated water. Polluted water directly affects the health of 1.2 billion people every year. Diseases borne by mosquitoes and other pests, such as malaria, kill another 1.5 to 2.7 million people per year because of inadequate water management.

Hard Water versus Soft Water

Hard water, found in various parts of the country, contains the minerals calcium and magnesium, which prevent soap from lathering well and deposit a sediment film on hair, clothing, pipes, dishes, and washtubs. Although hard water can be annoying, studies show that deaths from heart disease are lower in areas where the drinking water is hard, possibly due to its magnesium content. However, some health-care professionals believe that the calcium found in hard water is not good for the heart, arteries, or bones. Unfortunately, hard water deposits its calcium and other minerals on the outside of these body structures while it is the calcium found within these structures that is beneficial to the body.

Soft water can be naturally soft or it may be hard water that has been treated with sodium in order to remove the calcium and magnesium. The problem with artificially softened water is that it is more likely to dissolve the lining of pipes than hard water. This poses a significant threat where lead pipes are used. In addition, plastic and galvanized pipes are composed of cadmium, posing another threat of toxic poisoning. Although these two types of pipe are now rarely used, today's copper pipes can lead to dangerous levels of copper, iron, zinc, and arsenic entering the body through the use of soft water; more good reasons not to drink tap water.

Fluoridated Water

For many years now, controversy has raged over whether fluoride should be added to drinking water. Chemist and microbiologist Albert Schatz, Ph.D., has said about fluoridation ". . . it is the greatest fraud that has ever been perpetrated on more people than any other fraud has." Proponents say that fluoride occurs naturally and helps develop and maintain strong bones and teeth. Opponents have vastly differing views. Research reported in the *Journal of Dental Research* concluded that tooth decay rates in Western Europe, which is 98 percent unfluoridated, have declined as much as they have in the United States in recent decades. Indeed, it is only in the United States that the government champions fluoride. The Delaney Congressional Investigation Committee, the government body charged with monitoring additives and other substances in the food supply, has stated, "fluoridation is mass medication without parallel in the history of medicine." Dr. Robert Carton, former scientist at the EPA, has said, "Fluoride is

More Water Worries

The Federal Bureau of Investigation says that bioterrorist threats to the nation's drinking water are a possibility that must be considered. Many toxic biological organisms and chemical substances could be introduced to the water supply. No drinking water treatment products have been tested or certified for effectiveness in reducing chemical or biological health threats. However, commonly available water plant and home distillation, reverse osmosis, ultraviolet light, and fine filtration units may provide a protective barrier against many agents. Many biological organisms are inactivated by heat in household distillation units.

somewhat less toxic than arsenic and more toxic than lead, and you wouldn't want either of them in your mouth."

Chronic fluoride use has been linked to numerous health problems, including osteoporosis, arthritis, osteomalacia, and Alzheimer's disease. Five different studies since 1990 show that the incidence of hip fracture in older men and women is at least twice as high (some studies indicated as much as 87 percent higher) in areas with fluoridated water as compared with unfluoridated areas. Fluoride was found to be an equivocal carcinogen by the National Cancer Institute Toxicological Program. In addition, more than 150 symptoms and associations of hypothyroidism correlate with known symptoms of fluoride poisoning.

We still do not have solid research on the long-term effects of fluoride on the human body, though it has been in use for more than fifty years. The short-term effects, however, are frightening enough to sound an alarm.

The most common salts used to fluoridate the United States' water supply are hydrofluosilicic acid and sodium silicofluorides, waste products of the phosphate fertilizer industry. The resulting toxic waste cannot be dumped in oceans, rivers, or landfills, even if diluted, and it cannot be given away (it is a class I toxic waste), so it has to be neutralized at a cost of $1.40 or more per gallon.

If this same waste (with the heavy metals arsenic, cadmium, lead, and uranium also present) goes into the water we drink, the local water district will pay thirty-five to forty-five cents per gallon for transportation, and the industrial wastewater is suddenly considered benign. It can then be shipped, untreated, to go in drinking water. The naturally occurring form of fluoride, calcium fluoride, is not toxic—but this form of fluoride is not used to fluoridate water.

Today, more than 60 percent of the cities in the United States fluoridate their water supplies. In many states, it is required. Fluoridation has become the standard rather than the exception.

Individuals have different levels of tolerance for fluoride. In addition, many water sources have levels of fluoride higher than one part per million, the level generally recognized as safe and originally set as the acceptable limit by the EPA. After the EPA learned that water in many towns had natural fluoride levels much higher than this, the permissible fluoride level was raised—quadrupled, in fact—to four parts per million. And this is in addition to fluoride encountered from other sources. Fluoride is the thirteenth most widely distributed element on earth, so it can turn up just about anywhere—in vegetables and meats, for example. In addition, fluoride is found in many cola and fruit juices, in well-known cereals, in products using white grape juice, in toothpaste, and in the pesticide residue on fruits and vegetables, which further increases our exposure.

To remove fluoride from tap water, you can use a reverse osmosis, distillation, or activated alumina filtration system, which will eliminate almost all of the fluoride from the water.

DRINKING WATER REGULATORS

While the EPA is charged with the regulation of public water supplies that provide the sources for the majority of tap water, the U.S. Food and Drug Administration (FDA) has the responsibility of regulating bottled drinking water. The FDA defines the terms required for the description of bottled drinking waters in specific requirements last revised in April 1997. The choices for the consumer are now easier than in the past.

All terms that are legally necessary to describe bottled drinking water are discussed on page 135. Terms not defined or included there are marketing slogans added to entice consumers to buy the product. They can mean anything that the manufacturer of the product says they mean.

TESTING WATER

The U.S. Environmental Protection Agency (EPA), which is charged with overseeing the safety of the nation's water, supplies a toll-free phone number to help locate the nearest office or laboratory that does certified water testing so that you can find out exactly what is in your tap water. A number of labs will send a self-addressed container that allows you to put the filled bottle into a local mailbox. The cost of testing may be as low as $35 to $40 per tap, and results are usually available in two to three weeks. (See the Resources section for more information.)

The EPA also makes available a list entiled the *Recommended Maximum Contaminant Levels.* This can help you to understand information received from a testing lab about your water. Information on this and other educational material is available from NSF International and from the Water Quality Association. (See the Resources section.)

Grapefruit Seed Extract

Grapefruit seed extract is ideal as a safe and simple way to disinfect drinking water when camping, backpacking, traveling to foreign countries, or in any emergency situation where safe drinking water is not obtainable and boiling is not possible. Available water should first be filtered (at the least, let suspended water particles settle). Retain the clear water and add 10 drops of grapefruit seed extract per gallon of water. Shake or stir vigorously and let it sit for a few minutes. You may notice a slightly bitter taste, but this is just the inherent taste of the grapefruit seed extract. It is not harmful. Safe and easy to carry with you, grapefruit seed extract is actually a first-aid remedy with many uses.

WATER TREATMENT PROCESSES

There are a variety of ways of treating water to improve its quality. Some can be utilized at home, while some require larger or more complicated installations. Steam-distillation is one of the best. Distillation is the process of converting liquids into a vapor state by heating. The vapor cools and is condensed back into a liquid and stored. This process removes solids and other impurities, producing pure drinking water. Metals, including lead, cadmium, mercury, and aluminum, as well as other toxins are removed. Steam-distilled water is preferred (be sure the bottle states *steam-distilled*). Boiling water does not accomplish the same thing because all the harmful chemicals are left concentrated in the water. Consuming fresh, leafy green vegetables, grains, and other healthy foods will supply the necessary minerals that have been removed from water.

Water softeners offer another way to treat water. They use either sodium or potassium to exchange or substitute for the calcium and/or magnesium present in naturally "hard" water. The primary benefit of softening is in improved cleaning properties for the water and less mineral buildup inside household pipes and equipment.

Filtration is probably the most commonly used home treatment method. Filters use either an absorbing or screening material to physically remove or block contaminants from water at the faucet. There are many different types of filters and filter materials—varieties of carbon and activated carbon are the most common. Filters are often arranged in series so that the media materials that are most effective for specific types of contaminants can be used. The primary advantage is relative low cost and ease of use.

Water can also be treated with ultraviolet light to kill bacteria and viruses. Reverse osmosis is a high-tech method of purifying water in which water is forced through a semipermeable membrane while charged particles and larger molecules are repelled. It is the best system for treating water that is brackish (high in salt), high in nitrates, and loaded with inorganic heavy metals such as iron and lead. Reverse osmosis is also one of the best methods for producing quality water. A good source for reverse osmosis units for the home (including the shower) is Waterwise, which offers options combining both predistillation and postdistillation carbon filtrations for the highest level of quality and taste.

Each treatment method has its advantages and disadvantages, but using a combination of methods can result in the best overall quality drinking water. Even the quality and taste of distilled water can be improved by passing the water through a charcoal/carbon filter as a final step.

Before purchasing a water treatment unit, write, call, or visit the Web sites of NSF International or the Water Quality Association. (See the Resources section.) These nonprofit testing and certification organizations verify manufacturers' claims and certify that the materials used are nontoxic and structurally sound. Periodic unannounced audits of products are conducted to insure compliance with standards. Some of the manufacturers whose products meet the standards of these organizations include Waterwise, Inc., Pure Water, Inc., EcoWater Systems, and Rainsoft. (For more information, see the Resources section.)

CHAPTER SIXTEEN

HIGH-FIBER FOODS: THE BODY'S INTERNAL BROOM!

Retained debris in the colon leads to the absorption of toxins resulting in systemic intoxication (poisoning) . . . which can lead to more serious disorders.

—*Prescription for Nutritional Healing*

Adding the right type of fiber to the diet can reduce the risks of certain cancers, diabetes, heart disease, and bowel disorders such as irritable bowel syndrome and diverticulitis. Fiber helps to lower high blood cholesterol and stabilizes blood sugar levels. It also helps to prevent constipation and hemorrhoids and can assist weight loss by suppressing appetite.

More than 135,000 colon cancer cases are diagnosed each year in the United States, and the number is growing. Research has proven that the American diet, which relies heavily on processed foods, lacks sufficient fiber for colon health. The theory is that, in addition to keeping the large intestine (colon) swept clean, fiber collects carcinogens and binds to them so that they are easily removed from the body. While the most recent studies say that there may be no link between a high-fiber diet and a lowered incidence of colorectal cancer, we do know for certain that many high-fiber foods contain anticancer nutrients. Studies *have* proven that the incidence of colon cancer is lower in people who eat a diet low in meat and high in fiber-rich foods. Natural fiber has been removed from most refined foods, so the average American—who relies heavily on processed and refined food products—consumes a mere 12 grams of fiber daily. To put this in perspective, the National Cancer Institute recommends a daily intake of between 20 grams and 35 grams from a wide range of high-fiber foods.

Fiber supplements, in the forms of pills, raw bran, capsules, and drinks, are available for those who have difficulty eating high-fiber foods. A ground flaxseed supplement works for many people. However, fiber supplements should not be a substitute for fiber-rich foods, which also contain nutrients that help fight chronic disease.

TYPES OF FIBER

Found only in foods such as whole grains, fruits, vegetables, nuts, seeds, and legumes, fiber makes up the components of plant cell walls. There are two basic categories of dietary fiber: soluble and insoluble. Most plants contain some of each form. Both soluble and insoluble fiber are needed in the diet, as they have different health effects. Fiber is further classified as six distinct types: cellulose, hemicellulose, lignin, gums, mucilages, and pectins. All except lignin are complex carbohydrates. Cellulose, lignin, and pectin are further considered to be phytochemicals, substances manufactured in plants that have numerous health benefits. (See Chapter 7.)

Humans lack the enzymes and digestive juices needed to break down fiber, so much of it passes through the body without adding energy or calories. Some plant fibers, however, are fermented in the colon by "friendly" bacteria. Fermentation byproducts include certain fatty acids that have anticancer activity and produce energy for the liver and colon. Fiber's main job is to help the bowels function more efficiently by cleaning the intestines and adding more bulk to stool. Without correct bowel movements, toxins can build up and be carried through the body, resulting in a variety of illnesses.

Soluble Fiber

Soluble fiber (gums, mucilage, and pectin) dissolves and blends with water to form a gel in the gastrointestinal tract. Most of the fiber in plant cell walls is water-soluble. Soluble fiber promotes regular bowel movements and aids in weight loss by slowing down the passage of food and giving a full feeling.

Soluble fiber is useful in the management of diabetes, hypoglycemia, hyperglycemia, and other conditions that are affected by the quick breakdown of carbohydrates into glucose, a form of sugar. It retards the absorption of glucose, allowing the body to release it into the bloodstream gradually. In this way, it moderates blood sugar levels. Foods low in glycemic value (those that are converted into

An Apple a Day

One apple, eaten whole with the skin, has about 3.6 grams of fiber and is a tasty and natural way to assist proper bowel function. Recent research shows that apples help prevent lung disorders. There's more truth to the old saying, "An apple a day keeps the doctor away," than we ever realized. Apple pectin can be purchased in tablet or capsule form and is beneficial for many disorders.

blood sugar slowly) are whole grains, beans, seeds, soybeans and soy products, mushrooms, leafy vegetables, and vegetables such as cucumbers, zucchini, cabbage, and string beans. Foods that have been processed, however, such as canned vegetables and fruits, instant rice, or quick-cooking grain cereals, have been stripped of fiber and are not able to retard sudden rises in blood sugar. This is one reason why you should add raw foods to your diet as much as possible. They are filling and prevent overeating; plus, they have abundant nutrients and enzymes required to maintain health. Eating raw foods that are naturally high in fiber satisfies hunger, whereas nutritionally empty, processed foods leave the body craving even more food.

Soluble fiber also helps to lower elevated serum cholesterol and remove fat from the gastrointestinal tract. It is less effective than insoluble fiber at speeding elimination of waste, absorbing toxins, softening stools, and improving bowel disorders. One note of caution: soluble fiber can be metabolized by gas-forming bacteria in the colon. This is harmless, but if you have intestinal gas or flatus problems, avoid or test particular foods to see if they cause discomfort. Start by consuming small amounts and increase gradually to avoid a problem.

Good food sources of soluble fiber include barley, beans and peas, lentils, oat bran, fruits, and vegetables.

Insoluble Fiber

Plant cell walls that do not dissolve in water are collectively referred to as insoluble dietary fiber—commonly called "roughage." These components are cellulose, hemicellulose, and lignin. The main structural fiber of the plant cell wall is cellulose; hemicellulose ties the cellulose fibers together. Lignin is a woody substance in some plants that makes the plant cell walls rigid.

Consuming immoderate amounts of insoluble fiber may decrease the absorption of certain minerals, such as iron, calcium, and magnesium. Soluble fiber, on the other hand, does not block mineral absorption. Insoluble fiber does not break down during digestion. Though it does not dissolve in water, it can bind water, much like a sponge. For instance, wheat bran absorbs three times its weight in

water. This absorption causes bowel movements to be softer and to have greater bulk. The increased bulk places pressure against the intestinal walls, which eases and regulates movement through the intestines. As a result, insoluble fiber, unlike soluble fiber, speeds up transit time and gastric emptying.

Insoluble fiber appeases the appetite, reduces bacterial toxins, speeds the elimination of waste, absorbs toxins, softens stools, and improves bowel disorders. It is less effective in lowering serum cholesterol, speeding bile acid excretion, and reducing gas. Water-insoluble fiber does not give a full feeling for a prolonged period or stabilize blood sugar.

Food sources of insoluble fiber include whole grains, brown rice, nuts, vegetables, and fruits.

HOW FIBER PROMOTES HEALTH

Fiber helps to remove fat from the colon wall and unwanted metals and toxins from the body. In today's polluted environment, our bodies need help in excreting this overload.

Soluble fiber binds with bile acids and forces their excretion, which causes the body to make more bile acid. This process requires cholesterol, so the amount of cholesterol circulating in the blood is reduced. Some researchers theorize that the bile acids carried out of the intestines by some types of soluble fiber may act as cancer-promoters once they reach the colon. Thus, high-fiber consumption may be a trade-off between lowering cholesterol and increasing the risk of cancer. This could be offset, however, by the action of insoluble fiber in sweeping out the colon with regular bowel movements. The soluble fibers pectin (in fruits) and beta-glucan (in oat bran) are believed to absorb harmful fatty acids. Fiber is thought to interfere with cholesterol synthesis, or possibly to block the action of carcinogens.

Psyllium seed, which is all soluble fiber, acts as both a soluble fiber, lowering cholesterol levels, and an insoluble fiber, scrubbing through the intestines and cleaning them of potential carcinogens. Psyllium seed should be used only in a powder form that dissolves in liquid. The mixture must be drunk quickly because it thickens, which may slow its progress through the gastrointestinal tract and allow it to become stuck. Be sure the psyllium powder is thoroughly dissolved before swallowing it. Drinking a full glass of plain water immediately afterward will help ensure the psyllium mixture moves quickly into the colon.

Though rice bran contains mostly insoluble fiber and oat bran contains a type of soluble fiber called beta-glucan, both can reduce cholesterol. Rice bran may be a better source of dietary fiber than oat bran. When rice bran fiber is properly processed, it can contain 27 percent dietary fiber by weight, 20 percent insoluble and 7 percent soluble.

To increase your daily fiber intake, start by adding a few grams from a wide range of food sources and gradually increase the amount until stools are the proper consistency.

Loading up on fiber too quickly can cause gas, bloating, and abdominal pain. Be sure to increase your fluid intake accordingly to replace the water that fiber soaks up—at least eight glasses daily. Insufficient water can cause fiber to create blockage in the intestine, creating a very serious problem.

If you use a fiber supplement, do not take it at the same time as medications or other supplements. They will lose much of their effectiveness and strength because some fibers are so absorbent they will pick up the beneficial elements as well as the bad. Replace lost minerals that may be absorbed by fiber with a mineral supplement taken at another time. Fiber supplements of all types should be taken between meals, or at least one-half to one hour before meals. If taken during meals, fiber will bind with food nutrients and remove them from the body.

FOODS WITH THE HIGHEST FIBER CONTENT

Among foods that will add the greatest amount of useful fiber to your diet are whole-grain cereals and flours, brown rice, all types of bran, apricots, dried prunes, apples, and most other fruits. Be careful of oranges, however. They are highly acidic and can aggravate arthritis. Also, some people are allergic to oranges. Nuts, seeds, beans, lentils, peas, and vegetables (especially beets, broccoli, cabbage, carrots, cauliflower, carrots, and dark-green leafy vegetables) are also good sources of fiber. Be sure to eat several of these foods daily, as each fiber has its own function. Also, all fiber is not the same—for example, wheat fiber differs from apple fiber. Other good sources of fiber are bananas, blueberries, parsnips, raisins, raspberries, spinach, strawberries, and sweet potatoes. Table 16.1 below lists the fiber content of a number of good fiber sources.

A simple way to get more fiber from your food is to increase your intake of raw foods. Eating the skin and

TABLE 16.1 POWER EATING: A DOZEN HIGH-FIBER FOODS

The table below, adapted from an article in the Tufts University *Diet and Nutrition Letter*, lists some of the most powerful food sources of fiber, together with the number of grams of fiber they contain per serving.

FOOD	GRAMS OF FIBER
All-Bran cereal (⅓ cup)	8.5
Lentils, cooked (½ cup)	7.8
Black beans, cooked (½ cup)	7.5
Kidney beans, cooked (½ cup)	7.3
Lima beans, cooked (½ cup)	5.8
Chickpeas, cooked (½ cup)	5.3
Potato, baked with skin (1 medium)	4.8
Peas, raw (½ cup)	4.4
Oatmeal (1 cup cooked)	4.0
Pear, with skin (1 medium)	4.0
Apple, with skin (1 medium)	3.7
Brussels sprouts, raw (½ cup)	3.4
Peach, with skin (1 medium)	3.4

Fiber and Probiotics

Fiber can help keep the colon and bowels healthy by stripping them of harmful bacteria. At the same time, however, it removes some of the *friendly* bacteria in the colon that are necessary for good health. When consuming high-fiber foods, add to your diet a source of friendly bacteria, or probiotics, such as *Lactobacillus acidophilus*, *Lactobacillus bulgaricus*, or *Bifidobacterium bifidum*. These are commonly found in cultured dairy products, especially yogurt, and fermented foods. Milk-free friendly probiotic supplements such as Kyo-Dophilus from Wakunaga of America and Primadophilus from Nature's Way, are also available in health food stores.

membranes of vegetables and fruits ensures that you get every bit of fiber. Cooking may reduce the fiber content of foods by breaking down some fiber into its carbohydrate components. When you do cook vegetables, steam them only until they are tender but firm to the bite.

In addition, one or more of the following high-fiber foods should be part of daily meal planning:

- Oat bran, which helps to lower blood cholesterol.

- Cooked beans. One cup contains the same amount of soluble fiber as ⅓ cup of oat bran.

- Psyllium seed, which is an intestinal cleanser and stool softener. It is one of the most popular dietary fibers.

- Fennel seed, which helps to rid the intestinal tract of mucus.

- Flaxseeds, which help to protect against rheumatoid arthritis and atherosclerosis. They have the added benefit of supplying essential fatty acids.

FIBERS FOR SPECIFIC HEALTH PROBLEMS

Simply adding adequate amounts of the right fiber to the diet can eliminate or alleviate many common health problems, particularly as we age. Fiber is found in many foods, and you should eat several servings of fiber-rich food daily. You can easily incorporate the various types of fiber into your daily diet by including servings of whole-grain cereals and flours, brown rice, agar-agar, all kinds of bran, most fresh fruits, prunes, nuts, seeds (especially flaxseeds), beans, lentils, peas, and fresh raw vegetables. This is an inexpensive and natural way to give the body what it requires for good colon health and can eliminate the need for costly fiber supplements. If you really do need to take fiber supplements, do not take them at the same time as any other medications. The information that follows will help you to understand the different types of fiber and how you can use them to your best benefit.

Pectin

Pectin is useful in managing diabetes because it slows the absorption of food after meals. It removes unwanted metals and toxins and helps to lessen side effects of radiation therapy. Pectin also helps to lower cholesterol and to reduce the risk of heart disease and gallstones.

Food sources of pectin include apples, carrots, beets, berries, bananas, pears, prunes, plums, cabbage, citrus fruits, dried peas, grapes, and okra.

Cellulose

Found in the outer layer of fruits and vegetables, cellulose is useful for people with hemorrhoids, varicose veins, constipation, colitis, or diverticulitis. It also helps to get rid of cancer-causing substances lodged in the colon wall.

Food sources of cellulose include apples, apricots, asparagus, beans, beets, bran flakes, celery, mushrooms, oatmeal, onions, pears, cabbage, carrots, broccoli, peas, peanuts, whole grains, and Brazil nuts.

Hemicellulose

Less chemically complex than cellulose, hemicellulose aids in weight loss, relieves constipation, and lowers the risk of colon cancer by fighting carcinogens in the intestinal tract.

Food sources of hemicellulose include apples, beets, whole-grain breads and cereals, cabbage, Brussels sprouts, bananas, green beans, corn, peppers, broccoli, mustard greens, pears, eggplant, and radishes.

Lignin

Lignin helps to lower cholesterol levels, protects against colon cancer, and prevents gallstone formation. It binds with bile acids and removes them from the body. It is beneficial for people with diabetes.

Food sources of lignin include cabbage, cauliflower, carrots, barley, green beans, kale, parsley, peas, soybeans, whole grains, flaxseeds, Brazil nuts, peaches, tomatoes, spinach, strawberries, and potatoes.

Gums and Mucilages

Both gums and mucilages regulate blood glucose levels, aid in lowering cholesterol levels, and help in the removal of toxins.

Food sources of gums and mucilages include oatmeal, oat bran, sesame seeds, and beans and legumes.

CHAPTER SEVENTEEN

SPICES AND HERBS: FLAVOR ENHANCERS THAT HEAL

As for rosemary, I let it run all over my garden wall, not only because my bees love it, but because it is the herb sacred to remembrance and to friendship.

—Sir Thomas More (1478–1535), English politician, scholar, and writer

Herbs and spices can change the most ordinary food into a memorable meal and have been doing so for thousands of years. There are records of cinnamon being traded in the Middle East 2,000 years before the birth of Jesus. At one time, spices were more treasured than gold and were even used as currency between some countries. At the end of the fifteenth century, Europeans sent ships to circumnavigate the globe in search of precious herbs and spices, and, as a result, the "New World" opened up. Wars were won and lost, over and over, to claim control of the valuable spice territories. It is indeed fortunate that exotic herbs and spices are now readily available to help transform common recipes into uncommon delights!

In some cultures, the word *spice* and *herb* are interchangeable. Both have healing powers, but there are some differences. Herbs are plants that have culinary, medicinal, cosmetic, or fragrant properties. Most herbs grow in temperate regions and are derived from the fresh or dried leaves or other green parts of the plant, although other parts are occasionally used. Spices usually have a stronger scent than herbs and often have a piquant taste. They usually come from the flowers, seeds, fruit, roots, or bark of trees and shrubs grown in tropical or subtropical climates. Herbs and spices have been used for centuries as curatives for common ailments, as well as for their taste.

Many culinary herbs and spices that add flavor to recipes also have powerful medicinal properties. They are full of phytochemicals and antioxidants, which protect the body against diseases. Spices are all very low in calories. Herbs such as sage, rosemary, and thyme have even fewer calories than many spices. Yet just 1 teaspoon of paprika or chili powder provides as much as 16 percent of the daily requirement for vitamin A in the form of beta-carotene.

Use fresh or dried herbs creatively to cut back on cooking oil (fat) without sacrificing taste and to spark up restricted-diet recipes. Replace salt with oregano and sugar with allspice or anise, for instance. Choose whole-leaf dried herbs rather than ground ones, if possible. Then, to release their flavor, crumble them between your fingers just before adding them to dishes. Generally, herbs should be added toward the end of cooking because they are less potent and lose their flavor the longer they are heated. Bay leaves are the exception. If you are preparing a recipe that calls for bay leaves or other herbs that are to be removed before serving, place them in a stainless-steel tea ball or tie them in a bundle of several layers of cheesecloth and attach the tea ball or cheesecloth bundle to the handle of the pot to make removal easier. Herbs enhance foods best if used with a light touch, and release their flavor when soaked for ten to thirty minutes in some of the liquid to be used in a recipe.

Great combinations can make seasoning simple. Combine equal amounts of the following herb mixtures in small jars and keep them on hand for quick and easy seasoning. In most places, you can grow your own fresh herbs all year long in flowerpots on a windowsill. Generally, you have to use two to three times the amount of a fresh herb to have the same flavor impact as the same herb in dried form.

- For an Italian flavor, combine basil, marjoram, oregano, rosemary, and thyme.

- For an Asian flavor, combine anise, cinnamon, clove, fennel, ginger, and licorice root.

- For a Continental flavor, combine bay leaf, marjoram, tarragon, and thyme.

STORING HERBS

The appropriate method of storing herbs depends on whether they are dried or fresh. You can also freeze herbs, preserve them in oils, or use them in the form of herbal vinegars.

Dried Herbs

Light, oxygen, and moisture destroy the flavor and health-promoting potency of herbs' flavors and medicinal potency. Dried herbs last the longest if they are stored in opaque glass, dark-colored glass, or ceramic containers. Fill the containers to the top to minimize the amount of oxygen allowed in. As the herbs are used, add pieces of sterile rolled cotton to the containers to fill the empty space and, again, limit the amount of oxygen inside. If the herbs get wet, refrigerate them and use them within a few days. Also, to help keep out the small bugs that some herbs attract, add a few aromatic bay leaves and peppercorns to the containers.

If stored properly, aromatic herbs such as sage, rosemary, and thyme can retain their potency for more than a year. Nonaromatic herbs such as dill seed and nutmeg can last considerably longer. Never store dried herbs and spices close to a heat source or stovetop. This will cause them to lose their flavor and color.

Fresh Herbs

Fresh herbs are fragile, like all fresh produce. Wrap them in a damp dish towel and store them, dish towel and all, in a plastic bag in the refrigerator. This will keep them fresh for about two weeks.

Frozen Herbs

Certain herbs freeze exceptionally well. These include basil, chervil, chives, coriander, dill, fennel, mint, parsley, tarragon, and thyme. Freeze them whole or chopped, individually or in combinations. To make sure they retain their bright color, before freezing, swish the herbs' tops for a few seconds in boiling water, then quickly swish them in ice water. For best results, do not defrost the herbs before using. Add them directly to simmering soups, stews, and sauces, or blend them into salad dressings.

Oil-Preserved Herbs

Fresh herbal essences can be preserved in oil for several weeks. The oils can be used for stir-frying and in marinades and salad dressings. There are a number of different oils you can choose for preserving herbs. The mild, light flavors of corn, soy, safflower, and sunflower oils make an ideal base for any herb. The more flavorful herbs, such as rosemary and garlic, can hold their own with the heavier olive oil. The strong flavor of sesame oil overpowers anything but garlic. With the intricate taste of tarragon, try light peanut oil.

To make most herbal oils, fill a glass jar with chopped herbs and cover them with the desired oil. Let the mixture stand in a warm spot for a few hours, then strain the mix-

ture into a clean bottle, discarding the herbs, and store in the refrigerator. To make garlic oil, add two or three chopped or crushed cloves to one pint of olive oil. Steep the oil for four days, then strain, press the garlic, and add it back to the oil. Be careful when making garlic oil. If not handled properly, garlic oil (and garlic butters or garlic marinades) carry the risk of botulism. Be sure to keep all homemade garlic preparations refrigerated, and do not store them for longer than one month. If you dip the garlic in vinegar before adding it to the oil, this will destroy any mold and bacteria that might be present, and allow you to keep the garlic oil for up to a month if it is refrigerated. If this is not possible, it might be preferable to prepare a fresh batch each time you wish to use it.

Do not confuse herbal oils with herbal extracts. All oils should be stored in the refrigerator, with the exception of olive oil.

Herbal Vinegars

Herbal vinegar preparations are another good way to preserve fresh herbs. (Dried herbs make excellent vinegar, too.) These vinegars can be used to flavor a variety of foods, including soups, stews, ground meat dishes, gravies, stuffing, aspics, fruit and vegetable salads, salad dressings, and marinades. Most herbs, either alone or combined with other herbs, will produce fine vinegar. Use apple cider vinegar, wine vinegar, rice vinegar, balsamic vinegar, or malt vinegar as a base.

When making herbal vinegar, use only glass containers, preferably with nonmetal lids such as glass or plastic. If you must use a container with a metal lid, be sure to keep the lid from coming into contact with the vinegar to prevent a chemical reaction that might spoil the preparation. You can cover the inside of the lid with waxed paper. Fill the container with chopped or bruised (lightly crushed between the fingers) herbs, both stems and leaves, and add enough vinegar to cover. Cap the container tightly and let it stand in a sunny, warm spot for one to two weeks, shaking it occasionally. When the preparation is finished, or when you are ready to use it, strain the vinegar into fresh bottles and discard the herbs. Herbs placed in vinegar will keep for months if stored in a dark place such as the interior of a cupboard to protect the color of the herbs.

HERBS, SPICES, AND THEIR USES

The following are some of the most popular cooking herbs and spices, their flavor attributes, suggestions for using them, and lists of their known key nutrients, phytochemicals, and healing actions. For more in-depth information on which herbs to use for specific health disorders, refer to *Prescription for Herbal Healing* (Avery/Penguin Putnam, 2002).

Allspice

Allspice is the dried, unripe berry of a Caribbean evergreen tree. Its flavor is like a combination of cinnamon, pepper, juniper, and clove. Whole or ground berries can be used with sweet and savory foods. Add a few berries when making stock or stew; add ground allspice to mulled cider, fruit desserts, and pumpkin pie. Allspice is also called pimento and Jamaica pepper.

As a healing spice, allspice has anti-inflammatory, antioxidant, and anticancer properties. Oil from allspice berries is an effective pain reliever and may promote digestive enzyme activity. For toothache, apply allspice oil with a cotton swab directly to the tooth or gum. To make a digestive tea, use 1 to 2 teaspoons of allspice powder per cup of boiling water; steep for ten to twenty minutes, then strain.

Key nutrients in allspice include calcium, vitamin C, vitamin B_6, vitamin A, vitamin E, iron, magnesium, manganese, phosphorus, potassium, vitamin B_2 (riboflavin), vitamin B_1 (thiamine), zinc, and folate, and fiber. Phytochemicals include limonene, eugenol, alpha-pinene, and phytosterols.

Anise

Anise belongs to the parsley family. Its flavor is highly aromatic, sweet, and licoricelike. It is also called star anise and Chinese anise.

Traditionally, anise has been used to treat digestive problems, coughs, bronchitis, and asthma. The Chinese have used star anise for centuries to treat rheumatism. It is used also to soothe inflamed mucous membranes in nasal passages. Anise seeds can be chewed as a breath freshener. To help relieve emphysema, take 5 drops of anise oil in a teaspoon of honey a half-hour before meals. To make anise tea, use 1 teaspoon of gently crushed anise seeds per cup of boiling water; steep for ten to twenty minutes, then strain and drink.

Whole or ground anise seeds can be used in Asian dishes, soups, spice cakes, cookies, fruit, and other desserts.

Key nutrients in anise include calcium, iron, magnesium, phosphorus, potassium, manganese, zinc, vitamin C, vitamin B_6, vitamin A, vitamin E, vitamin B_1 (thiamine), vitamin B_2 (riboflavin), vitamin B_3 (niacin), pantothenic acid, and fiber. Phytochemicals include limonene, alpha-pinene, apigenin, bergapten, caffeic acid, chlorogenic acid, eugenol, linalol, myristicin, rutin, scopoletin, squalene, stigmasterol, amd umbelliferone.

Caution: Ingesting large doses of anise oil may cause nausea and vomiting.

Basil

Basil, a member of the mint family, is sweet and pungent, minty, and mildly peppery. It relieves a variety of digestive disorders, including stomach cramps, vomiting, and constipation. It may be used as a disinfectant, immune stimulant, and treatment for intestinal parasites, and is helpful to the lungs, spleen, and large intestines. According to Italian researchers, eating basil may reduce the risk of lung cancer. In large amounts, however, this herb can cause problems such as nervousness and rapid heartbeat, so use it sparingly.

As a culinary herb, basil perks up fresh-sliced tomatoes and cucumbers and goes well with chicken, fish, and pasta sauce. A staple in Italian cooking, it is the basic ingredient in pesto. To make basil tea, use 1 teaspoon of dried basil per ½ cup of boiling water; steep for five minutes, then strain and drink.

Key nutrients in basil include vitamin A, vitamin C, calcium, iron, magnesium, phosphorus, potassium, zinc, manganese, vitamin B_1 (thiamine), vitamin B_3 (niacin), pantothenic acid, folate, and fiber. Phytochemicals include eugenol.

Bay Leaves

Bay leaves are the dried leaves of the evergreen laurel tree. Also called laurel and sweet bay, their flavor is woody and astringent, with a subtle minty aroma. They are an aid to relaxation and help to manage stress. Bay is good for relieving migraines and for those with diabetes. It also has a beneficial effect on the stomach and intestinal tract. Bay leaf oil is antibacterial. To repel household pests naturally, spread some crushed bay leaves in kitchen cupboards and other infested areas. Also, place them in grain to deter insects. For a relaxing tea, use 1 to 2 teaspoons of crushed leaves per cup of boiling water. Strain the tea before drinking. One to 2 drops of bay oil can be added to regular black tea, honey, or brandy.

Bay leaves add flavor to meats, fish, poultry, vegetables, and stews. The leaves blend well with thyme. Remember to remove bay leaves after cooking and before serving your dish—they are tough and leathery, and very strong-tasting.

Key nutrients in bay leaves include calcium, iron, magnesium, phosphorus, potassium, zinc, manganese, vitamin C, vitamin A, vitamin B_6, vitamin E, vitamin B_2 (riboflavin), vitamin B_3 (niacin), folate, and fiber. Phytochemicals include carvone, limonene, caryophyllene, 1,8-cineole, alpha-pinene, eugenol, geraniol, kaempferol, linalol, perillyl alcohol, quercetin, and rutin.

Used as a seasoning, bay leaves are quite safe. However as with herbs, if you are pregnant, you should not take medicinal doses.

Caraway

Caraway seeds are most commonly known as the seeds that flavor rye bread. Their flavor is sharp and slightly bitter, with a sweet undertone.

Caraway helps to soothe stomach disorders and aid digestion. It stimulates the appetite and the production of breast milk. It helps in treating bronchitis, colic, and coughs. A powder made from the seeds and used in a poultice can speed the healing of bruises. Caraway can help relax smooth muscles, such as the uterus, for relief of menstrual cramps. To make caraway tea, use 2 to 3 teaspoons of crushed seeds per cup of boiling water; steep for ten to twenty minutes, then strain and drink. The seeds can also be chewed for medicinal benefit.

To use caraway in foods, add the seeds to breads, soups, salads, stews, cheeses, sauerkraut, pickling brines, and meat dishes. The caraway root can be eaten as a vegetable. The oil is used in canning and for flavoring meats.

Key nutrients in caraway include calcium, vitamin C, vitamin A, vitamin B_6, vitamin E, iron, magnesium, phosphorus, potassium, zinc, manganese, vitamin B_1 (thiamine), vitamin B_2 (riboflavin), vitamin B_3 (niacin), folate, and fiber. Phytochemicals include phytosterols, carvone, limonene, alpha-pinene, beta-carotene, linalol, myristic acid, myristicin, perillyl alcohol, quercetin, and tannin.

Used as a seasoning, caraway is quite safe. However as with most herbs, if you are pregnant, you should not use it in medicinal doses.

Cardamom

Cardamom is a member of the ginger family. Its flavor is grapefruit-like and floral, with a hint of menthol. Cardamom seeds or powder can be made into a tea or used with liquids as a digestive aid and gas remedy. It is good for the lungs and helps to relieve asthma and bronchitis. Cardamom also stimulates the appetite and is used by tribes on the Arabian Peninsula to boost energy.

Cardamom is used extensively in Scandinavian and Indian cuisines. It is often used in holiday breads. It goes well with fruit. Use it also in homemade curry powder and sweet rice pilafs, and with sweet vegetables such as winter squash, pumpkin, and sweet potatoes.

Key nutrients in cardamom include calcium, iron, magnesium, phosphorus, potassium, zinc, manganese, vitamin C, vitamin B_1 (thiamine), vitamin B_2 (riboflavin), vitamin B_3 (niacin), and fiber. Phytochemicals include limonene, 1,8-cineole, alpha-pinene, beta-sitosterol, geraniol, linalol, phytosterols, and stigmasterol.

Cayenne, African Pepper, Red Pepper, and Chilies

Cayenne is a member of the nightshade family. Its flavor is pungent and fiery. Capsaicin—the substance that burns the mouth and the active component in chili peppers—can relieve pain such as arthritis pain when applied topically, and may be useful in treating psoriasis. Capsaicin has been found to work as an anticoagulant, thus possibly helping to prevent heart attacks or strokes caused by the formation of clots in blood vessels. It stimulates the production of endorphins, the body's natural painkillers, and kills the stomach bacterium known to cause ulcers. In one British study, eating ⅗ teaspoon hot pepper sauce one time was found to raise the subjects' metabolic rate by 25 percent, causing them to burn an extra 45 calories in three hours. As an element of the diet, cayenne can be used liberally for its powerful antioxidant and cardiovascular benefits, and as an expectorant and decongestant. For a medicinal drink, mix ⅛ to ½ teaspoon of dry cayenne powder in water or juice. Sip in small increments to gauge your "heat" tolerance, and adjust the dosage accordingly. Cayenne is available also in capsule form in health food stores. To ease joint pain associated with arthritis and other inflammatory disorders, blend cayenne powder with enough pure wintergreen oil to make a paste and apply it topically to the affected area.

Cayenne pepper, made by grinding dried hot red peppers, is an important ingredient in hot sauces. Cayenne adds the spicy zip to many ethnic foods, such as Thai and Mexican food, and can be used in marinades and barbecue sauces.

Key nutrients in cayenne include vitamin A, vitamin C, vitamin B_6, vitamin E, vitamin B_1 (thiamine), vitamin B_2 (riboflavin), vitamin B_3 (niacin), calcium, iron, folate, potassium, phosphorus, magnesium, manganese, zinc, and fiber. Phytochemicals include carvone, caryophyllene, limonene, 1,8-cineole, alpha-carotene, beta-carotene, beta-ionone, caffeic acid, capsaicin, chlorogenic acid, cryptoxanthin, hesperidin, kaempferol, lutein, myristic acid, P-coumaric acid, phytosterols, quercetin, scopoletin, stigmasterol, tocopherols, and zeaxanthin.

A word of caution: When using cayenne, avoid letting it come into contact with your eyes and be careful with a shaker—if the powder hits the air, it can cause sneezing. If some gets in your eyes and burns, flush your eyes immediately with cool water.

Celery

Celery seed has a mild, slightly bitter celerylike taste. Like the root and leaves of the celery plant, they assist the flow of urine through the kidneys, aid the digestive system, and help to relieve the symptoms of arthritis, rheumatism, and gout. If you have any of these disorders, take ¼ cup of juice made from celery leaves and roots two to three times daily, or mix 6 to 8 drops of celery oil in a glass of water and drink twice daily. This will help to relieve symptoms and promote healing.

The seeds of this familiar vegetable enhance split-pea soup, fish, chowders, tomato sauces and soups, hot or cold potato dishes, and stuffing. The leaves, or celery "tops" from fresh celery, are good chopped and used in dishes while they are cooking.

Key nutrients in celery seed include calcium, iron, magnesium, phosphorus, potassium, zinc, manganese, vitamin C, vitamin B_6, vitamin A, vitamin E, vitamin B_1 (thiamine), vitamin B_2 (riboflavin), vitamin B_3 (niacin), folate, and fiber. Phytochemicals include phytosterols, carvone, limonene, alpha-pinene, apigenin, bergapten, beta-carotene, coumarin, eugenol, isoquercitrin, linalol, myristic acid, myristicin, psoralen, rutin, scopoletin, sinapic acid, thymol, umbelliferone, and xanthotoxin.

While celery seed is quite safe used as a seasoning, celery juice and celery oil are more concentrated, so you should not consume them if you are pregnant.

Chervil

Chervil has a flavor that is sweet and slightly aniselike. This herb can be used as a digestive aid, gas remedy, and appetite stimulant. It has an overall tonic effect. Some herbalists recommend it to lower blood pressure.

Because it is similar to parsley, chervil can be used with almost any dish, either as a garnish or as a flavoring. Use in combination with other herbs to bring out the flavor.

Key nutrients in chervil include calcium, iron, magnesium, phosphorus, potassium, zinc, manganese, vitamin C, vitamin A, vitamin B_6, vitamin E, vitamin B_1 (thiamine), vitamin B_2 (riboflavin), vitamin B_3 (niacin), folate, and fiber.

Chives

Chives have a flavor that is mild and onionlike. They stimulate the appetite, ease digestion, protect against heart disease and stroke, and help relieve gas. They may increase the body's ability to digest fat. Their high iron content helps in preventing iron-deficiency anemia. Fresh chives, which are easily grown at home, offer the greatest medicinal benefit. Cut chives just before using them to keep their vitamins, aroma, and flavor. When chives are heated, they lose their vitamin C content and digestive properties.

A milder substitute for onions, chives can be added to cream cheese, cottage cheese, or sour cream to make a spread or topping, or used as a garnish. They give zest to salads, soups, broths, stews, omelets, scrambled eggs, and cooked vegetables. Add the blossom as a milder, decorative touch to salads.

Key nutrients in chives include calcium, iron, magnesium, phosphorus, potassium, zinc, manganese, vitamin C, vitamin B_6, vitamin A, vitamin E, vitamin B_1 (thiamine), vitamin B_2 (riboflavin), vitamin B_3 (niacin), pantothenic acid, folate, and fiber. Phytochemicals include beta-carotene, caffeic acid, ferulic acid, kaempferol, myristic acid, P-coumaric acid, phytosterols, quercetin, and saponins.

Cinnamon and Cassia

Cinnamon has a flavor that is mildly strong, acidic, and sweet. Cassia technically comes from a different (though related) plant, but has similar properties and is often referred to as cinnamon as well. Like many kitchen herbs and spices, cinnamon has antiseptic properties; sprinkle the powder on minor cuts and scrapes (after cleaning the affected area thoroughly). It is a widely used digestive aid

that helps to relieve nausea, vomiting, diarrhea, and indigestion. It is beneficial for the heart, lungs, and kidneys. It has anticancer properties and has been shown in laboratory tests to stop the growth of liver cancer and melanoma cells. George Washington University studies show that cinnamon may lower blood pressure. Tufts University researchers have found that cinnamon more than doubles insulin's ability to metabolize blood sugar, which helps protect against diabetes. Doses of cinnamon tincture taken every fifteen minutes may help stop uterine bleeding. The propanoic acid in cinnamon stops the formation of stomach ulcers without interfering with the production of gastric acid.

Sprinkle powered cinnamon on toast, add it to cookie batter, or stir it into hot apple cider. Use it with winter squash, sweet potatoes, yams, carrots, and parsnips. Cinnamon is good in cakes, pies, muffins, and breads. It is also good for pickling. For a warm, sweet spicy drink, use ½ to ¾ teaspoon of powered cinnamon per cup of boiling water.

Key nutrients in cinnamon include calcium, iron, magnesium, phosphorus, potassium, zinc, manganese, vitamin C, vitamin B_6, vitamin A, vitamin B_1 (thiamine), vitamin B_2 (riboflavin), vitamin B_3 (niacin), folate, and fiber. Phytochemicals include phytosterols, caryophyllene, limonene, 1,8-cineole, alpha-pinene, beta-carotene, coumarin, eugenol, geraniol, linalol, tannin, and vanillin.

You should not ingest essential oil of cinnamon or apply it to your skin as it is strong and can be irritating.

Cloves

Cloves are the petals of the clove plant that have been picked and dried. Their flavor is strong, fruity, and sweet—almost hot. They are a digestive aid, kill intestinal parasites, and are helpful for relieving abdominal pain and symptoms of peptic ulcers. They have been used for their anticoagulant effects and as an anti-inflammatory against rheumatic diseases. Studies by one Danish researcher suggest that cloves make blood platelets less likely to stick together, which could help to prevent blood clots that lead to heart attacks and strokes. Taken as a hot tea, cloves can ease digestive complaints; use 1 teaspoon of powdered cloves per cup of boiling water and steep for ten to twenty minutes.

To use cloves in cooking, combine whole dried or ground cloves with other sweet spices in apple desserts, gingerbread, and pumpkin pie. Add their pungency to pea and bean soups, baked beans, chili, barbecue and tomato sauces, and sweet potatoes. Use "spikes" to flavor meats, pickles, fruits, and syrups.

Essential oil of cloves is anti-inflammatory, antimicrobial, analgesic, and antifungal. The oil also increases the effectiveness of acyclovir (Zovirax), a drug used to treat Bell's palsy, chronic fatigue syndrome, and herpes. Clove oil is well known for deadening the pain of toothache and dental treatment. To temporarily ease a toothache, apply a drop or two of clove oil with a cotton swab to the affected tooth and surrounding gum. To help stop vomiting, take 2 drops of clove oil mixed in 1 cup of water. Be aware that undiluted clove oil is potentially toxic in large doses. You should not use it at all if you are pregnant.

Key nutrients in cloves include calcium, iron, magnesium, phosphorus, potassium, zinc, manganese, vitamin C, vitamin B$_6$, vitamin A, and vitamin E, vitamin B$_1$ (thiamine), vitamin B$_2$ (riboflavin), vitamin B$_3$ (niacin), folate, and fiber. Phytochemicals include phytosterols, carvone, caryophyllene, beta-carotene, beta-sitosterol, ellagic acid, eugenol, gallic acid, kaempferol, linalol, stigmasterol, tannin, and vanillin.

Coriander and Cilantro

Coriander, also known as Chinese parsley and cilantro, is an essential ingredient in Mexican and Asian cooking. Its flavor is mild, sweet, and pungent—similar to lemon and sage. Generally, the term *coriander* refers to the seeds, while *cilantro* denotes the leaves.

Coriander helps to relieve indigestion, gas, and diarrhea. Externally, you can use powdered coriander in salves for muscle and joint pain and to disinfect minor cuts and scrapes (it kills bacteria and fungi). You can also make a tea using ½ teaspoon of powder or 1 teaspoon of lightly crushed seeds per cup of boiling water; steep for five minutes and then strain, if necessary, before drinking it.

Use both the leaves and seeds with poultry, fish, vegetables, and sauces. Also, add minced fresh leaves to green salads, salsas, avocado dip, corn, and black beans. Coriander is a key component of curry powder.

Key nutrients in coriander include calcium, iron, magnesium, phosphorus, potassium, zinc, manganese, vitamin C, vitamin B$_6$, vitamin A, vitamin E (in leaf only), vitamin B$_1$ (thiamine), vitamin B$_2$ (riboflavin), vitamin B$_3$ (niacin), folate, and fiber. Phytochemicals include carvone, caryophyllene, limonene, 1,8-cineole, alpha-pinene, apigenin, beta-carotene, beta-sitosterol, caffeic acid, chlorogenic acid, geraniol, isoquercitrin, linalol, myristic acid, myristicin, psoralen, quercetin, rutin, scopoletin, tannin, umbelliferone, and vanillic acid.

Cumin

Cumin is musty and earthy tasting, with grassy undertones. Traditionally, it has been used to relieve gas, to aid digestion, and to treat colic and headaches. It also has antioxidant properties. Preliminary studies from researchers in India suggest that cumin also has cancer-preventing properties. It may help to prevent blood clots that lead to heart attacks and strokes.

Whole or ground cumin seeds are one of the ingredients in chili powder and a chief ingredient in curry powder. Use cumin sparingly in stews, soups, sauces, and as a flavoring for cheeses, breads, and chutney.

Key nutrients in cumin include calcium, iron, magnesium, phosphorus, potassium, zinc, manganese, vitamin C,

vitamin B$_6$, vitamin A, vitamin E, vitamin B$_1$ (thiamine), vitamin B$_2$ (riboflavin), vitamin B$_3$ (niacin), folate, and fiber. Phytochemicals include phytosterols, caryophyllene, limonene, 1,8-cineole, alpha-pinene, beta-carotene, eugenol, linalol, luteolin, and tannin.

Dill

Dill has a delicate, lemony, celerylike flavor. This herb has been used for thousands of years as a digestive aid and gas remedy. It is good for the kidneys and spleen. It lowers blood pressure, improves poor appetite, and increases circulation. It also helps milk production in nursing mothers. Dill seed oil may help prevent infectious diarrhea, as it has been shown to check the growth of several bacteria that attack the intestinal tract. Chewing ½ to 1 teaspoon of seeds also freshens the breath. You can make dill tea by steeping 2 teaspoons of lightly crushed seeds in a cup of boiling water for ten minutes; then strain and drink.

Dill has long been used to pickle foods because it inhibits the growth of food-spoiling microorganisms. The seed is excellent sprinkled on seafood and stirred into cottage cheese, tofu, tuna, or potato salad. It perks up eggs and green salads. French cooks use dill seeds to flavor cakes, pastry, and sauces. Use the green leaves of the dill plant to complement the same foods.

Key nutrients in dill include calcium, iron, magnesium, phosphorus, potassium, zinc, manganese, vitamin C, vitamin A, vitamin B$_6$, vitamin E, vitamin B$_1$ (thiamine), vitamin B$_2$ (riboflavin), vitamin B$_3$ (niacin), folate, and fiber. Phytochemicals include carvone, limonene, alpha-pinene, tocopherols, bergapten, beta-sitosterol, caffeic acid, chlorogenic acid, esculetin, eugenol, ferulic acid, geraniol, kaempferol, linalol, myristic acid, myristicin, quercetin, scopoletin, stigmasterol, tannin, and umbelliferone.

Fennel

Fennel is a member of the carrot and parsley family that has a mild, licoricelike flavor milder than that of anise. It aids in digestion and helps to prevent gas. It also aids kidney and bladder function. It has a gentle laxative effect; helps to stimulate onset of menstruation; helps promote milk production in nursing mothers; and relieves infant colic (use a weak preparation for children under age two). It is beneficial for people with bronchitis, asthma, coughs, nausea, tuberculosis, and rheumatism. It is good for treating food poisoning, indigestion, and motion sickness. Either chew a handful of fennel seeds or make a tea by using 1 to 2 teaspoons of gently crushed seeds per cup of boiling water; steep for ten minutes, then strain and drink.

Fennel leaves, stalks, roots, and seeds can be used with fish, in Italian dishes and sauces, and in salads. You can add whole or ground seeds to breads and pickles. (See Chapter 9 for more information about fennel.)

Key nutrients in fennel include calcium, iron, magnesium, phosphorus, potassium, zinc, manganese, vitamin C, vitamin A, vitamin B_1 (thiamine), vitamin B_2 (riboflavin), vitamin B_3 (niacin), fiber, and folate. Phytochemicals include beta-carotene, alpha-pinene, bergapten, psoralen, beta-sitosterol, 1,8-cineole, caffeic acid, limonene, ferulic acid, isoquercitrin, kaempferol, linalol, myristicin, P-coumaric acid, pectin, phytosterols, quercetin, rutin, scopoletin, sinapic acid, stigmasterol, tocopherols, umbelliferone, vanillic acid, vanillin, and xanthotoxin.

Fennel is quite safe when used as a seasoning, but because of its menstruation-stimulating actions, it should not be used medicinally during pregnancy.

Fenugreek

Fenugreek is a member of the bean family. Its flavor is maplelike (the food industry uses it as a source of imitation maple flavor), with a bittersweet burnt taste and some flavor of celery. Fenugreek contains potent antioxidants that have beneficial effects on the chemistry of the liver and pancreas. Taken internally, fenugreek helps treat coughs and bronchitis. It makes an excellent tea for relieving intestinal irritation, or a gargle for soothing sore throat. It reduces mucus in sinus passages and relieves asthmatic conditions. Ground seeds also can be applied as a poultice to treat wounds or inflamed areas. A study done in India showed that the pulverized seeds of fenugreek lower blood sugar levels in people with diabetes.

Either the dried plant or its seeds can be used in breads, chutneys, and curry powder, or as a condiment. The sprouted seeds can be used as a vegetable or in salads.

Key nutrients in fenugreek include vitamin A, vitamin C, calcium, iron, potassium, phosphorous, magnesium, manganese, zinc, vitamin B_1 (thiamine), vitamin B_2 (riboflavin), vitamin B_3 (niacin), folate, and fiber. Phytochemicals include beta-carotene, beta-sitosterol, coumarin, kaempferol, luteolin, P-coumaric acid, quercetin, rutin, and saponins.

Fenugreek should be used sparingly or be avoided by people with diabetes or by pregnant women.

Garlic

Every study conducted on garlic has shown it to be one of the most powerful plant substances known. Garlic oil is helpful in the treatment of all heart disorders, high blood pressure, and fungal infections such as candidiasis. Garlic is also beneficial in combating all degenerative diseases. This wondrous herb's benefits to human health are so numerous that an entire chapter of the book is devoted to it. (See Chapter 20.)

Ginger

Ginger has a strong, spicy, sweet flavor. It is one of the most widely available and used medicinal herbs on the planet. It is a time-proven remedy for nausea, morning sickness, upset stomach, indigestion, vomiting, motion sickness, and cramps. British research has found ginger to be as effective as drugs at relieving nausea after surgery. Patients with rheumatoid arthritis and osteoarthritis studied at Denmark's Odense University got relief from pain and swelling after taking ginger daily for at least three months. Ginger can destroy bacteria, including *Salmonella*, which causes food poisoning, and has a chemical called zingibain that dissolves parasites and their eggs. Gingerol, an aromatic compound in ginger, promotes healing of inflammations and minor burns and may prevent transient ischemic attacks (TIAs), often referred to as "mini-strokes." Ginger also helps lower blood pressure, reduces fever, prevents internal blood clots, reduces cholesterol, aids circulation, and eases asthma symptoms. Ginger root tea eases sore throat pain and kills cold viruses; take ⅓ teaspoon ground ginger or 1 teaspoon fresh ginger root in food or drink three times a day. To prevent motion sickness, drink tea or juice mixed with ½ teaspoon ground ginger one-half hour before traveling.

The rhizomes, or underground stems, of the ginger plant are used fresh or in dried, ground form. Fresh ginger (peel the skin before grating or slicing the root) is a favorite in Asian dishes, marinades, and fruit salad dressings. Ground ginger lends a warm, spicy pungency to breads, cookies, spice cakes, and pumpkin pie. It also flavors soft drinks and candy.

Key nutrients in ginger include calcium, iron, magnesium, phosphorus, potassium, zinc, manganese, vitamin A, vitamin C, vitamin B_6, vitamin E, vitamin B_1 (thiamine), vitamin B_2 (riboflavin), vitamin B_3 (niacin), folate, and fiber. Phytochemicals include phytosterols, limonene, 1,8-cineole, gingerol, alpha-pinene, beta-carotene, beta-ionone, beta-sitosterol, caffeic acid, capsaicin, chlorogenic acid, curcumin, ferulic acid, geraniol, kaempferol, linalol, myrcetin, myristic acid, P-coumaric acid, quercetin, vanillic acid, and vanillin.

If you take anticoagulant (blood-thinning) drugs, avoid consuming large amounts of ginger, which could thin the blood further. Also, taking more than 3 grams of ginger at a time can cause stomach upset.

Horseradish

Horseradish, actually a cruciferous vegetable, is a relative of the radish and member of the mustard family. It is a root with a sharp, hot flavor that is usually grated and eaten raw or added to sauces as a condiment. It has anticancer properties and diuretic, digestive, and blood sugar–balancing actions. It is good for people with bronchial and lung disorders. It acts as an expectorant to loosen and remove mucus. For sore throats and coughs, add 1 tablespoon of grated fresh horseradish, 1 teaspoon of honey, and 1 teaspoon of ground cloves to a glass of warm water. Sip it slowly, or use as a gargle.

Horseradish complements cheeses, salad dressings, and vegetables. You can make fresh horseradish sauce by peeling and grinding the roots, then mixing them with vinegar. To make a healthy spread, blend fresh horseradish with yogurt.

Key nutrients in horseradish include vitamin C, calcium, fiber, iron, magnesium, manganese, vitamin B_3 (niacin), phosphorus, potassium, vitamin B_2 (riboflavin), vitamin B_1 (thiamine), and zinc. Phytochemicals include limonene, kaempferol, pectin, sinapic acid, tannin, and vanillic acid.

Marjoram

Marjoram is a member of the mint family that is similar to oregano, but with a milder, more delicate, sweeter flavor. It is also called wild marjoram and sweet marjoram.

Effective as a digestive aid, marjoram also helps reduce fever and relieve cold and flu symptoms (vomiting), jaundice, headaches, and insomnia. It's also used to ease menstrual cramps and prevent motion sickness. Laboratory studies show marjoram inhibits the growth of *Herpes simplex*, the virus that causes cold sores and genital herpes. For a tea, use 1 to 2 teaspoons of dried leaves and flower tops per cup of boiling water; steep for ten minutes, then strain and drink.

Marjoram is good in sauces and tomato-based dishes, green salads, stuffing, stews, and soups. It goes well with a variety of cooked vegetables, lentils, and beans. Both leaves and flower tops can be used, either fresh or dried.

Key nutrients in marjoram include calcium, iron, magnesium, phosphorus, potassium, zinc, manganese, vitamin C, vitamin B_6, vitamin A, vitamin E, vitamin B_1 (thiamine), vitamin B_2 (riboflavin), vitamin B_3 (niacin), folate, and fiber. Phytochemicals include carvone, caryophyllene, limonene, alpha-pinene, beta-carotene, beta-sitosterol, caffeic acid, eugenol, geraniol, linalol, phytosterols, saponins, tannin, and ursolic acid.

Mint

Mint, a member of the botanical family that includes basil and marjoram, comes in hundreds of varieties, though peppermint and spearmint are the most common. Its flavor is sweet and cooling. Mint is useful for easing insomnia, upset stomachs, and nervous tension. It helps the body break down fat by stimulating bile flow. Mint also has been shown to increase the number of phagocytes, cells that are capable of destroying pathogens, bacteria, and cancer cells.

For a fragrant zest, put fresh mint leaves in fruit salads and fruit soups, on new potatoes, in cold fruit beverages, on cooked carrots or peas, and on cold grain salads, such as tabbouleh. Mint also makes a refreshing herbal tea or an appetizing garnish.

Key nutrients in mint include vitamin C, vitamin A, vitamin B_6, vitamin E, calcium, magnesium, phosphorus, potassium, manganese, iron, vitamin B_1 (thiamine), vita-min B_2 (riboflavin), vitamin B_3 (niacin), pantothenic acid, folate, and fiber. Phytochemicals include limonene and hesperidin.

Mustard Seed

Both the leaves, known as mustard greens, and seeds of the mustard plant can be used in cooking. The oil from the seed is used as a condiment. This herb has a strong, hot, spicy flavor.

Mustard can help loosen and remove mucus and trigger bronchial gland secretion. Mustard oil diluted with rubbing alcohol and applied to the skin, helps increase blood flow to arthritic areas. For a cold, apply a plaster made with prepared powered mustard and cold water to the chest—the mustard's warming action can be soothing.

The whole and ground seeds liven up sauces, marinades, salad dressings, chutneys, pickles, and relishes.

Key nutrients in mustard include calcium, iron, magnesium, phosphorus, potassium, sodium, zinc, copper, manganese, selenium, vitamin C, vitamin B_6, vitamin A, vitamin E, vitamin B_1 (thiamine), vitamin B_2 (riboflavin), vitamin B_3 (niacin), folate, and fiber. Phytochemicals include phytosterols.

Caution: Prolonged use of mustard plasters can result in skin irritation.

Nutmeg

Nutmeg is the pit, or seed, of the fruit of the nutmeg tree, a tropical evergreen. Its flavor is piney and citruslike with a sweet and bitter, warm taste.

Oil of nutmeg is used to disguise the taste of various drugs and as a gastrointestinal stimulant. Both nutmeg and mace (the dried, ground outer coating of the nutmeg seed) are used to relieve gas and to ease nausea, vomiting, and diarrhea. Nutmeg has anti-inflammatory and antiviral properties and is an ingredient in True Man's Decoction, a traditional Chinese herbal tonic to dispel infection from the digestive tract and restore the body's fluid metabolism.

Available both whole and ground, nutmeg is commonly used in sweet foods such as puddings, cakes, and cookies—and sprinkled on eggnog. Nutmeg also complements vegetables, pasta, grains, and cheese. Mace can be used in the same way as nutmeg.

Key nutrients in nutmeg include vitamin C, vitamin A, vitamin B_6, vitamin E, calcium, iron, magnesium, phosphorus, potassium, zinc, copper, manganese, selenium, folate, and fiber. Phytochemicals include limonene, 1,8-cineole, eugenol, geraniol, kaempferol, linalol, myristic acid, myristicin, pectin, phytosterols, and quercetin.

Oregano

Also called wild marjoram and Mexican wild sage, oregano has a peppery flavor with a hint of sage and thyme. Chinese doctors have used oregano for centuries to treat fever, vomiting, diarrhea, and skin problems. It helps to loosen and remove mucus. It is a digestive aid and is thought to help get rid of intestinal parasites. Oregano is known to have powerful antioxidant and anticancer activity. In a study at Georgetown University, essential oil of oregano inhibited the growth of *Staphylococcus* (staph) bacteria in the test tube as effectively as antibiotics did. In a 1998 Cornell University study, oregano oil was found to destroy *Escherichia coli* (*E. coli*) and *Salmonella* bacteria, and even anthrax spores. At a meeting of the American Society of Microbiology, researchers reported that essential oil of oregano may destroy bacteria that cause pneumonia. Tests by a U.S. Department of Agriculture researcher show that oregano doubles the potency of insulin so that less is required to process sugar.

Used in bath oils, oregano helps relieve aches and stiff joints. The essential oil is also beneficial used in a diffuser or an aromatherapy lamp—or simply place a single drop on a cotton ball and sniff it three or four times daily. It will be absorbed directly into the sinuses. To make a spicy herbal infusion, add 1 or 2 teaspoons of dried oregano to a cup of boiling water; steep for ten minutes, then strain and drink.

Oregano is used in many Mexican and Italian dishes, including pizza and pasta sauces. Its distinctive flavor accents tomatoes, sweet peppers, zucchini, and eggplant. Oregano combines well with soups, tomato dishes, stews, and a variety of vegetables, too.

Key nutrients in oregano include calcium, potassium, phosphorus, iron, magnesium, manganese, zinc, copper, selenium, fiber, folate, vitamin A, vitamin C, vitamin B_6, and vitamin E. Phytochemicals include carvone, caryophyllene, limonene, 1,8-cineole, alpha-pinene, linalol, phytosterols, and thymol.

Paprika

Originally from Hungary, paprika is a pungent, savory powder made from ground dried mild red peppers. Sweet paprika is made from only the pepper pods. Hotter versions contain the ground seeds and ribs also. The phytosterols in paprika have cancer-preventive, anti-inflammatory, and immune-boosting properties.

Add paprika to meats, salads, relishes, eggs, and vinegar.

Key nutrients in paprika include vitamin A, vitamin B_6, vitamin C, vitamin E, calcium, iron, potassium, phosphorus, magnesium, manganese, zinc, copper, selenium, vitamin B_1 (thiamine), vitamin B_2 (riboflavin), vitamin B_3 (niacin), pantothenic acid, folate, and fiber. Phytochemicals include phytosterols.

Parsley

Parsley is a familiar herb with a mild, agreeable flavor that is used mostly as a garnish or seasoning. Dried parsley leaves, root, or seed taken as a tea or tincture, eases digestion, is a diuretic, helps in the secretion of urine, and acts as a mild laxative. It is also useful for detoxification and indigestion and helps the lungs and spleen. Munch fresh parsley sprigs to help freshen breath. Parsley has essential oils and one, apiole, is a kidney stimulant. These oils may stimulate uterine contractions, so pregnant women should not eat large quantities. Parsley is beneficial for genitourinary tract disorders, stones in the kidneys and bladder, nephritis, and other types of kidney disorders, as well as for the adrenal and thyroid glands. It is helpful for dieters because it has strong diuretic properties. When using parsley medicinally, do so sparingly because it is very powerful. For a soothing tea, use 2 teaspoons of the dried herb, or 1 teaspoon of lightly crushed seed per cup of boiling water; steep the tea for ten minutes, then strain and drink.

Parsley gives salads, soups, and stews flavor and nutrition. Do not cook parsley, as heat destroys valuable vitamins and minerals. Whenever possible, use fresh parsley, not dried parsley, in recipes. A new flat-leaf variety called Italian parsley is more nutritious and has a better flavor than curly leaf parsley. Parsley can be frozen if necessary; simply wash, dry, and chop, then place it in a sealed plastic bag. In the refrigerator, keep parsley fresh by sprinkling it with water or wrap it in a paper towel and refrigerate it in a plastic bag. Do not use large amounts in juices—it has powerful diuretic properties.

Key nutrients in parsley include vitamin A, vitamin E, vitamin C, calcium, iron, potassium, phosphorus, magnesium, manganese, selenium, copper, zinc, vitamin B_1 (thiamine), vitamin B_2 (riboflavin), vitamin B_3 (niacin), pantothenic acid, folate, and fiber. Phytochemicals include limonene, alpha-pinene, apigenin, tocopherols, bergapten, beta-carotene, caffeic acid, chlorogenic acid, geraniol, kaempferol, linalol, lutein, myristic acid, myristicin, naringenin, P-coumaric acid, phytosterols, psoralen, quercetin, rutin, sesquiphellandrene, and xanthotoxin.

Rosemary

Rosemary is a member of the mint family with a piney, savory, sweet flavor. It is a powerful antioxidant, antiseptic, and antispasmodic. Rosemary stimulates the appetite, aids digestion and circulation, and helps to prevent food poisoning. It relieves intestinal cramps and spasms and irritable bowel syndrome. As a diuretic and fungicide, it helps prevent yeast infections. It is useful in treating and helping prevent the onset of Alzheimer's disease. Studies at the University of Pennsylvania showed that rosemary's antioxidant action might impede tumor formation in animal mammary cells by inhibiting the binding of a known carcinogen. Researchers at Rutgers University found in laboratory tests that rosemary applied topically reduced the number of skin tumors by 64 percent. Its strong antioxidant actions make it an excellent food preservative, too; mix the crushed leaves with food that spoils easily. Rosemary is used to treat nasal and chest congestion and chronic circulatory problems. Used externally, it helps soothe sprains and bruises and disinfects wounds. For a healing tea, mix 1 teaspoon of rosemary in 1 cup of boiling water; steep for ten minutes, then strain and drink.

Rosemary's strong, assertive flavor makes it a difficult herb to combine with others. Use its leaves sparingly with vegetables, grains, soups, and stews. Or add it to olive oil for an Italian-style bread dip. Rosemary is good with root vegetables, such as potatoes and onions, and is often used to season lamb.

Key nutrients in rosemary include calcium, iron, magnesium, phosphorus, potassium, zinc, copper, manganese, vitamin C, vitamin B_6, vitamin A, vitamin E, vitamin B_1 (thiamine), vitamin B_2 (riboflavin), vitamin B_3 (niacin), pantothenic acid, folate, and fiber. Phytochemicals include limonene, carvone, caryophyllene, 1,8-cineole, alpha-pinene, apigenin, beta-carotene, beta-sitosterol, caffeic acid, carnosol, chlorogenic acid, geraniol, hesperidin, linalol, luteolin, pectin, phytosterols, squalene, tannin, thymol, and ursolic acid.

Saffron

By far the most expensive of the spices, saffron comes from the crocus family. The stigma, or top part of the flower that receives pollen, is powdered to add a bright yellow color and exotic taste to food. It takes more than 70,000 flowers to produce just one pound of saffron—hence its high price. The flavor is pleasantly spicy and slightly bitter.

Saffron acts as an antioxidant and stimulant to the circulatory system. Saffron has been shown to inhibit tumor growth in mice and to stimulate multiplication of T cells, important to the immune system. It may also help control blood pressure. It is used also as an expectorant and to relieve pain and aid digestion. To make a tea, use twelve stigmas or 2 teaspoons of saffron powder per cup of boiling water; steep for ten minutes, then strain and drink.

Saffron is used in rice dishes, sauces, soups, cakes, breads, dressings, and seafood. Usually just a pinch of saffron will do—dissolve it in warm water before adding it to the dish.

Key nutrients in saffron include calcium, iron, magnesium, phosphorus, potassium, zinc, manganese, selenium, vitamin A, vitamin B_6, vitamin C, vitamin E, vitamin B_1 (thiamine), vitamin B_2 (riboflavin), vitamin B_3 (niacin), folate, and fiber. Phytochemicals include beta-carotene, kaempferol, lycopene, myricetin, quercetin, and zeaxanthin.

Sage

Sage has a flavor that is intense, earthy, warm, and slightly bitter. It is known to have antioxidant and anticancer activities. It helps retard food spoilage as effectively as commercial food preservatives. Tests by a U.S. Department of

Agriculture researcher show that sage, like oregano, doubles the potency of insulin so that less is required to process sugar. Sage tea is used as a gargle to treat sore throats, canker sores, and bleeding gums. This herb contains a volatile oil, tannin, and can be bitter. Sage oil is composed of pinene, camphor, salveve, and cineol. To make sage tea, use 1 to 2 teaspoons of dried sage per cup of boiling water; steep for ten minutes, then strain and drink.

Best known as a seasoning for stuffing, sage leaves, whole or crushed, also go well with fish. Use it in eggplant and cheese dishes, and in beans, potatoes, vegetables, salads, chowders, biscuits, and cornbread.

Key nutrients in sage include calcium, iron, magnesium, phosphorus, potassium, zinc, manganese, selenium, vitamin C, vitamin B_6, vitamin A, vitamin E, vitamin B_1 (thiamine), vitamin B_2 (riboflavin), vitamin B_3 (niacin), folate, and fiber. Phytochemicals include camphor, cineol, phytosterols, salveve, and tannin.

Savory

Savory, a member of the mint family, is commonly grown in two species: summer savory and winter savory. Both have the same uses. The flavor is peppery and suggestive of thyme.

Savory relieves gas, diarrhea, and upset stomach. It also is useful as an expectorant. For a soothing tea, use 1 to 2 teaspoons of savory per cup of boiling water; steep for ten minutes, then strain and drink.

Savory goes well with bean dishes, soups, and stuffing. It enhances peas, cabbage, Brussels sprouts, and potatoes, too.

Key nutrients in savory include calcium, iron, magnesium, phosphorus, potassium, zinc, manganese, selenium, vitamin A, vitamin C, vitamin B_1 (thiamine), vitamin B_3 (niacin), and fiber. Phytochemicals include caryophyllene, limonene, alpha-pinene, geraniol, linalol, and thymol.

Tarragon

A prominent seasoning in French cooking, tarragon belongs to the daisy and dandelion family. It has a sweet flavor, with a hint of licorice.

Traditionally, tarragon has been used as an appetite stimulant, to ease digestion and toothache pain, and to stimulate urine flow. It helps to expel intestinal parasites and strengthen the stomach. Tarragon has cancer-preventive, anti-inflammatory, antioxidant, antiviral, and antitumor properties. It also promotes liver health and enhances immune function.

Tarragon is excellent with fish and adds a lively flavor to pasta dishes, tomatoes, chicken, red peppers, and potatoes. It also makes tasty vinaigrette.

Key nutrients in tarragon include calcium, iron, magnesium, phosphorus, potassium, zinc, manganese, selenium, vitamin C, vitamin B_6, vitamin A, vitamin E, vitamin B_1

(thiamine), vitamin B$_2$ (riboflavin), vitamin B$_3$ (niacin), folate, and fiber. Phytochemicals include carvone, limonene, 1,8-cineole, alpha-pinene, apigenin, beta-carotene, beta-sitosterol, caffeic acid, chlorogenic acid, coumarin, esculetin, eugenol, ferulic acid, gallic acid, geraniol, linalol, luteolin, naringenin, P-coumaric acid, phloroglucinol, phytosterols, quercetin, rutin, scopoletin, sinapic acid, squalene, stigmasterol, tannin, umbelliferone, and vanillic acid.

Thyme

Thyme is an herb with a woodsy, warm, slightly peppery flavor. The leaves and flower tops are used both fresh and dried. It has long been used as a digestive aid, cough and laryngitis remedy, and antiseptic. It is helpful in treating sore throat, laryngitis, and tonsillitis. Oil of thyme (thymol) has antibacterial, antifungal, and preservative actions, and is the main ingredient in Listerine mouthwash. The antifungal agent in thyme is good for relieving athlete's foot and yeast infections. Thyme is useful for upper respiratory and urinary tract infections. It has cancer-preventive, antioxidant, and anti-inflammatory actions. At a meeting of the American Society of Microbiology, researchers reported that essential oil of thyme may destroy bacteria that cause pneumonia. To make a tea, use 2 teaspoons of dried thyme per cup of boiling water; steep for ten minutes, then strain and drink.

Thyme blends well with many foods, including fish, tomato-based sauces, salad dressings, soups, vegetables, and cheeses.

Key nutrients in thyme include calcium, iron, magnesium, phosphorus, potassium, zinc, copper, manganese, vitamin C, vitamin B$_6$, vitamin A, vitamin B$_1$ (thiamine), vitamin B$_2$ (riboflavin), vitamin B$_3$ (niacin), pantothenic acid, folate, and fiber. Phytochemicals include carvone, limonene, alpha-pinene, apigenin, beta-carotene, caffeic acid, eugenol, ferulic acid, gallic acid, geraniol, kaempferol, linalol, luteolin, myristic acid, naringenin, P-coumaric acid, phytosterols, tannin, thymol, ursolic acid, and vanillic acid.

While thyme is quite safe used as a seasoning, it should not be used medicinally during pregnancy.

Turmeric

A close relative of ginger, turmeric is a naturally yellow-colored spice derived from the powdered roots of an East Indian plant. It is fragrant and slightly acrid and peppery, similar to ginger.

Turmeric is the primary anti-inflammatory herb of ayurvedic medicine. Its antibacterial action helps to retard food spoilage and treat wounds. It helps blood flow, reduces cholesterol levels, and improves blood vessel health.

Turmeric contains curcumin, a compound that reduces swelling, making it useful in treating inflammatory disorders such as arthritis. Researchers at the University of Texas in Houston have shown that turmeric inhibits cancer. It also inhibited the spread of HIV in laboratory tests. Traditionally, turmeric has been used as a digestive aid and a liver stimulant. It is also good for people with atherosclerosis, carpal tunnel syndrome, gallstones, cataracts, tendinitis, eczema, endometriosis, and bursitis. For a healing drink, use 1 teaspoon of turmeric powder per cup of warm soymilk. Turmeric also is available in capsule form in health food stores.

In food, turmeric is mainly used to flavor and lend color to curry powder, prepared mustard, dressings, cheeses, and butter.

Key nutrients in turmeric include calcium, iron, magnesium, phosphorus, potassium, zinc, copper, manganese, selenium, vitamin C, vitamin B$_6$, vitamin B$_1$ (thiamine), vitamin B$_2$ (riboflavin), vitamin B$_3$ (niacin), folate, and fiber. Phytochemicals include 1,8-cineole, beta-carotene, caffeic acid, curcumin, P-coumaric acid, phytosterols, and vanillic acid.

Turmeric is not recommended for people who have clotting disorders or who are on anticoagulant medication. And, since it increases bile production, you should not use it in medicinal amounts if you have gallstones or obstructed bile ducts.

Vanilla

A member of the orchid family, vanilla beans are long, slender seedpods that grow on climbing vines. The pods are picked just before maturity, then fermented and dried. The flavor is warm, delicate, and spicy.

Traditionally, vanilla has been used to invigorate and strengthen the body and promote healing, to relieve gas, and to treat abnormal menstruation. Vanilla's phytochemicals have cancer-preventive, anti-inflammatory, and antioxidant properties.

Vanilla can be used as the whole bean or in pure extract form. Take care to buy the pure extract, rather than an extract made from vanillin, a derivative product. If it is pure, it will state that on the bottle. (By law, pure vanilla extract must be 35 percent alcohol by volume.) For superior vanilla beans, look for those grown in Mexico, Indonesia, and Madagascar. Vanilla is used mainly to flavor desserts, confections, beverages, and sauces. It is a popular scent in perfumery as well.

Key nutrients in vanilla include calcium, magnesium, phosphorus, potassium, manganese, fiber, small amounts of vitamin B$_1$ (thiamine), vitamin B$_2$ (riboflavin), vitamin B$_3$ (niacin), pantothenic acid, and vitamin B$_6$. Phytochemicals include catechin, eugenol, tannin, vanillic acid, and vanillin.

CHAPTER EIGHTEEN

ORGANIC FOOD:
EXTRA LIFE INSURANCE

Call on God, but row away from the rocks.

—*Indian proverb*

In March 2000, the United States Food and Drug Administration (USDA) announced the approval of national organic standards, which means that supermarket food labeled *organic* must meet specific, consistent requirements. Under these rules, organic crops cannot be genetically engineered, irradiated, or fertilized with sewage sludge; farmland where crops are grown is prohibited from being treated with synthetic pesticides and herbicides for at least three years prior to harvest; and farm animals raised under organic standards cannot receive antibiotics or growth hormones. Accepting any less than these "standards" for our food seems foolhardy, if not irresponsible. (See Chapter 26.) Eating organic food and drinking quality water will cost more, but it can profoundly affect long-term health.

Reports show conflicting results when looking at the nutritional benefits of organic products. *Organic Consumers* says that thirty studies comparing the nutrient content of organic crops with conventional crops (using chemical fertilizers and pesticides) found that overall, organic crops had a higher nutrient content about 40 percent of the time, and were equal or higher 85 percent of the time. *The Journal of Alternative and Complementary Medicine* reviewed forty-one scientific studies from countries around the world and found that organic crops, on average, contained 19.3 percent more magnesium, 27 percent more vitamin C, 21 percent more iron, 13.6 percent more phosphorus, 26 percent more calcium, and 11 percent more copper. Crops such as spinach, lettuce, cabbage, and potatoes showed even higher nutritional superiority, consistently. Selenium, a key mineral that boosts the immune system and fights disease, is seriously lacking in the soil, worldwide. Regardless of the nutritional content (which is difficult to measure and compare), it's what organic food *doesn't* have—chemicals, pesticides, herbicides, and antibiotics—that make a convincing argument for paying extra money. Studies have revealed that some pesticides and herbicides can mimic the actions of estrogen in the body. Additionally, consumers consistently agree that organic food is superior in taste.

The public demand for organic foods is growing, even though some traditional farms are becoming even more reliant on pesticides, fertilizers, and hormones to increase crop yields. Organic farming is still a relatively small industry (about 10 percent of agriculture in the United States), but it is experiencing growth worldwide. A number of European nations expect 30 to 50 percent of their farms to go organic in the near future. The organic movement also includes meat, dairy, and egg sources.

Converting farmlands to organic takes time and money; however, when it is done correctly, organic farming can reduce (or eliminate) water pollution and conserve both water and soil on farms. Since synthetic input (chemicals) is prohibited, rotating crops and building soil must be done naturally, which is more labor-intensive. Organic farmers seek to optimize land, plant, and animal interactions; preserve the soil; and overall, contribute to sustainable agriculture. In general, they use organic manure and mulches to improve soil structure and they employ natural pest controls. Mixed and relay crops give continuous ground cover and expose farmland to less sun, wind, and rain erosion. Organic farmers are still learning the best ways to bring the soil back and maintain it. Marion Nestle, board member of Center for Science in the Public Interest has said, "Every time people choose organic food they are choosing the kind of world that they want to live in by voting with their fork." It seems that "organic" is a way of life, as well as a quality of food.

If it is not economically feasible or physically possible to buy only organic food or to plant your own garden, *Country Living's Healthy Living* recommends a list of top ten foods to buy organic, especially if there are children or there is a nursing mother in your household:

The "Ring of Poison"

Some pesticides that are banned for use in the United States are still permitted to be sold to other countries. These chemicals can then be reintroduced on food imported into the United States from those countries, creating what the environmental organization Greenpeace has dubbed a "ring of poison." Tests conducted on imported grapes and melons, for example, showed high concentrations of pesticides that are considered harmful and have been banned here. For this reason, it is far better to eat fruit and vegetables that are in season and purchased from a local source, or at least from a U.S. source.

- Baby food. Pesticides have been found in more than half of the baby foods tested. Commercial organic baby foods are available. Some brand names are Earth's Best, Well-Fed Baby, and Gerber's Tender Harvest.

- Rice. Rice is often heavily sprayed. Pesticide used on rice fields in the Sacramento River Valley of California has contaminated ground water there.

- Strawberries. These have been called the single most pesticide-laden produce in the United States. Out-of-season berries may be imported from countries where farmers use pesticides that have been banned in the United States.

- Grain and grain products. In 1994, the FDA found illegally high pesticides residue in some batches of a popular breakfast cereal. Two years later, residues from at least one pesticide were found in 91 percent of wheat samples tested.

- Dairy products. Many dairies inject cows with recombinant bovine growth hormone to boost milk production. Organic dairies do not use hormones or antibiotics.

- Corn. Processed foods made with corn are among the top foods likely to expose children to a unsafe doses of organophosphate residues.

- Bananas. Many bananas are produced using the pesticides benomyl, which has been linked to birth defects, and chlorpyrifos, a neurotoxin.

- Green beans. Tests have found residues of three different pesticides in conventional green bean baby food samples.

- Peaches. An FDA study found that 5 percent of the U.S. peach crop was contaminated with excessive amounts of pesticides.

- Apples. Apples often carry residues of pesticides, the fungicide captan, and the insecticide chlorpyrifos.

In addition, you can minimize your exposure to contaminants by handling and storing food properly. The section on pesticides in Chapter 26 gives detailed instructions for proper food handling and washing practices that can significantly reduce levels of these chemicals in nonorganic food.

It is possible that we do not yet know the long-range effect on the human body of contaminants on our food. If we purchase only the best clothing and cosmetics to put *on* our bodies, can we accept any less than the best for what we put *in* our bodies? Organically grown food is always the superior choice for the health-conscious consumer.

CHAPTER NINETEEN

IMPROVE DIGESTION AND MAXIMIZE NUTRITION: FOOD COMBINING GUIDE

Digestion, of all the bodily functions, is the one which exercises the greatest influence on the mental state of an individual.

—*Jean-Anthelme Brillat-Savarin (1755–1826), French politician and gourmet*

Correct food combinations are important for proper digestion and the utilization and assimilation of nutrients. If food is not digested properly, it can pass through the intestinal tract without being completely broken down, and catch in crevices where toxic wastes then putrefy. Without complete digestion, even the most powerful nutrients cannot be extracted and assimilated for use. Tiny particles may also pass into the bloodstream, where they can cause allergic reactions. Food that the body cannot utilize wastes energy and overworks organs. Additionally, the undigested food particles become soil for unhealthy bacteria that decompose and ferment in it. Even with a healthy diet, foods must be eaten in proper combinations for the body to assimilate the nutrients they contain. Correct food combining is especially important for people with hypoglycemia, diabetes, digestive disorders, and food allergies.

The body must work overtime to get rid of the toxins and poisons created by combining food incorrectly. Organs that are overworked cannot function properly. When they begin to falter, they generally give a warning signal, and if it is not heeded, the whole system may malfunction. Incomplete digestion and inefficient metabolism are prime causes of obesity, high cholesterol, and high and low blood sugar, to name a few.

Food combining is a very important part of meal planning. Only those very few people who have no digestive problems, chew food extremely well, and eat mostly vegetables and all-natural foods, may be able to achieve optimum health without following the rules of food combining.

SIMPLE RULES FOR FOOD COMBINING

The basic principles underlying the rules for food combining are extremely simple. They can be summed up in three statements:

1. Proteins, acidic fruits, and green vegetables can be eaten together.
2. Fats, starches, and green vegetables can be eaten together.
3. Starches and proteins, fats and proteins, and starches and acidic fruits should *not* be eaten together.

To see the reasoning behind these basic principles, it is necessary to understand some things about the nature of the different categories of foods.

PROTEIN

Our bodies contain more proteins than any other type of substance other than water. Proteins are the building blocks for all tissue and cells. They also provide energy and can be converted to fat.

All proteins are made up of substances called amino acids. There are some twenty-eight amino acids that are put together into various combinations to create all of the structural proteins in the body. Of these, eight are considered essential, which means that the body cannot manufacture them and so must get them from food.

Protein foods in general are meat, fish, beans, poultry, eggs, cheese, milk, yogurt, soy products, nuts, and seeds. Dietary protein sources are classified as either *complete* or *incomplete*. The incomplete proteins lack one or more of the eight essential amino acids. In general, animal sources such as meat and dairy products supply complete protein, whereas plant sources supply incomplete proteins. This does not necessarily mean, however, that animal products are always the best protein source. The high-fat content and toxins in animal products can lead to many health problems if consumed in excessive quantities. Meat is also hard on the digestive system and may take as much as twelve hours to break down. (See Chapter 29.)

Consuming excessive amounts of protein can damage the kidneys. Too much protein results in a buildup of nitrogen, which is eliminated as urea in the urine. For this reason, people with kidney disorders, like nephritis and chronic kidney infections, require a low-protein diet. Older adults also should go easy on protein-rich foods, as kidney function decreases with age. People with liver disease need to limit their protein intake as well. Excess protein also interferes with calcium metabolism, so people with osteoporosis should consume protein in moderation.

Pregnant women, on the other hand, need extra protein to build the developing baby's tissues, brain, and placenta, in addition to supplying their own needs. Two to five ounces of protein per day may be needed during the first five months of pregnancy, and after the fifth month, three to five ounces daily. After giving birth, if her baby is breast-fed, the mother may need as much as four to five ounces daily. This protein should come partly from vegetable sources, because there is a chance that pesticide and other chemical residue that build up in animal fats may be passed along to the baby through the placenta, and later via the breast milk.

The way to get complete protein from plant sources is to combine different foods whose amino acids complement one another. These foods lack one or more of the amino acids by themselves, but when combined, they make a complete protein, which is healthier and easier to digest than meat. The following food combinations will supply complete protein:

- Beans: Combine with cheese, corn, nuts, rice, seeds, or wheat.

- Cornmeal: Combine with cheese, eggs, fish, lima beans, milk, potatoes, red meat, soy products, or yeast.

- Legumes (beans, peas, or peanuts): Combine with any grain, nuts, or seeds.

- Rice: Combine with beans, cheese, nuts, seeds, or wheat.

- Vegetables: Combine with dairy products, grains, seeds, or nuts.

Any of the above combinations in meals constitute a complete protein without animal protein (except for the cheese). For instance, a meal of veggie chili or beans over brown rice gives you a complete protein. Eat bread with nut butters, or with nuts or seeds added to meals. All soybean products (tofu, cheese, soymilk, or tempeh) are complete proteins. The availability of complete proteins is limited unless foods are combined. Vegetables contain protein, but it would take a large amount of them to fulfill the body's protein needs.

Good Protein Combinations

All meat/protein meals combine best with other proteins or vegetables, except for vegetables with a high-starch con-

tent. All sources of protein also combine well with green vegetables, especially salads. It is best to eat only one major type of protein each meal.

Poor Protein Combinations

Proteins combine poorly with fats, starchy foods, and all fruit, especially sweet fruit. Eating protein foods with sugar or starches neutralizes the enzymes needed by each for digestion. Concentrated proteins and carbohydrates should not be eaten at the same meal, with nuts being the exception.

Drinking milk with protein neutralizes the acid needed to break down the protein. Though milk is a complete protein, it also contains fat and combines poorly with any food except other dairy products. It curdles in the stomach, then the curds coagulate around food particles and keep them from proper exposure to gastric juices. It delays digestion so that food putrefies in the digestive tract. Do not drink milk with food.

Meat and pasta are also a poor combination. Some additional examples of poor sugar/protein combinations are ice cream (sugar, milk, and eggs), yogurt with sugar, sweetened baked beans, milk shakes, chocolate milk, and any fruit combined with eggs, cheese, or meat.

VEGETABLES AND FRUITS

Vegetables are the most flexible food and combine well with all starches and proteins.

Fruit should be combined with other foods only if the other food is soured (fermented), such as yogurt and cottage cheese.

Acidic and sweet fruits are a poor combination, but acidic fruits can be eaten with nuts or cheese.

Sweet fruits should not be combined with breads, crackers, muffins, or any starchy foods. Remember, fruit contains a high percent of sugar, and because of this, it should not be eaten with protein, either. Sugar and protein do not go well together. Fruit eaten alone makes a good breakfast and has a cleansing effect on the body. It also provides quick energy. Sweet fruit is not good for individuals with hypoglycemia or diabetes.

Most important, remember not to eat sweet fruits with a protein meal—fruits should always be eaten alone. All melons should be eaten alone as they digest quickly and pass through the body easily. It is best not to combine fruits with vegetables. Apples are the only fruit that should be combined with vegetables.

SIMPLE CARBOHYDRATES

The category of carbohydrates comprises both sugars and starches. Sugars are simple carbohydrates and starches are complex carbohydrates. Simple carbohydrates are found in all forms and types of sugars, some juices, and in processed and refined grains (not whole grains).

Simple carbohydrates should be avoided altogether if possible. However, glucose, fructose, and galactose (which are also simple carbohydrates) are commonly found in our diets.

All sugars slow down digestion. The secretion of gastric juices needed for the breakdown of protein is almost stopped by sugar. Sugar breaks down in the intestine and proteins break down in the stomach. Because of this, if food containing sugar is eaten with meat, the sugar can be held up in the stomach by meat until it ferments and creates problems. The result is foul-smelling gas and stools, bloating, and even heartburn.

Dessert combines poorly with everything. Even fresh fruit should be avoided after a meal of protein or carbohydrates, as it will stay in the full stomach and ferment. To replace the craving for sugar, eat a protein snack. This will increase energy levels rather than creating feelings of tiredness or hunger.

Obesity, diabetes, and hypoglycemia are possible results of a diet high in simple carbohydrates (sugar). Sugar and fat lurk behind many health problems, with heart disease and cancer leading the list.

COMPLEX CARBOHYDRATES

Complex carbohydrates are the best type of carbohydrates to eat. They give a steady flow of energy. Complex carbohydrates are found in fresh vegetables, fresh fruits, beans, natural whole grains, and starchy foods like potatoes, rice, and pasta. They provide dietary fiber and have only one-third the calories found in fats and simple carbohydrates. Proteins and carbohydrates are rich in vitamins and minerals. Carbohydrates can be converted into fat and provide the body with energy and warmth. A constant flow of energy is supplied from complex carbohydrates, rather than the short-lived energy bursts from simple carbohydrates, such as sugar or starches. To avoid the high energy and fatigue cycle (ups and downs) of unregulated blood sugar levels from eating sugar, try eating a diet high in complex carbohydrates that avoids all refined, processed foods and all forms of sugar. This is more than a method to reduce or maintain a normal weight—it is a credo to be followed for basic good health.

Two important rules to follow that require only very minor changes in dietary habits are:

- Eat complex carbohydrates during the day, when you are hungry.

- Do not raid the refrigerator late at night or eat a heavy meal late in the evening.

ACIDITY AND ALKALINITY

A body that is more alkaline is a healthy body, whereas disease is associated with an overly acidic body.

TABLE 19.1 FOOD COMBINING AT A GLANCE

The following table will help to make proper food combining easy—just follow the icons:

😊 = Recommended combination

🙂 = Acceptable combination

☹ = Don't combine

Samples of items found in each of the groups in the table are:

- Vegetables: leafy greens, broccoli, cabbage, cauliflower, celery, green peas, tomatoes, sprouted seeds, and onions.

- Sweet fruits: custard apples, bananas, figs, dates, raisins, prunes, and dried fruits.

- Acidic fruits: apricots, lemons, limes, oranges, grapefruits, grapes, pineapples, pears, peaches, strawberries, raspberries, plums, and guavas.

- Starch: rice, whole grains, lentils, beans, potatoes, and noodles.

- Protein: meat, fish, poultry, cheese, eggs, yogurt, nuts, seeds, and soybeans.

- Fat: butter, margarine, lard, ghee, oils, olives, and cream.

FOOD GROUP	VEGETABLES	SWEET FRUIT	ACIDIC FRUIT	STARCH	PROTEIN	FAT
Vegetables	😊	☹	☹	😊	😊	😊
Sweet Fruit	☹	😊	☹	☹	☹	🙂
Acidic Fruit	☹	☹	😊	☹	🙂	🙂
Starch	😊	☹	☹	😊	☹	🙂
Protein	😊	☹	🙂	☹	😊	☹
Fat	😊	🙂	🙂	😊	☹	😊

Knowing the acidity or alkalinity of your body is important for making proper food choices. A simple test to assess your body's metabolism can provide a clue as to whether you are consuming excessive amounts of processed foods and simple carbohydrates.

Purchase nitrazine paper, available at any drugstore, and apply saliva or urine to the paper (or check both). Check before eating or at least one hour after eating. The paper will change colors to indicate if the body is overly acidic or alkaline. Water is neutral at pH 7.0. Below pH 7.0 is acid, above pH 7.0 is alkaline.

The ideal pH range for saliva and urine is 6.0 to 6.8—the body functions best when it is naturally mildly acidic. The best balance is low acidic and higher alkaline—and *balance* is the key. Values below pH 6.0 are too acidic, and above pH 6.8 are too alkaline.

Depending on your test results, you may want to alter the composition of your diet to bring your body's pH into the desirable range. If your body is extremely acidic or alkaline, omit acid-forming or alkaline-forming foods, as appropriate, from your diet until a new pH test is in the normal range.

Following is a summary of selected foods and the categories they fall into.

- Highly acidic fruits: cherries, cranberries, dates, dried fruits, grapefruit, kumquats, lemons, limes, oranges, persimmons, pineapples, pomegranates, raisins, sour apples, sour grapes, sour peaches, sour plums, tangerines, and tomatoes.

- Mildly acidic fruits: all berries, apricots, bananas, figs, grapes, huckleberries, kiwi fruit, loquats, mangoes, mulberries, nectarines, papayas, peaches, pears, strawberries, sweet apples, sweet fruits, sweet grapes, and sweet plums.

- Starch-free/sugar-free vegetables: all lettuces, all onions, asparagus, bamboo shoots, beet greens, bell peppers, broccoli, Brussels sprouts, cabbage, cauliflower, celery, Chinese cabbage, chives, collards, cucumbers, dandelion greens, eggplant, endive, fresh sprouts, garlic, kale, kohlrabi, leeks, okra, parsley, radishes, rhubarb, sauerkraut, scallions, spinach, string beans, Swiss chard, tomatoes, turnip greens, turnips, and watercress.

- Complex carbohydrates: all whole grains, brown rice, all vegetables, artichokes, avocados, banana squash, corn, peas, beans, lentils, fresh and dried fruits, hubbard squash, pastas, potatoes, yams, pumpkin, sweet potatoes, and water chestnuts.

- Acid-forming foods: beef, chicken, dairy products, eggs, fish, grains, lamb, pork (all forms), most nuts and seeds, turkey, veal, and all store-bought processed foods.

- Alkaline-forming foods: all melons, almonds, apricots, coconut, figs, grapes, honey, lemons, maple syrup, molasses, raisins, umeboshi plums, vegetables, and yogurt and other soured foods. Most fruits turn alkaline in the body.

If you find that your body is overly acidic, avoid acid-forming foods until your pH is back to normal. Similarly, if your body is too alkaline, avoid alkaline-forming foods. Keeping the proper balance is the key to every body function.

PART FIVE

SUPER FOODS

CHAPTER TWENTY

GARLIC: NATURE'S MIRACLE HEALER

Tomatoes and oregano make it Italian; wine and tarragon make it French; sour cream makes it Russian; lemon and cinnamon make it Greek; soy sauce makes it Chinese; garlic makes it good.

—Alice May Brock, American author, illustrator, and one-time restaurateur, The Back Room Rest (made famous in Arlo Guthrie's Alice's Restaurant*)*

Most of us have in our kitchens a humble yet powerful ally in the fight against a variety of health problems: *garlic.* Thousands of research papers have been published in the United States alone pointing to garlic's beneficial effect on heart disease, cancer, and infectious diseases. A meta-analysis by the University of North Carolina of eighteen studies on garlic showed that eating ten cloves of raw or cooked garlic weekly decreases the chances of colorectal cancer by 30 percent and stomach cancer risk by 50 percent.

Actually, garlic has been part of humanity's medicine chest for thousands of years. Touted since ancient times as a miraculous "cure-all," useful for everything from athlete's foot to warding off heart disease, garlic's medical reputation goes back at least to 1550 B.C.E. The Persians, the Medes, the Phoenicians, and the Babylonians all had extensive knowledge about garlic. The Talmud also contains references to the benefits of garlic.

Dubbed the "stinking rose," garlic belongs to the lily family and is related to onions, chives, shallots, and leeks. It is a perennial plant that is cultivated worldwide. Garlic is one of the most popular natural remedies of all time. Science, however, was slow to catch up with the wisdom of folklore. It wasn't until over a century ago that scientists began looking more closely at garlic, and in 1858 Louis Pasteur proved that it could kill bacteria.

Garlic research took a dramatic leap in 1983 when New York University Medical Center researchers showed in laboratory tests that garlic oil inhibited the development of skin cancers. Garlic's current popularity stems from an ever-growing body of evidence that it can be used to prevent and treat chronic diseases.

THE POWER OF THE "STINKING ROSE"

Garlic's many health benefits, as confirmed by scientific studies, are of three types: they help to treat infection, they protect circulation, and they fight various types of toxins.

Treating Infection

Fresh garlic is effective against bacteria, yeasts, and fungi. It is most effective against fungi and candida. Studies at the University of Oklahoma have shown that garlic juice is as strong as certain antifungal drugs, and it is certainly safer. According to research conducted at New Jersey Medical University, blood can kill fungi a half-hour after one or two cloves of fresh garlic are eaten.

Garlic is recommended for mild, recurring, or chronic infections that are not dangerous, such as infections of the mouth, ears, throat, stomach, or skin. It is effective against bronchitis, cystitis, thrush, colds, catarrh, and particularly candida. To treat vaginitis, women can use garlic slices as a vaginal suppository, or the juice as a douche.

Protecting Circulation

The ancient Greeks used garlic "to keep the arteries open." We now know that garlic reduces blood cholesterol levels, thus cutting the risk of heart attack. Researchers at Pennsylvania State University's College of Health and Human Development found in laboratory tests that garlic "inhibited fatty acid synthesis in liver cells by up to 64 percent and suppressed cholesterol synthesis by 87 percent."

Garlic provides protection from heart disease by preventing clots that can lead to heart attacks and strokes, and can reduce high blood pressure significantly. It can be of benefit to persons with diabetes who are especially susceptible to cardiovascular diseases. Garlic can significantly lower blood sugar levels.

Detoxifying

The sulfur and hydrogen compounds of garlic are potent toxic heavy metal chelators, binding and removing metals through excretions. These same compounds are effective protectants against oxidation and free-radical damage that can lead to disease and premature aging. A good book on this subject is *The Garlic Cure* by Charlie Fox, James Scheer, and Lynn Allison (McCleery and Sons, 2002).

Garlic's powerful compounds stimulate the immune system by increasing the potency of immune-system cells, which, in turn, help to fight microbes and cancer.

Researchers at California's Loma Linda University found that garlic activates enzymes in the liver to destroy aflatoxin, a strong carcinogen produced by a mold found in nuts, mainly peanuts and peanut butter. Their research also indicated that garlic may suppress the effects of cancer-causing agents in cigarette smoke, charbroiled meats, and air pollution.

SPECIFIC HEALTH BENEFITS FROM GARLIC

Beyond the general categories of health benefits outlined above, it is possible to summarize the specific actions of garlic and the conditions that it may benefit. The health-promoting actions of garlic include functioning as the following:

- Acidophilus growth stimulant
- Antibacterial agent
- Antifungal agent
- Antioxidant and antiaging agent
- Antiradiation treatment
- Antistress agent
- Antitumor agent
- Antiviral agent
- Heavy-metal chelation agent
- Immune-system enhancer
- Liver-protective agent

Specific health problems that may be helped by garlic include the following:

- Allergies
- Arthritis
- Asthma
- Atherosclerosis
- Bronchitis
- Cancer
- Canker sores
- Cardiovascular disease
- Carpal tunnel syndrome
- Circulation

- Colds/flu/persistent fever
- Diabetes
- Excessive sweating
- Excessive unexplained weight loss
- Fatigue
- Fungal diseases such as candidiasis and athlete's foot
- Gastrointestinal disorders
- Hemorrhoids
- High cholesterol
- High toxin levels
- High triglycerides
- Hypertension
- Hypoglycemia
- Impotence
- Pneumonia
- Sore throat
- Swallowing difficulty
- Swollen lymph nodes
- Vaginal discharge
- Varicose veins

Another of garlic's amazing abilities is that it can pep up breast milk for baby's benefit. In one recent study, mothers of eight nursing infants took either a garlic capsule or a flavorless capsule with no active ingredients. The babies showed a definite preference for the garlic-flavored milk, spending more time on the breast and sucking more often.

Research in England found that taking standardized garlic supplements during pregnancy may increase the birth weight of potentially growth-retarded babies, and may also lower the risk of preeclampsia, a potentially dangerous complication of pregnancy characterized by hypertension, swelling, and large amounts of protein in the urine.

GARLIC CHEMISTRY

Garlic has a complex biochemistry wrapped in a simple, compact package. It contains numerous phytochemicals, including seventy-five different sulfur compounds. The presence of these various compounds depend upon whether the garlic is fresh or aged, raw or cooked, natural or in a processed form (tablets, capsules, oils, or extracts). Recent research has focused on the compounds s-allyl cysteine (SAC), s-allyl mercaptocysteine (SAMC), and diallyl disulfide (DADS).

Crushing or slicing a garlic clove releases the enzyme alliinase. This substance in turn modifies another molecule, called alliin, into one known as allicin, which is the active component that gives garlic its aroma and flavor. By itself, allicin is a potent antioxidant that neutralizes cell-damaging free radicals. The garlic *must* be fresh, as the active ingredient is destroyed within one hour of crushing. Swallowing the clove intact will not permit the allicin to be converted into its active ingredient. Cooking, aging, and otherwise processing garlic causes allicin to break down into other compounds. During the aging process, alliin and allicin are converted to water-soluble, stable compounds that are virtually odorless. Because allicin decomposes immediately, it is not biologically available to the body and cannot be absorbed into the bloodstream.

HOW MUCH GARLIC?

The recommended minimum intake of fresh garlic is one to two cloves a day. A clove is one of the individual segments that make up a head of garlic. Most studies have focused on the healing powers of fresh, raw, or cooked garlic, and aged garlic extract (AGE), while only a relative few have tested dried or powdered garlic supplements. Kyolic Aged Garlic Extract from Wakunaga of America is a garlic extract that is standardized to contain a certain level of both SAC and SAMC. Unlike other aged garlic products, Kyolic contains the compound fructosyl arginine, which, in laboratory tests, proved to be as effective as vitamin C in its antioxidant activity. Researchers at Pennsylvania State University found that both fresh garlic and aged garlic extract were effective in curbing the spontaneous formation of nitrosamines, carcinogens absorbed from food and water. A study reported in *The Journal of Nutrition* showed that supplementation with aged garlic extract lowered oxidative stress in humans. Study volunteers (both smokers and nonsmokers) were given aged garlic extract once daily for fourteen days, and researchers concluded that supplementation with aged garlic may help prevent atherosclerosis and other diseases associated with oxidative stress. Aged garlic extract is odorless and tasteless for those worried about putting a strain on their social lives. Other garlic supplements include garlic oil and garlic powder in capsules or tablets.

Avoid consuming very large quantities of garlic if you take aspirin or anticoagulant drugs on a regular basis, because all three restrict clotting. Do not substitute garlic for any prescription medications without first talking to a health-care professional.

GARLIC REMEDIES FOR SPECIFIC HEALTH PROBLEMS

Ear Infections

Add two to four drops of warm (not hot) liquid garlic extract in each infected ear. Do not use the same dropper for both ears, as it can spread the infection. This remedy is especially helpful for children.

Eye Problems

Combine an equal amount of liquid garlic extract and pure water in an eyedropper and place two drops in each eye every four hours, as needed.

Finger or Toe Fungus

Place a cotton ball saturated with liquid garlic on the infected areas. Use an adhesive bandage or cotton sock to hold it in place. Change the saturated cotton daily.

Hemorrhoids

Insert liquid garlic into the rectum with a cotton swab, or insert a Kyolic capsule.

High Cholesterol

Eat two to four crushed fresh garlic cloves each day. Add garlic to salads, dressings, or anything else you like—but don't eat it alone as it may irritate the stomach lining. Or take four to six capsules of garlic extract daily for two months, then four daily thereafter.

Mosquito Repellent

Take four capsules of garlic extract with vitamins B_1 and B_{12} one hour before going outside.

Mouth Sores

Place 1 teaspoon of liquid garlic in your mouth, swish it around, then hold it for a few minutes before swallowing. For added healing, mix one capsule or four drops of goldenseal herbal extract to the liquid garlic.

Vaginal Yeast Infections

Douche with a solution of 1 tablespoon of liquid garlic in a quart of warm water.

For Pets

Place two drops of liquid garlic extract in the ears for ear mites.

COOKING WITH GARLIC

The beauty of garlic is its versatility as a medicine, spice, and food. It is culinary, as well as medicinal. Nearly all commercially grown garlic comes from California, Texas, Mexico, and Egypt. Of the 300 varieties grown worldwide, the Italian variety is the one generally found in supermarkets. It has either white or pinkish skin, depending on when it is harvested, and a strong flavor. The so-called elephant variety is not a true garlic, but a form of leek with larger cloves and milder flavor.

Key nutrients in raw garlic include calcium, iron, magnesium, phosphorus, potassium, zinc, copper, manganese, selenium, vitamin B_6, vitamin C, vitamin E, vitamin B_1 (thiamine), vitamin B_2 (riboflavin), vitamin B_3 (niacin), pantothenic acid, folate, and fiber. Phytochemicals include allicin, tocopherols, beta-carotene, beta-sitosterol, caffeic acid, chlorogenic acid, diallyl disulfide, ferulic acid, geraniol, kaempferol, linalol, P-coumaric acid, phloroglucinol, phytic acid, quercetin, rutin, s-allyl cysteine, s-allyl mercaptocysteine, saponin, sinapic acid, and stigmasterol.

Buy garlic loose, rather than packaged, to choose healthy bulbs. Look for plump, dry, solid bulbs that are free of soft spots. They should feel solid and heavy, and have tight, unbroken outer skin.

Garlic will keep for several weeks when stored in a covered container placed in a cool, dry spot—but do not refrigerate it. Garlic will sprout. The sprouts have a milder taste and can be used like scallions and chives.

Following are a few tips on capturing garlic's flavor, aroma, and health benefits in the kitchen:

- Do not pulverize raw garlic in a blender. This makes it bitter (beyond repair).

- To peel a garlic clove, place it on a cutting board and lay the flat side of a broad knife on top. Tap the knife sharply to split the peel, and the clove will pop out. If you need a lot of cloves, drop them in boiling water for a minute or two, then plunge into cold water, and the skins should slip off easily.

- To mince garlic by hand, use a sharp, heavy chef's knife. Chopping releases the most odoriferous compounds. Use whole cloves for a milder taste.

- Don't let garlic burn when sautéing or roasting. It turns sharp and bitter. Gently sauté cloves on low heat until they become transparent.

- Roast the cloves, or the whole head, to produce garlic that is quite sweet.

- Make a great sauce by puréeing together roasted garlic cloves with stock, and spiking it with tamari sauce and fresh rosemary, thyme, or basil.

- To give foods as much or as little garlic flavor as desired, look for pure garlic juice in a pump spray bottle from Garlic Valley Farms. It is available in health food stores and has many of the benefits of garlic cloves. Use it to make garlic bread, spray it on salads, or spritz it on cooked dishes such as vegetables, seafood, and pasta.

- For safety's sake, be sure to store chopped or crushed garlic oil blends in the refrigerator and use them within three weeks. Before placing garlic in oil, drop each clove in vinegar for a second to destroy mold, which is sometimes found on the cloves. Garlic can pick up botulism bacterium from the soil. If it does, covering the garlic in oil and leaving it at room temperature can allow the the botulism spores to sprout.

- To add garlic to your diet, try one or more of the following: Mix raw garlic with roasted red peppers and serve as an appetizer; add raw garlic to Caesar salad; add garlic to tomato sauce; sautée it with olive oil and parsley and serve over pasta; dice very finely and add to puréed cucumbers and yogurt for a cold soup; sprinkle it into a gratin; or mash it with black beans for burritos.

CHAPTER TWENTY-ONE

IMMORTAL MUSHROOMS

Does it follow that because there are toadstools which resemble mushrooms, both are dangerous?

—*Marianne Moore, twentieth-century American poet*

The 5,300-year-old "iceman" found in 1991 between Austria and Italy wore a well-preserved amulet of dried mushrooms around his neck. It seems that even during the Stone Age, earth's inhabitants recognized the power of this "fungus" growing in darkness. Ancient Chinese herbalists considered the reishi mushroom the most beneficial of all medicines and the emperors of Japan believed the reishi granted them immortality. Today, the Japanese government officially recognizes the reishi mushroom as a substance for treating cancer.

Reishi is only one of more than 38,000 varieties of mushrooms that flourish throughout the world. Some varieties are edible, others (often called toadstools) are highly toxic or even poisonous, and most grow in the wild. The culinary mushrooms sold in grocery stores are usually grown in special buildings, where the desired environment for cultivating mushrooms can be controlled. The French were the first to grow mushrooms as a crop in caves beginning in the seventeenth century.

Though stocked in the produce department of grocery stores, mushrooms are not really a vegetable, but a fungus. A fungus is an organism classified as a plant that does not have roots or leaves, and does not flower or bear seeds. It grows in darkness and reproduces by releasing spores that are spread by the wind, find an ideal place to grow, and begin the cycle again. Mushrooms are the above-ground fleshy, fruiting body of a fungus. Mushrooms, like all fungi (plural for fungus), do not have the chlorophyll necessary to turn light into energy. They are the last rung of the food chain and must obtain their nutrients from organic matter like dead leaves, wood, and other waste. Mushrooms are nature's recyclers—without them, the planet would pile up with dead, decaying matter.

MUSHROOM NUTRITION

Contrary to popular belief, mushrooms are highly nutritious. They supply protein, amino acids, B vitamins, copper, magnesium, vitamin C, potassium, phosphorous, folate, selenium, and iron. Mushrooms are among the few food sources rich in the trace mineral germanium, which is thought to promote efficient use of oxygen in the body and to protect against damage from free radicals. Some species of mushrooms even provide beta-carotene, a powerful antioxidant.

Despite their somewhat meaty texture, mushrooms are low in calories. A cup of raw mushrooms contains approximately 20 calories and little or no fat. Because the small amount of fat in mushrooms consists mainly of unsaturated fatty acids, such as linoleic acid, they may be the ideal food to lose weight and maintain a healthy heart and cardiovascular system.

HEALING MUSHROOMS

All edible mushrooms contain both medicinal and nutritional qualities. Scientific research indicates that the major actions of medicinal mushrooms are stimulating the immune system and protecting against cardiovascular disease, free radicals, mutagens, and toxins. Most medicinal mushrooms contain *polysaccharides* (complex sugar molecules) called beta-glucans that increase RNA and DNA in the bone marrow where immune cells, like lymphocytes, are made. The combination of compounds in mushrooms is believed to target the immune system and aid in neuron transmission, metabolism, and the transport of nutrients and oxygen. Three mushroom varieties—reishi, shiitake, and maitake—have been studied intensively and have proven to possess strong medicinal properties. All mushrooms must be cooked to get the nutritional value. The cell walls cannot be digested unless they are tenderized by heat.

BUYING MUSHROOMS

Most grocery stores today carry several varieties of mushrooms. Choose fresh varieties that show no sign of deterioration and are firm, plump, and dry to the touch. Also, select mushrooms with smooth, unwrinkled caps that are not frayed on the edges. Avoid mushrooms that are wet, black, bruised, or spotted with mold. Fresh mushrooms should smell like the woods. Avoid any mushrooms that smell of ammonia.

A word of caution: *Do not* pick and eat wild mushrooms. Only a trained mycologist (mushroom expert) can determine if a wild mushroom is safe to eat. Eating unidentified mushrooms picked in the wild could lead to serious illness and even death.

STORING MUSHROOMS

Most refrigerator vegetable bins do not provide adequate air circulation needed to keep mushrooms fresh. Store them unwashed and untrimmed in a loosely closed brown paper bag in the main compartment of the refrigerator. You can also place them in a shallow glass dish covered with a kitchen towel or lightly moistened paper towel. Leave prepackaged mushrooms unopened until you use them.

Dried mushrooms can be kept indefinitely at room temperature in a dry place, providing they are unopened and in their original packaging or an airtight container.

PREPARING AND CLEANING MUSHROOMS

The best method for cleaning fresh mushrooms is to gently wipe them clean with a damp paper towel. You can clean them also with a brief spritz from the spray attachment of the faucet, but be careful not to waterlog them. After mushrooms have been cleaned, cut off the tip of the stem if it is dried out. Mushrooms can be used whole or sliced. Slicing, however, causes fresh mushrooms to lose 33 percent of their vitamin B_2 (riboflavin). To prevent darkening, dip mushroom slices in lemon water. Cooked mushrooms give foods a delightful flavor, due to their large quantity of *natural* glutamic acid, the same flavor enhancer in monosodium glutamate (MSG). Unlike MSG, however, mushrooms contain very little sodium.

Dried mushrooms can be reconstituted by placing them in a pan of hot water for twenty to thirty minutes. Reserve the soaking liquid, filter it through cheesecloth or a coffee filter, and use it in stock.

Be aware that mushrooms will discolor aluminum cooking pans and utensils. However, the use of any aluminum pans or utensils is not recommended in any case.

MUSHROOM VARIETIES: THE "BIG THREE"

Maitake Mushrooms

Pronounced (my-TAH-key), this giant mushroom grows wild in northeastern Japan and is known as the "king of the mushrooms" because of its health benefits. Maitake (*Grifola frondosa*) contains protein, fiber, amino acids, vitamin C, vitamin B_{12}, vitamin B_2 (riboflavin), magnesium, potassium, phosphorus, and other nutrients.

The maitake mushroom also contains compounds called beta-glucans. Beta-glucans are one of the known active polysaccharide compounds that enhance the functioning of the immune system. In 1992, the U.S. National Cancer Institute, along with the Japanese National Institute of Health, reported that maitake extract exhibited anti-HIV activity. Maitake's anti-HIV effect prevents the HIV virus from destroying T cells. Extensive testing of maitake on cancer patients has shown a dramatic reduction of tumors and other symptoms. In one study, the side effects of chemotherapy (vomiting, loss of appetite, hair loss) were improved in 90 percent of the patients using maitakes.

Research has further confirmed maitake as an effective remedy for high blood pressure, diabetes, rheumatoid arthritis, high cholesterol, cardiovascular and liver disorders, candida, constipation, and obesity. In addition, maitake helps regulate endocrine functions. Current research is focusing on using maitake to treat Alzheimer's disease, osteoporosis, chronic fatigue syndrome, and hair loss.

The most efficient way to obtain the medicinal benefits is to take maitake extract in supplement form, as the essential nutritional ingredients are lost during the cooking process. Maitake caplets and D-fraction and MD-fraction extracts, beta-glucans derived from maitake that have anti-tumor activity, are available in health food stores. For increased health benefits when using the D-fraction extract, also take maitake caplets, as this will make the extract a whole food complex. The whole mushrooms are also available dried in grocery and health food stores, and can be added to foods such as soups and stews.

Reishi Mushrooms

This fungus is a hard, woodlike mushroom that contains more than 90 percent indigestible fiber. Reishi (RAY-she) is also called varnished conk, phantom mushroom, and ten-thousand-year mushroom. In China it is called *ling zhi*, which means "spirit plant." Reishi usually grows on oak trees and Japanese plum trees.

Reishi (*Ganoderma lucidum*) contains carbohydrates, fiber, amino acids, protein, steroids, triterpenes, lipids, alkaloids, polysaccharides, glucoside, coumarin glycoside, volatile oil, vitamin B_2 (riboflavin), and ascorbic acid. It also contains the minerals calcium, zinc, magnesium, copper, and germanium. Additionally, reishi contains ganoderic acid, which is a free-radical scavenger, giving reishi antioxidant powers. The polysaccharides in reishi mushrooms appear to activate a type of white blood cell known as a macrophage. These cells filter the blood, destroying cancer cells, viruses, bacteria, and other large particulate material. Macrophages also signal other white blood cells to seek out and destroy tumor cells.

Reishi is the most commonly used medicinal mushroom because of its proven health benefits. Clinical studies on humans for more than twenty years have shown that reishi reduces the side effects from radiation and chemotherapy, boosts overall health, promotes longevity, speeds recovery from illness, detoxifies and regenerates the liver, improves circulation and stamina, increases blood flow, reduces platelet aggregation, enhances the immune system, and reduces inflammation in the joints. Reishi is now used to treat an assortment of disorders, including cancer, myasthenia gravis, migraines, Candida infections, Epstein-Barr virus, anxiety, depression, insomnia, chronic fatigue syndrome, hepatitis, neuralgia, rheumatism, duodenal ulcers, heart disease, high blood pressure, bronchitis, neurasthenia, dizziness, insomnia, rhinitis, retinal pigmentary degeneration, muscular dystrophy, osteogenic hyperplasia, Alzheimer's disease, high cholesterol, hyperlipidemia, diabetes, high-altitude sickness, and symptoms associated with anorexia. Reishi's ability to block the release of histamines makes it a useful treatment for bronchial asthma and other allergic diseases. In the majority of the clinical studies, reishi was taken along with vitamin C to increase the absorption of the mushroom's polysaccharides.

Six different types of reishi, classified by color, have been identified. Each type has a different medicinal use:

- Red reishi has a bitter taste and is generally regarded as the most potent and medicinal of the reishi mushrooms. It is used to aid the internal organs, build vitality, and improve memory.

- Blue reishi has a sour taste. It improves eyesight and liver function and has a calming effect on the nerves.

- Purple reishi has a sweet taste. It enhances the function of the joints, muscles, and ears, and nourishes the complexion.

- Black reishi has a salty taste. It is used primarily to protect the kidneys.

- Yellow reishi has a sweet taste. It improves spleen function and has a calming effect.

- White reishi has a hot, pungent taste. It is used to assist lung function.

Reishi is found in tablet and liquid products the world over. Available forms of reishi include syrups, soups, teas, injections, tablets, tinctures, and extracts.

Shiitake Mushrooms

The shiitake (*Lentinus edodes*) mushroom is delicious and nutritious, and has a wonderful texture. Many vegetarians enjoy the shiitake (she-TAH-key) as a meat substitute. It grows in the wild in Asian countries on a variety of trees. Though it does not grow in the wild in the United States, shiitake is widely cultivated here.

Shiitake mushrooms contain protein, free amino acids, lipids, enzymes, polysaccharides, carbohydrates, fiber, vitamin B_{12}, vitamin B_2 (riboflavin), and vitamin C. They also contain ergosterol, a provitamin that is converted into vitamin D in the presence of sunlight. Cultured varieties of shiitake also contain the minerals calcium, manganese, magnesium, potassium, iron, phosphorus, and zinc.

Shiitake mushrooms are the source of two well-studied extracts with proven medicinal effects—*Lentinus edodes mycelium* (LEM) extract, and lentinan (a polysaccharide). These extracts have been proven to inhibit tumors and viruses. They help to regulate the immune system, ward off bacterial and parasitic infections, improve circulation, increase stamina, protect the liver, promote the production of antibodies to the hepatitis B virus, reduce the side effects from radiation and chemotherapy, and lower the levels of cholesterol and fat in the blood. Shiitake has been used to treat cancer, HIV/AIDS, herpes simplex, Epstein-Barr virus, environmental allergies, Candida infections, influenza, the common cold, bronchial inflammations, migraine, obesity, urinary incontinence, high blood pressure, and chronic high cholesterol.

Another shiitake extract, called KS-2, activates macrophages and induces the body to produce interferon, a powerful antiviral and anticancer substance. Although KS-2 is still being studied, it may prove to be the most valuable shiitake compound because of its high oral bioavailability.

Scientists have also isolated an amino acid, eritadenine, in shiitakes that may prove to be beneficial in the prevention of heart attack, stroke, and diabetes by lowering cholesterol, preventing blood clots, and regulating blood sugar levels.

Fresh and dried shiitake mushrooms are available in most grocery stores. They are easily cultivated at home. Fresh shiitake do not lose their nutrient value when cooked at high temperatures. To soften dried mushrooms, place them in water for a few minutes before using. Some ideas for using shiitakes include:

- Use them to enhance prepared foods and mixes, such as soups, stuffing, sauces, gravies, dips, and more.

- Marinate them for one hour in salad dressing, slice, and add to tossed salad.

- Include them in rice and other grain dishes for added flavor and nutrition.

- Mix them with other vegetables for stir-fries, fried rice, and other Asian-style dishes.

- Add them to omelets, scrambled eggs, or quiche.

- Make a shiitake sauce or gravy to dress up leftovers.

- Marinate and grill or skewer them with kabobs for summer barbecues.

- Slice them and add them to spaghetti sauce or use them as a pizza topping.

- Add them to fresh, frozen, or canned vegetables during cooking.

In addition to the whole mushrooms, there are many prepared shiitake products available in health food stores. LEM extract also is available in tablet or capsule form. Lentinan is poorly absorbed when taken orally, and must be injected under the supervision of a health-care provider.

OTHER MUSHROOM VARIETIES

In addition to the "big three" medicinal mushrooms listed above, there are many other types of mushrooms that have various health benefits.

ABM Mushrooms

Identified by the initials of its Latin name, *Agaricus blazei Murill*, the ABM mushroom grows in Brazil. Studies at Tokyo University showed the ABM to have a remarkable effect on the human immune system. When compared to other powerful medicinal mushrooms, including reishi and shiitake, ABM had the highest level of beta-glucan.

Button Mushrooms

The button mushroom (*Agaricus bisporus*) is the most commonly cultivated mushroom. It contains protein, carbohydrates, fiber, B vitamins, vitamin C, ergosterol, vitamin E, calcium, iron, magnesium, manganese, phosphorous, potassium, selenium, and zinc. A decoction of the dried fruiting bodies of the button mushroom is reported as useful in the treatment of diabetes.

Raw button mushrooms contain potentially carcinogenic compounds related to a class of chemicals called hydrazines. Cooking destroys them. You would have to consume extremely large quantities of raw button mushrooms over a long period of time for there to be a significant risk from this. Nonetheless, it is wise to eat only moderate amounts no more than three times a week. Button mushrooms also contain hemagglutinins, which laboratory studies indicate can interfere with protein absorption and produce lesions in the small intestine.

Chanterelle Mushrooms

The chanterelle mushroom (*Cantharellus cibarius*) grows on the ground around conifers and broadleaf trees and likes cool, damp climates. Chanterelles have a meaty texture and flavor and are prized as a culinary mushroom. They contain eight essential amino acids and vitamin A. Traditionally, chanterelles have been used to treat night blindness, ophthalmia, and dry skin. Laboratory studies show that an extract of the chanterelle can inhibit the growth of certain tumors.

Chanterelles are available by mail order and in gourmet grocery stores. They are sold canned and dried in European countries.

Cordyceps

Found in the highland regions of China, this mushroom, also known as caterpillar fungus, is one of the most valued medicinal fungi in Chinese medicine, and among the most potent. Cordyceps (*Cordyceps sinensis*, sometimes called simply ceps) is formed when a bladelike growth develops after fungal infestation of dead caterpillar larva. These bladelike growths are then harvested, cleaned, and dried in the sun.

Cordyceps contains water-soluble polysaccharides that work to stimulate the cells of the immune system. Traditionally, cordyceps has been used as a kidney purifier and to treat pneumonia, chronic bronchitis, pulmonary emphysema, and tuberculosis. Recent studies indicate that cordyceps helps to protect the kidneys from toxicity, lowers high cholesterol levels, treats impotence, inhibits tracheal muscle contractions, and relaxes the airways. Cornell University researchers found that an extract of cordyceps supported the function of helper T-cells by protecting them against immune-suppressing invaders.

Crimini Mushrooms

Crimini mushrooms are related to button mushrooms. They are light tan to medium brown in color and have a meatier, earthier taste. Crimini mushrooms contain protein, carbohydrates, vitamin A, vitamin C, calcium, phosphorous, and iron.

Enokitake Mushrooms

This white stringy variety of mushroom is commonly referred to as enoki. Enokitake (*Flammulina velutipes*) contains several types of amino acids, one of which—valine—inhibits the growth of certain cancers. Enokitake stimulates the immune system and fights viruses. Consumed on a regular basis, enokitake may help to prevent and/or heal gastroenteric ulcers and liver disease.

Mo-er Mushrooms

Also known as tree ear or wood ear, mo-er mushrooms are customarily added to Chinese dishes such as soups and stir-fries. The mo-er has a long history in traditional Chinese medicine as a longevity booster, a stomach tonic, and soothing to throat inflammation. Scientists have now isolated a compound in mo-er—adenosine—that acts as an anticoagulant. Adenosine also accounts for the blood-thinning properties in onions and garlic.

Morel Mushrooms

Morels (*Morchella esculenta*) resemble brown sponges on a thick stem. Morels contain the following amino acids: isoleucine, leucine, lysine, methionine, phenylalanine, threonine, and valine.

Oyster Mushrooms

Named for its oyster-shell shape, this mushroom grows on deciduous trees in the United States, Europe, and Asia. It has a high protein content and also supplies amino acids, vitamin B_1 (thiamine), vitamin B_2 (riboflavin), vitamin P, essential fatty acids, minerals, fiber, lipids, and carbohydrates.

Laboratory studies have demonstrated that oyster mushrooms possess antitumor activity and reduce cholesterol levels. When dried, they contain a high level of iron and may be an excellent blood-builder.

Oyster mushrooms are available by mail order and in gourmet grocery stores. They are easily cultivated at home.

Portobello Mushrooms

The portobello mushroom is related to the button mushroom. They are quite large in size, and can have caps up to six to eight inches in diameter. Portobello mushrooms contain protein, carbohydrates, fiber, vitamin A, vitamin C, calcium, phosphorous, and iron. They are a chef's favorite due to their delicate flavor and meaty texture.

Snow Fungus

Also known as trembling fungus and white fungus, this variety of mushroom prefers to grow on a wide variety of deciduous trees and is commonly cultivated in Asia. Snow fungus (*Tremella fuciformis)* grows in the wild in the southern United States and in warmer climates around the world.

Snow fungus contains polysaccharides A and B, along with an assortment of fatty acids. Testing on the polysaccharides has shown they are effective in treating leukopenia induced by radiation or chemotherapy cancer treatment, enhancing immune function, and stimulating white blood cell activity. Other studies indicate that these polysaccharides possess antitumor and antiradiation properties, provide resistance to chronic bronchitis, and aid in the healing of chronic hepatitis.

Turkey Tail Mushrooms

In Japan this mushroom is known as *kawaratake*, which means "mushroom by the riverbank," and in China it is known as *yun-zhi*, which means "cloud fungus." The English name is derived from the fact that its multicolored cap resembles the tail of a tom turkey. The turkey tail mushroom (*Trametes versicolor*) grows in the wild in overlapping groups on decaying logs.

Turkey tail mushrooms contain the polysaccharide PSK (polysaccharide Kureha), which has been tested in numerous human clinical studies. The results of these studies show that PSK (used orally and intravenously) increases interferon production and macrophage activity, has antioxidant activity, is effective against some cancers, and enhances the immune system. PSK is showing positive results in testing on patients with glomerulonephritis, sarcoidosis, idiopathic nephrotic syndrome, lupus, rheumatoid arthritis, multiple sclerosis, genital herpes, Behçet's disease, and dermatomyositis. Other studies suggest that PSK may help to lower cholesterol levels.

PSP, another polysaccharide extract from the turkey tail mushroom, has shown promise in reducing the symptoms of chemotherapy and in increasing the remission rates for certain types of cancer.

Many of the mushrooms described in this chapter can be found in your local market. Some, however, may be harder to locate. For recommended suppliers of mushroom and mushroom products, see the Resources section.

CHAPTER TWENTY-TWO

YOGURT AND KEFIR

Yogurt is the only animal-derived complete-protein source recommended for frequent use in the diet.

—Prescription for Nutritional Healing

The French call yogurt *le lait de la vie eternelle*, which means "the milk of eternal life." Yogurt has been a staple food in the Middle East, Southeastern Europe, and much of Asia since recorded history. It is mentioned in the Bible, in Buddhist texts, and in the Koran. Genghis Khan commanded his military to carry yogurt with them on long marches, and in his book *Diet and Diet Reform*, Mahatma Gandhi recommended yogurt as a staple to his people. Called different names in various cultures, the myriad of benefits from yogurt, teeming with friendly bacteria, was recognized long before science even knew what bacteria was.

Plain yogurt is simply milk of any kind (including soymilk), that has been thickened by "good" bacteria, such as *Lactobacillus acidophilus*, growing in it. These bacteria produce lactase, an enzyme that breaks down the natural milk sugar lactose, producing lactic acid, which curdles the milk and gives yogurt its tart flavor. The lactic-acid–producing bacteria also protect yogurt from harmful pathogenic microorganisms, giving it a longer shelf life. Yogurt is nutritionally superior to milk in many ways. Each 8-ounce serving contains 30 to 45 percent of the recommended daily calcium requirement. Yogurt has more digestible milk protein than milk. Even most lactose-intolerant people can eat yogurt without discomfort. Yogurt is an outstanding source of protein, calcium, potassium, vitamin B_6, vitamin B_{12}, vitamin B_3 (niacin), and folic acid. A serving of yogurt contains just as much potassium as a banana. There are few foods that have as many health benefits as yogurt.

Kefir is a cultured milk product that is similar to yogurt but has a smaller curd size than yogurt, is easier to digest, and has a more liquid consistency, like that of a thick beverage. It is cultured from gelatinous particles called grains, which contain a mixture of good bacteria and yeast. Additional beneficial bacteria in kefir that are not found in yogurt—*Lactobacillus caucasus*, *Leuconostoc* species, *Acetobacter* species, and some *Streptococcus* species—make kefir a valuable addition to the diet. The active yeast and bacteria in kefir aids digestion and helps to keep the colon environment clean and healthy.

Yogurt is an essential curative for anyone who is taking antibiotics, which destroy the "friendly bacteria" in the body. Many doctors recommend acidophilus yogurt (or acidophilus supplements) for patients on antibiotics. Antibiotics disrupt the balance of good and bad bacteria in the intestines, killing off the helpful organisms and allowing the others to prevail. Yogurt also helps to prevent diarrhea and yeast infections—which, if treated with more antibiotics, set up a recurring cycle.

Dr. Khem Shahani of the University of Nebraska has said that he finds yogurt to be more effective as a preventative than as a cure for diarrhea and dysentery: "By ingesting lactobacilli in food form after diarrheal stress, one can reduce diarrheal incidence."

The Long Island Jewish Medical Center in New York reports that eating a cup of yogurt with live cultures of *Lactobacillus acidophilus* every day can significantly cut the incidence of vaginal yeast infections, thrush, and vaginitis in women. *L. acidophilus* is not destroyed by the acidic gastric juices of the stomach, unlike two other forms of bacteria used for yogurt. The *L. acidophilus* resides on the intestinal walls, where it can destroy disease-causing bacteria, providing a deadly environment for *Salmonella*, *Listeria*, and other types of bacteria that can cause food poisoning. Yogurt contains high levels of a natural fatty hormonal substance called prostaglandin E_2 that antagonize hormones. These substances protect the lining of the stomach from toxins. Yogurt has been found to boost the immune function of animal and human cells, causing these cells to make more antibodies and create other disease-fighting cells. Yogurt fights infections two ways—by boosting the immune system and by killing harmful bacteria.

There is evidence that yogurt may help prevent cancer, primarily in the colon. A top researcher in Boston has found that acidophilus culture can help suppress activity in the colon that converts harmless chemicals into carcinogenic agents. In a Polish study, bowel cancer patients were fed a quart of yogurt every day for two months, resulting in a reduction of cancer in many patients. The U.S. National Cancer Institute determined that malignant tumors shrink in patients who consumed a steady diet of yogurt. Studies at the Harvard Medical School and the University of Chicago Medical School showed that yogurt is especially effective against vaginal cancer.

The bacteria in yogurt can also lower cholesterol levels in the blood, helping to reduce the chance of strokes and heart attacks. The bacteria fight dysentery, cholera, diarrhea, and other infections. The enzymes in yogurt suppress the putrefactive organisms in incompletely digested foods; incomplete digestion can trigger food allergies. Yogurt enzymes also prevent gas and bloating. Older adults, who tend not to produce sufficient amounts of digestive enzymes, can benefit from supplementing their diets with plain yogurt.

According to the U.S. Food and Drug Administration (FDA), each 110 grams of nonfat yogurt contains less than 0.5 grams of milk fat, low-fat yogurt contains between 0.5 and 2.0 grams of milk fat, and whole milk yogurt has approximately 3.5 grams of fat per 100 grams. An 8-ounce (1 cup) serving of nonfat yogurt contains only 110 calories, making it a very healthy addition to any diet.

FRESH OR FROZEN YOGURT?

Dennis Savaiano, a professor of nutrition at the University of Minnesota, conducted a study on sixteen lactose-intolerant men. He found that frozen yogurt caused gas and bloating due to lactose intolerance. Small companies often buy commercial yogurt, pasteurize it, and turn it into frozen yogurt. When the yogurt is pasteurized a second time or frozen, the beneficial bacteria that produce lactase are killed. Frozen yogurt is also generally high in fat and has added sugar.

The University of Nebraska conducted research with mice that showed yogurt bacteria slowed the growth of harmful bacteria by as much as 75 percent. The bacteria contained in active yogurt cultures also can suppress the growth of deadly cancer cells. These effects are found only in *fresh* yogurt. The bacteria in frozen yogurt do not have the same effect.

BUYING YOGURT

Not all yogurts are created equal. When purchasing yogurt, read labels carefully and be sure to choose "live" yogurt that does not contain added sugars, preservatives, or thickeners. Some manufacturers heat yogurt to add tartness and extend the shelf life of the product, which destroys most of the active cultures (the friendly bacteria)—and the healt benefits. Yogurt produced by heat processing

is required by the FDA to be labeled *heat-treated after culturing*. Manufacturers are also required to add either *Lactobacillus bulgaricus* or *Streptococcus thermophilus* bacteria, but are not required to specify if these cultures are living or active. Make sure the label includes the phrase *active yogurt cultures, living yogurt cultures,* or *contains active cultures.* Yogurt advertised as low fat and sugar-free may still contain flavorings, stabilizers, and other added chemicals. Plain low-fat yogurt is the healthiest and most digestible form.

Finally, purchase only yogurt that has an expiration date at least ten days ahead on the carton. If there is no date, do not purchase the product.

INCORPORATING YOGURT INTO YOUR DIET

There are many ways to incorporate yogurt and its health benefits into your diet. You can, of course, simply eat the yogurt plain. To increase the benefits of yogurt, mix in the contents of two capsules of acidophilus powder before consuming it. You can also add yogurt to fruit snacks. For a refreshing, healing beverage, replace ice cream shakes with mashed bananas and fresh berries blended into yogurt. Children love it!

To reduce calories and fat in salad dressings, potato salad, bean salad, cole slaw, pasta salads, tuna salad, and sandwich spreads, substitute a mixture of equal parts plain yogurt and soy mayonnaise for regular mayonnaise. Plain yogurt makes a good substitute in recipes calling for sour cream and is great on baked potatoes. Yogurt also can be substituted for buttermilk in waffles, pancakes, breads, muffins, biscuits, and in many other dishes. Experiment and try your own recipes. You should not substitute yogurt in cake mixes without adjusting the amount of leavening.

NONDAIRY YOGURT

Of special interest to vegans and people who are allergic to dairy products, yogurts made from soymilk are getting better all the time. Silk Cultured Soy, made by White Wave, is the tastiest and creamiest nondairy yogurt I have found. The product is sweetened with juices and comes in a variety of flavors.

MAKING YOGURT AT HOME—IT'S EASY, INEXPENSIVE, AND TASTES BETTER!

The benefits of homemade yogurt are numerous. It aids in neutralizing uric acid in the body and helps to prevent and combat digestive tract infections. Live yogurt cultures flourish in the digestive tract and have a natural antibiotic effect.

Fresh homemade yogurt contains bulgaricus and thermophilus cultures in high amounts. It has a smooth taste and a mild, nontangy flavor. All you will need is a yogurt maker, milk, and yogurt starter. Follow the directions that come with your yogurt maker.

If you use skim milk, low-fat milk, or nonfat milk, the resulting yogurt should have a soft consistency. If the yogurt is *too* soft, add powdered nonfat dry milk directly to the fluid milk before heating it. Use ⅓ to ½ cup of powder per quart of milk. This will make your yogurt thicker and creamier. The longer the yogurt remains in the machine, the firmer and more tart it will become. The curd and whey may eventually separate.

Make sure to get yogurt starter that is fresh, with an expiration date months ahead. The freeze-dried yogurt starter Yogourmet, available in health food stores, makes a good, firm yogurt. You can also use commercial yogurt as starter, but make sure that the product contains live cultures and has not been entirely pasteurized to prolong its shelf life. Only unpasteurized, unflavored yogurt contains live cultures.

Following are some yogurt-making do's and don'ts and other tips:

- Do not heat the milk for too long or on too high a temperature. This will produce a poor-quality yogurt.

- Never use an electric mixer. If the yogurt turns out too liquid because the culture used was not strong enough or there were antibiotics in the milk, try using this liquid yogurt in dressings or fruit drinks—or simply drink it as is.

- Most health food stores carry yogurt thermometers, needed for accurate temperature control, as well as automatic yogurt makers. (Many yogurt makers come with their own thermometers.) Compared to purchasing yogurt, investing $25 to $35 in an automatic yogurt maker can save a great deal of money over the years.

- When you are ready to place the yogurt in jars, fill them to the rim before refrigerating. If there is no room for excess air, the yogurt can be preserved for a longer period of time.

- For a thicker and smoother texture, strain the yogurt through a white cotton cloth before refrigerating it. Don't waste the strained-off liquid—drink it. This is whey, and it contains live cultures.

- If there is a watery substance on the top of your yogurt after refrigeration, you can either mix it in or pour it off before eating the yogurt.

- If you want to flavor your yogurt, do so after it has been refrigerated for several hours or right before eating it.

- Always save 4 tablespoons of plain yogurt to make the next batch. Yogurt takes eight to ten hours to develop with yogurt culture, but only three to five hours using fresh yogurt from the last batch.

If you would like to try making yogurt without a specially designed yogurt maker, that is a relatively simple process also, though not as easily managed without the special equipment, of course. See Homemade Yogurt under Yogurt Recipes below.

FLAVORING YOGURT

Homemade yogurt is far superior in taste and texture to what you can buy. It is creamier, lighter, and not as tart. Even plain, the cool creamy taste is good. If using yogurt for health reasons, eat it first thing in the morning and a couple hours after dinner. It works best on an empty stomach.

There are also many healthy ways of flavoring yogurt, should you wish to do so. Add 1 tablespoon of one or more of the following to 8 ounces of fresh yogurt:

- Frozen juice concentrate—apple, orange, pineapple, or any other juice concentrate of your choice.

- Dietetic or all-fruit jam, preserves, or jelly.

- Juice nectar—pear, apricot, or peach.

- Molasses or pure maple syrup.

- Applesauce with a dash of cinnamon and raisins.

- Natural cereal.

- Honey with a teaspoon of vanilla.

- Barley malt sweetener (to taste).

YOGURT CHEESE

Yogurt "cheese" can replace high-fat ingredients such as cream cheese, mayonnaise, or sour cream. It is made by draining the whey (the liquid portion) from plain nonfat or low-fat yogurt. You can do this by simply putting it in a yogurt strainer, a drip coffee filter, or a cheesecloth-lined strainer positioned over a bowl. Leave the entire setup in the refrigerator for three and a half to twenty-four hours (the longer the time, the firmer the cheese). When it reaches the desired consistency, either use it or store it in an airtight container in the refrigerator.

YOGURT RECIPES

HOMEMADE YOGURT

This is a basic, old-fashioned recipe. Before you begin, you will need a good thermometer to maintain appropriate temperatures.

> 1 quart raw, skim, goat, cow, or 2 percent homogenized milk (use 1 cup of 2 percent to 3 cups of skim for a richer taste)
>
> 3–4 tablespoons noninstant, nonfat dried milk powder (optional; for a firmer texture)
>
> 4 tablespoons unflavored, unpasteurized yogurt from the previous batch of yogurt or 2–3 tablespoons of yogurt starter, as directed on the product label

1. Place the milk in a large, heavy saucepan.
2. If you are using the nonfat milk powder, in a small bowl, make a paste from a small amount of the milk and the milk powder. Add this back to the rest of the milk.
3. Heat the saucepan over low heat to scald the milk: Bring it *just* to the boiling point. It should be steaming with bubbles on top but *not* boiling.
4. Keep the milk at 140°F to 150°F for ten minutes to destroy any unwanted organisms in the milk. Remove from the heat and let it cool to 100°F, which will be warm to the touch.
5. Mix the yogurt or yogurt starter (the culture) into the milk. Make sure it is smooth and without lumps—do not beat it, but mix gently and thoroughly.
6. Pour the mixture into clean jars (scald them first by filling them with boiling water, then pouring out the water) and cover. Keep the jars at 110°F until the desired thickness is achieved, usually six to eight hours (keep in mind that it will thicken further in the refrigerator). If the yogurt is too hot or too cold, it will not develop. Some suggestions for places to keep yogurt at 110°F include:

   - In a heavy skillet with a few inches of water over a pilot light.
   - In a preheated oven at 110°F (use an oven thermometer for accuracy).
   - An electric frying pan with the water level as high as possible on the yogurt cups, kept on lowest heat.

   Test any of these locations with a thermometer before using them to make yogurt. Do not allow the yogurt to overincubate (continue at 110°F for too long) or the whey and the curd will separate, leaving a watery layer on top of a thick, solid layer of curds. Once this separation occurs, it cannot be reversed (although you can use the solid layer as yogurt cheese; see page 174).
7. When the yogurt is done, place it in the refrigerator. It will continue to thicken after it is refrigerated. Wait until it is thoroughly cooled before eating it. This usually takes at least two hours.

Variation: Add 1 tablespoon of unsweetened gelatin in place of dried milk powder for thicker yogurt and increased protein.

LOW-FAT MIRACLE SPREAD

Use this spread in place of butter or margarine in all recipes, or simply use it as a spread.

> 1 tub unsaturated unhydrogenated soft safflower margarine
> ½ cup unrefined canola oil
> ½ cup plain yogurt, preferably homemade

1. Blend all of the ingredients at low speed with a hand mixer or food processor until well mixed and creamy.
2. Spoon into a tub and refrigerate.

YOGURT DRESSING

The dressing is good as a nacho dip.

> ½ cup soy or eggless mayonnaise
> ½ cup plain yogurt, preferably homemade
> 1 finely mashed garlic clove
> 1 tablespoon chili sauce or hot sauce
> Barley malt sweetener to taste
> Lemon juice or vinegar to taste

Place all of the ingredients in a medium-sized bowl and mix together well. As a dressing, it can be used immediately. To use as a dip, chill for at least one hour first.

YOGURT AVOCADO DRESSING

This dressing is good for people with low blood sugar.

> 1 cup plain yogurt, preferably homemade
> ½ teaspoon finely mashed garlic clove or 1 dash garlic powder
> 1 mashed avocado
> 1 teaspoon fresh lemon juice
> 1 dash of sea salt (optional)

Place all of the ingredients in a small bowl and beat until thick. Serve it over crisp lettuce or use it as a dip. It's also good on baked potatoes.

YOGURT CREAM CHEESE

This is a tasty low-fat substitute for cream cheese and sour cream.

> 1 quart homemade nonfat plain yogurt

1. Line a strainer with three layers of cheesecloth and fill with the yogurt.
2. Place the strainer in a bowl in the refrigerator to drain overnight. A creamy textured cheese that can be used as cream cheese will be ready the next morning.

Variation: Add a packet of organic dry onion soup mix to make a dip or a topping for baked potatoes. Or make a spread by mixing this creamy cheese with any type of fruit, chopped nuts, raisins, or herbs of your choice.

COLD CUCUMBER SOUP

This soup can also be used as a salad dressing.

> 32 ounces plain yogurt, preferably homemade
> 10 ounces cold quality water (you can use less or omit for a thicker consistency)
> 2 large diced cucumbers (peel if waxed or not organic)
> ½ cup chopped parsley
> 2 garlic cloves finely chopped
> ½ teaspoon sea salt (optional)

Place all of the ingredients in a large bowl and mix together well. Chill. Serve cool or cold.

THE STOPPER

This recipe is good for relieving diarrhea in infants and adults.

> 3 bananas
> 1 pint plain yogurt, preferably homemade
> 1 tablespoon ground flaxseeds, cooked rice,
>   or oat bran

1. Purée the bananas in a blender.
2. Add the yogurt and flaxseeds, rice, or oat bran and mix on low speed to blend.

Variation: Use puréed carrots in place of the bananas.

DILL YOGURT CREAM SAUCE

Use this sauce over tofu patties, fish, sliced cucumber or tomato, green vegetable salads, and boiled whole new potatoes. It's great on potato skins, too.

> 3 cups plain yogurt, preferably homemade
> 6 scallions, finely chopped
> 1 bunch finely chopped fresh dill or 2 tablespoons
>   dried dill
> ¼ cup apple cider vinegar
> ½ teaspoon horseradish powder or 1 tablespoon
>   grated fresh horseradish
> 2 teaspoons sea salt (optional)
> 1 dash cayenne pepper (optional)

Place all of the ingredients in a medium-sized bowl and mix together well. Store in the refrigerator in a jar with a tight-fitting lid.

CHAPTER TWENTY-THREE

SPROUTS: THE NUTRITIOUS GARDEN ANYONE CAN GROW

Don't judge each day by the harvest you reap, but by the seeds you plant.

—*Robert Louis Stevenson, nineteenth-century British writer*

Sprouts are edible seeds that have just germinated. Chinese nobles ate sprouted seeds for healing and rejuvenation more than 5,000 years ago. Captain Cook sailed the seas for a decade without losing one shipmate to scurvy (which was common in those times) because of a daily ration of malt made from sprouted beans. Sprouts, a virtual explosion of life, should be an important part of the diet. They supply fresh greens year-round when grocery bins are filled with vegetables from faraway places that may have been chemically treated or irradiated to retain freshness and appearance. There is nothing simpler to grow than a sprout. This chapter will open your eyes to the many varieties of sprouts available, as well as to necessary precautions to keep them free from bacteria and mold.

Sprouts have, pound for pound, the largest amount of nutrients of any food. Sprouting increases the vitamin content of seeds significantly. The vitamin C value of wheatgrass is 600 percent in the early sprouting phase and all sprouts contain more vitamin C than oranges by weight. Sprouts are also a tremendous source of antioxidants, vitamin A, B vitamins, vitamin E, calcium, potassium, magnesium, iron, selenium, and zinc. The sprouted seeds of some legumes, like lentils, peanuts, and soybeans, contain complete protein, as do many seeds.

All seeds contain enzyme inhibitors that allow them to remain dormant and be stored for years. Once exposed to moisture and temperature, the enzyme inhibitors are neutralized and the seeds come to life. In this embryonic stage, sprouts are bursting with nutrients. They are essentially a predigested food.

Most types of seeds can be sprouted, but the most popular and commonly available are grain, nut, and legume seeds. Eating sprouts is a good way to supplement your diet with food enzymes that are critical for literally every biochemical reaction that takes place in the body. Incorporating sprouts into your diet may significantly enhance your health, energy, and longevity. Sprouts are filling and are low in calories. They make interesting edible garnishes and condiments.

Typically, sprouts are added to salads and sandwiches, but with a little imagination, you can incorporate them into just about any dish. A variety of sprouts can be mixed together to make a complete salad. A plate layered with sprouts makes an attractive base for serving salads and hot dishes alike.

Sprouts fall into two categories: those made from seeds that produce chlorophyll and develop a green leaf and those that do not. Chlorophyll-producing sprouts include radish, cabbage, fenugreek, mustard, broccoli, cress, and other vegetable sprouts. These sprouts are generally consumed raw on sandwiches and in salads. Broccoli sprouts may be the number-one beneficial sprouts. They contain more nutrients than broccoli florets.

Legume and grain seeds do not develop a leaf when sprouted. Legume seeds contain natural toxins that serve as a defensive measure, which aids the immune system. Large legume seeds, such as garbanzo, kidney bean, mung bean, and soybean sprouts, should be lightly cooked prior to serving to destroy natural toxins and facilitate ease of digestion. Smaller legumes, such as alfalfa and adzuki bean, do not lend themselves well to cooking and so should not be consumed raw in large quantities on a regular basis.

The best way to get super-fresh, wholesome sprouts is to grow them at home. Supermarket and salad bar sprouts may contain mold or be contaminated in other ways, or simply may not be fresh. Sprouts should be eaten fresh and kept for only two or three days in the refrigerator. It's easy as well as fun to grow sprouts, and the satisfaction of getting first-quality, organic produce is greatly rewarding. As with all living food, organic is always best. Whatever the source of sprouts, they should be well rinsed before you consume them.

Precautions for Safe Sprouting

A large number of outbreaks of foodborne illness in the 1990s that were associated with sprouts prompted the United States Food and Drug Administration (FDA) to issue guidance documents geared to enhance their safety. The conditions under which sprouts are produced commercially are ideal for the rapid growth of bacteria, and if pathogens are present on or in the seeds being sprouted, these conditions are likely to encourage bacterial proliferation. The FDA now closely monitors the safety of sprouts and the adoption of prevention practices recommended in the guidance documents, and considers enforcement actions against producers who do not have preventive controls in place. Home-grown sprouts also can contain mold and bacteria. Cooking sprouts significantly reduces the risk of problems. Children, older adults, and people with weakened immune systems have a higher than normal risk of developing serious illness due to foodborne disease and may wish to request that raw sprouts not be included in their food in restaurants, and may prefer to eat sprouts only if they have been cooked. All sprouts should be rinsed thoroughly before they are cooked or eaten. Cooking sprouts is the preferred method.

BUYING AND STORING SPROUTS

Most grocery stores carry packaged alfalfa and loose mung beans, while farmer's markets, health food stores, and gourmet shops may offer a few of the more unusual sprouts, such as radish, sunflower, and clover. Fresh sprouts have a wonderful, clean aroma. When purchasing sprouts, look for firm, crisp stalks with intensely green leaves. As sprouts age, their tops lose their rich color and sometimes darken. Examine the roots, as they show the first signs of aging. If they are brown or dry, do not purchase them. Mung bean sprouts should be plump, with the husks still attached and not too long (over three inches), since this is a sign of age. The smaller sprouts are more crisp and tender. Many Asian markets display mung bean sprouts in water-filled containers.

Sprouts should be stored in the refrigerator in a glass jar or rigid plastic container. Plastic bags will suffocate the plant, which is still living. Sprouts purchased in aerated plastic boxes can be stored in their original containers. For homegrown sprouts, place the sprout basket directly in the refrigerator with its top on, which will ensure that the sprouts remain sufficiently humid. Frost-free refrigerators tend to be very dry, so it may be necessary to mist sprouts with a pump spray or plant mister to keep them moist. Sprouts should not be stored for more than three to five days, depending upon the hardiness of the variety. While delicate in appearance, alfalfa, fenugreek, turnip, and mustard are the most vigorous.

Sprouts purchased loose, such as mung bean, should be soaked before using. Wilted sprouts can be revived by soaking in cold water for ten minutes. Gently swirl sprouts in a basin of cold water, skimming any hulls off the top using a tea strainer. Remove them from the water and pat them dry with paper towels before using them. Canned mung beans should be rinsed to remove excess sodium. Soaking canned mung beans in cold water will brighten their flavor and restore their crisp texture.

GROWING YOUR OWN SPROUTS

Many more varieties of sprouts can be grown at home than can be purchased from retailers. Growing sprouts at home is always preferable to purchasing them, as the risk of mold or contamination is much lower. It is easy to do.

Supplies to Get Started

A green thumb isn't necessary to grow these delicious greens at home. The following are a number of basic approaches to sprouting:

- A large, wide-mouthed jar works well for most bean seeds and smaller seeds, such as radish, cabbage, and alfalfa. The mouth of the jar can be covered with a fine mesh screen or piece of cheesecloth held in place with a strong rubber band. Some varieties of seeds, especially the taller sprouts such as sunflower, require more room than a jar offers to achieve uniform growth. Another drawback of the jar method is that the draining and air circulation are poor, and that can result in mold if not done properly. Sprouts in a jar must be rinsed daily—do not let them dry out, as this will prevent sprouting. After rinsing the sprouts, place the jar upside down on a drain board until the next rinsing. Rinsing once daily is sufficient.

- A basket-type sprouter allows the sprouts to obtain their full height and produces uniform growth among sprouts. Basket sprouters are often referred to as vertical sprouters. In general, the yield of sprouts is higher with this method. An unvarnished bamboo basket with a small, tight weave can be fashioned into an efficient sprouter. Depending on the circumference of the basket and the size of the seeds, you can sprout up to 6 to 7 tablespoons of seed in a basket. You will need to create a "greenhouse tent" over the homemade basket. This can easily be accomplished by placing a document-sized locking plastic bag over the basket during the growth stage of the sprouts. The "greenhouse tent" will keep the sprouts moist and prevent them from drying out. You should also elevate the basket using small wooden dowels to accommodate airflow under the basket.

- A colander can be used to make sprouts—just make sure the grid is small enough so that the seeds won't fall through. Purchase a colander made of a natural material or plastic. Do not use an aluminum colander, since the relationship between Alzheimer's disease and aluminum deposits in the brain is well documented.

- Vegetable sprouting kits can be purchased from most health food stores or from companies that specialize in seeds and sprouting equipment. (See the Resources section for some recommended sources.) Most seeds can be sprouted using a vertical sprouter. Larger seeds, such as buckwheat and sunflower, tend to perform better in a basket with a larger weave.

- Sprout bags made from natural fibers of the flax plant are the easiest to use and work well for bean and grain seeds. They are not suitable for sprouts that develop chlorophyll, since they don't permit sufficient light into the bag.

Ready, Set, SPROUT

Whichever type of system you use, the procedure for growing sprouts is essentially the same. If you are growing sprouts in a jar, use 2 tablespoons of seed. An eight-inch basket type sprouter will accommodate 5 tablespoons of seed, while a bag can sprout up to 2 cups of seeds. First, rinse the seeds. Most seeds (except for chia, alfalfa, cress, oat, or mustard seeds) should then be soaked by placing them in a quart jar and covering them with several inches of cold water. Most seeds require soaking overnight, but smaller seeds require only a few hours of soaking. For an additional nutritional boost, add a few drops of liquid kelp or two leaves of dry or fresh kelp to the water during soaking. The seeds will absorb the nutrients in the kelp. If you are using dry or fresh kelp, be sure to remove it after soaking and before sprouting.

After the seeds have been soaked, drain the water, rinse the seeds in fresh water, drain the seeds again, and then place them in whatever vessel you will be using to sprout them. The sprouting bag or basket should be moistened before you add the seeds. Handle sprouters "gently." Rapid movement may cause awkward shifting of sprouting seeds, breaking the tender shoots and causing spoilage.

From this point on, it is very important that the seeds remain moist. If they dry out, they may still sprout, but they will not develop to their full potential. Gently rinse and drain the seeds twice a day. Use either distilled water with trace minerals added or a good quality filtered water, since the sprouts will absorb the water. (The rinse water contains nutrients—save it and use it to water houseplants or use it in soup stock.)

As the seeds begin to germinate, soak them in cold water to remove the hulls. Using a tea strainer, skim hulls off the water as they float to the top. This will help to prevent premature spoilage. The germination stage is critical to the development of sprouts. In nature, Mother Earth keeps the seeds warm and moist. Light isn't necessary for germination, but the seeds must be kept warm and moist or they will be ruined.

If you are using a jar, cover it with a towel and place it near a sunny window, on a seventy-degree angle or thereabouts. If you are using the basket method, go ahead and place the "greenhouse tent" over the basket at this stage. A bag sprouter can be dipped in a basin of warm quality water then hung on a hook to drain.

Once the seeds have germinated, place chlorophyll-forming sprouts in a sunny window. Since grain and bean seeds do not produce chlorophyll, it isn't necessary to place them in a window. Continue to rinse the sprouts twice daily until they reach maturity.

However you decide to make your sprouts, the following tips will ensure the healthiest, freshest sprouts possible:

- Purchase only high-quality, organic seeds that have not been treated with pesticides or other chemicals.

- Grain seeds such as quinoa, barley, millet, and oats must be obtained from farm seed companies in their unhusked, whole-seed form. Grain sprouts will turn an ordinary loaf of bread into a hearty, full-bodied loaf of bread.

- Use only quality water for soaking and rinsing seeds— either distilled water with trace minerals added or a good quality filtered water.

- Wire-mesh screening is best for draining small seeds. Switch to screening with larger openings for better drainage of bigger sprouts.

- If you are using a jar, a piece of cheesecloth secured with a rubber band around the top can be used in place of a lid if a lid is not available. Do not use a lid that is not intended for sprouting, because sprouts need air.

For specifics on growing specific types of sprouts, see Table 23.1 on page 180.

TYPES OF SPROUTS

Adzuki Sprouts

Adzuki beans are a smaller cousin of Chinese mung beans. The small lentil-shaped bean produces a thin feathery sprout that has a full, rich flavor. They add texture and flavor to salads and sandwiches or can be added to stir-fry dishes. When cooking adzuki sprouts, leave them in the pan just long enough to warm them, as they can get mushy very quickly. Eating adzuki sprouts can help to control blood sugar levels. Adzuki beans sprout in five to seven days.

Alfalfa Sprouts

Alfalfa is probably the most well-known sprout. The word *alfalfa* is derived from Arabic and, roughly translated, means "father of all foods." Alfalfa's list of therapeutic values is noteworthy. It has been used as a remedy for arthritis, diabetes, ulcers, and high cholesterol, and contains estrogenlike compounds that can reduce the risk of breast

TABLE 23.1 SPROUTING TIMES

The following table will help you to become familiar with the different seeds and their sprouting times.

SEED	AMOUNT OF SEEDS	SPROUTING TIME	NUMBER OF RINSES	MATURE HEIGHT	YIELD
Adzuki beans	½ cup	6 days	4	1 inch	2 cups
Alfalfa (for salads)	2 tablespoons	4 days	2	1–2 inches	1 quart
Alfalfa (for baking)	¼ cup	2 hours	2	⅛ inch	1½ cups
Beans (kidney, lima, fava, green, and pinto)	1 cup	6 days	4	2 inches	4 cups
Chia	2 tablespoons	4 days	1	1½ inches	3 cups
Cress	1 tablespoons	4 days	2	1½ inches	1½ cups
Fenugreek	¼ cup	5 days	2	3 inches	4 cups
Garbanzo beans (chickpeas)	1 cup	4 days	5	½–1 inch	3 cups
Guar beans (soak for 36 hours before sprouting)	1 cup	5 days	4	2–3 inches	4 cups
Lentils	1 cup	4 days	2	1 inch	6 cups
Millet	1 cup	3 days	3	¼ inch	2 cups
Mung beans	1 cup	4 days	4	2–3 inches	4 cups
Peas	1½ cups	4 days	2	½–1 inch	4 cups
Radish	1 tablespoon	5 days	2	½–1 inch	2 cups
Red clover	3 tablespoons	5 days	2	½ inch	1 quart
Soybeans	1 cup	5 days	8	½–¾ inch	5 cups
Sunflower	1 cup	2 days	10	½ inch	3 cups
Wheat	1 cup	4 days	3	½ inch	4 cups

cancer. The sprouts are rich in chlorophyll, magnesium, manganese, and protein. They have a full-flavored, nutty taste, and are best consumed raw. Alfalfa sprouts within four to seven days. The seed jackets tend to cling to the sprouts but they can be rinsed to remove most of the hulls. They are sensitive to heat and direct light, so sprout them in a cool, shady area with indirect light.

Buckwheat Sprouts

Buckwheat is not a true grain but an herb. The sprouts have the largest leaf of any sprout and the seed is hard and must be removed before eating. The seeds mature in about nine to ten days. Around day six, immerse the entire sprouting basket into a basin of room-temperature water. Gently swishing the basket around will cause many of the seed hulls to fall off. Shake off excess water and allow them to continue to sprout for a few more days. Harvest them when 80 to 90 percent of the hulls have fallen off. The remaining hulls will have to be removed by hand, but it's worth the extra work. Buckwheat sprouts are long and slender, with a crunchy texture and a mild flavor that is similar to Bibb or Boston lettuce. They are loaded with B vitamins, magnesium, and phosphorus. They are very easy to digest and aid in metabolizing fats.

Cabbage Sprouts

Cabbage sprouts have a robust, peppery flavor similar to that of the mature vegetable. The thin, grasslike sprouts

have a small green leaf at the top. Be sure to rinse them twice a day to prevent the seed jackets from developing mold. The seeds of kale, rutabaga, turnip, and black mustard, also members of the cabbage family, produce sprouts that are similar in flavor and texture.

Chia, Cress, Flaxseed, and Psyllium Seed Sprouts

Chia, cress, flax, and psyllium are considered gelatinous seeds. They are extremely nutritious but require a little extra effort to sprout because of their mucilaginous nature. Integrating them in a basket with other seeds, such as alfalfa, kale, and clover, is the easiest way to enjoy these unique sprouts. Other sprouting methods involve using clay sprouters or sprouting on top of a bag or an inverted basket. With lots of bright-green leaves, they are visually appealing and dress up any salad. Their mucilage content helps to cleanse the intestinal tract and promote bowel health. Flaxseed sprouts should be harvested when they reach about one-quarter inch in height, since allowing them to grow too long will result in a very bitter and unpalatable sprout. Chia and cress sprouts are very spicy, while psyllium has a nutty flavor. Gelatinous seeds only require one hour of soaking time.

China Red Pea Sprouts

China red pea is a mild-flavored sprout with a chewy texture. The sprouts can reach five to eight inches in height and are topped with large, beautiful green leaves that have

Our Fine Feathered Friends Love Sprouts!

"Sprouted seeds, grains, and legumes can enhance a bird's diet by adding a nutritious supply of vitamins, minerals, enzymes, chlorophyll, and high quality protein," according to Alicia McWatters, Ph.D., CNC. Owners know that pet birds need greens for a healthy diet, but many birds resist eating them. Most will eagerly devour sprouts, though, if given the chance. The Sproutpeople have organic sprouting mixes combined especially for birds. When making sprouts for birds, it is important to be extremely scrupulous about cleanliness and avoid even the slightest chance of bacterial contamination, since birds are extremely sensitive to bacterial disease.

a flavor similar to buckwheat lettuce. The stalks are high in fiber. The germination rate is about 99 percent, and they reach maturity within seven to ten days. Frequent rinsing will wash away the hulls, which are prone to decay.

Clover Sprouts

Clover is related to alfalfa and the much-sought-after four-leaf clover. There are many types of clover, but the most commonly available are red and crimson. Clover seeds are small, hard seeds that easily sprout and mature within six days. Like alfalfa, they are sensitive to heat. They have a pungent taste and a delicate threadlike texture. Crimson clover has a large leaf and readily sheds its hull. Clover sprouts contain an abundant supply of easily absorbable calcium and magnesium. Clover can tone and relax the nervous system and work as an antispasmodic. These sprouts also help detoxify the body and purify the blood.

Fennel Sprouts

Fennel seeds sprout within two to three days but it takes from ten to fourteen days to reach maturity. It's well worth the wait. Fennel's sweet, warm flavor enhances breads, salads, or grain dishes. The sprouts are very strong and aromatic, and a little goes a long way. Fennel sprouts are very easy to digest, and the seeds, as well as the sprouts, can be eaten.

Fenugreek Sprouts

Fenugreek is an aromatic sprout with a unique flavor that is similar to celery, yet bitter. It is best to mix fenugreek sprouts with other sprouts such as alfalfa. The stem of the sprout is green and about four inches long, with a rich emerald-green, oval leaf. Fenugreek sprouts are a rich source of vitamin A and iron. They aid digestion and lower blood sugar.

Lentil Sprouts

Lentils are medium-sized legumes and sprout within four to five days. The mature sprout will have a one- to two-inch tail with a "bean" on top. They have a fresh, mild flavor and crisp texture. Lentil sprouts are rich in potassium, silicon, and phosphorous, and trace elements important to optimum health.

Mung Bean Sprouts

Mung bean sprouts are a staple in Asian cuisine and are commonly found at salad bars. Mung bean sprouts are fairly large, with a crisp, crunchy texture. Their mild flavor lends itself to a variety of uses, including soups and casseroles. The hulls should be removed prior to eating by soaking in a basin of room temperature quality water; the hulls will float to the surface where they can be skimmed off the top. Home-sprouted mung beans look different from the plump, white stalks on the commercial market. Commercial growers achieve this effect by applying ethylene gas, a naturally occurring plant hormone that hastens ripening. To approximate this effect, place sprouts in a bag with a green banana and allow the banana to turn yellow. As the banana ripens, it will emit ethylene gas that will enhance the size and color of the mung bean sprouts.

Onion and Garlic Sprouts

Onion and garlic seeds can be sprouted, and, just like the bulbs, they have powerful healing qualities. The sprouts are chock-full of vitamins, minerals, and enzymes necessary for cellular growth. They take about two weeks to sprout, but it is well worth the wait. They have a pungent, flavorful taste and make a great addition to salads or homemade dressings. Garlic and onion sprouts have a natural antibiotic effect on the body, making it more resistant to bacteria and parasites. They also act to purify the blood and cleanse the liver.

Radish Sprouts

Radish sprouts are slender and threadlike, with a fiery hot flavor similar that of to the vegetable but even spicier. It is best to mix radish sprouts with milder sprouts to tone down their heat. Radish seeds sprout easily within five days. The sprouts develop tiny hairs called cilia, which are often confused with mold. The cilia are formed to seek water, so they are an indication that the sprouts need more vigorous rinsing. There are several varieties of radish that can be sprouted, including daikon, which is sometimes marketed as *kaiware*. China rose radish sprouts, which have brilliant leaves with reddish stalks, make a stunning presentation on a salad. Radish sprouts can help clear the sinuses and ease respiratory problems.

Soybean Sprouts

Soybean sprouts have a strong flavor and a firm, crunchy texture. They should be lightly cooked for ease of digestion and to eliminate natural toxins. They are a terrific source of protein, second only to alfalfa. Eating the sprouts can help to lower cholesterol and regulate blood sugar levels.

Sunflower Sprouts

Sunflowers are among the most familiar garden plants, and throughout history, they have been used for medicinal purposes. Literally every part of the plant has some therapeutic use. Often referred to as the king of sprouts, sunflower sprouts can reach six or seven inches in height and have large, succulent leaves. They contain more protein per serving than spinach! They also contain ample supplies of iron that promote healthy blood cells and calcium necessary for the development and maintenance of healthy teeth and bones. They are one of the only plant sources of vitamin D, which is necessary for controlling the metabolism of calcium and phosphorus in bone building and tooth formation. It is also valuable in treating heart conditions. Their robust, almost meaty flavor and crisp texture make them versatile enough for salads as well as for cooked dishes. The seeds germinate easily and mature within ten days. Just like the gigantic sunflower plant that follows the sun's progression from east to west, the sprouts require plenty of sunlight to sprout. They also require lots of water. The black oil sprouting variety has the best germination rate and the hulls fall off naturally.

Wheatgrass

Wheatgrass is one of the most highly nutritious foods on the planet and is easy to grow. Fill a large tray (like the type used for bedding plants) with soil and plant the seeds. Cover the tray with plastic and place it on a windowsill until the first sign of green appears. Then remove the plastic, water as needed, and watch the fresh greens grow. Wheatgrass juice is used throughout the world for healing many diseases, is an excellent tonic, and is good for all intestinal disorders. Be sure to watch for signs of mold; if it appears, cut back on watering and rinse the sprouts well before using them.

SERVING SPROUTS

Sprouts can be cooked or served raw as a plain vegetable. Use sprouts with the seeds (but not the hulls) attached. If you cook sprouts, take care not to overcook them, as this will destroy their crispness. Cook them just long enough to remove the raw flavor. All sprouts (with the exception of alfalfa) are appetizing when cooked.

To sauté sprouts, place a small amount of oil in a pan and add the sprouts plus a small amount of water or tamari sauce. Cover the pan and cook for ten minutes (some people prefer to cook sprouts for only five to eight minutes). Minced onion or mushrooms browned in the oil add flavor, as do shredded carrots, turnips, and cabbage.

You can also steam sprouts or brown them in a small amount of oil.

Cooked sprouts can be added to any vegetable combination for casserole dishes and are popular in stir-fried vegetables. They are a great addition to dress up plain salads and scrambled eggs or omelets. Add them to potato salad or rice, use them in sandwich spreads, or mix them with soft cheese for dips.

SPROUT RECIPES

SPROUT SALAD

This salad is high in all nutrients and is especially good for people with cancer, arthritis, and colon disorders. (If you have a colon disorder, be sure to chew the seeds well.)

> 1 pound mixed bean sprouts and alfalfa sprouts, rinsed thoroughly
> 1 apple or onion, chopped
> 1 stalk celery, chopped
> 1 cup shredded carrots
> 1 cup shredded turnip
> 1 cup shredded red cabbage
> ½ cucumber, chopped
> ½ cup raisins
> ½ cup sesame or sunflower seeds

1. Place all of the ingredients in a medium-sized bowl.
2. Toss lightly with Good Things House Dressing (below) or any other dressing of your choice, and serve.

GOOD THINGS HOUSE DRESSING

This is an all-purpose dressing that supplies unsaturated fatty acids. Lecithin is a wonderful brain food that is high in choline, inositol, and B vitamins. It is an emulsifier that holds water and oil in suspension so they will not separate.

> 3 cups apple cider or balsamic vinegar
> 1 cup honey or 2 teaspoons barley malt sweetener
> 1 cup water
> 3 packages Hain's dry Italian dressing mix or 6 tablespoons dry Italian seasonings
> 3 tablespoons minced dried onions
> 2 tablespoons dried parsley
> ½ teaspoon powdered garlic or granules
> 1 tablespoon liquid lecithin
> 11 cups expeller-pressed pure virgin olive, canola, or other vegetable oil of your choice

1. Place all of the ingredients, except the oil, in a gallon jar. Shake well.

2. Fill the rest of the jar with oil (olive oil is the best for lowering cholesterol) and shake again. Store in the refrigerator and shake before each use.

AVOCADO DREAMING SANDWICH

This is a great-tasting sandwich that is easy to make.

   1 1-inch thick slice cream cheese or yogurt cheese (see pages 174–75)
   ½ avocado

   1 piece whole-grain pocket bread or regular whole-grain bread
   1 onion, sliced
   1 tomato, sliced
   1 handful alfalfa sprouts, rinsed thoroughly

1. Mash the cream cheese or yogurt cheese and the avocado together.
2. Spread the cheese mixture in pocket bread or on sliced bread. Top with the onion, tomato, and sprouts, and serve.

CHAPTER TWENTY-FOUR

SOY FOODS: A COMPLETE PROTEIN SOURCE

Nutritionally, the humble soybean is a 5-carat diamond in the rough.

—*Anonymous*

No other single food has as many uses or is as versatile as the common soybean. Soybeans are a complete protein source, and provide more protein than any other legume. Because of their bland flavor and high nutrient content, soybeans can be made into many different nutritious foods. As a whole, Americans have not acquired a taste for the naturally processed forms of soybeans found in the traditional Asian diet, such as tofu, miso, tempeh, tamari, and soymilk. However, the "next generation" of manufactured soy foods is increasingly popular. These are highly refined products such as soy ice cream, cheese, yogurt, oil, burgers, and frozen desserts. Commercial applications for soybeans range from soap to paint to earth-friendly printing ink.

Though the United States grows half of the world's soybeans (as a crop, soy is second in importance only to corn), most of them are ground into meal for animal feed or exported, particularly to Japan, where the soybean is a principal food. Soy protein has been used for decades as a meat extender. It also is added to numerous foods as a thickener and emulsifier. Textured vegetable protein, known as TVP, which is made from defatted soy flour, is used in simulated meat products, such as veggie burgers. TVP is the most concentrated source of soy protein, with as much as 23 grams per ounce. Several manufacturers, such as Lumen Foods (Heartline Meatless Meats), have a good textured protein product made entirely from soybeans. The meatlike texture works well in casseroles, stews, and soups.

ACTIONS AND USES OF SOY

Soybeans have been an important part of the Asian diet since ancient times. In China, this common legume is considered a sacred grain. The Chinese word for soybean means "greater bean." Today, scientists are learning through research what Asian populations have known for centuries: The ordinary soybean is a healing food.

Soybeans have the highest concentrations of protease inhibitors of any food. Proteases are protein-digesting enzymes whose secretion by tumor cells likely plays a role in the metastasis (spread) of some forms of cancer. Because protease inhibitors counteract these enzymes, consuming soybeans (and other types of beans) may help to fight cancer.

The American Heart Association recommends adding soy to the daily diet to reduce high cholesterol. Researchers in Finland reported in the *American Journal of Cardiology* that soybean extracts known as sterols lower cholesterol by limiting its absorption in the intestines. The cardiac benefits are so notable that the U.S. Food and Drug Administration (FDA) allows products containing at least 6.25 grams of soy protein per serving to carry this claim: "Diets low in saturated fat and cholesterol that include 25 grams of soy protein a day may reduce the risk of heart disease." A study reported in the *American Journal of Clinical Nutrition* reported that men who ate a low-fat diet and relied on soy as their main protein source for five weeks saw their levels of low-density lipoprotein (LDL, or "bad" cholesterol) decrease by as much as 14 percent and levels of high-density lipoprotein (HDL, or "good") cholesterol increase by as much as 8 percent. The FDA concluded, based on evidence from more than fifty studies, that ingesting 25 grams of soy protein a day can lower cholesterol by as much as 10 percent.

Lately, this miracle food has come under attack, and reports are confusing. The balance of research from health experts still supports soy as an important and beneficial food. Like any food, it should not be eaten in excess. Consuming large amounts of soy daily may lead to mineral deficiencies. It is also possible soy can depress thyroid function. However, it is safe to consume large amounts of fermented products such as tempeh and miso.

In addition to being low in saturated fat and containing high-quality protein; fiber; complex carbohydrates; vitamins; and minerals, such as calcium and iron, soybeans provide an abundance of phytochemicals. As you've learned, phytochemicals are naturally occurring compounds in plants that can have medicinal and disease-preventing properties.

One group of phytochemicals unique to soybeans is soy isoflavones. On the molecular level, they are similar to the female hormone estrogen, yet different enough to be called weak estrogens. They are also antioxidants. Genistein and daidzein are the two primary isoflavones in soybeans. Extensive studies have shown that these isoflavones can help to guard against various cancers, prevent bone loss, and lower cholesterol. Soy foods have varying concentrations of isoflavones depending on the amount of soy used to make them and how the beans were processed; some highly processed products do not contain nutritionally significant amounts. Traditional soy products—tofu, soymilk, tempeh, and miso—have ample amounts of isoflavones.

Genistein works against cancer by blocking blood vessels that supply blood to tumors. When cancer cells are deprived of nourishment, they cannot grow or spread. Isoflavones have been shown to check the growth of tumors by interfering with enzyme activity involved in breaking down male steroid hormones, such as testosterone. For women, isoflavones are antiestrogenic; by binding to estrogen receptors in the body, they block the body's own stronger estrogens from exerting stimulating effects on breast and uterine tissue. This can help to inhibit the development and spread of estrogen-related cancers.

SOYBEAN NUTRITION

The soybean is a self-contained protein factory. Through the action of bacteria living in its roots, the soy plant can make its own nitrogen fertilizer to stimulate protein production. Research conducted at the Massachusetts Institute of Technology has shown that the soybean produces such high-quality protein that it can supply the essential amino acids the body needs daily. Soybean protein is high in quantity, as well: one-half cup of cooked soybeans contains 14 grams of protein.

The nutrients in soybeans are fiber, protein, calcium, iron, magnesium, phosphorus, potassium, sodium, zinc, copper, manganese, vitamin C, vitamin B_1 (thiamine), vitamin B_2 (riboflavin), vitamin B_3 (niacin), pantothenic acid, vitamin B_6, folate, lipids, and amino acids. Phytochemicals include daidzein, genistein, glycitin, glycitein, ipriflavone, beta-sitosterol, gamma-sitosterol, stigmasterol, Bowman-Birk inhibitor, lignin, phenolic acids, phytic acids, saponins, lecithin, and protease inhibitors.

TYPES OF SOY FOODS

Whole Soybeans

Soybeans can be either green (fresh) or dry. Green soybeans are harvested just before maturity, when the beans are still green, and have a sweet flavor. Green soybeans can be enjoyed as a snack, served as a main vegetable dish, stir-fried, or added to soups and salads. They can be boiled in the pod (which is not eaten), or shelled. They are also sometimes called *edamame*.

The Humble Soybean Gets First Prize

In numerous studies, soybeans have exhibited the ability to do the following:

- Block enzymes that promote tumor growth.
- Protect cells from oxidative damage that can be a precursor to cancer and other diseases.
- Inhibit and suppress the growth of prostate, breast, lung, colon, and skin cancer cells.
- Help to lower cholesterol without affecting levels of "good" cholesterol, which is beneficial in preventing stroke and coronary artery disease.
- Reduce the loss of protein in the urine of persons suffering from nephritic syndrome, a kidney disorder.
- Aid in preventing heart attacks and strokes by maintaining clot-forming cells in a passive state.
- Regulate and stabilize estrogen levels, which helps to manage symptoms of menopause. (Genistein's behavior closely resembles that of estrogen in the human body. But because it is significantly weaker than human estrogen, it is not likely to be involved in estrogen-related cancer. Some researchers believe soy protein may become a widely accepted alternative to estrogen replacement therapy.)
- Help to retain bone mass, which guards against osteoporosis, by reducing excretion of calcium through the urinary tract.
- Boost the immune system.
- Reduce hypertension by interfering with the production of certain enzymes that elevate blood pressure.
- Improve digestive function by helping with the breakdown and absorption of fats, and by stimulating the growth of "friendly" bacteria in the intestinal tract.

Some Asian markets stock fresh green soybeans; however, they are most likely to be found in the frozen food section of natural foods stores. Refrigerate fresh soybeans and use them within two days. Frozen, they will keep for several months.

Dry soybeans, which are light tan, yellow, or black, are fully mature beans. They are hard and take the longest of the legumes to cook—at least three hours, even after being soaked overnight. Once cooked, they have a strong bean flavor. Use them in soups, stews, and casseroles. They can also be ground up and made into burgers and loaves.

Natural foods stores and supermarkets generally carry whole dry soybeans. They can be purchased prepackaged or in bulk. They have a long shelf life when kept in an airtight container.

Soymilk

Soymilk is the dissolved liquid pressed from whole soybeans that have been soaked, cooked, and ground. The creamy milk can serve the same purposes as cow's milk—but with added advantages. It is a boon for people who are lactose intolerant or allergic to cow's milk. You can buy soymilk in several flavors, including chocolate, carob, and vanilla, and in lower-fat versions. You also can make your own soymilk. Some brands of soymilk are fortified with calcium, vitamins, and minerals. They may also contain a natural sweetener, oil, and/or a thickener. Plain, regular soymilk by itself has a nutty flavor and is loaded with nutrients. Eight ounces has 10 grams of protein and 80 milligrams of calcium, plus iron, B vitamins, and complex carbohydrates. Street vendors in China and Japan sell soymilk made fresh daily. It is usually served sweetened as a beverage or flavored with soy sauce, onions, and vegetables as a savory soup.

Use soymilk straight as an invigorating drink; over hot or cold cereal; as the base for cream sauces, cream soups, and shakes; in pancake and waffle mixes; or as a substitute for condensed milk in custards and pies. Children over one year of age can enjoy homemade or manufactured soymilk. Commercial soymilk-based infant formulas are available for babies less than a year old.

Previously available only in health food stores and specialty food shops, soymilk now is sold in many supermarkets. You will find soymilk usually packaged in aseptic, or nonrefrigerated, containers in either 8-ounce or 1-quart sizes. Unopened, the package gives soymilk a long shelf life. Once opened, however, the soymilk must be refrigerated and used within five days. Some stores also sell refrigerated soymilk in plastic containers. You also can buy powdered soymilk and mix it with water. Refrigerate both the mixture and the soymilk powder. The powder can be stored in the freezer, too.

Tofu

Also known as soybean curd, tofu is becoming a popular staple in this country. This completely flavorless, cheese-

---

Make Your Own Soymilk

Fresh soymilk can be made at home with a specially designed appliance such as the Miracle Exclusives' Miracle Soy Wonder Soy Milk Maker. Two quarts of milk from soaked soybeans is ready in a little over twenty minutes. The machine cooks and grinds the beans and makes a nutritious drink. If you drink a lot of soymilk, making it yourself is quite economical, as each batch will cost only a fraction of the price of packaged soymilk.

---

like food is made by adding a coagulant to fresh, hot soymilk, which curdles the liquid. The curd then is formed into cubes. Typically, the curdling ingredient is either nigari, a substance found in sea salt, or calcium sulfate, a natural mineral. Tofu made with calcium sulfate is exceptionally high in calcium, with as much as 130 milligrams in a 4-ounce serving. Acidic foods such as lemon juice or vinegar also can create curds.

Tofu is a significant source of protein, and it has ample amounts of B vitamins, potassium, and iron. It is cholesterol-free and low in calories, carbohydrates, saturated fat, and sodium. And it is easily chewed and digested. Tofu makes an excellent food for vegetarians, infants, growing children, older adults, people on sodium-restricted diets, and anyone with a sensitive stomach.

Tofu's blandness is also its greatest asset. In recipes, it can become whatever flavor you want. Add it to chili and it tastes like chili; mix it with cocoa and a sweetener and it doubles for chocolate pudding or pie filling. No other food can substitute as tofu can for mayonnaise, sour cream, cream cheese, dips, low-calorie dressings, meat, eggs, cheese, sandwich spreads, and much more. Tofutti Better Than Cream Cheese is a great nondairy product for vegetarians and lactose-intolerant people. And tofu can be sautéed, stir-fried, grilled, or baked. You can even make tofu desserts including cream pies, puddings, shakes, and cheesecake. This food is so healthful and its potential uses so numerous that an entire chapter of the book is devoted to it. (See Chapter 25.)

Miso

Miso (pronounced mee-so) is produced when soybeans and a grain, usually rice or barley, are combined with salt and a mold culture, then fermented in wooden vats for up to three years. The resulting paste, which is rich in B vitamins and protein, is an essential condiment in Japan and China. Rather than starting their day with coffee, most Japanese get a nutritional boost from a cup of hot miso soup. Miso can be used to season and enrich all types of soups and stews, whether clear or creamed. It also can add nutrition and flavor to sauces, gravies, salad dressings, dips, sandwich spreads, casseroles, and vegetables. You can even marinate tofu in miso.

Unpasteurized miso contains live cultures and has abundant lactic-acid-forming bacteria, protein, and enzymes that aid digestion. Also, the antioxidants in fermented soy foods—such as miso—are more easily absorbed than those in unfermented soybeans and soy products.

To get miso's health benefits and full flavor, buy the unpasteurized kind packaged in either plastic tubs or in plastic bags sold in the refrigerated sections of health food stores. Miso found on the dry-goods shelves is pasteurized and, therefore, lacks the health-promoting live cultures found in unpasteurized miso.

The addition of other ingredients and variations in the length of aging produce types of miso that differ in color, flavor, and texture. *Mugi* is the most popular for seasoning. It is made from fermented barley, soybeans, and sea salt. *Hatcho* is made only with soybeans and sea salt and has a stronger flavor. *Kome,* the mildest miso, is made from a fermented sweet brown rice, soybeans, and sea salt. *Genmai* miso is made from soybeans and the husked grains of roasted brown rice.

Unpasteurized, naturally aged miso should be stored in the refrigerator in a glass jar or ceramic crock. Like fine wine, miso gets better with age and, kept cold, will be good for several years. Should a white mold appear on the miso's surface, simply scrape it off. As the mold is harmless, you can even add it back into the miso.

When using miso, do not boil it, but add it at the end of cooking to preserve all its enzymes and nutrients. Use miso sparingly, as it is very salty.

Tempeh

Tempeh (pronounced TEM-pay) originated in Indonesia, where it is a staple food, eaten with rice as a main meal or alone as a snack. To make tempeh, whole, cooked soybeans are blended with rice or grains. This mixture is then injected with a culture and fermented for twenty-four hours to form a dense, chewy cake. Tempeh is much higher in fiber than most other soy-based products because it is made from the whole bean. It also is high in protein. Like tofu, it picks up the flavors of whatever it is seasoned or cooked with. However, it does have a flavor of its own, which is nutty and reminiscent of mushrooms.

Tempeh is available in the refrigerated section of natural foods stores. It should be firm to the touch and have "veins," a grayish-white, threadlike substance resulting from fermentation that binds the tempeh into firm cakes. Black patches on the tempeh do not mean it is spoiled, just that the good bacteria are still at work. Trim this part off before cooking. Tempeh should be kept refrigerated. It will stay fresh for about ten days and can also be frozen.

Use tempeh to make fillings for potpies, steamed buns, or squashes; add it to soups, stews, chili, tacos, casseroles, and stir-fry dishes; or in recipes that call for meat or poultry. For best results, steam, simmer, or brown tempeh before adding it to a dish.

TABLE 24.1 FOOD PRODUCTS FROM SOYBEANS

The following table gives a quick reference to the many and varied soy foods available.

Miso	Soybeans fermented into a paste. It has a meaty taste, excellent for seasonings or as a soup base.
Natto	A bacterially fermented soybean.
Soy flour	Soybeans ground into flour. Substitute part of the wheat flour in a recipe with soy flour to increase protein content.
Soy grits	The oil is extracted from the soybeans; the residue is coarsely ground.
Soy oil	The oil is extracted from the bean.
Soymilk	A liquid extracted from the soybean that is meant to be used in place of milk.
Tamari	Naturally aged and fermented soy sauce.
Tempeh	A mold-fermented soy patty.
Tofu	Curdled soymilk, using a mineral coagulant, and pressed into a cake.

Soy Oil

Milling the soybean into meal for animal food produces soy oil, an important but little known ingredient in our diet. Most likely when a product label says simply "vegetable oil," it really contains soy oil. Most commercially sold baked, fried, frozen, canned, imitation dairy, and processed meat foods contain soy oil. Free of cholesterol and saturated fat, soy oil is a good source of healthy omega-3 fatty acids, which are believed to help prevent heart disease. Use soy oil in recipes as a substitute for other types of vegetable oil. The high smoking point of soy oil means that foods may be fried at high temperatures virtually smoke-free. Other soy oil byproducts include lecithin, which helps to keep mixed foods blended; vitamin E, used to make supplements; and sterols, which pharmaceutical companies use to make supplemental sex hormones.

Tamari Sauce

The naturally fermented, dark-brown liquid called tamari or shoyu is true soy sauce. Tamari is made by mixing cooked soybeans with a grain and a mold, then allowing the mixture to ferment in salty brine from twelve to eighteen months.

You will find natural shoyu or tamari in Asian markets and health food stores, packaged in glass containers. Use tamari as you would soy sauce in rice and vegetable dishes, soups, casseroles, marinades, and stir-fries. Do not boil tamari sauce—add it at the end of cooking to preserve all its enzymes and nutrients. A little bit goes a long way, as it is salty and very high in sodium.

Other Soy Foods

In addition to the major soy foods described above, there are a number of lesser known ones. These include the following:

- Natto. Made from fermented, cooked whole soybeans that are mixed with a bacteria culture and aged in plastic bags, natto can be used over rice, in miso soups, and with vegetables.

- Soy cheese. Made from soymilk, it has a creamy texture and can be substituted for dairy sour cream or cheese.

- Soy fiber. Okara, soy bran, and soy isolate are generous sources of high-quality dietary fiber. The pulp left when the liquid is pressed from the soybean, okara has a coconut flavor that works well in granola and cookies. Soy bran is the fibrous material extracted from soybean hulls. It is used as a food ingredient. Soy isolate is concentrated soy protein in fiber form.

- Roasted soy nuts and soy-nut butter. Similar to peanuts, soy nuts are sold as a crunchy snack food. They are made from roasted whole soybeans. Soy-nut butter, an alternative for those allergic to peanuts, is produced by crushing soy nuts and blending them with soy oil. Soy Wonder makes a delicious nut spread.

- Soy mayonnaise. With 70 percent fewer calories than regular mayonnaise, this is good on sandwiches, on veggie burgers, or as a base for a dip. Nayonaise, made by Nasoya, is one brand of soy mayonnaise.

SOY RECIPES

SOY BURGERS

These burgers are healthy and taste great!

> 1 cup cooked, mashed soy beans
> 1 cup uncooked oats
> 1 cup shredded carrots
> 1 onion, chopped
> 1 green pepper, finely chopped
> 2 teaspoons dried or fresh oregano
> 1 teaspoon garlic powder
> 1 teaspoon sea salt or other seasoning of your choice
> 1 cup grated soy cheese or other cheese of your choice
> 1 teaspoon dried or 2 teaspoons fresh minced basil

1. In a large bowl, mix all of the ingredients together well. The batter should be quite stiff.
2. Roll the batter into a balls that are slightly larger than a golf ball. Flatten them to ½-inch thick.
3. Fry in hot oil until crisp.

Variation: For cheeseburgers, just before serving, put a slice of cheese on top. Broil for a few seconds until the cheese melts.

CAROB TOFU CHEESECAKE

Everybody loves this dessert! It's delicious and easy to make.

> 3 cups tofu or 1½ cups tofu plus 1½ cups cream cheese

> ½ cup liquid fructose or honey
> 2 bananas
> ½ to 1 cup carob powder, depending on desired taste and darkness
> 1 tablespoon lemon juice
> ⅓ cup nonfat powdered soymilk or cow's milk (optional; add it if you like a firmer-textured cheesecake)
> crumbled sugar-free cookies or graham crackers to line the pan

1. Blend the tofu, fructose, bananas, carob, and lemon juice together in a food processor at medium speed until smooth. If you like it firmer, add the powdered milk. (The mixture will not be firm until frozen.)
2. Lightly oil or butter a 9-inch cake pan. Place a ½-inch layer of crumbled cookies in the pan. Pour the tofu mixture over the cookies.
3. Put the pan in the freezer until the cake is firm, at least two hours. Take the cake out of the freezer a half-hour before serving.

Variations: (1) Before freezing, top with carob chips and/or nuts if desired. (2) Before freezing, top with fruit topping made from preserves or cooked-down fruit and honey or fresh fruit such as strawberries, blueberries, or peaches. (3) Blend in ½ to 1 cup of preserves in place of carob powder and liquid fructose.

EGGLESS EGG SALAD

Even without the eggs, this dish is high in protein.

> 1 pound tofu, cubed
> ½ onion, minced
> 1 stalk celery, chopped
> ¼ cup chopped sweet honey pickles or pickle relish
> 1 teaspoon chopped parsley
> ½ teaspoon dill
> ¼ teaspoon mustard
> ¼ teaspoon turmeric
> ¼ teaspoon celery seed
> 1 dash sea salt or seasoning of your choice, to taste
> 2 tablespoons Tofu Eggless Mayonnaise (see below)

1. In a large mixing bowl, toss all of the ingredients together lightly.
2. Chill and serve on a bed of greens, stuffed in pocket bread, or on a slice of whole-grain bread.

Variation: In place of pure mayonnaise, use equal parts of plain yogurt and mayonnaise with a little honey or other sweetener added.

TOFU EGGLESS MAYONNAISE

This healthy spread is easy to make, and is good for people with heart disorders.

½ pound tofu
¾ cup cold-pressed oil
3 tablespoons yogurt
2 teaspoons lemon juice or apple cider vinegar
2 teaspoons prepared mustard
1 teaspoon tamari
1 teaspoon seasoning of your choice
1 dash of cayenne
3 tablespoons honey or ½ teaspoon barley malt
   sweetener (optional)
2 tablespoons sesame tahini (optional)
1 teaspoon horseradish powder (optional)
1 teaspoon liquid lecithin (optional)
1 dash granulated or powdered garlic (optional)

1. In a blender, mix all of the ingredients at medium speed until smooth.
2. Store in the refrigerator. If the mayonnaise separates, just stir again. Use within two weeks.

SCRAMBLED TOFU

This makes a fast breakfast or a quick hot protein dish for any meal.

1 tablespoon expeller-pressed vegetable oil
½ cup chopped onion
½ cup chopped green pepper
½ cup sliced mushrooms
1 pound drained, crumbled tofu
1 tablespoon tamari
1 teaspoon basil
¼ teaspoon garlic powder
1 dash of sea salt (optional)

1. Place the oil in a skillet and sauté the onion, pepper, and mushrooms.
2. Add the rest of the ingredients and continue to sauté until tofu starts to brown. Serve hot with whole-grain toast.

LOW-FAT NO-CHOLESTEROL PUMPKIN PIE

This version of the Thanksgiving classic is high in protein and good for people with high cholesterol.

1 pound drained tofu
2 cups plain canned pumpkin (not pumpkin-pie
   filling)
½ cup fructose or honey or 1 tablespoon barley
   malt concentrate or 1 cup barley malt syrup
   or rice syrup
2 tablespoons arrowroot powder
2 teaspoons ground cinnamon
½ teaspoon ground allspice
½ teaspoon ground ginger
½ teaspoon ground nutmeg
9-inch unbaked pie shell

1. Preheat the oven to 400°F.
2. In a blender or food processor, mix all of the ingredients thoroughly. Pour the mixture into the pie shell.
3. Bake for fifteen minutes. Reduce temperature to 350°F and bake an additional fifty to fifty-five minutes. The pie is done when a toothpick comes out clean after being inserted in the center of the pie. Let cool and serve topped with chopped or halved pecans.

LOW-FAT SOUR CREAM

This recipe makes a one-cup serving with only 3 grams of fat.

½ pound tofu
2 tablespoons lemon juice
3 tablespoons canola oil

1. In a blender or food processor, blend the tofu and lemon juice until creamy.
2. While mixing, gradually add the oil through the feeder tube and continue to process until the mixture is thick. If it is too thick, blend in a little quality water, as needed.

CHAPTER TWENTY-FIVE

TOFU: THE VERSATILE PROTEIN

Prince Liu An (179–122 B.C.E.), grandson of the founder of the Han dynasty, developed tofu while searching for a substance to help him achieve immortality.

—Chinese legend

Tofu, also known as bean curd, is fast becoming a popular staple. It first hit U.S. supermarkets in 1958. Tofu is produced by pulverizing soybeans, boiling the mash, and adding calcium or sea salt to coagulate the curds. Soy, a legume, contains all eight essential amino acids as well as vitamins and minerals. Tofu was made in northern China as early as 220 A.D., according to archeologists. In 1878, a San Francisco firm began making tofu in the United States, primarily for the growing number of Chinese immigrants in that area. Now, most supermarkets carry tofu in the produce section, and it can also be found in health food stores and Asian markets.

Eating a single serving of tofu daily has been linked to reducing the risk of heart disease, cancer, osteoporosis, and kidney disease. It can lower cholesterol levels and may help to promote bone health. The combination of tofu, fish oil, fiber, vitamin D, and a low-fat diet may lower the risk of developing breast cancer, the major cancer killer of American women. At an American Cancer Society seminar, Dr. Stephen Barnes, a biochemist at the University of Alabama said, "Experimental studies involving thirty rats indicated that isoflavones, naturally occurring substances found in soybeans and tofu, seemed to reduce the rate of mammary cancer by half." The active soybean agents were also referred to as *phytoestrogens* because they block the activity of cancer-inducing estrogen in much the same way as the synthetic drug tamoxifen (a synthetic hormone) does. These phytoestrogens are also found in regular soybeans, soymilk, soy flour, and miso (soybean paste).

Tofu is an excellent food for babies, and is good for growing children, vegetarians, and older adults, because it has a high protein content and is easily digested. It is good for sensitive stomachs and is lactose-free.

Having no flavor of its own, tofu can take on the flavor of whatever other foods it is prepared with. It is therefore extremely versatile—it can be used as a substitute for mayonnaise, sour cream, cream cheese in cheesecake, dips, low-calorie dressings, meat, cheese, sandwich spreads, and much more.

TOFU NUTRITION

The type of soybean used to produce tofu determines the precise nutritional content of the tofu, but in general ½ cup (or ½ pound) of tofu contains the following:

- Calories: 86
- Protein: 9.4 grams
- Fat: 5 grams
- Calcium: 154 milligrams
- Iron: 2 milligrams
- Potassium: 50 milligrams
- Sodium: 8 milligrams

Tofu is low in calories, fat, and carbohydrates, and is rich in calcium and potassium. In equal servings, tofu has 25 to 50 percent fewer calories than beef and 40 percent fewer calories than eggs. It also contains a wealth of valuable phytochemicals.

FORMS OF TOFU

There are different types of tofu, primarily distinguished from one another by their texture.

Silken tofu, or Japanese-style tofu, ranges from the softest to medium-soft.

Chinese-style, or hard-pressed tofu, is medium-firm to dense-firm.

The medium-firm tofu is good for slicing, freezing, and cubing. The softer form may be used the same way but it has to be drained and squeezed dry, and it does not hold its shape as well. It is best in recipes that require blending, such as mayonnaise and cheesecake. You can make tofu firmer by placing paper towels on the top and bottom of the tofu and placing a heavy chopping board on it for fifteen minutes or longer.

BUYING AND STORING TOFU

Look for tofu in the produce, deli, or dairy section of your supermarket, or in natural foods stores. It is packaged in water-filled tubs, vacuum packs, or aseptic containers. Some Asian markets sell tofu in bulk. Tofu is perishable, so be sure to check the expiration date on the package and to keep it refrigerated after opening. Tofu in aseptic packaging will keep for a long time, but also needs to be refrigerated after being opened.

Always buy tofu in sealed containers. Tofu blocks floating in open containers of water are susceptible to bacterial contamination and may cause food poisoning. After the package is opened, tofu should be stored in distilled water that is changed daily. You should consume it within a week after you open the package. Rinse the tofu before placing it in the fresh water. Fresh tofu has a delicately sweet scent. If it starts to smell a little sour before you can use it all, boil it for twenty minutes. This will renew the tofu and plump it up.

You can also freeze tofu. Frozen tofu has a meaty texture that resembles ground beef in recipes, such as chili, spaghetti, sloppy Joes, and the like. It must be properly frozen to be good. Drain the chunk of tofu well and take a paper towel and squeeze out all the excess liquid. Let it sit for a few minutes and pat it dry again. Cut it into half-inch chunks, place them on a cookie sheet, and freeze for three to four hours. Once the tofu is frozen, move the chunks into a freezer bag. It will keep for up to five months. Once defrosted, the tofu will have a meaty, chewy texture and caramel color. Marinated, defrosted frozen tofu that is baked or grilled will taste much like tender meat.

CREATIVE WAYS TO USE TOFU

Tofu is an incredibly versatile food. It makes a great dip—just add a packet of Hain's or Mayacamas dry soup mix (or any dry soup mix of your choice) to 1 pound of blended soft tofu and refrigerate it for a few hours. Onion, mushroom, vegetable, and even cheese soup mix is easy and delicious mixed with tofu. Another idea is to use dried minced onion or chopped chives, or dried vegetables, and season it with garlic granules, cayenne pepper, dried parsley, and a little miso or vegetable bouillon granules. For a guacamole dip, blend the tofu, ripe avocados, salsa sauce, a touch of garlic powder, and a little lemon juice. For jalapeño dip, omit the avocados and add chopped onion and jalapeño peppers and a tablespoon of oil. Always chill dips before serving them to flavor the entire dish. Experiment and create your own favorite dips. Just add blended tofu and seasoning, plus desired flavors, like dill, chive, curry, or garlic.

You can make a "lighter" meat loaf by adding crumbled tofu to the meat mixture.

Use tofu as a nutritious replacement for sour cream, cream cheese, ricotta, and similar dairy products.

Sandwich spreads are easy to make using blended tofu and adding chopped nuts, pimiento, pickle relish, and sweetener, if desired. If you do not wish to make your own spreads, there are products such as Vegenaise available on the market. They are usually found in the refrigerated section of health food stores. Tofu mayonnaise has no cholesterol, dairy, or eggs, and contains far fewer calories, less fat, and more protein than regular mayonnaise.

To cut down on giving nut butters to children, mix nut butters and/or jelly with an equal amount of mashed tofu for a healthier sandwiches.

If you are allergic to eggs or if you are a strict vegetarian, you can use tofu to make a substitute for scrambled eggs. (See the recipe on page 189.) There are also products, such as Tofu Scramble, available that make this easier. Scrambled tofu is low in calories, has no cholesterol, is quick and easy to fix, and tastes incredibly good.

Tofu works well with marinade. You should always marinate tofu in a stainless steel or glass container. If you are marinating cubes, use a flat dish and turn the cubes several times while they are marinating. If you are using frozen tofu, press the marinade into the tofu with your hands every so often. Do not let marinating tofu stand out at room temperature longer than an hour. After one hour, refrigerate it.

To use frozen tofu, just thaw and crumble. Added to recipes, it resembles meat in texture and takes on the flavor of the food it is cooked with. Remember, tofu itself has virtually no flavor, so taste dishes you add it to, because it may need more seasoning than usual.

For baby foods, add tofu to a blender along with other foods, like fresh fruit, vegetables, or canned baby foods. This will assure there is enough protein and calcium in the baby's diet.

If you are too busy to prepare your own homemade soy-based foods, there are many products available that you can buy in your local market or health food store, including soy cream cheese, ice cream, sour cream, cheese slices, frozen macaroni, hot dogs, cheese, and many more, including frozen dishes. Tofutti is one company that produces a lot of foods that are soy based.

In addition to the suggestions above, the recipes that follow will give you some easy and appetizing ways to use tofu.

TOFU RECIPES

NUTRITIOUS GRAVY

This delicious brown gravy is packed with protein.

   ½ cup tofu, mashed until there are no lumps
   1½ cups water
   1 package Hain's or Mayacamas brown gravy mix

1. In a saucepan, blend the mashed tofu with water.
2. Add Hain's or Mayacamas brown gravy mix and cook over medium heat, stirring constantly, until thickened. Serve over browned, sliced tofu patties, mashed or baked potatoes, or brown rice.

Variation: Sauté ½ pound sliced mushrooms and onions and add them to the gravy. Just before serving, add 1 cup plain yogurt and serve over noodles Stroganoff-style. Or, to make chicken Marsala, substitute ½ cup Marsala cooking wine for ½ cup of the water and add sautéed mushrooms to the gravy and ladle over free-range chicken.

GRILLED TOFU SANDWICHES

These make a tasty lunch that is a great source of protein for vegetarians.

> 8 ounces firm tofu, drained and sliced
> 2 tablespoons miso or tamari sauce
> 1 tablespoon expeller-pressed vegetable oil
> 1 tablespoon soy mayonnaise
> 4 slices whole-grain bread
> 1 or 2 scallions, finely chopped

1. Mix oil and miso together, and spread mixture on tofu slices. (If you are using tamari, marinate the tofu for one hour in the sauce.)
2. Preheat the broiler.
3. Lightly oil a cookie sheet. Place the tofu slices on the cookie sheet and broil, without turning, for about eight to ten minutes, until hot.
4. Spread half of the soy mayonnaise on one slice of the bread, sprinkle with half of the scallions, top with half of the broiled tofu slices, and close with another slice of bread. Repeat this procedure for the second sandwich.

Variations: (1) Prepare open-faced sandwiches topped with sautéed sliced mushrooms and onions with barbecue sauce or Hain's or Mayacamas prepared dry gravy mix. (2) Substitute a slice of onion and tomato for the scallions.

EASY TOFU MAYONNAISE

This spread is egg- and dairy-free—and delicious.

> 6 ounces tofu, drained and patted dry
> 1 tablespoon lemon juice
> 2 tablespoons canola or safflower oil
> 1 teaspoon mustard
> 1–2 teaspoons honey
> ½ teaspoon sea salt (optional)

In a blender, purée all the ingredients until smooth. Store in the refrigerator.

Variations: Add pickled relish, fennel, chopped onion, a dash of horseradish powder, or fresh-grated horseradish powder for a tasty sauce.

CREAMY ITALIAN DRESSING

A creamy dressing that's better than any containing dairy products.

> ½ pound drained tofu
> 4 tablespoons virgin olive oil
> 2 tablespoons balsamic or apple cider vinegar
> 1 teaspoon sea salt (optional)

> ½ teaspoon dried onion flakes or 1 tablespoon minced fresh onion (optional)
> 4 cloves garlic, minced, or ½ teaspoon garlic powder (not garlic salt)
> 2 tablespoons honey or sweet pickled relish
> 1 teaspoon Italian seasoning or 1 packet Hain's Italian seasoning mix
> ¼ teaspoon barley malt sweetener (optional)

1. In a blender, combine the tofu and olive oil, and, if desired, sea salt and/or onion flakes.
2. Fold in the garlic, honey or relish, Italian seasoning, and, if desired, barley malt sweetener. Store in the refrigerator.

COTTAGE TOFU SALAD

This is great used either as a salad or a dressing.

> 1 pound drained tofu, crumbled
> 2 tablespoons olive oil
> 1½ teaspoons apple cider vinegar
> 1½ teaspoons lemon juice
> 1 teaspoon sea salt (optional)
> 1 tablespoon chopped fresh parsley
> 1½ teaspoon dried chives
> ¼ teaspoon dill weed

1. In a blender or food processor, blend ½ cup of the tofu, olive oil, vinegar, lemon juice, and, if desired, sea salt.
2. Place the remaining tofu, parsley, chives, and dill in a mixing bowl. Add the dressing and toss lightly. Use it as a sandwich spread or serve on a bed of lettuce and tomato as a salad.

TOFU WHIPPED CREAM I

Use this as a festive dairy-free topping.

> ⅓ pound soft tofu
> ¼ cup expeller-pressed vegetable oil
> 4 tablespoons honey
> ½ tablespoon lemon juice
> ½ teaspoon vanilla

In a blender or food processor, blend all of the ingredients until light and fluffy. Chill. Store in the refrigerator.

TOFU WHIPPED CREAM II

Here's another variant of the classic dessert topping.

> 2 cakes firm tofu, drained and patted dry
> 6 ounces soymilk, almond milk, rice milk, or cow's milk
> 6 tablespoons rice or barley malt syrup or honey

In a blender, process of all the ingredients until soft peaks develop. Chill until ready to serve as a whipped cream topping for fresh fruits or pies.

PART SIX

PROCEED WITH CAUTION

CHAPTER TWENTY-SIX

THREATS TO HEALTH: WHEN FOOD, WATER, AIR, AND EARTH GET SCARY

I have sinned against the wisdom of the creator and, justly, I have been punished. I wanted to improve His work because, in my blindness, I believed that a link in the astonishing chain of laws that govern and constantly renew life on the surface of the Earth had been forgotten. It seemed to me that weak and insignificant man had to redress this oversight.

—*Justus von Liebig, author of* Organic Chemistry in Its Application to Agriculture and Physiology *and the "Father of Chemical Agriculture" (1803–1873)*

Beyond any reasonable doubt, the quality of life on planet Earth is dependent upon the surrounding environment. Everything looks like it's connected because it *is* connected. Humankind, at a very late date, is discovering just how that connection affects our health, individually and globally.

Intelligence and the ability to create tools and weapons elevated humans to the very top of the food chain, where we are generally safe from predators other than ourselves. Thousands of years later, people discovered the "sciences," giving us a great ability to control and manipulate our environment. Science did not, however, bestow the ability to see into the future and the effects these changes would have on Earth and its inhabitants (hindsight is always 20/20). Global warming. Smog. Soil and water tainted by pesticides. Lead, arsenic, and radon poisoning. Food, water, and air contaminated by bacteria and viruses. The very source of life, the oceans, polluted. Not by acts of God, but by the effects of humankind's seemingly innocent alteration of the environment. It seemed like such a tiny finger dipped in the cosmic pie. And now life, as we know it, can be brought to its knees by organisms so small they cannot be seen by the human eye. Even those at the top of the food chain, we have learned, are still totally dependent upon the bottommost link. No matter how clever or advanced (or arrogant) we become, life still comes down to three things—food, air, and water.

Scientific "advances" alarm and enthrall us at the same time. Folks are not so quick to trust information given by people with something to sell. We are beginning to wonder: Is food that is microwaved, irradiated, or genetically modified still nutritious, or even safe? When the stuff under the sink and on the lawn that kills bugs and weeds winds up in the drinking water (along with 4.5 billion other pounds nationwide), what happens and what can be done about it? Are food additives and preservatives harmful, and exactly why *are* they added? How can we protect our families from foodborne illnesses? This chapter will provide you with information on potential health hazards from the processes used to grow, harvest, handle, and cook food, and their effects on health and the environment.

ENVIRONMENTAL DANGERS

There are many negative environmental factors that affect the food chain for humans and animals. Possessing some knowledge of these influences can arm us with safeguards to protect our well-being and that of our families. When applicable, the discussions in this section also advise you of an available "dietary fix" for a given environmental hazard.

The Air—the Effects of Ozone

Ozone is a gas composed of three atoms of oxygen that forms in the Earth's upper atmosphere and also on the surface. Ten to thirty miles above the Earth's surface, there is a protective layer of ozone that helps to shield us from harmful ultraviolet rays from the sun. Ozone that forms closer to the Earth's surface, however, is considered a pollutant, and can harm both our food and our health. It is created when ultraviolet light from the sun causes a chemical reaction with pollutants from car exhaust, power plant emissions, and industrial waste.

The Air Quality Index (AQI), posted daily, measures concentrates of five air pollutants: ozone, sulfur dioxide, particulate matter, carbon monoxide, the nitrogen dioxide. Over half the population of the United States lives in areas where the AQI exceeds and violates federal health standards at least once a year. We know that ozone exposure can aggravate respiratory conditions, reduce lung function and the ability to exercise, and, in extreme instances, cause coughing or chest pains. What you may not know is that ozone is corrosive and can damage plants and trees—even destroy agricultural crops and some forest vegetation.

In addition to having respiratory effects, research indicates that exposure to ozone and other airborne pollutants is associated with a higher incidence of heart attack and deaths from heart disease. Inhaling tiny particles emitted by power plants, factories, cars, and trucks, may kill as many as fifty thousand Americans a year. Scientists believe that this may cause subtle abnormalities in the heart's ability to vary its rhythm in response to changing demands, such as the need to beat faster during exercise or more slowly while sleeping. A study by Harvard University researchers found that people who have diabetes are more likely than to be hospitalized when air quality is poor.

The Fix

If you have diabetes or any type of cardiovascular problem, check local air quality indexes daily and stay indoors when pollution levels rise. In addition, the U.S. Environmental Protection Agency (EPA) recommends the following:

- If there is a haze, a smog alert, or if it is very windy, keep doors and windows closed. Do not run, walk, or bicycle along busy roads. Smog levels are lowest in the early morning and evening, so schedule any exercise at that time.

- When outside air quality is good, open your windows and doors to allow the air in your home to mix with air from outside. This dilutes the concentration of trapped airborne particles.

- Buy good air filters for your home. A high-efficiency particulate air (HEPA) filter can lower particulate levels in your home by as much as 76 percent.

- Use an exhaust fan when cooking: Broiling and sautéing can cause indoor particle levels to soar. Install and use a fan that vents to the outside and that is approved for kitchen use.

- Upgrade your vacuum. A model equipped with a HEPA filter will capture more small airborne particles. If a HEPA filter vacuum is not affordable, try switching to vacuum bags labeled *microfiltration*. They are costlier but can cut particulate levels considerably.

- Ban smoking in your home. The smoke contains noxious particles, which is why secondhand smoke is so dangerous. If you smoke, quit. Ask friends to light up outside.

- Do not allow a car to run inside a garage, particularly if the garage is attached to your house. This can cause high levels of noxious fumes to build up. Modern cars should not need to warm up for longer than it takes for you to fasten your seat belt. If you feel you must allow your car's engine to run a bit to warm up, do so in the street or driveway.

The Dietary Fix

Eating foods high in antioxidants and phytochemicals (a minimum of three to five servings of fruits and vegetables daily) combats any assault on the heart and lungs, as well as the immune system. Because particles of pollutants may be deposited on food crops, wash all fruits and vegetables thoroughly before eating them.

Ground Zero—Soil and Mineral Depletion

That which is soil now was once mountains, crushed by ice floes and ground slowly down into the many kinds of dirt found planetwide. There were abundant minerals in the early soil that can now be found only in areas that are impossible to cultivate. Eons of farming and grazing have removed these minerals from the soil more rapidly than they can be replaced by nature.

There are some sixty minerals, including trace minerals, present in human blood. It stands to reason that most of them must have some function in the body. Most important, these minerals can be obtained only through food, herbs, and supplements. Minerals like selenium, iron, zinc, and magnesium, are vital to the immune system of humans and animals. Studies suggest that mineral deficiencies can contribute to heart disease, cystic fibrosis, and attention deficit disorder. Without minerals, vitamins cannot work efficiently. Selenium deficiency has been linked with cancer and many other health problems. Mineral levels in food, in turn, depend on the quality of the soil where that food is produced. In an alarming trend, an analysis comparing the mineral contents of fruit and vegetables in the United States from 1939 to 1991 showed drops ranging from 16 to 59 percent. Another analysis on soil mineral depletion presented to the Earth Summit in Rio de Janeiro in 1992 by the U.S. senate showed North America at 85 percent, South America at 75 percent, Europe at 72 percent, Asia at 76 percent, Africa at 74 percent, and Australia at 55 percent of 1939 levels.

To ensure an adequate supply of the full spectrum of minerals through diet, adults (and especially children) can consume seaweed, chlorella, or spirulina, in addition to fish, seeds, nuts, and brewer's yeast. In addition, purchase organic produce whenever possible. The mineral content is generally higher in organically grown fruits and vegetables that have been raised in enriched soil without pesticides. Since most American's diets are deficient in minerals, supplements are likely to be needed to compensate.

Climbing Toxic Waste Levels

The U.S. Public Interest Research Group (USPIRG) reported in 2002 that the U.S. Environmental Protection Agency (EPA) documented that toxic waste generated by U.S. industry jumped more than 25 percent in 2000. Released directly into the air, land, and water were 7.1 billion pounds of toxic waste, along with another 38 billion pounds of toxins classified as "managed." Chemicals like dioxins and mercury persist in the ecosystem, increasing the chances of exposure. These toxins accumulate in the body and can have detrimental health effects. Companies reported releasing 12 million pounds of these persistent chemicals in 2000 and generated nearly 72 million pounds of waste containing these chemicals.

Dioxins are created in industrial processes that burn or use chlorine or chlorinated materials. They are linked to damage to the nervous, immune, and reproductive systems, and are known to be carcinogenic. These toxic chemicals accumulate in the body and persist in the environment.

Industry reported releasing 4.3 million pounds of mercury and mercury compounds into the American environment and generating 4.9 million pounds of mercury compounds in toxic waste in 2000. To gain some perspective on how potentially dangerous this is, consider that depositing a single teaspoon of mercury each year in a twenty-acre lake can contaminate the lake to the point that fish from it are unsafe to eat. A 2001 report by USPIRG and the Environmental Working Group, a not-for-profit research organization, found that fish contamination is already so high that eating fish such as bluefish, grouper, king mackerel, shark, swordfish, and tilefish can expose a pregnant woman to levels of mercury that could threaten a developing fetus.

Lead and Other Heavy Metals

People ingest lead, one of the most toxic metals known, due to water treatment procedures, industrial releases, older plumbing systems, lead-based paint, and other sources associated with old housing. It is in some ceramic-ware glazes (it turns chalky after washing) and lead crystal dishes and glassware. It is also in the soil. Even at low levels, lead is not excreted by the body but is instead absorbed directly from the blood into other tissues. It is stored in the bones and continues to build up over a lifetime. If present in toxic amounts, it can damage the heart, kidneys, liver, and nervous system.

Children are particularly at risk from lead exposure. Children's bodies absorb 25 to 40 percent more lead per pound than adults. The U.S. Centers for Disease Control and Prevention (CDC) estimate that nearly 1 million American children aged one to five years old are affected by lead poisoning. The use of lead in paint, gasoline, and some other products was banned in 1970, but children can still be exposed through paint chips in older homes, lead in dirt, and from plumbing soldered with lead. The chemicals used to fluoridate many municipal water supplies can also increase children's absorption of lead.

The most disturbing information about lead poisoning comes from Roger D. Masters, Ph.D., a researcher and professor at Dartmouth College in Hanover, New Hampshire, who is an expert on the effects of toxic metals on human behavior. According to Dr. Masters, "Communities with a higher percentage of children having blood lead over 10 mg/dL [milligrams per deciliter] are significantly more likely to have higher rates of violent crime and higher rates of educational failure . . . High lead intake is often a factor among children who are hyperactive (ADHD)." Instead of using methylphenidate (Ritalin) to treat ADHD, specialists at the Pfeiffer Treatment Center in Naperville, Illinois, have found that treatments to reduce levels of lead and other toxins provide lasting improvement without medication. Even low levels of lead in the body can be associated with decreased intelligence, decreased growth and stature, and impaired hearing.

The Fix

Chelation, a process that cleans out toxins, can be helpful for removing heavy metals from the body. This is a process in which certain substances, known as chelators, are introduced into the body to bind with molecules of toxic debris and so pull them out of the body. Quality water (not tap water) naturally chelates some toxins due to its magnetic and trace mineral properties. Many clinics offer chelation treatments performed on an outpatient basis by medical doctors using dimercaptosuccinic acid (DMSA), a drug that has been approved by the U.S. Food and Drug Administration (FDA). There have been some reported problems with DMSA treatment. There are also oral chelation supplements and formulas available at health food stores; however, one must be relatively healthy to sustain the process. If lead poisoning is suspected, hair analysis may be better than blood testing for determining the extent.

The Dietary Fix

Eat generous amounts of beans, broccoli, Brussels sprouts, cauliflower, eggs, garlic, kale, legumes, onions, and spinach, all of which help the body to get rid of lead. Make sure that your diet is low in fat and contains enough calcium, iron, and zinc so that your body does not mistakenly absorb lead instead of these minerals. A sufficient calcium intake helps to prevent lead from being deposited in body tissues.

Mercury and Autism

Mercury toxicity is a suspected cause of a steep rise—a tenfold increase between 1984 and 1994—in diagnosed cases of autism in children around the world, according to some scientists. Specifically, the culprit is thimerosal, a mercury-based compound used as a preservative in vaccines commonly administered to babies and infants. Thimerosal-free vaccines are available. If you have a child who will be receiving vaccinations, ask for and make sure thimerosal-free vaccines are used.

Kelp, with its essential minerals (especially calcium and magnesium), helps remove unwanted metal deposits.

The body absorbs more lead if it is nutritionally depleted. People with lower intakes of vitamins C and E and iron absorb and accumulate more lead in their bodies. If you cannot get enough through diet, take supplements of vitamin C (choose a mineral ascorbate form) and vitamin E daily to provide maximum protection against lead accumulation.

Pesticides

Pesticides of concern include insecticides, fungicides, herbicides, rodenticides, and other agricultural chemicals. In a brochure entitled *Beyond Pesticides*, the National Coalition Against the Misuse of Pesticides defines pesticides as "anything that kill a pest (insect, weed, fungi, rodent, etc.), whether a chemical or biological agent." More than 4.5 billion pounds of active pesticide ingredients are applied a year throughout the United States alone. Agriculture accounts for 77 percent of the pesticides used in this country, industry and government for 12 percent, and private homes and gardens for 11 percent.

Pesticides have been linked to cancer, birth defects, reproductive problems, neurotoxicity, and kidney and liver damage, and are known irritants. At least 107 different active ingredients in pesticides are believed to cause cancer in animals or humans. Pesticides seep through the ground and into the nation's lakes, streams, and rivers, and then flow into the ocean. Many are potentially toxic to birds, fish and aquatic organisms, and bees. Some pesticides that are banned for use in the United States can nevertheless be sold to other countries and then reintroduced on food imported into the United States from those countries, creating what has been dubbed a "ring of poison."

Scientists at Tulane University in New Orleans wanted to know if pesticide chemicals become more dangerous when combined. They tested four chemicals for their ability to increase estrogen production. When two were paired, the potency rose by 160 to 1,600 times, surprising even the researchers. Other researchers suspect testicular and breast cancer in humans might eventually be traced to these chemicals.

A pesticide report by the National Research Council (NRC) warns the public that chemical pesticides can seriously affect children's health. "The federal government's decision-making process for pesticides does not pay sufficient attention to the protection of human health, especially the health of infants and children," according to Philip Landrigan, M.D., who chaired the NRC committee. In a 1995 report, three major baby food manufacturers were tested for pesticides residue. Trace amounts of sixteen pesticides were found in eight of the brand name foods tested. Though levels were low, the report questioned whether government standards are tough enough to protect children. Children face long-term threats from environmental toxins, which can potentially affect their growth, development, and immunity to disease.

Maverick scientist Devra Lee Davis, Ph.D., a leading epidemiologist and researcher on environmental health and chronic disease, believes that a vast number of man-made chemicals, including pesticides that are used on crops and lawns as well as chemicals used in cosmetics and in plastic bottles, behave in the body like hormones, mimicking estrogen or blocking testosterone. In the United States, testicular cancer has doubled in the past three decades and prostate cancer has doubled in the last decade. Davis believes that this is at least partly due to the soup of hormone-disrupting pollutants in the environment. The same is true for breast cancer.

Pesticides also are involved in many cases of direct poisoning due to accidental ingestion. The majority of such cases involve children. In 1993, The American Association for Poison Control reported more than 64,000 poisonings from pesticides, with a large percentage involving kids under six. Of chemicals commonly brought into the home, mothballs, flea foggers, and roach sprays are the main sources of exposure.

The Fix

Chemical pesticides, though government-approved, cannot be described as safe. All pesticides are by definition toxins or they would not kill pests. Take this risk very seriously.

If you feel you must use any kind of over-the-counter pesticide in your home, read and follow the manufacturer's directions carefully. Keep it away from all food, even packaged foods. Do not expose pregnant women, small children, infants, or pets to the chemical. Avoid hanging pest strips, which constantly release pesticide into the air and contain known and suspected carcinogens. You should *never* use such products in the kitchen. Be aware that any kind of bug spray you may use will accumulate on carpet and linoleum and that vapors can rise and settle on toys and other objects used by children. Children's toys can accumulate enough pesticides to be dangerous to their fragile systems. Before spraying (or having a professional

Most and Least Contaminated Fruits and Vegetables

The FDA conducted testing of produce available for sale in the United States to determine pesticide contamination. Based on this research, they produced the following list of the fruits and vegetables most likely to be contaminated:

- Celery (81 percent)
- Grapes (from Chile; 79 percent)
- Cantaloupe (from Mexico; 76 percent)
- Cherries (71 percent)
- Peaches (71 percent)
- Strawberries (70 percent)

- Apricots (64 percent)
- Sweet bell peppers (64 percent)
- Apples (61 percent)
- Spinach (50 percent)
- Cucumbers (40 percent)

The twelve least contaminated fruits and vegetables were avocados, corn, onions, sweet potatoes, cauliflower, Brussels sprouts, U.S. grapes, bananas, plums, green onions, watermelon, and broccoli.

spray) pesticides in your home, put toys away in a sealed container. At night, store toys in a toy box or in a closet with a tight-fitting door if your home has been sprayed recently. If spraying pesticides indoors, use only small amounts in cracks and crevices. Ventilate the room both while spraying and afterward.

Increasing numbers of localities are now engaging in aerial spraying of pesticides for mosquito control. If this is done in your area, keep all household members indoors, with doors and windows closed and air-conditioning turned *off*, during the spraying and for twenty-four hours afterward. Close up the house tightly. Do not allow children to play outside for several days after the spraying if their play area is highly vegetated. If possible, cover gardens or any food-growing areas.

The Dietary Fix

The best way to approach the problem of pesticide residues in foods is to avoid them as much as possible. Whenever possible, buy certified organic produce, which is likely to contain lower levels of pesticide residues. Avoid purchasing imported foods, which may contain residues of pesticides whose use is banned or severely restricted in the United States. Buy locally and avoid purchasing out-of-season produce that must be transported long distances or stored for long periods of time. (Avoiding pesticides is one of the most compelling reasons to pick up a hoe and start that organic garden.) Many cities have a municipality garden plot where families can plant food together. Make sure to use only quality water that is free of pesticides for drinking and cooking.

The way you prepare food can help to reduce possible exposure to pesticide residues. Washing hard-skinned produce in a mild soapy solution and rinsing with plain water afterward will reduce surface residue levels. Adding a small amount of vinegar or citric acid to the water will help to dissolve pesticides that are otherwise insoluble.

Remove the outer leaves of leafy vegetables, such as cabbage and lettuce, and discard them, as these have probably received the most recent pesticide applications.

Peel wax coatings, which can trap pesticide residues. Also, fungicides may be added to waxes to help prevent spoilage during transit. It is better to peel such produce, even though this also reduces the vitamin content.

Cooking destroys many pesticide residues, although in some cases, it creates dangerous breakdown chemicals.

Do not eat citrus peels. Use only organically grown citrus fruits when using the peels for zest to flavor food.

Another strategy for minimizing exposure to pesticides is to adopt a diet heavy in organic fruits and vegetables and low in animal fat. Pesticides and other toxins are stored in the fatty tissue of food animals.

FOODBORNE ILLNESS

Food-related diseases are numerous and are caused by biological and nonbiological agents. *Salmonella* (in eggs and poultry), *Escherichia coli* (*E. coli*, in apple juice and alfalfa sprouts), *Listeria monocytogenes* (in cheese and hotdogs), *Campylobacter* (in undercoked poultry or meat, raw milk, and contaminated water), *Shigella*, *Clostridium perfringens*, *Staphylococcus aureus*, and *Vibrio vulnificus* are common bacterial foodborne illnesses that affect an estimated 76 million people each year in the United States. More than 300,000 people are hospitalized and over 5,000 die from food-related illnesses. The very young, the very old, and the immune-compromised are the most susceptible to foodborne illnesses. Children are by far the most susceptible to microbiological pollution in food and water because they have less resistance to disease-causing organisms and, for their weight, drink about twice as much water as adults do. In addition, some infections have shown a resistance to antibiotics, possibly due to increased human and farm use of antibiotics, and are more dangerous than ever.

Less than 2 percent of imported fruits and vegetables are inspected by the FDA, which leaves the potential for new pathogens to get in. Manure, which harbors *E. coli* and *Salmonella,* is often substituted for chemical fertilizer on both organic and conventional crops.

Symptoms of Food Posioning

The typical symptoms of foodborne contagion are vomiting, diarrhea, and abdominal pain. Look for high temperatures, a stiff neck, and dry mouth. If digestive symptoms last more than three days, you should see a physician. Sometimes nonspecific symptoms and neurological symptoms occur due to food poisoning. Suspect foodborne illness if symptoms come on within a short time after you consume raw or poorly cooked food (especially eggs, meat, or fish), unpasteurized milk or juices, home-canned goods, fresh produce, or soft cheeses from unpasteurized milk.

The Fix

The best approach to food poisoning is prevention, which means careful handling and proper preparation of foods. Before handling food, wash your hands well with hot, soapy water for at least twenty seconds. Repeat this often, and always wash your hands between handling meat and produce.

Use only pasturized milk and fruit products.

Cook all meats well, and use a thermometer to verify that they are sufficiently cooked. Beef, lamb, and veal should reach an internal temperature of 145°F (rare) to 175°F (well-done); chicken and turkey, 165°F; ground meat, 160°F to 180°F (well done); and pork, 160°F to 170°F (reheat ham to 140°F); and casseroles and egg dishes, 160°F. Reheat leftovers to 165°F. Eggs should be refrigerated and cooked until yolks are firm—cook foods containing eggs thoroughly.

Refrigerate perishables as soon as you get them home. Defrost meat in the refrigerator, not on the counter. For safe, rapid defrosting, place the meat in a sealed plastic bag and surround the bag with cool water. Meat should defrost within thirty minutes.

Wash raw produce before eating it. Use a soft scrub-brush whenever possible.

When peeling fruits and vegetables, wash the rind *and* the knife before cutting the fruit—otherwise, the knife could transfer bacteria (or pesticide residue) from the peeling or rind to the interior of the fruit or vegetable.

Wash cutting boards thoroughly after cutting meat and before cutting fruit and vegetables. It is wise to keep two separate cutting boards, one for meat and one for plant food. Wooden boards may be microwaved to kill bacteria. Plastic boards can be run through a dishwasher cycle. Both may be washed with a bleach solution made by adding ¼ cup of bleach to a sinkful of water.

The Risk of Raw Sprouts

Based on increasing reports, the FDA has issued statements saying that eating raw sprouts can pose a risk of foodborne illness. Fortunately, cooking sprouts can significantly reduce this risk. (See Chapter 23 for instructions for cooking sprouts.) Check sandwiches and salads prepared out of the home for the presence of raw sprouts and consider requesting sprouts not be put in food. Bacteria may be present in the seed, so home-grown sprouts can also present a risk. Children under age twelve, older adults, and people with immune deficiencies should stay away from all sprouts, whether raw or cooked.

The sink is a breeding ground for bacteria from different sources. Make sure it is clean before washing fruits and vegetables in it. Wash countertops and sinks with a little bleach and water. Bleach dishcloths and sponges often or run them through a dishwasher cycle where high temperatures help kill bacteria. Sponges are not recommended for use as they may harbor high amounts of bacteria.

Refrigerate leftovers immediately after a meal is finished. Don't worry about whether it is hot. It is better, however, to transfer hot food into a fresh room-temperature container before refrigerating it so that it cools more quickly. Keep your refrigerator at 50°F. Check it periodically with a thermometer to verify the temperature. Marinated foods may still contain growing bacteria. Throw used marinades out.

Even with all these precautions, the risk of foodborne illness cannot be completely eliminated. Many common toxins in food cannot be destroyed by heat—boiling does not kill everything. Freezing does not kill bacteria.

COOKWARE

Aluminum pots and pans are controversial cooking vessels. Food cooked in aluminum reacts with the metal to form aluminum salts that have been associated with dementia, Alzheimer's disease, and impaired visual motor coordination. Studies that revealed aluminum deposits in the brains of people who had died of Alzheimer's disease first raised these concerns. This theory has never been conclusively proven, but it may be worth consideration. Newer, anodized versions, in which electrochemical baths seal the surface of the aluminum, are scratch-resistant and deemed safer.

Another source of potential concern with cookware are nonstick coatings. Although these have different brand names, they are all fundamentally the same type of substance. At high heats, these coatings release polytetrafluoroethlyene (PTFE) fumes, which are potentially toxic. While there may not be obvious or dramatic effects on people, pet bird owners have known for years that exposure to PTFE gas can kill a bird within seconds, raising the question of what effects this has on the human body as well, especially with long-term use. Nonstick finishes also scratch easily and particles of the plastic can get into food.

Stainless steel (do not clean abrasively), glass, cast iron, and terra cotta (without a lead-based glaze) are good alternative choices for cookware.

FOOD ADDITIVES

To make processed food products more marketable, manufacturers frequently place preservatives and other additives in them. There are at least 3,000 food additives currently in use, of which some 2,000 are synthetic. They are used to enhance color, texture, or taste; to facilitate food preparation; and to extend shelf life. It is estimated that the average American consumes about 5 pounds of additives a year. A diet high in processed foods would increase that amount significantly. In small doses, these additives seem harmless enough, even though the body must detoxify them if they are not immediately excreted. It is the cumulative buildup of additives, along with other pollutants within the cells of the body, that has researchers concerned. Many additives that were once considered safe were ultimately removed from the market when they were later proven unsafe for human consumption. Vegetarians should also note that many additives are derived from meat, fish, or fowl. Additives in processed food are yet one more reason to enjoy a fresh-food diet.

Additives and artificial ingredients add little or no nutritional value to food, whereas "fortification" may increase nutrient content. Preservatives serve as antimicrobials or antioxidants, or both. Antimicrobials prevent the growth of molds, yeasts, and bacteria. As antioxidants, they keep food from browning, becoming rancid, or developing black spots.

A growing number of scientists are convinced that the compounds termed excitotoxins, including monosodium glutamate (MSG), hydrolyzed vegetable protein, and aspartame (NutraSweet) play a role in neurological disorders such as dementia (including Alzheimer's disease), learning disorders in children, and Parkinson's disease. Other additives generally given the thumbs-down by nutritionists until more tests are done are the fake fat olestra (Olean), artificial colors, and preservatives including sodium nitrates, sulfites, butylated hydroxyanisole (BHA), and butylated hydroxytoluene (BHT).

MSG

MSG is a food additive that enhances flavors in food while having virtually no flavor of its own. How it adds flavor to other foods is not fully understood, but people do experience a more intense flavor from food containing MSG. Many scientists believe that MSG stimulates glutamate receptors in the tongue to augment meatlike flavors. It is a simple, inexpensive way for the food industry to enhance flavors, mask unwanted tastes, and hide undesirable flavors in foods.

MSG is the sodium salt of the amino acid glutamic acid and a form of glutamate. It is sold as a fine white crystalline substance, similar in appearance to salt or sugar. Asians originally used a seaweed broth to obtain the flavor-enhancing effects of MSG. MSG is now made by a fermenting process using tapioca starch, sugar beets, sugar cane (the main raw material), or molasses. Ajinomoto, a main manufacturer of MSG, predicted an estimated worldwide demand of 1.5 million tons in 2001.

Glutamate is found in many living things. It occurs naturally in our bodies and in protein-containing foods, such as cheese, milk, meat, peas, tomatoes, and mushrooms. Every time a food containing protein is ingested, there is a certain amount of MSG. This natural form found in food is not the problem, however. It is the pure synthetic crystalline MSG that creates havoc. The use of MSG has increased dramatically over the years and has spread to soups, sauces, and salad dressings in restaurants; many canned, frozen, and prepared foods found in local supermarkets; and even cheese, ice cream, cookies, and candy. One form of MSG is autolyzed yeast, which can appear on food product labels as "yeast extract." Other sources of "hidden" MSG include hydrolyzed milk proteins, which may be labeled "sodium caseinate," "calcium caseinate," or "casein." Hydrolyzed casein (milk) protein may be offensive to vegetarians because it contains hidden milk protein, which is also a potentially lethal allergen. Other label items to be wary of are "natural flavor" and "kombu extract." These additives are often found in frozen dairy products, like ice cream and yogurt, as well as in hot chocolate mixes, breads, and processed meats.

Is MSG Harmful?

MSG-sensitivity is a sensitivity to a toxic substance, rather than an allergic reaction. People's tolerance for MSG varies. The use of MSG is controversial because of reports of adverse reactions, from slight to extreme, experienced by people who have eaten foods that contain it. Reported reactions include migraine headaches; rapid heart beat; burning sensation in the back of the neck, forearms, and chest; numbness in the back of the neck radiating to the arms and back; tingling, warmth, and weakness in the face, temples, upper back, neck, and arms; seizures; weakness; dizziness, panic attacks, or anxiety; nausea; diarrhea; mood changes; sleep problems; skin flushing; excessive sweating; chest pain; facial pressure; and hyperactivity. Physician George R. Schwartz, M.D., coauthor of *In Bad Taste: The MSG Symptom Complex* (Health Press, 1999), maintains that MSG could be responsible for ailments seemingly far removed from digestive distress. He contends that it has been implicated in damage to the central nervous system, endocrine organ disorders, cardiac arrest, and illness in other parts of the body.

In otherwise healthy MSG-intolerant people, the symptoms of MSG intolerance tend to occur within one hour and up to forty-eight hours after eating 3 grams or more of MSG on an empty stomach or without other food. Severe, poorly controlled asthma may be a predisposing medical condition for the MSG complex. The level of vitamin B_6 in a person's body may play a role in glutamate metabolism, and the possible impact of marginal vitamin B_6 intake is being considered in research.

Research on the role of glutamate (the group of chemicals that includes MSG) in the nervous system suggests a relationship between elevated brain glutamate levels and neurodegenerative disease such as Alzheimer's disease and amytrophic lateral sclerosis (ALS, or Lou Gehrig's disease). In addition, there is evidence that glutamic acid kills brain cells and causes neuroendocrine disorders in laboratory animals. Several books and television news shows have reported widespread and sometimes life-threatening adverse reactions to MSG, claiming that even small amounts of manufactured glutamates may cause adverse reactions in some people.

MSG Labeling

Since 1958, the FDA has designated MSG as a generally regarded as safe (GRAS) ingredient. Under current FDA regulations, when MSG is added to a food, it must be identified as "monosodium glutamate" in the label's ingredient list. Each ingredient used to make a food must be declared by its name in this list.

While technically MSG is only one of several forms of free glutamate used in foods, consumers frequently use the term MSG to mean all free glutamate. For this reason, the FDA considers foods whose labels say "No MSG" or "No Added MSG" to be misleading if the food contains ingredients that are sources of free glutamates, such as hydrolyzed protein.

The Fix

If you suspect you have an adverse reaction to MSG, avoid the food sources at home and in restaurants. Learn the following terms, which indicate potential food sources of MSG, and look for them on food labels:

- Definite sources of MSG are hydrolyzed protein, sodium caseinate, calcium caseinate, autolyzed yeast, yeast extract, and gelatin.

- Possible sources of MSG are textured protein, carrageenan, vegetable gum, natural flavoring, seasonings or spices, flavorings, chicken, beef, pork, smoke flavorings, bouillon, broth or stock, barley malt, malt extract, malt flavoring, aspartame, whey protein, whey protein isolate or concentrate, powdered milk, soy protein, soy

protein isolate or concentrate, soy sauce, or soy extract. AuxiGro WP Plant Metabolic Primer, a product that contains processed free glutamic acid (MSG), has been approved for spraying on grapes, including grapes to be used for producing wine.

Sodium Nitrite and Nitrate

Sodium nitrite and nitrate, used as preservatives and color fixatives in cured meats and fish products, inhibit the growth of bacterial spores that cause botulism. Safety concerns with nitrites are that the salts can react with derivatives (amines) in food to produce nitrosamines, many of which are known to cause cancer. Sodium nitrite can lessen the blood's ability to carry oxygen and, if enough is ingested, respiratory failure is a danger.

BHA and BHT

BHA and BHT, used as a preservatives in dry foods, are in almost every processed food, from cereals and rice to potato chips. These chemicals are also used in making plastic packaging material, milk cartons, wax paper, and others. Both have caused severe allergic reactions and been linked to cancerous tumors in animals.

Sulfites

Sulfites, used primarily as antioxidants to reduce the discoloration of fruits and vegetables, to inhibit bacterial growth in wine, and to prevent "black spots" on shrimp and lobster, can produce adverse allergic reactions in many individuals who are sulfite-sensitive, particularly people with asthma. Sulfites are still found in some cooked and processed foods, including baked goods, condiments, potatoes, and beverages such as hard cider, fruit and vegetable juices, and tea. The FDA estimates that one out of a hundred people is sulfite-sensitive. This sensitivity may develop at any point in life. Symptoms include difficulty breathing, stomach ache, and hives after consuming food products containing sulfites. If you suspect you are sensitive, watch also for labels that say sulfur dioxide, sodium sulfite, sodium and potassium bisulfite, and sodium and potassium metabisulfite. Foods served in restaurants, especially potato products, and even some canned foods contain sulfites. Bottled lemon juice often contains sodium bisulfite. Read packaged food labels and avoid processed foods that contain sulfites. If you have asthma make sure to take your inhaler along when you are eating out. If you have had a severe allergic reaction in the past, also carry an antihistamine or self-administered injectable epinephrine kit.

ANTIBIOTICS IN LIVESTOCK

According to a recent report, about 70 percent of the antibiotics used in the United States each year are not used to

Mad Cow Disease

Bovine spongiform encephalopathy (BSE), known popularly as mad cow disease, is a chronic degenerative disorder affecting the central nervous system of cattle. It is believed that eating meat products from affected animals can cause a disorder in people called variant Creutzfeldt-Jakob disease (vCID). Both BSE and vCID may not cause obvious symptoms for up to twenty years after the original infection and both are always fatal. A three-year study at Harvard University determined that the chances of BSE entering the United States and threatening consumers are "extremely low." However, the U.S. Department of Agriculture (USDA) tests only some 5,000 cows for BSE annually. Joint efforts of the USDA and the FDA so far seem to have been responsible for keeping BSE out of this country. These organizations say that they have a "multiple firewall" system (including feed bans, import controls, and a surveillance program) that can keep it from spreading. While experts say no cows in the United States currently have mad cow disease, a similar disorder known as wasting disease has been found in the wild deer and elk in South Dakota, Colorado, Montana, Wyoming, Oklahoma, Wisconsin, Nebraska, and parts of Canada. At the present time, there is no "fix" for BSE.

cure illness, but are fed to healthy pigs, chickens, and cattle to speed their growth and prevent disease. When animals are given low does of antibiotics, only some of the bacteria in their bodies are killed. The more resistant bacteria survive, multiply, and pass on their strength to future generations of bacteria. *Salmonella* and *Campylobacter* are becoming increasingly resistant to antibiotics, resulting in more severe illnesses and more deaths. This raises the specter of infections that cannot be treated successfully with antibiotics.

Almost 3 million pounds of antibiotics are prescribed to Americans annually. All too often they are prescribed and/or used inappropriately. While the use of antibiotics in human medicine is probably the biggest contributor to antibiotic resistance, the contribution of animal use is being considered to the extent that the American Medical Association has adopted a resolution urging that the nonmedical use of antibiotics in animals should be terminated or phased out. The FDA has announced plans to ban the use of two antibiotics commonly used in chickens and turkeys, saying the use increases the danger that humans may become infected with antibiotic-resistant germs. The U.S. Centers for Disease Control and Prevention (CDC) and the World Health Organization (WHO) have been advocating a ban, but agriculture and pharmaceutical interests have blocked it, according to published reports.

The Fix

Build up your immune system with a nutrition-rich diet and avoid taking antibiotics unless your doctor determines it is absolutely necessary. Many antibiotics are incorrectly prescribed for viral infections, like flu and colds, which antibiotics cannot help. Opt to forgo antibiotics unless absolutely necessary.

Whenever possible, purchase organic meat or meat from range-fed animals. Grass-fed cows produce beef that is leaner, has a superior ratio of omega-6 to omega-3 fatty acids, and possesses more natural minerals and vitamins. Hormones and residues of pesticides from feed grains in

grain-fed animals are another reason to limit the amount of meat in your diet and purchase only free-range beef. Dioxins, polychlorinated biphenyls (PCBs), and other hormone-disrupting chemicals from the environment also become concentrated in animal fat. Consider replacing meat with soy products, grains, legumes, fruits, and vegetables.

FOOD IRRADIATION

Irradiation is a process by which foods are exposed briefly to a radiant energy source (gamma rays or electron beams) at an irradiation facility. It can kill harmful bacteria, reducing potential hazards to consumers. It reduces spoilage, bacteria, levels of insects and parasites, and delays ripening in some fruits and vegetables. Irradiated food must be labeled with the international symbol for irradiation.

While organizations like the World Health Organization and the American Medical Association endorse irradiation, there are consumer activists who feel emphasis should be placed on raising healthier livestock and uncontaminated fruits and vegetables. Detractors also say that irradiation kills bacteria by blowing up their genes, which can create free-radical molecules that, in turn, contribute to disease and the aging process. They also say there is a possibility that irradiation will lead to new strains of radiation-resistant bacteria.

Price is another issue—irradiation increases the cost of food production, which is always passed on to the consumer. In the opinion of Jack Challem, a nutrition reporter and author, "Irradiation is just another way of tampering with a food supply that has already been tampered with far too much."

GENETICALLY MODIFIED (BIOENGINEERED) CROPS

Bioengineering refers to new methods of plant breeding that permit scientists to alter the genetic makeup of food crops by introducing a copy of a gene (DNA) for a specific trait. The gene can be copied from any organism (plant, animal, or microbe), thus providing plant breeders with a source of potentially useful genes and traits that would not be available by conventional breeding methods. Proponents say that bioengeering can result in increased resistance to pests, herbicides, and viruses; thicker skin; enhanced fresh market value due to an extended ripening process; and higher yields due to more rapid plant growth. A list of genetically altered foods from *Gene Exchange,* a publication of the Union of Concerned Scientists, in 1996 showed all new gene sources were from bacteria or viruses.

Concerns about genetically engineered foods include the following: they may have as-yet-unknown long-term health effects; they may result in damage to the ecosystem, the creation of new allergens and toxins, and unpredictable combinations of genetic material, with unknown effects; and they may decrease the nutritional value of food. John D. Fagan, Ph.D., a member of the coalition Citizens for Health, observed, "Many scientists believe that the genetic manipulation of the food supply could set off a chain reaction throughout the entire ecosystem, upsetting the delicate balance in nature for generations to come . . . genetic pollution cannot be cleaned up or contained."

The Fix

Genetically altered foods do not have to be labeled or identified. It appears that consumers have no choice in whether or not to consume them. It may be years, or even decades, before the effects on the environment and humans can be assessed. This is just one more reason to consider creating an organic home garden.

MICROWAVE COOKING

More than 90 percent of American homes use microwave ovens to prepare food. Microwaves are a form of electromagnetic energy like radio or light waves. The oven contains a magnetron, in which electrons are affected by magnetic and electric fields and produce micro wavelength radiation that interacts with the molecules in food. In addition to emitting radiation, most health food experts agree that microwaves change the cellular structure of food. Wave energy changes polarity from positive to negative with each cycle. In microwaves, these polarity changes happen millions of times each second. As microwaves generated from the magnetron bombard food, they cause polar molecules to rotate at the same frequency, millions of times a second. The agitation creates molecular friction that then heats food.

No government or FDA studies have proven that current microwaves are harmful to food or health. However, independent studies have concluded that microwave cooking does change the nutrients in food. Changes have also been detected in human blood samples from people ingesting microwaved food. Dr. Lita Lee, in a May 2001 article entitled *Health Effects of Microwaves and Microwave Ovens,* maintains that every microwave oven leaks some electromagnetic radiation, harms food, and converts substances cooked in it into dangerous organotoxic and carcinogenic products. Similar studies concur. Not enough is known about the effects of chemically altered food to say that microwaves are not harmful to humans.

The Fix

Until more is known, it might be safer to "nuke" food only when a "quick fix" is necessary, rather than on a daily basis. With modern machines, the leakage of radiation is unlikely unless the unit has been damaged. Even so, as a precaution, do not stand close to the oven while it is on. A few electromagnetic field experts recommend staying several feet away. The heat generated in microwave ovens can also drive molecules from plastic containers and wraps directly into food. Use only glass or ceramic containers to heat food and cover them with waxed paper or paper towels rather than with plastic wrap.

Caution: Microwaving baby's milk (especially breast milk) may destroy some of its protective properties. It also converts certain transamino acids into synthetic cis-isomers, which are not biologically active. In tests, one of the amino acids was converted to its D-isomer, which is known to be toxic to the nervous system and poisonous to the kidneys. Also, microwaves heat food unevenly, and the outside of the bottle does not always reflect the temperature inside. If at all possible, do not use a microwave oven to heat baby's milk. If you have no choice, be sure to check the temperature of the milk on your wrist before feeding it to a baby.

CHAPTER TWENTY-SEVEN

SUGAR BY ANY OTHER NAME . . .

There is no sugar cane that is sweet at both ends.

—*Chinese proverb*

The average American consumes about 150 pounds of sugar each year. This accounts for 550 to 650 calories a day, or almost three pounds per week. In 2001, Americans spent $21 billion on candy alone—more than the gross national products of Lithuania, Costa Rica, and Mozambique combined, according to the *Tufts University Health and Nutrition Letter*. The empty calories in sugar contribute directly to overweight, diabetes, tooth decay, and overall poor health. One in twenty of the world's adult population now has some form of diabetes, a disease associated with obesity, poor eating habits, and a sedentary lifestyle. More than half of American adults are overweight. The U.S. Centers for Disease Control and Prevention (CDC) relates that the incidence of type 2 diabetes (formerly known as adult-onset diabetes) has risen by 33 percent in the past decade and three out of every fifty American adults currently have this diet-related condition. Complications related to diabetes are the sixth leading cause of death in the United States.

Excess sugar consumption can suppress the immune system; upset the body's mineral balance; produce an acidic stomach; and cause hyperactivity, anxiety, concentration difficulties, and heart disease (by raising insulin levels), as well as fatigue, weight gain, depression, and arthritis. According to Nancy Appleton, Ph.D., author of *Lick the Sugar Habit* (Avery/Penguin Putnam, 1996), there are seventy-eight metabolic consequences to eating sugar. Dietary sugars feed harmful intestinal yeasts, toxic organisms, fungi, and all forms of cellular cancer. Bill Misner Ph.D., sports nutritionist and author, has said, "Because sugar is devoid of vitamins, minerals, fiber, and has such a deteriorating effect on the endocrine system, major researchers and major health organizations (American Dietetic Association and American Diabetic Association) agree that sugar consumption in America is one of the three major causes of degenerative disease." The rise in type 2 diabetes cases in young people is so great that experts are calling it an "emerging epidemic."

Numerous studies since 1984 have indicated that a high-sugar diet may be a major contributing factor to the incidence of *Candida vulvovaginitis* (yeast infection). One of the major drawbacks of sugar is that it raises insulin levels, inhibiting the release of growth hormones and in turn depressing immune function. Lowered immune function combined with the better growth environment for bacterial and plant organisms created by the presence of sugar pose a double risk for Candida. A study published in the *Journal of Reproductive Medicine* found that the intake of sugar, dairy products, and artificial sweeteners correlated positively with the incidence of vaginal yeast infections. When these foods were omitted from the diet, more than 90 percent of the subjects in the study were free of yeast infections for over a year. Sugar intake and the resulting rise in insulin levels may also be a cause of kidney stones by inducing an increased release of calcium into the urine.

Sugar is the number-one additive used by the food industry. Natural sugars are carbohydrates, which supply the body with the energy it needs to function. Carbohydrates can be divided into three categories: monosaccharides (simple sugars), disaccharides (double sugars), and polysaccharides (starches and fibers, including those found in breads and potatoes). The U.S. Food and Drug Administration (FDA) estimates that the average American consumes about 18 percent of dietary calories from simple sugars and two-thirds of that amount comes from added sugars in processed foods, rather than from naturally occurring sugars in fruits, vegetables, and dairy products.

As little as 2 teaspoons of sugar changes the blood chemistry so that the body is no longer in homeostasis—the balanced state where it functions best. After the body digests sugar, the mineral balance also changes. For example, blood calcium levels may increase and those of phosphorus may decrease. When the blood level of a mineral increases dramatically, the body is thrown off balance, as

Other Names for Sugar

If you see any of the following terms on the label of a food product, the product contains some form of sugar:

- Barley malt
- Beet sugar
- Blackstrap molasses
- Brown sugar
- Cane sugar
- Caramel
- Corn fructose
- Corn sweetener
- Corn syrup
- Date sugar
- Demerara sugar

- Dextrin
- Dextrose
- Fructose
- Fruit fructose
- Glucose
- Grape sugar
- Grape sweetener
- Herbal sweetener
- High fructose corn syrup
- Honey
- Invert sugar

- Lactose
- Maltose
- Mannitol
- Maple syrup
- Molasses
- Polydextrose
- Raw sugar
- Sorbitol
- Sorghum
- Sucrose
- Turbinado

While some forms of sugar are better than others, if you want to reduce your overall consumption of sugar, you should cut back on foods that contain any of the above ingredients.

---

minerals function efficiently only in balance with one another. When the levels of minerals in the bloodstream decrease, the body may no longer have enough to work synergistically with enzymes, which are mineral-dependent also. Enzymes are needed to digest food, and undigested food putrefies. The undigested, putrefied food then irritates the gastrointestinal tract and tiny particles can even get into the bloodstream, leading to allergic reactions, headaches, dizziness, fatigue, or mood changes such as anger or depression. It can go to the bones, joints, and tissues and cause stiffness and arthritis. If the putrefied food particles travel to the skin, via the blood, they can cause acne, psoriasis, or other skin problems. In addition, the white blood cells become overworked and exhausted when allergic reactions summon them forth as a result of continuous consumption of offending foods.

There are many different sources of sugar and sweeteners, with many different names. Some are more healthful than others, depending on how they affect the body and what other nutrients, if any, they contain.

ACESULFAME-K

Acesulfame-K is also known by the brand names Sunette and Sweet One. This is a sweetener of white, odorless crystals made from acetoacetic acid, which is 200 times sweeter than table sugar. Acesulfame-K can tolerate high temperatures without breaking down into other chemical compounds and can be used both for cooking hot foods and in cold foods and drinks.

Acesulfame-K gained FDA approval in 1988 under the Sunette brand name. Used in chewing gum, instant coffee,

tea, dry beverage mixes, gelatins, and nondairy creamers, it leaves no aftertaste. It is not metabolized, so it has no calories. The Center for Science in the Public Interest objects to acesulfame-K, saying that it has caused tumors in laboratory rats. The FDA concluded that those tumors had occurred spontaneously.

ASPARTAME

Approved in 1981 and more commonly known by the brand names NutraSweet and Equal, aspartame is found in thousands of processed foods, from colas to breath mints. It is now one of the most widely used artificial sweeteners in the United States. This sweetener is made up of a combination of the amino acids phenylalanine and aspartic acid, plus methanol.

The methanol (or wood alcohol) in aspartame is known to be poisonous even in small amounts and quickly breaks down into formaldehyde (which is a known carcinogen) and other possibly harmful compounds when subjected to heat. The temperatures reached in hot beverages, including coffee and tea, might be high enough to cause this action. Although the FDA states that exposure to methanol through aspartame consumption is not "of sufficient quantity to be of toxicological concern," the cumulative effects of high doses of aspartame are unknown.

Since its approval, critics have charged that aspartame can cause a myriad of adverse health effects. Numerous individuals have reported suffering neurological and other complaints—including headaches, dizziness, muscle spasms, seizures, nausea, and cramps—after consuming aspartame. People with asthma or other respiratory disorders may be particularly sensitive to aspartame. Do *not* use aspartame if you have phenylketonuria (PKU). You probably should not use it if you or are pregnant or lactating.

BARLEY MALT

Barley malt is a naturally sweet substance that comes in powder and syrup concentrate forms. It is very good for people who are on weight-loss diets or who have diabetes or hypoglycemia. Barley malt provides trace amounts of the nutrients vitamin A, vitamin C, calcium, and iron. In cooking and baking, barley malt can be substituted for sugar. It is highly concentrated; a dash (1/8 teaspoon) has only 3 calories and replaces 2 teaspoons of sugar.

Barley malt sweetener is an excellent sugar substitute. It tastes just like sugar, without the aftertaste often associated with sugar substitutes. Because it contains calcium-saccharate and hydrolyzed soy protein, however, people who are sensitive to monosodium glutamate (MSG) should use it with caution. Plain barley malt would probably be a better choice.

BLACKSTRAP MOLASSES

Blackstrap molasses is a byproduct of the sugar-refining process. To refine sugar cane into table sugar, the boiled, concentrated cane juice is spun in a centrifuge that collects sugar crystals. The uncrystallized syrup that remains is molasses. As the centrifuge process is repeated, the molasses produced becomes darker and thicker. The final grade of molasses produced is called blackstrap molasses. It contains about 50 percent sugar, as well as the minerals and vitamins separated during refining. Blackstrap molasses is rich in iron and minerals and lacks none of the essential nutrients that other forms of sugar are often deficient in. It is one of the best natural sweeteners and is even used in infant formulas. (See Chapter 33.)

BROWN RICE SYRUP

Brown rice syrup is a sweetener made by fermenting brown rice and boiling the resulting mixture until it becomes thick syrup. It is similar in texture to honey. This is another good sweetener for people with diabetes. Another form of brown rice sweetener is marketed under the name of DevanSweet. It is produced by a special air-drying process that granulates the syrup into crystals, retaining many of the grain's valuable nutrients.

EVAPORATED CANE JUICE

Evaporated cane juice is sold under the brand name Sucanat. This product consists of 100-percent evaporated sugar cane juice that is grown organically and contains no preservatives or additives. Naturally brown in color, it contains all the nutrients present in whole sugar cane.

FRUCTOSE

Fructose, or levulose, is a monosaccharide that is found in honey and fruit (except for grapes). Other names found on food product labels that indicate the presence of fructose are corn fructose, high-fructose corn syrup, fruit fructose, fruit sugar, invert sugar syrup (a mixture of glucose and fructose), beet sugar, brown sugar, turbinado sugar, raw sugar, tupelo honey, honey, and unpasteurized honey. If consumed together with other forms of sugar, such as glucose or sucrose (table sugar), fructose may aggravate high blood levels of triglycerides (blood fats) and cause losses of the essential mineral chromium.

The consumption of fructose in the form of high-fructose corn syrup in commercially prepared foods and beverages has increased nearly two and one-half times over the last twenty years. Because of the dangers associated with chromium loss due to high-fructose corn syrup, many researchers recommend reducing your consumption of processed foods containing this sweetener. When you eat fruit, the fiber and water that whole fruit contains dilute the fructose and make it safe.

FRUITSOURCE

This is a relatively new sweetener that comes in granular and syrup form and is available at most natural foods stores. It is derived from grapes and whole-grain rice and is delicious. Because it contains pectin, it can also be used to replace some of the fat in baked goods. It is widely used in commercial baking under the brand name Fruitrim. Use it like honey or any type of sugar.

GLUCOSE

Also a monosaccharide, glucose is also known as grape sugar, dextrose, corn syrup, corn sweetener, or glucose syrup. Glucose is the form of sugar burned by all of the body's cells for energy, and it is needed for brain function. Complex carbohydrates and starches found in food such as greens, vegetables, and fruits are broken down into glucose during digestion. In some circumstances, glucose can be derived from the breakdown of protein and fat.

If glucose is consumed in the forms mentioned above, rather than being derived by the body through the breakdown of complex carbohydrates, it causes blood sugar levels to go up (causing a very quick increase in energy) and then to drop just as quickly, resulting in a feeling of fatigue.

HONEY

Honey is natural syrup produced by bees. It is made up of glucose, fructose, and water, with trace amounts of vitamins and minerals, enzymes, pollen, and propolis. Because honey is not processed or cooked in preparation for sale, it contains all of its vitamins and minerals in their natural proportions.

Propolis is a natural resin occurring in the buds of certain plants that is collected by bees for repair of the honeycomb in the hive. Scientific studies indicate that propolis slows down the reproduction of some viruses. Bee propolis can be purchased with a small amount of honey or alone. It is available in health food stores.

LACTOSE

Lactose is a disaccharide found in milk. Approximately 80 percent of the adult population of the world does not produce enough of the the enzyme lactase, which is needed to digest lactose. There are aids to help the digestion of lactose found in a number of enzyme formulas that include lactase to make up for this deficiency.

MALTOSE

A disaccharide manufactured from starch, maltose is found in malted syrup, maltodextrin, dextrin, and dextrose. Maltose occurs naturally in germinating seeds.

SACCHARIN

Saccharin is most commonly known by a number of different brand names, including Sweet'N Low, Sprinkle Sweet, Sugar Twin, and Sweet 10. It is made of a chemical similar to acesulfame-K. Saccharin does not taste good when used in baking. It has a bitter aftertaste, and its safety continues to be under review.

Available for nearly a century, saccharin is truly an artificial sweetener—it comes from petroleum. About 300 times sweeter than sugar, it cannot be digested and therefore has no calories. Although the FDA proposed and nearly enacted a ban on saccharin after studies suggested a link between it and bladder tumors in rats, it was saved by public demand, to be left on the market. Federal regulations do require, however, that products containing saccharin be labeled. Do not use it if you are pregnant or nursing, and do not give it to a child.

SORBITOL, MANNITOL, AND XYLITOL

These are naturally occurring sugar alcohols. When used in large quantities, they can cause diarrhea and abdominal discomfort. Individuals with blood-sugar sensitivity conditions such as hypoglycemia and diabetes can safely use sugar alcohols in moderation because they do not cause a rise in insulin levels. Stevia (see below) is a better choice.

SORGHUM MOLASSES

Sorghum molasses is produced from a plant related to the millet family that is processed in a similar way to sugar cane. The stalks of the plant are crushed to separate out the

---

Some Sweet Alternatives to Sugar

The following sweeteners are the best sweeteners to use:

- Barley malt
- Barley syrup
- Beet sugar
- Blackstrap molasses
- Rice syrup
- Herbal sweeteners such as stevia

Any of these sweeteners is preferred over refined and artificially manufactured sweeteners. When whole foods containing any of these sweeteners are consumed, they also provide vitamins, minerals, and proteins that stabilize blood sugar and aid digestion.

---

sap, which is then boiled to produce syrup. Sorghum molasses is similar to maple syrup, but has a milder flavor.

STEVIA

Stevia, an herb also known as honeyleaf, is one of the best natural sweeteners available. It is not only completely safe, but actually has healing properties. Made from the leaves of a member of the chrysanthemum family that is native to South America and Asia, stevia is thirty to forty times sweeter than sugar and has been used for centuries. Stevia is the most common calorie-free sweetener in Japan, and is used in soft drinks as well as in baked goods, candies, gums, ice cream, and cereals. In the United States, it is considered an herbal product. Stevia does not affect blood sugar metabolism and is good for people who want to lose weight.

Refining the stevia leaf produces a white powder extract called stevioside, which is 100 to 300 times sweeter than table sugar. Just ¼ to ½ teaspoon of stevioside can substitute for 1 cup of table sugar.

Both stevia and stevioside are safe for use in cooking and baking. Liquid extracts and concentrates of stevia are strong, so small amounts sweeten effectively. Stevia is the sweetener of choice for people with many types of illness, including blood-sugar disorders. It is also available in pill form.

SUCROSE

Sucrose is a disaccharide that contains equal parts fructose and glucose. Sucrose is most commonly known as table sugar. Sucrose is also known as cane, beet, turbinado, confectioner's and powdered sugar, as well as sugar syrup, brown sugar, and glaze. This sugar is produced from sugar cane or sugar beets. When consumed, it adds empty calories and causes blood sugar levels to rise quickly, prompting a release of insulin that just as rapidly sends levels crashing again.

Remember, sugar is found in almost all processed foods like sodas, fruit drinks, frozen dinners, breads, cereals, and canned foods. High-fructose corn sweetener is the most popular with food processors because it is inexpensive. Learn to read labels and be familiar with the different names for sugar to know how much you are really consuming. You are likely to be surprised.

For optimum good health, it is extremely important to keep your sugar consumption as low as possible. Ideally, you should omit it from your diet or at least cut it way back. The next time a television commercial tries to sell the ideal of buying a candy bar for that sudden burst of energy, consider this: The liver can store only about 150 grams (a little over 5 ounces) of glycogen, the form in which sugar from food is saved to burn for energy. Any excess is then turned into fat globules. While "fat globules" might not sound particularly bad, they come together to become what we call a spare tire, thunder thighs, and flabby forearms.

To diminish cravings for sugar, consume more whole grains, squash, sweet potatoes, apples, and bananas. Use desserts sweetened with barley malt or rice syrup or powdered barley concentrate. Dried fruit, apricots, dates, figs, and raisins make good sweeteners for whole-grain cereals. Chop and cook them with the cereal or mash and purée them for baking and use in recipes calling for sugar. Soak them in boiling water before using to soften and rehydrate them.

CHAPTER TWENTY-EIGHT

DIETARY FAT: THE GOOD, THE BAD, THE UGLY

Don't dig your grave with your own knife and fork.

—*English proverb*

There are "good" and "bad" fats in foods—some toxic, some neutral, and some that are essential to good health. Dietary fats provide a concentrated energy source as well as the building blocks for cell membranes and a variety of hormones. All animal and plant fat can be broken down into fatty acids, glycerin, and water. Fats and lipids (another descriptive name for fat-soluble natural compounds) are better energy sources than protein or carbohydrates.

Quality unprocessed fats are also necessary in the diet because they carry the fat-soluble vitamins A, D, E, and K to the body's tissues. Vitamin A, an important antioxidant, prevents night blindness; enhances immunity; guards against cancer, heart disease, and strokes; and is important for the maintenance of healthy skin, mucous membranes, hair, bones, and teeth. Vitamin D is necessary for the absorption of calcium and phosphorus in the intestinal tract and plays a significant role in growth in children, as well as in building strong bones and teeth. It is also important in the prevention and treatment of breast and colon cancer, osteoarthritis, and osteoporosis, and enhances immunity. Vitamin E is a wonderfully active antioxidant that serves in many ways. It protects against cancer and cardiovascular disease, improves circulation, assists tissue repair, promotes blood clotting, reduces blood pressure, and supports healthy skin and hair, to name just a few of its benefits. Vitamin K, believed to promote longevity, is essential for bone formation and growth and the absorption of calcium. It also promotes healthy liver function and plays a role in the conversion of glucose into glycogen, the form in which glucose is stored in the liver.

Fats have the highest caloric density of the three major types of nutrients—9 calories per gram. Protein and carbohydrates, on the other hand, have only 4 calories per gram. One tablespoon of oil contains 120 calories. Fats act as an intestinal lubricant and help to build tissues and body cells. They stay in the digestive tract for longer periods, giving a full, satisfied feeling after a meal. They also are used to generate body heat. Fats soothe the nerves and provide the basis for myelin, the protective shield that covers

nerve cells. Fat is found in all body cells in combination with other nutrients. Essential fatty acids are an important link in the health chain.

Excess fat, however, can be a problem. It is stored in the liver, in arteries around the heart, and in all tissue. Cancer of the breast, prostate, and colon, not to mention obesity, and an increased risk of heart attack, are linked to high fat consumption. The typical American diet consists of 40 to 50 percent calories from fat, a primary cause for the rise in all of these disorders.

ESSENTIAL FATTY ACIDS

All fats are composed of building blocks called fatty acids. Some of these can be synthesized in the body, while others cannot. The ones that the body cannot make, and that therefore must be obtained through the diet (a characteristic they share with many vitamins), are known as *essential fatty acids* (EFAs). They are sometimes also referred to as vitamin F.

All animals and humans require essential fatty acids. There are two known essential fatty acids: alpha-linolenic acid (ALA), which is a member of the family designated omega-3 fatty acids, and linoleic acid, which is one of the omega-6 fatty acids. Another fatty acid, arachidonic acid (AA), also an omega-6 fatty acid, was once thought to be an essential fatty acid, but researchers have since learned that ALA and LA can be converted into AA in the liver. By weight, more EFAs are required by the body than any other type of fat or other nutrient that is considered essential. Every single cell, organ, and tissue requires a daily supply of EFAs.

Deficiencies of essential fatty acids are common today. There are a number of reasons for this, including:

- A diet high in saturated fats.

- Consumption of processed vegetable oils containing trans-fatty acids, which prevent the proper formation of linoleic acid.

- Excessive alcohol consumption.

- Diabetes.

- Aging.

- Lack of magnesium, zinc, and vitamins E, C, and B_6 (pyridoxine).

- Viral infections.

- Cancer, and the chemotherapy and radiation therapy used to treat it.

- Smoking.

- Exposure to environmental toxins.

- The use of certain drugs.

A study conducted at the University of Maryland found that people who consumed large amounts of trans-fatty acids (TFAs; more about them later in this chapter), found in margarine, cooking fats, bread, cakes, French fries, pretzels, chips, frostings, puddings, and other highly processed foods, were likely to be deficient in EFAs. The body needs EFAs, *not* TFAs.

TYPES OF FATS

Dietary fats are divided into different categories depending on the types of fatty acids that predominate in their makeup. There are four basic types of dietary fats: monounsaturated fats, polyunsaturated fats, saturated fats, and trans-fats.

Polyunsaturated and Monounsaturated Fats

Polyunsaturated fats (and their close relations, monounsaturated fats) are the "good fats." These fats are liquid and remain that way—ready for use at room *or* refrigerated temperature. Both of the essential fatty acids, alpha-linolenic acid and linoleic acid, are polyunsaturates. They are found primarily in nuts, vegetables, seeds, fish, soybeans, and seed and nut oils, such as walnut oil.

Polyunsaturated fats are found in the following foods:

Cod liver oil	Primrose oil
Corn oil	Safflower oil
Cottonseed oil	Sesame oil
Fish	Some soft margarines
Flax oil	Soy oil
Pecans	Sunflower seeds
Pine nuts	Wheat germ oil

If polyunsaturated oils are overprocessed, many benefits are lost. For that reason, use only cold- or expeller-pressed oils. Polyunsaturated oils should never be heated or used for cooking. We will now look in detail at the major categories of polyunsaturated fatty acids.

Omega-3 Fatty Acids

The essential omega-3 fatty acid, alpha-linolenic acid, promotes brain and eye development, is good for arthritis, helps to prevent abnormal heart rhythms, improves immune function, and reduces blood clotting. In addition to alpha-linolenic acid, there are two other common omega-3 fatty acids, docosahexanoic acid (DHA) and eicosapentaenoic acid (EPA). Fish are generally considered to be the richest source of these fatty acids, but the content varies depending on the species of fish. Cold-water marine (ocean) fish have a higher fat content and thus contain the largest amounts of DHA and EPA.

All dark-green leafy vegetables also contain omega-3 fatty acids, as do some plant-derived oils. The vegetable oils that contain the highest amount of omega-3 EFAs include:

- Pumpkinseed oil

- Flaxseed oil

- Canola oil

- Soybean oil

- Walnut oil

In *Fats That Heal, Fats That Kill* (Alive Books, 1999), author Udo Erasmus quotes unofficial observations by clinicians that 95 percent of the population is deficient in omega-3 fatty acids. Omega-3 fatty acids have the ability to thin the blood. Blood clots can cause heart attacks and stroke; the omega-3 fatty acids in fish help to prevent dangerous blood clotting by reducing the tendency of blood platelets to clump.

Omega-3 EFAs help to keep blood clots from forming in the arteries and can lower cholesterol levels, reducing the chance of heart problems. They are also known to reduce joint inflammation in people with arthritis, and are good for female disorders and breast disease. The beneficial attributes of these "good" fats are numerous, among them are the following:

- They are helpful for all forms of arthritis, including rheumatoid arthritis.

- They help to control viral infection.

- They reduce blood cholesterol and triglyceride levels.

- They lower the risk of heart attack, stroke, and hardening of the arteries.

- They improve psoriasis.

- They improve immune response.

- They lower harmful effects of body chemicals called prostaglandins, thus helping to prevent breast cancer.

- They can reduce the severity of migraine headaches.

- They improve brain function.

- They improve the functioning of the glandular system.

To add the essential fatty acid ALA to your diet, consume canola, walnut, or flaxseed oil daily. It is best to purchase unrefined oils. Keep them in the refrigerator. Do not heat these oils, as heating destroys the nutrients. Instead, use them in salad dressings. Also consume at least one serving of dark-green leafy vegetables daily to meet your omega-3 requirements.

Fish and fish oil are probably the best source of DHA and EPA. Fish from cold, deep waters have the highest content of these oils, with Atlantic mackerel, Atlantic herring, salmon, and albacore tuna being among the highest. (See Chapter 14.) Rather than using fish oil supplements, consume more fish. Marine fish from cold, deep waters are less likely to contain undesirable contaminants than are lake fish. In general, a 4-ounce serving of fish supplies about 1,400 milligrams of omega-3 oils. Three 500-milligram capsules of fish oil supply a total of 1,500 milligram. Avoid using high doses of cod liver oil as a source of fish oil, since its high content of vitamins A and D can be toxic—take only 1 teaspoon daily. Do not consume alcoholic beverages if you are taking cod liver oil. If you are a vegetarian and do not want to consume fish or fish oil, add flaxseed oil to your diet.

Flaxseed oil has the highest content of the omega-3 ALA (58 percent), about twice as much as fish oil. Flaxseed oil is also less expensive and more stable than fish oil. Adding about 2 tablespoons of flaxseed oil or ground flaxseeds to your diet each day will give you a generous supply of the essential omega-3 fatty acids. Both flaxseeds and flaxseed oil (sometimes also called linseed oil) can be found in health food stores. Keep flaxseeds in a tightly sealed container and grind them just before you use them, as ground flaxseeds become rancid quickly. Omega-Life, Inc., markets a fortified flaxseed product that is very rich in the omega-3s.

If you are taking blood-thinning medication, whether prescription drug or an over-the-counter agent like aspirin, avoid taking large amounts of omega-3 in supplement form. It may be better to take supplemental EFAs and avoid aspirin, as too much aspirin can have negative side effects. Always discuss any change in medication with your physician first, however.

Omega-6 Fatty Acids

The essential omega-6 fatty acid linoleic acid lowers total blood cholesterol levels as well as levels of low-density lipoprotein (LDL, or "bad") cholesterol.

Omega-6s are obtained from many vegetable oils and they are important, but many scientists feel that the ratio of omega-6 to omega-3 fatty acids is also significant. The human brain and brain tissues of other mammals contain an omega-6 to omega-3 ratio of 1 to 1. In other cells of the body, the ratio is between 3 to 1 and 5 to 1. Because omega-3s are lacking, comparatively, in the fats and oils most commonly used in this country, the typical American consumes these fats in a ratio of 20 to 1—or more.

Help for Arthritis

In one Danish study, subjects with rheumatoid arthritis experienced a significant decrease in pain, swollen joints, and morning stiffness after six months of eating 4 ounces of fish daily. The omega-3 fatty acids in fish lead to the suppression of inflammatory prostaglandins. Cold-water fish such as salmon, sardines, and halibut are best; flaxseed oil, borage oil, walnuts and pecans, tofu, and green leafy vegetables are other food sources. The omega-6 fatty acids, which can fuel the production of inflammatory prostaglandins and are present in corn, cottonseed, safflower, and sunflower oil, are overabundant in most diets. The inflammatory response can be triggered if the ratio of omega-3 to omega-6 fats in the body is out of balance. A practical approach to arthritis therefore is to lessen your intake of potentially inflammatory omega-6 oils and to increase your intake of the omega-3 oils, whether through diet alone or diet plus supplements.

Increasing omega-3 consumption while controlling intake of omega-6s (and also eliminating saturated fat and trans-fats) is one of the most overlooked steps to optimal health.

Omega-9 Fatty Acids

Omega-9 fatty acid, or oleic acid, is not an *essential* fatty acid, because humans can produce limited amounts. It is found in almost all natural fats. Large concentrations are found in avocados, macadamia nuts, apricot seeds, almonds, and olive oil. Omega-9 helps to prevent cancer and boosts the immune system. It can also dilute omega-6s, thereby containing the damaging effects of excessive inflammatory responses and helping to restore a healthy ratio of omega-3 to omega-6 fats in the body.

Monounsaturated Fats

Monounsaturated fats, cousins to polyunsaturated fats, are found in a number of foods. Like most polyunsaturates, they come from plant-based sources. This form of fat is desirable because it does not affect blood cholesterol levels—in fact, it may actually improve them—so monounsaturated fats are acceptable for people with cholesterol problems. Monounsaturated oils are liquid at room temperature but can become cloudy or semi-solid when refrigerated.

Monounsaturated fats are found in the following foods:

- Almonds
- Avocados
- Canola oil
- Cashews
- Hazelnuts
- Olive oil (in soft or solid form)
- Peanuts
- Pecans

Monounsaturated fats can be used for cooking; however, like all good fats, it is best to avoid subjecting them to heat. As with polyunsaturates, choose cold- or expeller-pressed oils.

Saturated Fats

Saturated fats come principally from animal sources such as meat and dairy products, and are normally solid at room temperature (think of the marbling in cuts of meat). They have been implicated in many serious health problems, including heart disorders and hardening of the arteries. Simply stated, hardened fats mean hardened arteries.

Saturated fats are "bad fats" because they replace "good fats" in the body's cellular structure when there is a deficiency of good fats in the diet. A critical balance in cell-membrane structure is necessary for these membranes to block the entrance of harmful materials and admit beneficial materials into the cells. If saturated fats are used instead of the unsaturated ones to construct cell membranes, this cellular function is disrupted—and all other cellular functions are disrupted along with it. A high intake of saturated fats has been shown to elevate serum cholesterol and to contribute to heart disease and many forms of cancer. They slow the liver's ability to remove artery-clogging LDL (low-density lipoproteins) from the blood. However, monounsaturated and polyunsaturated fats aid in removing LDL ("bad fats") from the bloodstream.

Beware of labels stating "no cholesterol." The cholesterol content in foods is not the most significant factor in elevated blood cholesterol levels. Rather, it is the saturated fat content of food that contributes most to the body's production of cholesterol. Elevated cholesterol in the bloodstream due to overconsumption of saturated fats can damage the coronary arteries, creating a risk of heart attack. Research suggests that the body has trouble metabolizing molecules of saturated fat when it has been exposed to extremely high heat, as occurs in the process known as hydrogenation, and that it may be carcinogenic. Saturated fats are found in the following foods:

- Bacon
- Beef
- Butter
- Cheese and processed cheese food
- Chocolate
- Coconut oils

- Coconut
- Lard
- Milk/cream
- Palm kernel oil
- Palm oil
- Pork
- Poultry (mainly in the skin)

Because they have been implicated in many health problems, you should keep your consumption of saturated fats, particularly those from animal sources, to a minimum.

Coconut Oil

Coconut oil is one of the few plant-based oils that contains significant concentrations of saturated fat. Its use has been controversial due to a forty-year-old study that said it raised blood cholesterol. It is worth noting, however, that the study in question used *hydrogenated* coconut oil. While coconut oil does contain saturated fat, it is easily digestible and converted into quick energy. In addition, nearly 50 percent of the fatty acid in natural coconut oil is lauric acid, which has adverse effects on a variety of microorganisms, including yeast, bacteria, fungi, and viruses. It is not necessary to avoid all coconut oil, but do not consume it in the hydrogenated form, which is found in most processed foods.

Trans-Fats and Hydrogenation

Trans-monounsaturated fatty acids, or trans-fats, are formed when oils are subjected to the heat of a process known as *hydrogenation*. While trans-fats are a form of monounsaturated fat, they appear to act like saturated fat within the body. Trans-fats are a great concern because there is no requirement that the trans-fat content of products be identified on food labels. This makes it difficult, if not impossible, to accurately determine the amount of trans-fats in your diet.

Most margarines and solid vegetable shortening—essentially, any vegetable-based oil or fat that is firm at room temperature—contain trans-fats because they have undergone hydrogenation. Hydrogenated oils are ingredients to *avoid*. Hydrogenation chemically alters oils by bombarding their molecules with hydrogen atoms that, in effect, saturate the unsaturated fats. This is done to make liquid oils solid at room temperature. However, since the hydrogen atoms attach themselves to the oil molecules in a different way than those in naturally saturated fats, the resulting fats are called *trans-fats*.

When fat is hydrogenated (hardened) to prolong shelf life, it destroys the essential fatty acids. Many, if not most foods, on supermarket shelves contain some amount of hydrogenated oils. These oils are almost impossible for the system to assimilate. Consuming many foods that have been fried in hydrogenated oil, like those from fast-food and other restaurants, can lead to a deficiency of good fats.

Soybean oil accounts for more than 80 percent of oil consumption in the United States, or more than 12 million tons a year. Half of that amount is partially hydrogenated oil. Both saturated and unsaturated fatty acids are present in all vegetable and animal fats. Liquid soybean oil—like liquid corn, olive, and safflower oil—contains only 15 percent saturated fats. But partially hydrogenating soybean oil, as is done to make solid vegetable shortenings such as Crisco, increases the level of saturated fat (and fat that behaves like saturated fat in the body) to 25 percent.

Oils: The Best and the Worst at a Glance

The Best:

- Olive
- Canola
- Walnut
- Safflower
- Avocado
- Almond
- Rice bran
- Sesame
- Flaxseed

The Worst:

- Coconut
- Peanut
- Palm
- Palm Kernel
- Cottonseed

Since 1930, the increased use of pasteurized dairy products and hydrogenated oils has increased in direct proportion to the number of deaths from heart attack. The March 1998 issue of Harvard University's *Women's Health Watch* reported that in one major study, a 2 percent increase in calories from trans-fats was associated with a 93 percent increase in the risk of coronary artery disease, the precursor to heart attack. In addition, possibly as a result of the prevalence of hydrogenated soybean oil in processed foods, soybean oil is fast becoming a common allergenic food.

Monounsaturated or polyunsaturated oils should replace trans-fats in the diet. If you must use margarine, softer or liquid margarines that are free of trans-fats, or that at least list liquid poly- or monounsaturated oils as the first ingredient, are better for health. Nonhydrogenated margarines are available in health food stores if not in your supermarket. Spectrum Spread, produced by Spectrum Naturals, is a butter substitute made with canola oil that is 94 percent saturated fat free and contains no trans-fats. It cannot be used in frying, but can be used just like butter on bread, rolls, toast, vegetables, and other cooked foods to add the taste of butter. Before buying any type of margarine, look carefully at the ingredients. The first ingredient listed is the one found in the greatest amount. If the first ingredient is "liquid oil," it is a better product to use. If the first ingredient is "hydrogenated oil," leave it alone. The best margarine is derived from vegetables, safflower, soy, or corn oil. Soft margarine is hydrogenated less, leaving more of the natural oils intact. It is lower in hard trans-fats.

THE BEST OILS

Considering all of this information, and all of the choices available, which type of oil is the best single source of dietary fat? Virgin olive oil. Olive oil has cholesterol-lowering benefits and helps to control blood pressure and diabetes. Olive oil contains a whopping 74 percent monounsaturated fat, 14 percent saturated fat, and 8 percent polyunsaturated fat. The *Journal of the National Cancer Institute* reported in a study that

women who consumed olive oil more than once a day had a 25 percent lower incidence of breast cancer than those who did not. Unrefined olive oil should be kept refrigerated. Olive oil is especially good for salad dressing and herb/oil mixtures, but is not the best oil to fry food with.

Canola is very low in saturated fat and high in monounsaturated fat, which experts believe are superior to polyunsaturated fats for lowering cholesterol. Canola contains 59 percent monounsaturated fat, 30 percent polyunsaturated fat, and 7 percent saturated fat. It contains up to 10 percent of the essential omega-3 fat alpha-linolenic acid, which is important to cell membrane structures and in the synthesis of metabolically active substances like prostaglandins. Prostaglandins are hormonelike substances that regulate some body processes, including blood pressure, immune function, and response to allergies.

High-oleic safflower and high-oleic sunflower oils are monounsaturated oils created from normally high-polyunsaturated safflower and sunflower oils. High-oleic safflower oil contains 75 percent monounsaturated fat, 14 percent polyunsaturated fat, and 6 percent saturated fat. High-oleic sunflower oil contains 84 percent monounsaturated fat, 10 percent saturated fat, and 4 percent polyunsaturated fat.

HOW OILS ARE EXTRACTED AND PROCESSED

Oils are extracted and processed in various ways. The methods used to produce an oil affect its quality and price, and can also affect flavor and other characteristics. Be aware of how oils are processed, the ingredients they contain, and what has been removed, and watch out for "refining." A product may be advertised as unsaturated, but manufacturers don't have to say whether it contains any trans-fatty acids. These act like saturated fats in the body.

Following are summaries of the extraction and processing methods to which oils may be subjected.

Expeller-Pressing

In this method, a screw- or expeller-type press is used to crush the seeds. The seeds are pushed against a metal press head in a continually rotating movement, and a spiral-shaped auger moves the seeds forward in a manner similar to a meat grinder. The oil is squeezed out of the seed by the pressure. This pressed oil may be filtered, then bottled as "cold-pressed," natural, crude, or unrefined oil. This pressing process takes only a few minutes and is carried out at temperatures of 185°F to 203°F. This pressed oil is the best type to purchase.

Modified Atmospheric Packing

A new method of processing oils that is gaining preference from quality oil manufacturers combines expeller-pressing with lower than normal temperatures and exclusion of light and oxygen during the pressing and packing processes. Known as modified atmospheric packing, it allows

TABLE 28.1 CONCENTRATIONS OF DIFFERENT TYPES OF FATTY ACIDS IN SELECTED OILS

Virtually all fats and oils contain some combination of polyunsaturated, monounsaturated, and saturated fatty acids. They tend to be referred to as one of these types based upon which kind of fatty acid is the predominant one. The table that follows will allow you to compare different oils and the proportions of types of fats that they contain.

Highest in Polyunsaturated Fats (Reduce Both "Bad" LDL and "Good" HDL Cholesterol)

TYPE OF OIL	PERCENTAGE POLYUNSATURATED	PERCENTAGE MONOUNSATURATED	PERCENTAGE SATURATED	COMMENTS
Safflower	75	12	9	Contains immune-boosting vitamin E.
Sunflower	66	20	10	Contains immune-boosting vitamin E.
Walnut	63	23	10	Rich in omega-3 fatty acids and vitamin E. Not good for frying.
Wheat germ	62	15	19	
Corn	59	24	13	A good all-purpose oil, unless you are allergic to corn.
Soybean	58	23	14	Contains linoleic acid, which is converted to the same fatty acids found in fish oil. High in vitamin E.
Cottonseed	52	18	26	A cotton byproduct found in most commercially baked goods. Can have a number of negative effects, including enhancing the potential of aflatoxins and irritating the digestive tract. Not recommended.

Highest in Monounsaturated Fats (Lower "Bad" LDL Cholesterol without Lowering "Good" HDL Cholesterol)

TYPE OF OIL	PERCENTAGE MONOUNSATURATED	PERCENTAGE POLYUNSATURATED	PERCENTAGE SATURATED	COMMENTS
Olive	74	8	14	Has cholesterol-lowering benefits and may help to control blood pressure and diabetes. Virgin olive oil is best. Good for salad dressings and vinegar/herb oils.
Avocado	71	13	12	Can contribute to a healthy monounsaturated intake.
Almond	70	17	8	The high price, required refrigeration, and strong taste make them less popular. They are good skin moisturizers.
Apricot	60	29	6	
Canola	59	30	7	Has a high percentage of monounsaturated fats that may have the same blood-fat and blood-pressure-lowering benefits as fish oil. Canola oil is second best to olive oil and has a milkier flavor.
Peanut	46	32	17	May promote atherosclerosis. More likely than other oils to be contaminated with aflatoxins.
Sesame	40	42	14	Unrefined types do not withstand high cooking temperatures well, but refined types do. This is still a good oil to use for salad dressings.

Highest in Saturated Fats (Linked to Elevated Blood Cholesterol, Heart Disease, and Cancer; Not Recommended)

TYPE OF OIL	PERCENTAGE SATURATED	PERCENTAGE POLYUNSATURATED	PERCENTAGE MONOUNSATURATED	COMMENTS
Coconut	87	2	6	Not generally recommended, especially in hydrogenated form.
Palm kernel	82	2	11	Not recommended.
Butter	50	3	23	Contains a relatively high percentage of monounsaturated fats for this category, but still not recommended.
Palm	49	9	37	Contains a relatively high percentage of monounsaturated fats for this category, but still not recommended.

temperatures of only 86°F to 91°F during processing. A number of companies, including Barlean's Organic Oils, Omega Nutrition, and Spectrum Naturals are utilizing this process under their own trade names; Bio-Electron Process, Omegaflo, and Spectra-Vac, respectively.

Refining

This process involves mixing the oil with caustic soda (sodium hydroxide [NaOH]), which is a very corrosive base. A mixture of NaOH and sodium carbonate (Na_2CO_3)

may also be used. The oil and the base are agitated and then separated, removing the free fatty acids from the oil. Phospholipids, which are proteinlike substances, and minerals are also removed in this process. The oil still contains pigments, usually yellow or red. The refining temperature is around 167°F.

Degumming

Degumming involves the removal of proteinlike compounds, complex carbohydrates, and true gums from the oil. Lecithin is isolated (much of it is then sold separately in the form of nutritional supplements). Degumming also removes chlorophyll, calcium, magnesium, iron, and copper from the oil. Degumming is carried out at 140°F.

Solvent Extraction

In solvent extraction, the oil is removed from the seed by dissolving it out of the seed meal using a solvent (such as hexane) at temperatures of 131°F to 149°F. Traces of the solvent remain in oils produced this way. Expeller-pressed and solvent-extracted oils are sometimes combined and sold as "unrefined" oil. Unrefined oil is treated with several processes, including degumming, bleaching, refining, and deodorizing.

Supercritical Fluid Extraction

Supercritical fluid extraction is one of the newer processes used to extract oils. It uses high-pressure chambers for the processing of seed meal. The process allows lower temperatures to be used. However, it is more damaging to polyunsaturated oils than solvent extraction because it causes increased chemical instability, altered fatty acid profiles, and decreased mineral content.

Bleaching

Chlorophyll, beta-carotene, and traces of soap have been removed from some oils by the use of filters, acid-treated activated clay, and/or fuller's earth. Natural polycyclic and aromatic substances are also removed in this process.

Supermarket Process

Refined oils found in supermarkets have several synthetic antioxidants added to them to replace the natural vitamin E and beta-carotene, which are removed during refining. This list of substances includes butylated hydroxytoluene (BHT), butylated hydroxyanisole (BHA), propyl gallate, tertiary butylhydroquinone (TBHQ), citric acid, and methylsilicone. A defoamer is added, and the oil is then bottled and sold.

Deodorization

To deodorize oils, aromatic oils and free fatty acids are removed by steam-distillation and the exclusion of air during this process. Pungent odors and unpleasant tastes not present in the natural seed before processing are also removed. Deodorization takes place at extreme temperatures of 464°F to 518°F for thirty to sixty minutes. The oil then becomes tasteless and cannot be distinguished from oils derived from other sources treated in a similar manner. Vitamin-and-mineral-deficient oils are the result of this

treatment. The oil can still be sold as "cold-pressed" because no external heat was applied during the pressing of the oil. Understanding the difference between true "cold-pressed" oil and oils that have been subjected to other processes is very important.

VITAMIN E: THE PROTECTOR

Vitamin E helps to protect the body's cell membranes from the free-radical damage that can take place if you consume oils that are heated or rancid. Pesticides, herbicides, chemicals, and other foreign substances are stored in the fatty tissues of animals. The more animal and dairy products consumed, the more chemical toxins are ingested. Carcinogenic substances cannot be avoided if the wrong foods are eaten consistently—and animal fat is one of the worst!

If you take any kind of fish oil supplement, be sure to take a vitamin E supplement along with it. This will help to protect your cells and keep the fish oil from turning rancid in your body. Carlson Labs has an excellent salmon oil supplement in capsule form that has vitamin E added for protection. It is wise to take a vitamin E supplement before consuming any type of fatty food.

OIL DO'S AND DON'TS

When choosing and using any type of fats and oils, keep the following hints in mind:

- Purchase only unrefined cold- or expeller-pressed oils.
- Avoid hardened (hydrogenated) oils.
- Never reuse oil that has been used for frying.
- Before opening, store all oils in a cool, dark cupboard.
- Refrigerate all oils after opening.
- Never consume any oil that smells rancid.
- Olive oil maintains a longer shelf life than most oils.
- Do not let oils heat to the smoking point.
- To sauté or stir-fry foods, add 2 tablespoons of quality water to the cooking oil, before heating the oil.

Since fats and oils are a necessary and vital part of the diet, it is important to know these simple guidelines for using them.

TOXIC SUBSTANCES IN OILS

There are many toxic substances in some oils. Even canola oil, generally one of the healthier oils, contains erucic acid, which may damage heart tissue in very high doses. During the 1960s, canola oil that contained 40 percent erucic acid was marketed. Now, with improved government standards, canola oil contains only 5 percent. This oil is a good choice now that new standards are in effect. Castor oil contains 80 percent ricinoleic acid, which causes the body to throw off this oil, and everything else in the intestines, quickly.

Peanut oil may contain carcinogenic substances, as peanuts are grown in damp places and may be contaminated by fungus. Aflatoxins, which are produced by a type of fungus, are found primarily in peanuts and corn, but traces may be found in many other grains. Aflatoxins have been implicated in liver cancer.

Peanut oil—even though it is a majority monounsaturated oil and contains only 17 percent fats—appears to promote arteriosclerosis, or hardening of the arteries, according to Dragoslava Vesselinovitch, D.V.M., M.S., emeritus professor of pathology at the University of Chicago.

Cottonseed oil contains up to 1.2 percent of a cyclopropene fatty acid that has a toxic effect on the liver and gallbladder. It also interferes with the functioning of needed essential fatty acids. This oil enhances the potential of the cancer-causing aflatoxins in the body. Cottonseed also contains gossypol, a substance containing benzene rings, which may irritate the digestive tract. This oil may also cause shortness of breath and water retention in the lungs. Cottonseed also has the highest content of pesticide residues.

Be very careful to not use rancid oils. Heating oils to high temperatures produces free radicals that damage the body. Choose oils that come in dark containers to protect them from light and heat, and store them in the refrigerator.

REDUCING UNHEALTHY FATS

A study reported in the *American Journal of Clinical Nutrition* said that eating olive oil lowered levels of harmful LDLs even more than eating a low-fat diet, without changing the level of beneficial HDLs. A tablespoon of olive oil contains an average of almost 10 grams of monounsaturated fat. The same amount of monounsaturates can be derived from the following nutritious alternatives:

- 4 teaspoons unrefined canola oil
- 1½ tablespoons raw almond butter
- ½ fresh avocado
- ½ cup raw almonds
- 3 tablespoons raw hazelnuts
- 2 tablespoons raw macadamia nuts
- ¼ cup raw pecans
- ½ cup raw pistachios

In a study conducted at the University of Manitoba, young men fed a diet of canola products experienced lower serum cholesterol levels. The oil supplied nearly all the fat in the diet and 38 percent of all the energy requirements.

Canola oil is derived from the rapeseed plant, and, like olive oil, it is high in monounsaturated fat and helps to prevent heart disease. Unlike olive oil, canola oil has no distinct flavor, so it is a good choice if you do not enjoy the flavor of olive oil.

Remember the following when changing your diet to eliminate unhealthy fats in favor of healthy fats:

- Avoid saturated fats. Saturated fats are those that are solid or semisolid at room temperature—for example, butter, lard or the fat marbling in meats.

- Eat fish or take supplemental fish oil. Fish contain unsaturated omega-3 fatty acids that aid in lowering cholesterol.

- Use unsaturated fats. These are fats that are liquid or very soft at room temperature, like vegetable oils.

Use vegetable oils, but make sure they are cold- or expeller-pressed (unhydrogenated). These are readily available from health food stores. Virgin or crude unrefined oils like olive oil are also good.

Consume broiled fish containing high amounts of omega-3 fatty acids. Have at least three servings per week. Instead of buying bottled salad dressings, make your own dressings at home using one of the healthy oils.

Beware of any product labeled *saturated fats* or that contains coconut and/or palm kernel oils. If a product label doesn't list the source of vegetable oils, avoid it. Coconut and palm kernel oils are higher in saturated fat than animal fat, but they are often listed on product labels as vegetable oils.

Red meat, salad dressings, butter, some margarines, shortening, and oils are the most concentrated sources of fat. All fried foods should be avoided; they cause premature aging and contribute to obesity and chronic disorders such as arthritis and cardiovascular disease. Isn't this reason enough to avoid saturated fats or at least cut back on their consumption to once weekly instead of daily?

Begin to improve your health by removing red meat from your diet. If you do occasionally eat red meat, avoid marbled cuts of beef and hamburgers, and trim all fat from the edge of the meat before cooking. If you use ground turkey, grind it at home, using only skinless breast meat. The ground turkey sold in supermarkets generally contains about 14 grams of fat in just 4 ounces of meat.

To further declare war on fat, reduce your consumption of the following items—or eliminate them from your diet altogether:

- Aerosolized whipped cream
- Bacon
- Black olives
- Bologna

- Butter
- Cakes
- Cereals*
- Chocolate
- Chow mein noodles
- Cocoa
- Coconut
- Coconut oil
- Cookies*
- Corned beef
- Crab
- Crackers*
- Cream
- Cream cheese
- Creamy dressings
- Duck
- Egg yolks
- Fried foods
- Goose
- Gravies
- Ground turkey
- Hamburger
- Hot dogs
- Hydrogenated margarine
- Ice cream
- Imitation dairy products
- Lamb
- Lard
- Liver sausage

- Lobster
- Luncheon meats
- Mayonnaise
- Microwave popcorn
- Most chips
- Muffin mixes*
- Nondairy creamers
- Organ meats such as liver
- Packaged potatoes
- Packaged rice
- Palm kernel oil
- Palm oil
- Peanut butter
- Peanuts
- Pork
- Poultry skin
- Processed granola
- Refried beans*
- Salami
- Sardines
- Sausages
- Shellfish
- Shrimp
- Smoked meats
- Soft cheese
- Spare ribs
- Toaster pastries
- Whole milk
- Yellow cheeses

Above items marked with an asterisk (*) may be eaten if they are homemade and the fat content is controlled. Cake, muffin, and pancake mixes found in health food stores and natural markets, such as those produced by Fearn or Arrowhead Mills, have all-natural ingredients to which you can add a healthy sweetener and oil.

Read labels carefully, and learn to understand them. For example, the term "light" (or "lite") may refer to texture

rather than to the product's fat content. The following are a number of terms that signal a product that should be *avoided:*

- Au gratin
- Breaded
- Buttery/buttered
- Cheese/cheese sauce
- Cream/cream sauce/ creamed/creamy

- Fried (any form)
- Gravy
- Hollandaise
- Rich
- Scalloped

The following, in contrast, are terms that point to lower fat products. Look for the following:

- Broiled
- Grilled
- Poached

- Roasted
- Steamed
- Stir-fried

Instead of high-fat meals featuring meat as the main course, eat high-protein, low-fat meals such as lentil and bean soups, vegetable soups, pasta and vegetables, brown rice with steamed vegetables, spaghetti with soy chunks, meatless veggie chili, beans and brown rice, and tofu dishes. Top vegetable dishes with sesame seeds or raw nuts. For an occasional meat dish, have turkey or chicken breast, or choose poached or broiled fish instead.

Table 28.2 offers some suggestions for healthier foods that can be substituted for the higher fat foods typical of the American diet.

Be on the lookout for the fat in foods and in your diet as a whole. You should not only focus on improving the quality of the fats you eat, but be aware of how many of the calories in your diet come from fat. The goal is 10 percent fat, no more than 15 percent fat. Read labels carefully! Use the following formula to find the percentage of calories from fat in foods:

1. Look at the label on the product for the grams of fat and the number of calories per serving.
2. Multiply the number of fat grams by 9. This is the number of fat calories.
3. Take the calculated number and divide by the number of calories per serving listed on the label. The answer will be less than 1.
4. To get the percent of calories from the fat, multiply this number by 100.

For example, a cracker product's label says that one serving contains 70 calories and 4 grams of fat. Multiply 4 (the number of fat grams) by 9 (the number of calories per fat gram) to get 36. This is the number of calories from fat per serving. Divide 36 by 70 (the number of calories per serving) to get 0.514; then multiply by 100 to get 51.4. This is the fat calorie percentage—it means that 51.4 percent, or

TABLE 28.2 SENSIBLE ALTERNATIVES

Instead of the items in the left-hand column, try substituting the suggestion in the right-hand column.

TYPICAL AMERICAN DIET	HEALTHY ALTERNATIVE
Beef	Broiled fish, turkey breast, or beans (in casseroles, stews, and tacos)
Bologna	Baked turkey breast
Breaded and fried fish	Haddock, broiled
Canned biscuits	Homemade biscuits made with plain low-fat yogurt, whole-wheat flour, aluminum-free baking powder, and canola oil
Commercial canned soups	Homemade soups or Health Valley or Hain's brand soups
Commercial fried chicken	Home-roasted chicken. One 3.9-ounce serving of commercial fried chicken breast can contain as much as 22.3 grams of fat, whereas the same amount of skinless home-roasted chicken breast contains only approximately 4.1 grams of fat.
Danish pastry	Whole-grain muffin
Fried potatoes	Baked potatoes, not topped with butter or sour cream. Try topping with plain yogurt or seasoning and a little sesame or canola oil.
Hamburgers	Soy or veggie burgers
Ice cream	Frozen fruit juice or sherbet
One whole egg	Two egg whites or egg substitute
Potato chips	Plain popcorn
Tuna canned in oil	Tuna canned in water
Vegetables with cheese sauce	Vegetables with lemon juice

more than half, of the calories per serving of the crackers is due to the fat content!

A less precise but very easy method for testing the fat in foods such as crackers is to simply rub the item on a paper napkin. A grease mark indicates a high fat content. And in commercial processed foods such as crackers, the fat content is usually from some type of oil that is harmful, such as hydrogenated oils or palm or coconut oils.

Beware of cereals and granolas that are labeled as "healthy." Although they are advertised to be great for health, many are loaded with fat, as well as with salt and sugar. Many granola products also contain unhealthy tropical oils, and the nuts in them are high in fat as well, neither of which is desirable in a breakfast. Breakfast should have a good source of fiber, protein, complex carbohydrates, and vitamins, with a few calories from small amounts of fat. The calories from fat should be no more than 10 percent.

Lunch also can be loaded with disguised fats. Adding cheese to a sandwich can not only increase the calorie content by 100 calories per slice, but can give you an additional 66 calories' worth of dietary fat. Processed luncheon meats are full of fat and sodium, too. Even luncheon meat made from turkey can be high in fat calories. To cut down on fat in lunches, try eating skinless turkey breast or tuna that is packed in water instead of oil and use low-fat mayonnaise.

Other suggestions for reducing the amount of fat in your diet include the following:

- Use raw apple cider vinegar and oil in place of creamy salad dressings.

- Add flavor without fat to baked potatoes using plain yogurt and chives. Or mash tofu with a little low-fat (egg-free) mayonnaise, and add herbs for seasoning.

- Replace the oil in most recipes with plain low-fat yogurt.

- Steam or stir-fry vegetables. Or cook sliced vegetables with mushrooms in their own juices instead of in butter or oil. Mushrooms, onions, and garlic add flavor.

- Sauté foods in canola oil with a tablespoon of water added to prevent the oil from getting too hot. Or substitute vegetable broth or bouillon for oil.

- Try poaching instead of frying firm-fleshed fish. Use 4 parts water and 1 part lemon juice and herbs. Cook chicken in a blend of 4 parts water to 1 part tamari sauce and/or pineapple juice for an excellent flavor. Add fresh or granulated garlic to everything you poach, for flavor enhancement and health.

- Substitute turkey for chicken. Skinless turkey contains about one-third less fat than skinless chicken.

- When baking chicken, turkey, or fish, place the food on a rack so that it doesn't cook in the fat drippings. Cover the pan to keep the food moist instead of basting with fatty drippings or oil. Trim all fat and remove the skin before cooking poultry.

- Remove fat from soups, meat stocks, chili, and stew by refrigerating them for a few hours. Fat is then easily skimmed off the top.

- For low-fat sauces, purée vegetables or use potato flakes as the thickening base. Arrowroot is also a good thickener.

- In sauces that call for cream, substitute nonfat dry milk or plain low-fat yogurt. Yogurt can be substituted for sour cream in most recipes.

- Substitute mashed tofu for ricotta and cottage cheese in recipes.

- When serving potatoes or steamed vegetables, replace butter with sesame or olive oil and top with chives. Butter melts and looks like other oils when placed on cooked potatoes or other vegetables.

- Use egg-free safflower or soy mayonnaise, available in health food stores and natural foods markets.

- Consume oil-free breads such as macrobiotic bread. These are available in health food stores.

- Avoid all processed meats, such as hot dogs, luncheon meats, sausage, and bacon, which are very high in saturated fats as well as in sodium.

- When making muffins, cornbread, biscuits, and the like, use low-fat plain yogurt in place of butter or oil.

- To grease baking pans and casserole dishes, use liquid lecithin in place of oil.

- Replace one whole egg with two egg whites, or use arrowroot powder or egg replacement in recipes.

- Use walnuts in place of peanuts.

- Use crackers made without oil.

FAT REPLACEMENTS IN PROCESSED FOODS

In theory, the perfect fat replacement would be one that contributes everything that healthy fats do, but without the unwanted calories, saturated fat, and cholesterol. The question remains: Can reduced-fat products actually lower overall calorie intake and have a significant impact on the total fat intake?

Fat replacements can help reduce a food's fat and calorie levels while maintaining some of the desirable qualities fat brings to food, such as mouth feel, texture, and flavor. Under U.S. Food and Drug Administration (FDA) regulations, fat replacements usually fall into one of two categories: food additives or generally recognized as safe (GRAS) substances. Each has its own set of regulatory requirements.

Fat replacements may be carbohydrate-, protein-, or fat-based substances. The first to hit the market used carbohydrate as the main ingredient. Avicel, for example, is a cellulose gel introduced in the mid-1960s as a food stabilizer. Carrageenan, a seaweed derivative, was approved for use as an emulsifier, stabilizer, and thickener in food in 1961. Its use as a fat replacement became popular in the early 1990s. Polydextrose (Litesse) came on the market in 1981 as a humectant, a substance that helps food products to retain moisture. Other substances in this category include dextrins, maltodextrins, fiber, gums, starch, and modified food starch. The FDA has affirmed many carbohydrate-based fat replacements as GRAS.

Although originally intended to perform certain technical functions in food that would improve overall quality, some carbohydrate-based fat replacements are now used specifically to reduce the calorie content of foods. They provide from 0 to 4 calories per gram. They are used in a variety of foods, including dairy-type products, sauces, frozen desserts, salad dressings, processed meats, baked goods, spreads, chewing gum, and sweets.

Protein-based fat substitutes came along in the early 1990s. These and fat-based replacements were designed specifically to replace fat in foods. One form, microparticulated protein product (MPP) is made from whey protein or milk and egg protein. Examples of this type of product are Simplesse and Trailblazer. These fat replacements provide 1 to 4 calories per gram, depending on the water content, and are approved for use in frozen dessert-type foods. The FDA has agreed that whey-based MPP conforms to FDA definitions of whey protein concentrate, such as a fat replacement, Dairy-Lo, a GRAS substance. Therefore, whey-based MPP can be used in other foods, including reduced-fat versions of butter, sour cream, cheese, yogurt, salad dressing, margarine, mayonnaise, baked goods, coffee creamer, soups, and sauces.

Another type of protein-based fat replacement, called protein blends, combine animal or vegetable protein, gums, food starch, and water. They are made with FDA-approved ingredients and are used in frozen desserts and baked goods.

Olestra

Olestra (sold under the brand name Olean) is an example of a fat-based fat replacement. The FDA approved olestra, which is made by Procter & Gamble, in January 1996, for use in potato chips, crackers, tortilla chips, and other savory snacks. Frito-Lay had the first products on the market under the brand name WOW! potato chips and tortilla chips.

Olestra has properties similar to those of naturally occurring fat, but it provides 0 calories and no fat. That is because olestra is undigestible; it passes through the digestive tract but is not absorbed into the body. This is due to its unique molecular structure: a center unit of sucrose (sugar) with six, seven, or eight fatty acids attached. Olestra's configuration also makes it possible for the substance to be exposed to high temperatures, such as frying—a quality most other fat replacements lack.

Olestra has its drawbacks. Studies show that it causes intestinal cramps and loose stools in some individuals. Also, according to clinical tests, olestra reduces the absorption of fat-soluble nutrients, such as vitamins A, D, E, and K and carotenoids, from foods that are eaten at the same time as olestra-containing products. Tests by Procter & Gamble show that no reduction in absorption of fat-soluble vitamins occurs when vitamins are added to compensate for lack of absorption caused by eating foods containing olestra. To address these concerns, the FDA approved olestra on condition that vitamins A, D, E, and K be added to olestra-containing foods and that Procter & Gamble continue studies on consumption and long-term effects of olestra.

Concern with olestra's drawbacks led one of olestra's critics, the Center for Science in the Public Interest—a nonprofit consumer advocacy organization—to file an objection to the FDA's approval, which was rejected.

Other Fat Replacements

Some other fat-based replacements are being considered or developed. Salatrim (which stands for *short and long-chain* acid *triglyceride molecules*) is the generic name for a family of reduced-calorie fats that are only partially absorbed in the body. Salatrim provides 5 calories per gram. A petition seeking FDA's affirmation that Salatrim is GRAS was filed in June 1994. An example of its use is in Hershey's semisweet chocolate-flavored reduced-fat baking chips. Caprenin, another Procter & Gamble product, is a 5-calorie-per-gram fat substitute for cocoa butter in candy bars. A petition seeking FDA's affirmation that Caprenin is GRAS was filed in 1991. Emulsifiers are fat-based substances that are used with water to replace all or part of the shortening content in cake mixes, cookies, icings, and dairy products. They contain the same number of calories per weight as regular fat, but less is used, resulting in fat and calorie reductions.

Dialkyl dihexadecylmalonate (DDM) is a fat-based substance that is not absorbed by the body and can be used in frying and baking. Frito-Lay has been studying this fat substitute since 1986, although it has not yet petitioned the FDA for approval. Also on the horizon is a fat substitute made by combining starches and/or gums with small amounts of oil. Opta Food Ingredients Inc., received an exclusive license for such a process, called Fantesk, from the U.S. Department of Agriculture (USDA). This fat replacement would give foods the taste and texture of regular fat but provides less than 0.5 grams of fat per serving.

Even with advances such as these, it is still best to consume small amounts of healthy natural fats as part of a balanced diet of nutritious whole foods.

CHAPTER TWENTY-NINE

MEAT AND DAIRY PRODUCTS

Cheese and salt meat . . . should be sparingly eat.

—*Benjamin Franklin, American politician, writer, and scientist*

Red meat and whole-fat dairy products have a lot in common. Both are high in fat and carry a possibility of bacterial and chemical contamination. It is commonly accepted today that limiting or eliminating red meat in the diet and using skim or no milk products may be healthy practices for most people.

RETHINKING MEAT

The Farm Animal Reform Movement (FARM) reported that in the year 2000, 1.32 million—or 54 percent—of all deaths in the United States were attributable to diseases for which the consumption of animal products represents a substantial risk factor, according to a panel of physicians specializing in diet and health.

Heart Disease, Cancer, and Kidney Disease

As long ago as 1961, the *Journal of the American Medical Association* reported that eating a vegetarian diet could prevent an estimated 90 to 97 percent of heart disease cases. One major reason for the negative effects of eating meat is its fat content. A high intake of fat is associated with an increased risk of both cancer and heart disease. Fat is marbled all through meat, particularly red meat, and so cannot be completely removed. Red meat is a staple in American diets, which may be part of the reason why heart disease and cancer are the leading causes of death in the United States.

Carnivores (animals that eat meat) have unique digestive characteristics. They chew in an up-and-down motion, and only briefly, to chop up their food, then swallow it immediately so that it is broken down as it moves through the digestive tract. This has evolved because animal flesh decays very quickly, and the byproducts from decay could rapidly poison the bloodstream if it remained in the body for too long. The digestive system of carnivores is, therefore, relatively short so that food can move through it quickly. Carnivorous animals have an "almost unlimited

capacity to handle saturated fats and cholesterol," according to Dr. William Collins of the New York Maimonides Medical Center.

In herbivores (animals that live on herbs, grasses, and plants that are coarse, fibrous, and bulky), food is first digested in the mouth by ptyalin, an enzyme found in saliva. To be broken down, grasses and plants must be chewed well and thoroughly mixed with ptyalin. Herbivores have molar teeth that they use to grind their food with a side-to-side motion. Grass-eating animals do not have claws or sharp teeth. They drink by sucking water up, as compared with the lapping action performed by carnivores. As they do not eat rapidly decaying food like carnivores, their food needs longer to pass through the digestive system to be broken down. Herbivores have digestive systems that are up to ten to twelve times the length of their own bodies.

Studies have shown that eating a meat-based diet is very harmful to animals that normally eat grass and other plants. If a rabbit is fed a half pound of meat daily, its blood vessels become caked with fat and atherosclerosis develops in as little as two months. Like that of the rabbit, the human digestive system is not designed to digest meat.

Human and anthropoid apes (orangutans, chimpanzees, and gorillas) have very similar digestive organs. Anthropoid apes primarily eat fruits and nuts. They have molars to grind and chew food, and their saliva contains ptyalin to digest grass and plants. Their intestines are twelve times the length of their bodies, for the gradual digestion of fruits and vegetables.

Humans have characteristics much like those of these fruit-and-nut eaters. The human digestive system, tooth and jaw structure, and bodily functions are completely different from those of carnivorous animals. Just like those of the apes, the human digestive system is twelve times the length of the body. Physiologically, therefore, humans are not carnivores. Our anatomy, digestive system, and instincts are suited to a diet of fruits, nuts, grains, and vegetables.

A twenty-five year study of 25,000 Seventh Day Adventists, who are predominantly vegetarians, compared them with a group of nonvegetarians matched by age and sex. The Adventist men were found to have half the cancer death rate of their meat-eating counterparts. Adventist women had only two-thirds the cancer death rate of non-Adventist women. The Adventists also live longer. In another study, a group of members of the Church of Jesus Christ of Latter-Day Saints (LDS, also known as Mormons), another group who eat little meat, also had a 50-percent lower incidence of cancer than the general population.

The New England Journal of Medicine reported on an analysis of the diet of more than 88,000 women over a six-year period. Those who ate the most animal fat were nearly twice as likely to develop colon cancer as those who ate the least. Women who ate red meat as a main course every day were *two and half times* more likely to develop the disease than those who ate little or none.

Urea and uric acid, nitrogen compounds, are the most prominent wastes that collect in the body as a result of eating meat. Beefsteak contains approximately 15 grams of uric acid per pound. The kidneys have to work three times as hard to eliminate toxic nitrogen compounds from a meat-based diet than from a vegetarian diet. A young body can handle the extra work of processing meat with no outward signs of harm, but as the body ages, the kidneys can wear out and fail to work efficiently. Kidney disease is a frequent result. In 1906 and 1907, Dr. Irving Fisher of Yale University conducted endurance tests between vegetarians and meat eaters and found that vegetarians had nearly twice the stamina of the meat eaters. In summary, the human digestive system was not designed to digest meat.

Many people who advocate eating meat do so because of its protein content. The human body does need to get protein through the diet, specifically the eight essential amino acids. Meat is not the only complete protein containing all eight amino acids, however. Soybeans and products made from soybeans, such as tofu, tempeh, and soymilk, are complete proteins. They provide all the amino acids humans need. Rice and legumes together also make complete proteins. So not only is the human body not designed to digest meat, it has no real nutritional need of it.

Antibiotics

Nearly 50 percent of all the antibiotics produced in our country are fed to animals to increase their growth and prevent bacterial disease. This continued low-level use of antibiotics increases the risk of breeding super-drug-resistant bacteria that may be transmitted from the animal to meat consumers. Bacteria can build up a tolerance to antibiotics, finally reaching a point where the drug is ineffective. The Humane Farming Association reports that "veal and hogs are infected with mutant bacteria, requiring lots of antibiotics."

In 1998, news services across the country reported on the findings from the U.S. Centers for Disease Control and Prevention (CDC) that indicated an increase in drug-resistance from 6 percent of *Salmonella* bacteria samples in 1979 to 34 percent of samples in 1996. One strain of *Salmonella* has become resistant to the five most commonly used antibiotics (ampicillin, chloramphenicol, streptomycin, sulfonamides, and tetracycline) and has become a major cause of illness in humans and animals in Europe, especially the United Kingdom.

Tetracycline, an antibiotic added to chicken feed, was linked to an outbreak of severe food poisoning by Minnesota health officials. The chickens harbored a highly resistant strain of *Salmonella* bacteria that was passed on to the people who consumed the meat. Several victims had to be hospitalized. This has led many health professionals to petition the U.S. Food and Drug Administration (FDA) to ban the use of antibiotics in chicken and cattle feed. But lobbyists representing the poultry, beef, and pharmaceutical industries have been successful in protesting the ban so far.

Antibiotics given to cattle, hogs, chickens, and sheep can produce other problems in people as well. These secondary antibiotics contribute to candidiasis and all forms of yeast infections. Over a period of time, if ingested in sufficient quantities, antibiotics destroy the "friendly" bacteria in the intestines, which are vital for protecting the body against infection.

Raw meat is in a state of continual decay. It will contaminate everything it comes into contact with, including the cook's hands, cutting boards, and any other surface it touches. The bacteria in raw meat is not always killed if the meat is undercooked, barbecued, or roasted, and may become a source of infection to the unwary consumer.

Hormones

Hormones fed to cattle to speed growth and increase milk production are possible culprits behind the increases in female disorders like severe hot flashes, painful menses, breast lumps, premature breast growth in young girls, and even cancer of the uterus and breast. Anabolic steroids, whose dangers have been well recorded, are also used to increase growth rates in cattle. One estimate suggests that 80 percent of cattle raised in U.S. feedlots are being given growth hormones. These hormones can cause premature aging and impotence in men.

Chickens often retain estrogen pellets that they are given to promote growth and plumpness. Most retailers fail to remove these pellets because they add weight.

Other Potential Contaminants

Another downside of eating meat lies in the residues of pesticides and other chemicals it often contains. These toxins tend to be concentrated in animals' fatty tissues—and, of course, meat contains a lot of fat. They are also present in animal livers, since the liver is the organ of detoxification. These dangerous chemicals may contribute to cancer and other illnesses. Eating meat may also increase the risk of getting cancer because potentially carcinogenic preservatives like nitrites and nitrates are added to mask green discoloration that happens as the meat ages.

Other dangers can develop during cooking, especially charcoal-broiling. In 2 pounds of charcoal-broiled steak there is as much benzopyrene, a known carcinogen (cancer-causing agent), as in 600 cigarettes. In one study, mice fed benzopyrene developed stomach tumors and leukemia. Even if meat is not charcoal broiled, searing the meat at high temperatures to seal in the juices results in the formation of methylcholanthrene, another potentially carcinogenic substance.

Besides other contaminants in meat, animals going to slaughter experience radical biochemical changes. Blood levels of stress hormones, particularly adrenaline, increase drastically when they experience other animals around them dying and struggling to stay alive. These high amounts of hormones remain in the tissues of the meat and are later ingested by meat consumers. The Nutrition Institute of America reports, "The flesh of an animal carcass is loaded with toxic blood and other waste byproducts."

Animals raised for meat are often infected with diseases that either go undetected or are ignored by meat processors or inspectors. If an animal has cancer or a tumor, the diseased part of the animal is cut away, and the rest of the body is sold in parts. Yet it is possible that the disease may have circulated throughout the animal. Worse yet, the diseased parts may be incorporated into mixed meats such as hot dogs or luncheon meats. In addition to the 8,964 million animals reported in USDA's 2001 slaughter reports, another 888.5 million, or 9 percent of the total, suffered lingering deaths from disease, malnutrition, injury, or suffocation associated with today's factory farming practices.

Dangers to humans from feeding and processing practices were brought under great scrutiny with the 1996 outbreak of bovine spongiform encephalopathy (BSE) or transmissible spongiform encephalopathy (TSE) in cattle in British beef herds. The popular press quickly labeled these disorders "mad cow disease." The disease causes the structure of brain tissue to change to a spongelike form and the condition is ultimately fatal. A similar disease, known as scrapie, is found in sheep, and variations have also been found in elk, mink, deer, and goats in both the United States and Canada. The human version of the disease is called kuru. The 1996 outbreak, which came ten years after the initial identification of the diseases as the cause of the death of British cattle, was related to the deaths of twenty-one British citizens from Creutzfeldt-Jakob disease (CJD), a progressive and ultimately terminal neurological disorder. During the time of the outbreak, British medical authorities announced a possible link between BSE and CJD in humans. The British deaths were believed to be caused by eating meat from cattle infected with BSE. One possible cause of the disease in cattle appears to be the practice of mixing cattle byproducts into stockyard cattle feed. It was the use of infected stockyard renderings (ground parts of animal meat, fat, and bone from leftover byproducts of meat production) in feed mixer that was believed to have triggered the BSE epidemic in England.

But I *Like* Meat!

Removing red meat from the diet is one definite way to improve your health. However, I am not advocating strict vegetarianism as a way of life for everyone. If you cannot, or do not wish to, eat a vegetarian diet, there are still things you can do to minimize the risks posed by eating meat.

Unfortunately, much of the meat on our tables has been adversely affected by improper handling and processing. If you eat meat, consume only organically raised, range-fed beef and free-range poultry and eggs. Some markets now offer beef that is raised without hormones, antibiotics, and other harmful substances.

Avoid eating ground beef and marbled cuts of beef. Always trim all possible fat before cooking. Remove the skin and fat from poultry. As a substitute for ground beef, eat ground turkey—and grind it yourself at home (or have the butcher grind it at the store), using only skinless breast. When cooking meat (or fish), keep it on a rack and out of the drippings. Use paper towels and a disinfectant to clean anything that comes into contact with raw meat or poultry. Sponges or cloth towels are extremely difficult to sterilize. It is too tempting to reuse them before laundering.

Quorn, a meat-mimicking food from the mushroom family (mycoprotein), contains all eight essential amino acids, but has more fiber than meat, fewer calories, less fat, and no cholesterol. The texture of mycoprotein is more like that of beef or chicken than that of soy or grain products. Quorn is good for vegetarians or people seeking a meat replacement; however, vegans (people who consume no animal products at all) will not find it acceptable because it does contain egg white and milk protein.

DAIRY PRODUCTS

Pasteurized and homogenized milk have a high fat content and, conversely, a low calcium content. They retain toxins that are concentrated in the fat. No other animal on this earth drinks milk as a natural element of the diet after being weaned.

Lactase is an enzyme produced by the small intestines of young children that is needed to digest lactose (milk sugar), which is found in milk and dairy products. Lactase production generally declines with age. Most adults, and some children, are unable to digest the lactose found in milk, a condition known as lactose intolerance. According to the *Nutrition Action Health Letter,* almost 70 percent of the

Casein Intolerance—A Hidden Problem?

Casein is the principal protein found in the milk of all mammals. Usually found combined with calcium in milk to form calcium caseinate, casein can also be found as small particles, called caseinogen, suspended in liquid milk. In individuals with an intolerance to casein in milk (and casein or casein derivatives in prepared food products), the immune system produces antibodies to attack the invading casein molecules.

In the past, caseinate has been added to some products while appearing on the label only as *hydrolyzed protein* or *hydrolyzed animal protein.* James E. Gern and Hugh A. Sampson, research physicians at the Johns Hopkins University School of Medicine in Baltimore, have charged that meat processors were incorporating sodium caseinate, a milk derivative, in hot dogs and bologna but failing to identify that ingredient for the benefit of individuals whose allergic reactions to dairy substances could be serious. Many products labeled "nondairy" actually contain sodium caseinate, misleading consumers who are sensitive to milk and dairy products. Among the vulnerable are those who have been diagnosed as lactose-intolerant and who lack the enzymes to digest dairy products. Manufacturers are not required to list ingredients that make up less than one-half of 1 percent by weight of a product, but even in that small an amount, they can cause problems for people with severe allergies.

If you have any questions about a food product that are not answered on the label, ask the manufacturer directly. If you are a vegetarian who chooses to eliminate dairy products from your diet, you should be careful of this "hidden" milk product also. Be on the alert for any of the following ingredients: butter, casein, cheese, galactose, lactose, milk, milk solids, natural ingredients, nondairy (this does not necessarily mean milk-free), and sodium caseinate. Tuna (canned tuna may also contain hidden milk products), or yogurt.

Other good reasons to eliminate dairy foods from your diet include the following:

- Ovarian cancer has been linked to dairy products (the problem is the milk sugar, not the milk fat).
- Cataracts are associated with galactose (a component of milk sugar).
- Food allergies to milk and dairy products are common and can cause a wide range of elusive symptoms.
- Dairy products can be contaminated with traces of antibiotics.
- Cow's milk products are extremely low in iron and may actually promote iron deficiency.
- Two glasses of whole milk contain about the same amount of cholesterol as one 3-ounce beefsteak.

Finally, many promoters of dairy products say that they are important for preventing (or even reversing) osteoporosis. This is simply not true. Dairy products are relatively concentrated sources of calcium, which is important for strong bones, but if you eat a balanced diet with plenty of fresh green vegetables, you can get plenty of calcium without the potential risks of dairy foods.

If you are not yet convinced that adopting a diet without meat and dairy products would be good for you, consider the following list of common complaints that can be directly linked to the consumption of these foods: acne, allergies, anger, bedwetting, body odor, colic, colitis attacks, congestion, runny nose, constipation, depression, dermatitis, diarrhea, dry scaly skin, edema, excess mucus, fatigue, gas and bloating, headaches, heart disorders, hemorrhoids, hives, hormone imbalance, hot flashes, hyperactivity, impaired digestion, impotence, irritability, malabsorption, obesity, seborrhea, and sinusitis. It is apparent that a reduction of meat and dairy products in the diet will lead to a longer and healthier life.

world's population cannot tolerate lactose and develop such symptoms as gas, bloating, and diarrhea if they consume milk. Cheese and soured products may be tolerated in small amounts, because cheese has only about 2 percent lactose and the lactose in soured products, like yogurt, is already partly predigested by the fermenting bacteria.

As with meat, there can be problems with contamination of milk and dairy products. In 1986, milk cows were quarantined and milk products recalled in eight states after the products were found to contain dangerous amounts of heptachlor, a substance that has been banned from use in the United States for years, but is still manufactured here. Genetically engineered recombinant bovine growth hor-

mone (BGH), which is injected into cows to force them to produce more milk, is banned in Canada and Europe, but is still used in 4 to 5 percent of all U.S. dairy cows. Scientists have warned that this controversial hormone can result in significantly higher levels (400 to 500 percent or more) of the potent chemical hormone insulinlike growth factor (IGF-1) in the milk of injected cows and in dairy products made from that milk, and that this could translate into an increased risk of breast, prostate, and colon cancer in those who eat these foods.

There is evidence that babies fed on cow's milk are more likely to develop diabetes later in life than those who are not, according to an article published in the British medical

Safe Keeping of Meat and Dairy Products

If you choose to make some meat and dairy products a part of your diet, it is important to do so safely. Because of their relatively high fat content, these foods are particularly prone to spoilage. The table below indicates how long uncooked meat and dairy products can safely be stored in both the refrigerator and the freezer, according to the Food Marketing Institute and the U.S. Department of Agriculture.

FOOD PRODUCT	MAXIMUM STORAGE TIME	
	IN REFRIGERATOR	IN FREEZER
MEAT AND MEAT PRODUCTS		
Beef		
ground	1–2 days	3–4 months
steaks and roasts	3–5 days	6–12 months
Chicken		
giblets	1–2 days	3–3 months
parts	1–2 days	9 months
whole	1–2 days	12 months
Luncheon meat	3–5 days	1–2 months
Pork		
chops	3–5 days	4–6 months
ground	1–2 days	3–4 months
roasts	3–5 days	4–6 months
Sausage	1–2 days	2–3 days
DAIRY PRODUCTS		
Cheese	3–4 weeks	Can be frozen for a matter of months, but freezing will affect texture and taste.
Eggs		
fresh, in shell	3 weeks	Not recommended.
hard-boiled	1 week	Not recommended.
Ice cream	Not recommended	1 month.
Milk	5 days	1 month

journal *Lancet* in October 1996. According to Neal D. Barnard, M.D., president of the Physicians Committee for Responsible Medicine, epidemiologic studies in various countries show a strong correlation between the use of dairy products and the incidence of type 1 diabetes.

Crohn's disease may be triggered by bacteria in milk, *Mycobacterium paratuberculosis*, that do not die during the pasteurization process, according to researcher John Hermon-Taylor of St. George's Hospital Medical School, one of Britain's largest hospitals.

CHAPTER THIRTY

CAFFEINE

Good coffee is like friendship—rich and warm and strong.

—*Pan American Coffee ad*

Caffeine is the most popular natural stimulant on planet Earth. Eight out of ten people consume it in one form or another every day. Beverages containing caffeine, primarily colas and coffee in the United States and tea in much of the rest of the world, are second in popularity only to water.

Historically, the Turks were the first people to adopt coffee as a drink, which they enhanced with exotic spices. Throughout history, coffee has been banned, declared sacred, baptized, blessed, and cursed—and, under Turkish law, a woman could divorce her husband if he failed to provide her with a daily quota of coffee.

Caffeine is a substance readily found in nature in the leaves, berries, seeds, or bark of more than 100 plant species. The use of caffeine from plants is estimated to date back to the Stone Age. Paleolithic humans chewed the leaves, seeds, and bark from caffeine-containing plants to increase energy and elevate moods.

Discoveries in Ethiopia indicate that a mixture of raw coffee beans and fat was used for food more than 2,000 years ago. The earliest brewing of teas and coffee as a beverage, a form in which a higher concentration of caffeine is available, is believed to have begun 4,800 years ago. Chinese legend dates the brewing of tea to about 2737 B.C.E. and attributes the discovery to the emperor Shen Nung.

The primary natural sources of caffeine today are tea leaves, coffee beans, kola nuts, yerba maté leaves, and cacao beans (the source of cocoa for chocolate). Cocoa contains a much smaller concentration of caffeine than coffee or tea. However, cacao beans also contain theobromine, another purine family compound, in a concentration seven times greater than that of caffeine in coffee. Because of the concentration of theobromine, the caffeinelike effects of cocoa are still significant.

HOW CAFFEINE WORKS

The identification and isolation of caffeine as a substance is a very recent occurrence. Caffeine was separated and identified from coffee in 1820 and from tea in 1827. Shortly thereafter, experiments determined that the stimulant effect of both coffee and tea came from caffeine.

Caffeine is a member of the uric acid/purine group of chemical compounds. This chemical group consists of the compounds adenine, caffeine, guanine, 1-methylxanthine, paraxanthine, purine, theobromine, theophylline, and xanthine. Two of the compounds in this group, adenine and guanine, are two of the four compounds that make up the four basic letters of the genetic alphabet contained in DNA. Caffeine's similarity to adenine and guanine is a possible cause for concern, as it is believed these substances may be associated with birth defects.

Caffeine is also a member of the alkaloid family of nitrogen-containing organic compounds produced by plants. Many members of the alkaloid group are pharmacologically active substances. In addition to caffeine, these include atropine, cocaine, morphine, nicotine, and quinine.

Caffeine's ability to increase alertness is actually an indirect result. The caffeine molecule very closely mimics the structure of adenosine, a sleep-promoting compound classified as a neuromodulator (a body chemical that induces nerve cells to increase or decrease the rate at which they fire). The body produces adenosine when the nervous system is activated. A buildup of adenosine starts a chemical reaction that signals the firing of neurons to slow down and sets the stage for rest or sleep. Body chemicals such as hormones and neurotransmitters exert their effects by binding to sites called receptors on specific types of body cells, triggering the cells in question to start (or stop) performing a certain activity. In the case of adenosine, it binds to receptors on nerve cells and causes them to fire more slowly, inducing rest. Because it mimics adenosine, caffeine can bind to adenosine receptor sites within the body. This blocks an actual adenosine molecule from binding to that site. Thus, caffeine prevents the signal for rest from occurring.

A major pharmacological use of caffeine is to accelerate the action of other drugs. When analgesics (painkillers) are combined with caffeine, they can be taken in smaller doses than the analgesics alone, and be just as effective; 30 to 40

> ## Theophylline and Synthetic Caffeine
>
> Theophylline is a compound related to caffeine. It has a greater stimulatory effect on heart rate and breathing than caffeine does, and it is one of the most commonly prescribed drugs for the treatment of diseases that cause breathing difficulty, such as asthma, bronchitis, and emphysema. The theophylline used as a pharmaceutical drug is produced from the caffeine contained in coffee. Because a great quantity of caffeine is created as a byproduct of the decaffeination of coffee and tea, there has been no demand for the development of synthetic caffeine.

percent less analgesic is needed to produce the same results when it is combined with caffeine. Caffeine is also used in the formulas of certain diuretic medications and allergy and cold compounds, and in drugs used in the treatment of migraine headaches, bronchial asthma, and sleep apnea in newborn infants. Caffeine is also used alone as an antidrowsiness, antisleep stimulant.

CAFFEINE'S EFFECTS ON HEALTH

In spite of their great popularity, products containing caffeine should be consumed with caution. The use of caffeine has been associated with many health problems. Studies seem to agree that drinking two or three cups of coffee a day is generally no reason for concern, except for pregnant women, nursing mothers, people with heart problems, and, of course, people with a sensitivity to caffeine.

A research team in the United States and Sweden found that the consumption of as little as one to three cups of coffee a day by a pregnant woman was associated with a 30 percent higher rate of miscarriage. Because it is a natural diuretic, caffeine consumption has been linked to calcium loss and decreased bone mineral density, a precursor of osteoporosis, in women. Carbonated caffeinated soft drinks are also high in phosphates, which further cause the body to eliminate calcium as they are excreted, even if the body must rob calcium from the bones to do this. Oftentimes the sugar that comes with the caffeine "fix" contributes to obesity, tooth decay, and nutritional deficiencies, particularly in youngsters. The importance of this becomes more obvious when you consider that boys and men between the ages of twelve and twenty-nine consume an *average* of 160 gallons of caffeinated soft drinks a year—that's almost 2 quarts a day.

Studies have linked caffeine use to abnormal heart rhythms, stroke, heart disease, type 2 diabetes, first-trimester miscarriages, abnormal fetal development and low birth weight in infants, adverse drug interactions, anxiety and panic attacks, bladder irritation, certain types of cancer, higher cholesterol levels, fibroids and fibrocystic breast disease, heartburn, hypertension, osteoporosis, prostate irritation, sleep disorders, and ulcers.

Although flawed data from some early scientific studies led to overly broad negative conclusions, it is nevertheless true that most people should monitor their use of caffeine, and people with sensitivities to caffeine and/or other specific health problems or conditions should limit it or avoid it altogether. If you have been consuming large amounts of caffeine, remember that it is a drug and consider its possible effect on any health problems you may have or be at risk for.

The sections that follow address the role of caffeine in particular health concerns and situations.

CAFFEINE PRECAUTIONS

As noted earlier, caffeine in general should be approached with caution. For people with certain specific health concerns, this is particularly important. Following are discussions of a number of caffeine-related disorders and circumstances that call for special awareness of the effects of caffeine.

Acidosis

Cocoa, coffee, and tea are all acid-forming foods. If you have acidosis (systemwide hyperacidity) or a hiatal hernia, or if you suffer from any kind of heartburn, eliminate these drinks from your diet.

Acne and Rosacea

According to some experts, caffeine-containing foods and beverages can cause or worsen acne. This may be more of an inference by association, however, as the link between the aggravation of rosacea (sometimes called adult acne), a type of skin inflammation in adults not related to acne, can be traced to food sensitivities or allergies associated with caffeine-containing foods. It is also possible that the processed sugar in caffeinated soft drinks aggravates acne.

Others claim that acne and rosacea are not worsened by the caffeine contained in certain foods but by the flushing effect of ingesting hot beverages, which can make the conditions look worse.

Attention Deficit Hyperactivity Disorder

The symptoms of hyperactivity or anxiety, fearfulness, and attention difficulties associated with attention deficit hyperactivity disorder (ADHD) are amplified by the effects of a poor diet that is overloaded with caffeine and/or sugar. If you or your child suffers from ADHD, remove any such foods from the menu.

Chemical Contamination of Coffee

As you sip your morning cup, you should consider that coffee is the third most heavily sprayed crop in the world, behind cotton and tobacco. Synthetic chemical pesticides, herbicides, and fertilizers are sprayed on 70 percent of the world's coffee crops.

According to conventional coffee growers, the heat of coffee roasting destroys all but about 10 percent of the chemical residue remaining on green coffee beans after harvesting. The U.S. Food and Drug Administration (FDA) considers a 90-percent reduction in residue acceptable. However, some researchers have reported different findings. One study, using more sophisticated methodologies than the studies the FDA standards are based upon, found that the levels of one DDT byproduct were the same for roasted and green beans from one sample.

If you choose to drink coffee, for the best protection from chemical contamination from a cup of coffee, consider using only organically grown coffee beans. If you drink decaffeinated coffee, use only organically grown coffee that has been decaffeinated by a Swiss or other water process. Most manufacturers remove the caffeine from coffee beans by bathing them in trichloroethylene and methylene chloride. The Swiss water process can eliminate the risk of exposure to these chemicals.

Breastfeeding

Almost all drugs enter a nursing mother's milk. Caffeine is considered in the same class as tobacco, alcohol, medicines, and drugs for breastfeeding mothers: All of these substances pass into breast milk and may be harmful to infants. Some of the possible effects of caffeine on nursing babies are a rapid heart rate, restlessness, irritability, crying, and poor sleep.

Cancer

The excessive consumption of caffeine and/or artificial sweeteners has been identified as a risk factor for bladder and kidney cancer. A high intake of coffee is indicated as one of the risk factors for prostate cancer. If you have any of these conditions, or have a family history that indicates you may be at increased risk for them, avoid caffeine.

Cardiovascular Disease

The stimulant effect of caffeine is generally detrimental for people with cardiovascular disease. The use of caffeine can increase both heart rate and blood pressure, and may contribute to strokes. If you have a history of any of these disorders, you should avoid caffeine.

Chronic Fatigue Syndrome

Stimulants such as caffeine in coffee, tea, and soft drinks may provide a quick energy boost, so it may be tempting for people with chronic fatigue syndrome to consume them. The stimulant effect of caffeine is only temporary, however, and you may actually experience an increase in fatigue when it wears off. If you have chronic fatigue syndrome, it is better to avoid using any artificial stimulants.

Colitis, Crohn's Disease, and Irritable Bowel Syndrome

Caffeine has a laxative effect and can irritate the digestive tract. It can therefore increase the pain and intensity of attacks of colitis, Crohn's disease, or irritable bowel syndrome. If you suffer from any of these problems, eliminating caffeine from your diet will likely be beneficial.

Depression

Animal studies have shown that the regular consumption of large amounts of caffeine can actually have the opposite effect of stimulation experienced at lower usage levels—that is, high doses can act as a depressant. If you have a history of depression, limit your caffeine consumption to a very low level or avoid it altogether.

Diarrhea

Caffeine's laxative effect can aggravate and prolong a bout of diarrhea. As long as you are suffering from diarrhea, avoid any foods and beverages that contain caffeine.

Diverticulitis

The caffeine in chocolate, coffee, tea, and some soft drinks can overstimulate the colon and interfere with digestion. If you have diverticulitis, eliminate caffeine from your diet.

HIV/AIDS

An immune system that is suppressed by infection with human immunodeficiency virus (HIV) or acquired immunodeficiency syndrome (AIDS) is taxed by overuse of caffeine, sugar, or any other stimulant. If you have either of these conditions, eliminate from your diet any colas or other food or drinks that contain caffeine.

Liver Disease

The liver has the greatest role of any organ in the metabolism of caffeine. The consumption of caffeine, therefore, increases liver activity and places additional stress on that vital organ, particularly if liver function is already impaired. If you have cirrhosis of the liver, a hepatitis infection, or any other liver disorder, help your liver out by avoiding foods and beverages containing caffeine.

Pregnancy

Caffeine is a substance to be avoided, if not eliminated entirely, if you are pregnant or are attempting to become pregnant. Research indicates that caffeine consumption can increase the chance of having a miscarriage and/or a low-birth-weight baby. Although more research is needed, preliminary studies show that the use of even low levels of coffee, tea, or caffeine-containing sodas can decrease the chances of becoming pregnant as well. Avoid or strictly limit your consumption of coffee, tea, chocolate, and soft drinks, as well as caffeine-containing medications, during this time.

IS CAFFEINE REALLY ADDICTIVE?

Almost all of the research that has been done on caffeine agrees that it is definitely physically addictive. It is a mood-altering central nervous system stimulant. Though milder in its effects, caffeine manipulates the same neurochemical channels that amphetamines, cocaine, and heroin do. Overuse of caffeine can result in a variety of symptoms, including irregular heartbeat, sleeplessness, headaches, nervousness, tremors, irritability, and depression. Withdrawing from heavy caffeine use can cause symptoms, too, principally a nagging headache that is unaffected by aspirin or other over-the-counter painkillers, as well as fatigue, muscle pain, lethargy, and feelings of depression. To break a caffeine addiction, therefore, it is best to cut down gradually to avoid an uncomfortable withdrawal period. Decaffeinated coffee, which has only 5 milligrams of caffeine compared with a regular brewed cup, which has 135 milligrams, might be an option. However, there are studies underway that suggest that decaffeinated coffee may increase the risk of rheumatoid arthritis in older women. Decaffeinated tea and caffeine-free soft drinks are also available.

CHAPTER THIRTY-ONE

CHOLESTEROL: CAN'T LIVE WITH IT— CAN'T LIVE WITHOUT IT

Cholesterol is not the evil molecule it is made out to be. There clearly appears to be a risk for cholesterols that are too low.

—*Joseph Mercola, D.O., physician and author*

There are many misconceptions about cholesterol, particularly that all cholesterol is bad for you. In truth, cholesterol is an essential part of every cell structure in the human body, and is vital for proper brain and nerve function. It is also the basis for the manufacture of sex hormones. Most cholesterol is manufactured in the liver, then transported through the bloodstream to where it is needed in the body. It is a fatty substance, and, because blood is mostly water, it latches on to molecules called lipoproteins to hitch a ride throughout the body.

There are two types of lipoproteins—low-density and high-density. Low-density lipoproteins (LDLs) carry cholesterol from the liver to the places where it is needed. Because they also encourage the deposit of cholesterol in the arteries, these are the "bad cholesterol" doctors warn us about. Very low-density lipoprotein (VLDL) increases the risk of coronary artery disease (CAD). High-density lipoproteins (HDLs) are the "good cholesterol." HDLs carry unneeded cholesterol away from the cells and back to the liver, where it is broken down and removed from the body. *Total cholesterol* refers to the overall level of cholesterol in the blood, including LDLs, HDLs, and VLDLs.

If the body's systems are functioning as they should, the activity of LDLs and HDLs, and cholesterol levels, remain in balance. However, if there is too much cholesterol for the HDLs to pick up promptly, or if there are not enough HDLs to do the job, cholesterol may form plaque that sticks to artery walls and can eventually lead to heart disease. Cholesterol levels are greatly influenced by diet, but they are also affected by genetic makeup.

Other fats, called triglycerides, are also carried in the blood in the form of lipoproteins. The role of triglycerides in the development of coronary disease is unclear. However, health-care professionals may be concerned and may want to run more tests if blood tests show that an individual has very high levels of triglycerides—generally, more than 400 milligrams per deciliter (mg/dL) of blood. This is because fasting triglyceride tests are an indirect measure of VLDL.

THE PROBLEM OF HIGH CHOLESTEROL

Cholesterol in the bloodstream is *serum cholesterol;* the cholesterol present in the food we eat is *dietary cholesterol.* The two are related, but are not the same thing. Eating lots of foods that are high in dietary cholesterol can raise the levels of serum cholesterol, but even if you ate no cholesterol-containing foods at all, you would still have serum cholesterol—your body needs it and your liver manufactures it. When serum cholesterol levels rise above normal limits and stay high, however, some cholesterol is left behind in the arteries. Over time, this waxy substance, known as plaque, builds up on artery walls and reduces or blocks the flow of blood. This condition is atherosclerosis, narrowing and hardening of the arteries due to the accumulation of fatty plaques. Organs that rely on the affected arteries may become damaged because the reduced flow of blood to them means that they cannot receive the oxygen or nutrients they need. If a coronary artery (one of the arteries that feeds the heart) becomes completely blocked, the result is a heart attack; if blood flow to the brain is blocked, a stroke occurs.

Some risk factors for high cholesterol and the dangers associated with it include the following:

- Age. Levels of LDLs usually increase with age.

- Gender. Until age forty-five, men generally have higher total cholesterol levels than women. Also, up to about this age, women tend to have higher HDL levels. After menopause, women's total cholesterol rises and levels of protective HDLs drop.

- Family history. If immediate family members have undesirable cholesterol levels and cardiovascular problems, the risks increase.

In addition, there are a number of disorders and other factors that can increase risk, including the following:

- Diabetes. This condition can increase triglycerides and decrease HDLs. Diabetes accelerates the development of atherosclerosis, which in turn increases the risk of heart attack.

- High blood pressure. The increased pressure against the walls of blood vessels can damage them and can accelerate the development of atherosclerosis.

- Inactivity. A sedentary lifestyle is associated with higher LDLs and lower HDLs as components of total cholesterol. Aerobic and even moderate exercise is a natural way to increase HDLs, but you should consult with a health-care provider before beginning *any* new exercise program.

- Obesity. Excess weight is associated with higher levels of VLDLs and triglycerides, and lower levels of HDLs.

- Smoking. This damages the walls of the blood vessels, making them prone to accumulate fatty deposits. It may also lower HDL levels by as much as 15 percent.

- Stress and sustained tension. This induces the secretion of hormones that cause undesirable shifts in cholesterol, HDL, and LDL levels, among other things. Try to avoid stress and sustained tension. Learn stress-management techniques to help you deal with stresses that you cannot avoid.

Certain drugs also can elevate cholesterol levels. These include steroids, high-dose oral contraceptives, furosemide (Lasix) and other diuretics, and levodopa (L-dopa, sold under the brand names Dopar, Larodopa, and Sinemet), which is used to treat Parkinson's disease. Beta-blockers, often prescribed to control high blood pressure, can cause unfavorable changes in the ratio of LDL to HDL in the blood. If you are taking any of these medications—or any medications—check with your physician concerning how they might affect your cholesterol levels.

Even drinking coffee—in particular, unfiltered coffee—can have an effect on cholesterol levels. An article in the *American Journal of Epidemiology* reported that drinking six cups of unfiltered coffee daily was significantly associated with an increase in total cholesterol, LDL cholesterol, and triglycerides, but *not* HDL cholesterol. Their results pointed to coffee oils as the main cholesterol-raising culprit, so it would seem that filtered coffee does not have as detrimental effect as boiled or unfiltered coffee.

CHOLESTEROL TESTING

There are opposing theories about the importance of high serum cholesterol levels. Some medical practitioners believe that it has little to do with heart disease and that a direct correlation has never been fully established. Studies in India, Guatemala, Poland, and the United States claim to have proven that there is no relationship between atherosclerosis and cholesterol levels. However, it is probably best to take cholesterol levels seriously and to con-

sider other tests that may help to assess the likelihood of developing heart disease.

Most medical professionals recommend that all adults twenty years of age and older have their total cholesterol and HDL levels measured at least once every five years. For people without coronary artery disease (CAD), a total blood cholesterol level of less than 200 mg/dL is considered desirable; 200 to 239 mg/dL is classified as borderline-high; and 240 mg/dL or more is high. An HDL level of less than 35 mg/dL is defined as low and is considered a risk factor for CAD.

A lipoprotein analysis, which measures LDL as well as HDL, is recommended for people who have, or are considered to be at very high risk of developing, CAD. The goal of cholesterol-lowering therapy for high-risk individuals is LDL cholesterol of about 130 mg/dL; for those with established CAD, the optimum LDL cholesterol is 100 mg/dL or lower.

Cholesterol testing requires a small sample of blood taken by pricking a fingertip. It can be done in a physician's office or at a commercial laboratory. There are also home test kits available. The Advanced Care Cholesterol Kit, manufactured by Johnson & Johnson, is available in drugstores without prescription and gives a reading in fifteen minutes. Because cholesterol levels can vary from day to day by as much as 20 to 40 mg/dL, you should take at least two samples a week or more apart.

LOWERING CHOLESTEROL WITH DIET AND NUTRITION

Meat, dairy, and fried foods are the primary sources of "bad" dietary cholesterol. Fruits and vegetables, on the other hand, are totally free of cholesterol.

Foods to Include in the Diet

Foods that are good for lowering cholesterol include the following:

- Apples
- Bananas
- Barley
- Carrots
- Cold-water fish
- Flaxseed oil
- Garlic
- Grapefruit and citrus fruits
- Lentils
- Nuts and seeds
- Oat bran
- Olive oil
- Onions
- Sea vegetables
- Soybeans and other dried beans
- Whole grains

Soluble fiber regulates the body's production and elimination of cholesterol. In a study reported in the *American Journal of Clinical Nutrition*, in which participants were given 5.1 grams of psyllium a day, researchers concluded that this treatment "produced significant net reductions in serum total and LDL-cholesterol concentrations in men and women with primary hypercholesterolemia [high serum cholesterol]. Psyllium therapy is an effective adjunct to diet therapy and may provide an alternative to drug therapy for some patients." Make sure to take in plenty of fiber in the form of fruits, vegetables, and whole grains. Water-soluble dietary fiber is particularly important in reducing serum cholesterol. It is found in barley, beans, brown rice, fruits, glucomannan, guar gum, and oats. Oat bran and brown rice bran are the best grains for lowering cholesterol.

The best nuts are raw, unsalted walnuts, pecans, peanuts, macadamia nuts, and almonds. In one study, eating almonds cut cholesterol levels by 16 points over a four-week period.

Foods to Avoid

Reduce the amount of saturated fat and cholesterol in your diet. Saturated fats include all animal fats plus coconut and palm kernel oils. Also eliminate hydrogenated fats and hardened fats and oils such as margarine, lard, and butter. (Margarine that contains plant sterols is a healthier option.) Use only unrefined cold- or expeller-pressed vegetable oils that are liquid at room temperature, such as olive, soybean, flaxseed, primrose, and black currant seed oil. Pure virgin olive oil, which appears to help reduce serum cholesterol, is especially recommended. You can consume nonfat milk, low-fat cottage cheese, and skinless white poultry meat (preferably turkey), but in moderation only. Avoid all fried foods (except for stir-fried foods prepared at home with healthy oils). Many fast-food restaurants use beef tallow (fat) to make their hamburgers, fish, chicken, and French fries. These fried foods contain high amounts of saturated fats and cholesterol. Worse, the fat they contain has been subjected to high temperatures, which results in oxidation and the formation of free radicals. Heating fat, especially frying food in fat, also produces toxic trans-fatty acids, which behave like saturated fat in clogging the arteries and raising blood cholesterol levels.

The foods highest in cholesterol are liver, pork and pork products, lobster, lard, kidneys, bacon, shrimp, sweetbreads, sausage, oysters, brains, caviar, egg yolks, and shellfish. Foods to eliminate from your diet or approach with caution include any fatty or greasy foods, most dairy products, eggs (limit them to three weekly), hot dogs, potato chips and all other refined junk foods, alcohol, cakes, candy, carbonated drinks, coffee, gravies, nondairy creamers, pies, white pasta, processed and refined foods, refined carbohydrates, tea, and white bread. Also avoid exposure to tobacco smoke, including secondhand smoke.

To lower cholesterol levels, and to keep them down, go on a monthly spirulina fast, using carrot and celery juice or lemon and steam-distilled water. (See Chapter 4.) Drink fresh juices, especially carrot, celery, and beet juices. Carrot juice helps to flush out fat from the bile in the liver.

To help regulate cholesterol levels, make sure you get plenty of vitamin B_3 (niacin), which reduces cholesterol, whether through diet or supplementation. Good food sources of vitamin B_3 include brewer's yeast, wheat bran, bulgur wheat, wheat germ, buckwheat, sesame and sunflower seeds, green peas, halibut, tuna, canned pink salmon, marine fish, peaches, and wild and brown rice. If you have any kind of liver disorder, you should take vitamin B_3 supplements with caution, but food sources are fine. Also beneficial for lowering cholesterol are fish oil, lecithin, cholestin (red yeast rice products), soy foods, zinc, chromium, calcium, and citrus pectin. Barley broth, which is high in potassium, can be sipped throughout the day for high blood pressure and all heart disorders. There are also a number of herbs that can be helpful, including hawthorn berry and the Ayurvedic herb guggulow. In two-year study on rabbits, guggulow significantly lowered cholesterol and blood fats, as well as protected against atherosclerosis-induced artery damage.

CHOLESTEROL-BUSTERS

In addition to the general dietary recommendations outlined above, you should be aware of a number of foods with such powerful positive effects that they deserve to be in a category of their own.

Garlic

Studies have shown that eating just one-half clove of garlic per day can decrease cholesterol levels. In one study, researchers found that allicin, an active component in garlic, blocks the action of bacterial enzymes by reacting with thiols, a crucial component of some enzymes that participate in the synthesis of cholesterol. If you find the taste or smell of garlic offensive, use Kyolic aged, deodorized garlic capsules. Research has shown that using this product, which has been studied more than any other garlic product on the market, yields good results.

Ginger

Israeli researchers found that standardized ginger extract has dramatic effects on cardiovascular health. It lowers cholesterol levels and also prevents the oxidation of LDL, which contributes to cholesterol deposits on artery walls.

Soy Foods

Experts believe that natural soy compounds called isoflavones act like human hormones that regulate cholesterol levels. A 1998 study concluded that the regular consumption of soy isoflavones might reduce total cholesterol levels by up to 10 percent. Sources of soy protein are soymilk, tempeh, tofu, and textured soy protein.

Fish

Research has shown over and over that people who often eat omega-3-rich fish have a lower risk of heart disease than those who don't eat it as often. In addition to lowering triglyceride levels, research suggests that omega-3s make the blood more slippery and less likely to clot. The American Heart Association recommends eating fish two or three times a week.

Plant/Vegetable Oils

The FDA has concluded that compounds known as plant sterol and stanol esters found in vegetable oils and certain other oil-bearing plant foods may reduce the risk of coronary artery disease. Scientific studies show that an intake of 1.3 grams of plant sterol esters or 3.4 grams of plant stanol esters per day is needed for a significant cholesterol-lowering effect. Plant sterols block dietary cholesterol from being absorbed by the intestine, according to endocrinologist Tu T. Nguyen, M.D., a researcher with the Mayo Clinic. The best dietary sources of plant sterol and stanol esters are vegetable oils (particularly olive oil), avocados, olives, seeds, nuts, and sterol-enriched foods. Walnuts, peanuts, pecans, and macadamia nuts are high in monounsaturated fats and have been cited as effective in lowering cholesterol as well.

Citrus Fruits

Citrus pectin is a plant fiber found in the white part of the rind of citrus fruits that has cholesterol-lowering properties and inhibits cholesterol from forming plaques in the arteries. A study reported in the *Journal of Clinical Cardiology* found that supplementation with citrus pectin significantly decreased blood cholesterol levels.

Chromium

The trace mineral chromium (in the form called chromium picolinate) seems to have significant cholesterol-lowering abilities, according to researchers who analyzed data from five previous studies involving more than 300 people. The *Journal of the American College of Nutrition* reported that total cholesterol levels in subjects who took chromium supplements fell more than 20 points on average, going from more than 220 mg/dL to less than 200 mg/dL. Supplementation with 1,000 micrograms (mcg) per day had the greatest effect, though doses as low as 200 micrograms daily did significantly lower blood cholesterol.

Exercise

Finally, if you want to lower your cholesterol level, get regular moderate exercise. Exercise is essential for proper function of the gallbladder and other organs. It increases the transport of oxygen to all the cells and improves circulation. Deep-breathing exercises also help to stimulate the gallbladder and liver. (Consult with a health-care provider before beginning any new exercise program.)

CHOLESTEROL-LOWERING MEDICATIONS— PROCEED WITH CAUTION

The 1993 guidelines of the National Cholesterol Education Program (NCEP) as to which people should be considered eligible for the type of cholesterol medications known as statins were relaxed in 2001. This could triple the number of people younger than age forty-five who might be considered candidates for this type of treatment and increase the number of older Americans eligible by 130 percent. People with LDL cholesterol levels of 130 mg/dL and above plus two other known risk factors for heart disease are now considered candidates for medication; the previous guidelines had set a threshold of 160 mg/dL plus two other risk factors.

An article in the *Archives of Internal Medicine* reported that the overuse and under use of the statins may be widespread, risking side effects in some people and failing to stop heart disease in others. Of more than 29,000 primary care patients from Boston's Brigham and Women's Hospital and associated sites, 1,575 took statins during 1996. This number included patients with heart disease as well as 1,080 without documented disease who were taking the medication as primary preventive therapy. Fewer than one in three of these people actually met the NCEP guidelines in effect at the time, the researchers wrote. In addition, about half of the more than 500 people who were on statin therapy because of known heart disease met the guidelines, meaning that 47 percent of the group was overtreated. When evaluating another 1,459 patients who had coronary artery disease but were not on statin medications, the investigators found that 88 percent met criteria for being able to receive a statin and thus were undertreated. In the study, the people found most likely to be overmedicated were those at least seventy years old, those without other cardiac risk factors, and those who had fewer than two risk factors for heart disease. The authors concluded, "The amazing thing about these new recommendations [increasing the pool of patients eligible for statin therapy] is that they completely ignore the previously published evidence that are quite clear in documenting that the actual cholesterol level itself is not the most important risk factor. It is actually the ratio between the level of total cholesterol and HDL."

People with elevated LDL and people with existing heart problems may reduce their risk of dying from heart disease by taking statins. However, statins themselves are far from risk-free. Depending on the specific statin, side effects may include hepatitis, gastrointestinal upset, jaundice, a variety of blood complications, liver problems, reduced platelet levels, and anemia. Most physicians recommend periodic testing of liver function. The maker of one formerly popular cholesterol-lowering drug, cerivastatin (Baycol), which had been prescribed for 700,000 Americans and 6 million people worldwide, voluntarily took it off the market because the FDA attributed thirty-one deaths to its use. Of the people who died, twenty-nine had kidney failure.

The lifetime expense, risk of liver and kidney damage, and other side effects of cholesterol-lowering drugs are good reasons why controlling cholesterol through diet and exercise should be a first-line defense. These drugs should be used only as a last resort. For people who must take statins, some physicians recommend supplementing with coenzyme Q_{10} to help offset some of the risks of these drugs.

CHAPTER THIRTY-TWO

SOME SAVORY SUBSTITUTIONS: NATURALLY GOOD NUTRIENTS

The products discussed in this chapter can be incorporated into your recipes in place of foods that are not as healthy. For instance, use arrowroot powder or kuzu to replace cornstarch to thicken sauces, gravies, and fruits—it's great in pies and cobblers, too. Unlike cornstarch, it does not have to be boiled to thicken, so arrowroot is ideal for Asian-style stir-fry dishes and heat-sensitive fruits. It is also a good substitution for people who are allergic to corn products. This chapter is devoted to pointing out a wealth of substitution ideas and other easy ways of making your diet—and yourself—healthier.

AGAR-AGAR

Also called kanten, agar-agar is a sea vegetable that grows abundantly in Japan's coastal waters, is high in trace minerals, and has a mild laxative action. It is available in bars, flaked, or powdered. One teaspoon of powdered agar-agar can be sprinkled over stewed prunes to aid regular bowel movements. It produces a clear, firm jelly and is suitable for vegetarians who choose not to use gelatin products.

APPLESAUCE

Rather than buy commercial versions, make your own applesauce. Simply core and cut up the apples, leaving the skins on, and purée them in a food processor. Add a little honey to sweeten, a little cinnamon for flavor, and, if you wish, a little lemon juice to help it stay fresh longer. Apples can be frozen in this form until needed for a recipe. To make apple butter, put the puréed apples with honey to desired sweetness in a roasting pan. Place several cinnamon sticks on top (or sprinkle with powdered cinnamon) and bake at 250°F, for six to nine hours, until desired thickness is reached. Preserve it in a jar, stored in the refrigerator, for delicious homemade apple butter.

ARROWROOT POWDER

The arrowroot plant is a starchy tropical herb. The rhizomes (underground stems) are used to make a powder. It is easily digested, even by infants, and can be used to thicken soups, gravies, fruit desserts, and fruit pies. Arrowroot can be substituted for cornstarch in any recipe. Since it thickens before it boils, do not overcook it. As the food cools to room temperature, it will thicken even more, so be careful not to use too much.

BAKING POWDER

Baking powder is used to make items such as pancakes, muffins, cookies, and other baked goods rise. Made of starch and acid, baking powder reacts immediately upon contact with a liquid. There are different types of baking powder available, and some are healthier than others.

The best baking powder to use is tartrate baking powder, composed of tartaric acid and cream of tartar (a combination of yeast and grape compounds derived from the sediment deposited in wine casks as a result of fermentation). Tartrate baking powder acts quickly, so batter should be used immediately after the baking powder is mixed into it.

Phosphate baking powder, another type of baking powder, is made of calcium and sodium phosphates. This type of baking powder poses a potential health problem because of its high sodium content. Another problematic type of baking powder is double-acting baking powder, which cannot be recommended because it contains sodium aluminum sulfate. Aluminum collects in the brain stem and has been associated with neurological disorders, including Alzheimer's disease. Some people who have died from Alzheimer's have been found to have unusually large deposits of aluminum in their brains. There are aluminum-free baking powders, such as Rumford Baking Powder, available in health food stores that can be used in place of products that contain aluminum. Read labels carefully when selecting baking powder.

BAKING SODA

Baking soda also is used as a leavening agent to help baked goods rise. It is not healthy for consumption due to its high sodium content. However, it *is* an excellent nontoxic cleanser for use in the kitchen and bathroom and is also a good deodorizer, especially for the refrigerator. Use it to clean fixtures, countertops, and sinks, and be sure to rinse well. Baking soda makes a great cleaning product for people with extreme sensitivities and chemical allergies.

As a substitute for baking soda, use a low-sodium, aluminum-free baking powder such as Rumford's, using two parts baking powder in place of one part soda.

BARLEY MALT CONCENTRATE

Barley malt concentrate is a sweetener that is especially good for people with diabetes and for those who are watching their calorie intake. It comes in a powder form, and is highly concentrated, although 1 teaspoon contains only three calories. It takes only a few grains to sweeten a cup of tea and leaves no bitter aftertaste. You can also use it as a substitute for sugar in recipes for baked goods.

BLACKSTRAP MOLASSES

Blackstrap molasses is very high in minerals and iron. Add this as a source of power to your diet. The iron in blackstrap molasses is easily assimilated and is good in infant formula. Blackstrap molasses and barley malt are the two best sweeteners. Crude blackstrap molasses has been used as a treatment for arthritis.

BLUE CORN

Blue corn has a high protein content, a unique color, and an unusual flavor. It is generally ground into a meal and made into chips, muffins, pancakes, tortillas, and other baked goods. The chips are now often available in local supermarkets.

BREWER'S YEAST

A one-celled plant and a very high-powered food, brewer's yeast makes an excellent addition to the daily diet. It is extremely high in B vitamins and can be added to cereals and other foods. The most popular way to take it is in drinks, juices, and shakes. Many people like the powdered form on popcorn.

Brewer's yeast consists of 50 percent protein, is very high in vitamin B_{12}, and contains the vital trace minerals selenium and chromium, which are lacking in highly pro-

cessed foods. It is also rich in nucleic acids, including RNA, which is a necessary building block for the body. Brewer's yeast comes in several forms: powder, flake, and tablet. The flaked yeast dissolves instantly and is good in casseroles, baked bean dishes, nut butters, spreads, vegetables soups, and other dishes. It does not require refrigeration and has a long shelf life. Store it in a tightly closed container in a dark place.

Note: Do not confuse brewer's yeast, which is available in health food stores, with baker's yeast. Never consume baker's yeast raw. People who suffer from gout (a form of arthritis) or yeast infections (Candida) should avoid brewer's yeast, as well as all other types of yeast and fermented foods. If you are introducing yeast into your diet for the first time, beware of bloating and flatulence. You can minimize or avoid such discomfort if you start with just a small amount of yeast, less than a teaspoon daily, and gradually increase the amount you consume.

CAROB

Carob is a fruit from a Mediterranean evergreen tree. It grows like a pod. It is also known as honey locust or St. John's bread. John the Baptist supposedly sustained his life in the wilderness by using carob. High in calcium, B vitamins, magnesium, and pectin, it can be used in place of chocolate, which is known to be high in caffeine, in all recipes. Carob is low in fat, so it does not need preservatives like BHA and BHT, which are added to chocolate as a preservative for fats. It has little sodium and no oxalic acid and contains 8 percent protein. It comes in a variety of forms—powder, chips or drops, liquid, and candy.

CAYENNE PEPPER

Cayenne pepper is great for circulation, the heart, respiratory system, lungs, and the colon. It makes an excellent substitute for black pepper. Remember, it is very hot, so use it sparingly.

CEREAL

Replace boxed processed cereals with granola or with whole, flaked, or cracked grain, either cooked or raw. Any of these substitutions will give you more vitamins, minerals, and fiber, while eliminating the excessive amounts of sugar, salt, and food additives so prevalent in processed foods. As a substitute for commercial hot cereals, soak whole grains overnight. In the morning, cook them lightly in the same water with a little honey or a bit of seasoning and herbs. The nutrients are not lost if you boil grains in this manner. Or place the grain in a thermal bottle or jar, cover with the appropriate amount of boiling water, tighten the lid, and allow to sit overnight. In the morning, the hot cereal should be ready to eat.

COFFEE AND TEA

If at all possible, avoid coffee, Chinese teas (except for green tea), and other caffeinated teas. Replace these with herbal teas, including kukicha tea, and cereal beverages. If you must drink coffee, substitute organically grown coffee for the commercial brands; as a crop, coffee is heavily sprayed with pesticides and residues can persist in the ground coffee.

COOKWARE

Do not use aluminum or coated nonstick cookware. Instead, do your cooking in stainless steel, iron, glass, or ceramic (such as CorningWare) cookware.

DRIED FRUIT

Instead of commercial varieties of dried fruit, such as prunes and apricots, buy organically grown, unsulfured ones that contain no preservatives.

FLOUR

In the place of refined white flour, substitute whole-wheat flour, rye flour, corn flour, oat flour, rice flour, or whole-wheat pastry flour. In the milling process, white flour loses most of the nutrients the wheat orginally contained, and it promotes the secretion of excess mucus that can clog up the system. Therefore, it is best to eliminate white flour from your diet entirely. It is best to throw out all white, processed food products in your kitchen.

FRUCTOSE

Derived from fruits and honey, fructose is a form of sugar that is a better choice than processed white sugar. Only half as much fructose as ordinary table sugar need be used to provide the same amount of sweetness, so you get a 50-percent savings in calories by using fructose. However, it is generally more expensive than sugar. Some people with blood sugar problems can handle it in small amounts, but most cannot. Fructose does not require digestion; like white sugar, it is absorbed directly into the bloodstream. Some people claim that metabolizing fructose requires little insulin and that it therefore is the ideal sugar for people with diabetes or hypoglycemia; however, most nutritionists do not recommend it for anyone who has blood sugar problems. It does not work as well as white sugar in bread or cookie recipes, as it absorbs the liquids and can make the baked goods dry. Fructose is great in pies, though, and it dissolves better in cold beverages than white sugar.

GINGER

Ginger is a root vegetable. The pulp and juice are used in many food preparations, especially Asian-style dishes. Grated fresh ginger is preferable to powdered ginger. Try adding it to stir-fry recipes.

Ginger has been found to inhibit the production of immune system compounds called cytokines. Cytokines are neurochemicals that function as a kind of molecular memory that conditions the nervous system to produce pain and tension. Since ginger inhibits the production of cytokines, it reduces pain and swelling. Ginger also reduces inflammation, stimulates blood circulation, and eases indigestion and nausea.

Interestingly, ginger is also an extremely potent snail and slug repellent. You can use it to protect plants by spreading it on the ground around the plants as a barrier; it will stop snails, slugs, or ants from crossing. This property may have evolved to protect the ginger plant from attack by insects; many spicy herbal flavors were developed by plants to protect themselves from insects.

NONFAT POWDERED MILK

If you are using milk in cooking, nonfat powdered milk is the product to use. It costs less, does not spoil, and has a natural sweetness. It can be used in make-ahead recipes for biscuit mix, pancake mix, or any other recipe that calls for milk. Soymilk also comes in a powdered form.

KUZU

Kuzu is a root starch than makes an excellent thickener for soups and sauces. Similar to arrowroot or cornstarch, it must be dissolved in cold liquid and the mixture stirred while it heats, thickening as it reaches the boiling point. It has an alkalizing effect on the body. One tablespoon of kuzu will thicken 1 cup of liquid to the consistency of Chinese vegetable sauce; adding 2½ tablespoons of kuzu to 1 cup of liquid yields a puddinglike consistency, which resembles soft tofu when it cools. As a remedy, kuzu can be used in two ways: salty and runny like a thick broth, or with juices such as papaya and apple. It can make apple juice kuzu thick, like a pudding.

KUKICHA TEA

Kukicha tea (also called twig tea), made from the pruning of naturally grown tea bushes, is an excellent substitute for ordinary black tea. It is a soothing beverage known for its distinctive nutty taste. Kukicha tea aids digestion and has been sipped with meals for centuries.

LECITHIN

Lecithin is a beneficial addition to the daily diet, especially for older adults and anyone with a weight problem. It is high in choline and inositol, which helps brain function, and is a natural emulsifier. It aids in keeping cholesterol levels down and protects the cardiovascular system.

Lecithin is available in three forms: granules, capsules, and liquids. The liquid form is much more versatile, and only a small amount is needed. Add it to baked goods in place of part of the oil called for in a recipe. Use it to make saturated-fat-free gravies, fudge, icings, and any recipe where you want a smooth finished product. As an emulsifier, it aids in the mixing of oil and liquid, as in gravies and dressings; it keeps the ingredients from separating so that the oil does not rise to the top. Liquid lecithin is an oil, which should be refrigerated after the container is opened. Also, the liquid can be used to oil baking pans. The granules are mild-flavored and can even be eaten without any preparation. Sprinkle them over foods, such as cereal and casseroles, or mix them into soups, juices, pancake batter, or baking dough. Lecithin capsules are convenient to use when traveling.

MILLET

Millet is a grain that is "king of the cereals." Extremely high in protein, millet is very easy to prepare. (See Chapter 11.) I suggest incorporating millet into your diet twice a week. Millet is a great dietary asset for people with sugar problems. Add cut-up dried fruit to millet and cook it as a cereal. Unlike fresh fruits, which must be digested quickly and should not be held up in the stomach with other foods, dried fruits can be consumed with cereal. Cooked millet makes an excellent first cereal for babies (alternate it with brown rice cereals). It is easily digested and has a very mild flavor. Uncooked millet can also be ground to make a flour.

MISO

Miso is a paste made from soybeans that have been aged in wooden barrels for three years. It contains living enzymes that aid digestion. There are different types of miso: kome, genmai, hacho, mugi, and a light, sweet type used in desserts.

Mugi, made from soy and barley, is the most popular miso for seasoning. Hacho is stronger and is made with soybeans without barley. Kome is the mildest in flavor, made with brown rice used in place of barley. Genmai is made from brown rice and soybeans.

Miso is good added to dips, spreads, sauces, soups, and stews. It has a slightly meaty taste and makes a good seasoning.

Do not boil miso. Like tamari sauce, add it at the end of the cooking to preserve all the enzymes and nutrients. It should be stored in a cool place and generally is not refrigerated because refrigeration destroys the living enzymes. Mold sometimes forms on top of miso, but this is simply an indication of its living quality. Just cut off the mold and discard—it is not harmful.

Miso is used in macrobiotic diets. There are several good books out on this wonderful product.

PASTA

Avoid eating white pasta—whether spaghetti, macaroni, shells, noodles, or any other shape. White pasta is made with refined flour. Instead, use whole-grain pastas. To avoid having whole-grain pasta become pasty, allow at least 5 quarts of rapidly boiling water per pound of pasta, and run the cooked pasta under hot, not cold, water before draining and serving.

PEANUT BUTTER

Instead of commercial peanut butter products, eat fresh-ground nut butters or an unhydrogenated peanut butter like the ones available at health food stores. The same suggestion applies to cashew, sesame, and almond butters.

RICE

There are many different types of rice available. The best is brown rice. Try substituting brown rice for potatoes with meals. It is by far one of the most nutritious foods that can be found, and is very high in the B-complex vitamins. There are three types of brown rice. Short-grain brown rice is higher in nutritional value and lower in calories than the long-grain type, but it clumps together more than the long-grain variety. You may wish to use long-grain brown rice for company meals and short-grain brown rice for everyday use.

Another good type of rice is sweet rice, which is slightly softer, sweeter, and stickier than the other varieties. Sweet rice has been used traditionally in Japan to make special holiday cakes. When toasted, sweet rice puffs up like popcorn.

Never eat processed white rice. If you dislike the flavor of brown rice or sweet rice, use basmati rice instead. (For more information about rice, see Chapter 11.)

RICE MALT SYRUP

Rice malt syrup is a good natural sweetener that can be used in place of sugar. It is available in health food stores.

SEA SALT

In general, adding salt to foods is *not* recommended. However, if you feel you need to use even a small amount of salt, use sea salt in place of iodized or white table salt. Sea salt contains an abundance of minerals. It is produced by the evaporation of seawater.

SNACKS

Instead of snacking on chips, try raw nuts or sesame seeds, sunflower seeds, and/or pumpkinseeds. Be careful when purchasing nuts and seeds, especially sesame seeds. Be sure they have been kept under refrigeration or are nitrogen-packed; otherwise, there is a risk that the oils they contain may have become rancid. Consuming rancid oils depletes the body of many vital nutrients and puts stress on the liver.

SOFT DRINKS

Instead of commercial carbonated soft drinks, drink fruit juices, mineral water, or iced herbal teas sweetened with fructose or honey. These can be found in health food stores.

SUGAR

Cane sugar, corn syrup, dextrose, glucose, and sucrose are all items that should be eliminated from your diet, whether on their own or as ingredients in food products or recipes. In recipes, you can replace ordinary white sugar with uncooked, unfiltered raw honey, using ½ cup honey instead of 1 cup of sugar and reducing the amount of liquid called for in the recipe by ¼ cup (if the recipe calls for no liquid ingredients, add 3 tablespoons of flour). Or you can substitute pure maple syrup, unsulfured molasses, or fruit juices, purées, and juice concentrates. Undiluted apple juice concentrate is good in a lot of recipes where sweetener is called for, such as in cobblers and pies, and is also good in other dishes and baked goods. Other acceptable substitutes for sugar are barley malt syrup, rice malt syrup, and, to a lesser extent, fructose.

TAHINI

Tahini is a fine paste made by grinding sesame seeds, with all the nutrients intact. It is rich in vitamins, minerals, protein, and essential fatty acids. Tahini is also very high in calcium. It is a wonderful addition to sauces and salad dressings. It also makes an excellent substitute for butter; spread it on crackers or whole-grain bread, then top with sesame seeds or jam. Or blend tahini with cooked chickpeas; add lemon juice, a crushed clove of garlic, and olive oil for a highly nutritious dip or spread. If tahini is not available at your local supermarket, it can be found at health food stores and natural foods markets.

TAMARI SAUCE

Tamari (also called shoyu) is the true form of soy sauce. Derived from soybeans, it is an excellent source of protein. You can purchase tamari sauce at health food stores and in many supermarkets. Choose a product made without added monosodium glutamate (MSG).

Use tamari in place of commercially produced soy sauce. Tamari is a superior choice because it is naturally fermented and preserved, whereas commercial soy sauce typically contains preservatives and other additives, including MSG. When browning onions or mushrooms, try using tamari sauce instead of oil or butter. The flavor is excellent. Add tamari to dishes like soups, casseroles, nutburgers, and stir-fried vegetables. Always add tamari at the end of the cooking process to protect the valuable enzymes and nutrients it contains. It has a naturally salty flavor, so do not use any sea salt when seasoning with tamari.

TEMPEH

Tempeh (pronounced TEM-pay) is a staple food in Indonesia. It is produced by fermenting presoaked and cooked soybeans (and sometimes a grain) with a culture called rhizopus (a starter culture grown on hibiscus leaves that is inoculated with hulled soybeans). High in protein, tempeh can be used as a healthier alternative to meat. Tempeh is good sautéed in a little oil or tamari sauce. It is often mixed in with vegetable dishes, grains, and casseroles. If gray or dark spots appear on the tempeh, it is not a sign of spoilage. Just trim off the spots and use the rest.

TOFU

Tofu is derived from soybeans, and is known as bean curd. It is white, cheeselike in texture, and very high in protein and B vitamins. Tofu has a bland taste, but takes on the flavor of any food that it is combined with. Tofu is also excellent sliced, patted dry, dipped in tamari sauce, and soaked a few minutes, then dipped in sesame seeds and sautéed. It is a good meat substitute with any meal and readily takes the place of ground beef or hamburger. It can also be used as a substitute for dairy products such as cream and cheese.

Once the package is opened, tofu will keep for approximately two weeks if stored, covered with water, in a bowl or jar in the refrigerator. After you open the package, drain off the water and immediately cover the tofu with fresh water. Before using tofu in recipes like cream-cheese frosting or tofu cheesecake, always drain it and pat dry. (For more information about tofu, see Chapter 25.)

UMEBOSHI PLUM

Umeboshi, also known as salt plums, come originally from Japan. The plums are pickled in salt for two about months, sometimes with beefsteak or chiso leaves, which gives them a bright color. Then they are aged for several years. Umeboshi have a salty-sour taste and are good in salad dressings, spreads, and dips. They can also be cooked with grains, beans, and vegetable dishes.

Eating umeboshi helps to reduce excess acidity or alkalinity in the body. Make sure that any umeboshi you purchase have not been doctored with other ingredients: Only plums, water, salt, and, perhaps, chiso or beefsteak leaves should be listed in the ingredients.

Quick Reference to Healthy Equivalents

Eating more healthfully doesn't mean having to give up all of the recipes you currently love. With a few small adjustments and substitutions, you can make most recipes more wholesome. Use the following table to find healthy equivalents that will work in most recipes, as well as helping you to find substitutes for ingredients you may not have on hand. For some items, there is more than one suggested substitution.

Conventional Ingredient	Healthy Equivalents
1 oz baking chocolate	• 3 tbsps carob powder + 2 tbsp water • 3 tbsp carob chips
1 tsp baking powder	• 1 tsp aluminum-free baking powder • 1 tsp tartrate baking powder • 1 tsp cream of tartar • 2 tsp arrowroot powder
1 tsp baking soda	• 1 tsp aluminum-free baking powder • 1 tsp tartrate baking powder • 1 tsp cream of tartar • 2 tsp arrowroot powder
1 cup beef bouillon	• 1 tbsp miso in 1 cup water • 1 cup vegetable broth • 1 pkg Hain's dry onion or vegetable soup mix in 1 cup water • 1 cup Vegex all-vegetable bouillon • 1 cup Morga vegetable broth mix
1 tbsp butter	• 1 tbsp sesame oil • 1 tsp vegetable oil • 1 tbsp tahini (sesame seed paste)
1 cup buttermilk	• 1 cup plain low-fat plain yogurt • 1 cup Tofutti sour cream • 1 cup Tofutti cream cheese • 1 cup rice or soy milk with 1 tbsp lemon juice or vinegar added • ½ cup tofu + ½ cup plain yogurt, blended • 1 cup cottage cheese, blended until smooth
1 tbsp cocoa powder	• 1 tbsp carob powder + add any sweetener gradually in small increments, as carob is far less bitter than unsweetened cocoa
1 tbsp cornstarch	• 1 tbsp arrowroot (be aware it thickens when cool, rather than while cooking, as cornstarch does) • 1 tbsp agar-agar • 1 tbsp instant tapioca • 1 tbsp kudzu
½ cup cottage cheese	• ½ cup tofu, mashed
1 egg (in baked recipes)	• 2 egg whites • ½ tsp baking powder + tbsp soy flour • 1 tbsp arrowroot powder • 3 tbsp Jolly Joan egg substitute
2 egg whites	• 2 tbsp unflavored gelatin dissolved in 2 tbsp water, whipped, chilled, and whipped again
1 clove fresh garlic	• ¼ tsp garlic powder
1 lb ground beef	• 1 lb ground nuts, soy granules, tofu, or textured vegetable protein, flavored to taste with miso, tamari, or vegetable bouillon
1 tbsp lard	• 1 tbsp unrefined cold-pressed or expeller-pressed vegetable oils (except for coconut, palm, palm kernel, or cottonseed oil)
1 tbsp margarine	• 1 tbsp sesame oil • 1 tbsp vegetable oil • 1 tbsp tahini (sesame seed paste)

(continued)

Quick Reference to Healthy Equivalents (cont.)

1 cup milk	• 4 tbsp powdered soy milk in 1 cup water
	• 1 cup almond or other nut milk
	• 1 cup soymilk
	• 1 cup coconut milk
	• 1 cup fresh fruit juice of your choice
	• 1 cup rice milk
1 cup sour cream (1 cup)	• 1 cup plain low-fat plain yogurt
	• 1 cup Tofutti sour cream
	• 1 cup Tofutti cream cheese
	• 1 cup rice or soy milk with 1 tbsp lemon juice or vinegar added
	• ½ cup tofu + cup plain yogurt, blended
	• 1 cup cottage cheese, blended until smooth
1 cup vegetable shortening (in baking)	• 1 cup unrefined cold-pressed or expeller-pressed vegetable oils (except for coconut, palm, palm kernel, or cottonseed oil)
1 tbsp white flour (used to thicken sauces, not in baking)	• 1½ tsp cornstarch
	• 1½ tsp arrowroot powder
	• 1 tbsp quick-cooking tapioca
	• 1½ tsp whole-grain flour
	• 1 tbsp oat flour
	• 1 tbsp soy flour
1 cup white sugar	• ½ cup honey in uncooked recipes; in baking, use ¾ cup honey and decrease other liquid by ¼ cup (if there is no other liquid in the recipe, add ¼ cup flour or the equivalent for each ¾ cup honey)
	• ½ cup maple syrup
	• ½ cup apple juice concentrate
	• ½ cup barley malt concentrate
	• ½ cup barley malt syrup
	• ½ cup rice syrup
	• ¼ cup raisin juice, soaked and blended
	• 1 cup raw sugar
	• 1 cup date sugar
	• 2 bananas, mashed and blended

VINEGAR

Instead of using white distilled vinegar, substitute pure apple cider vinegar, rice vinegar, or balsamic vinegar.

WHEAT AND CORN GERM

Wheat germ and corn germ can be used as a healthier substitute for bread crumbs in most recipes. Wheat germ can also be sprinkled on foods such as cereals to give an added nutritional boost. When buying wheat germ, make sure the product is fresh and vacuum-packed. If it is not vacuum-packed, it should be refrigerated and have either a packing or "use by" date on the label. Wheat germ turns rancid rapidly. In fact, it is almost impossible to purchase fresh, untoasted wheat germ that has not become rancid at least to some degree. If it is toasted, it has a longer shelf life. To avoid the problem of rancidity, use wheat germ that has been toasted and vacuum-packed.

Corn germ is very high in nutrients, sometimes even higher than wheat germ. Try using corn germ in recipes like corn bread, or as breading for chicken and fish.

YEAST

Yeast is a general term for microscopic fungi that feed on sugar and starches in the batter of baked goods. This produces carbon dioxide gas that causes batter or dough to rise. Active dry yeast, rapid yeast, and compressed yeast cakes are all made up of similar strains of yeast. When purchasing yeast check to make sure it does not contain preservatives like butylated hydroxyanisole (BHA). BHA has been found to cause cancer in tests on laboratory animals. Do not confuse baker's yeast with brewer's yeast; these are very different products.

YOGURT

Yogurt is generally made from cow's milk, but can also be made from goat's milk or soymilk. It has a custardlike consistency with a slightly sour taste. Yogurt can sometimes be used in place of sour cream in recipes. It also can be mixed with fruit and granola and used to make dressings and power shakes.

Yogurt has a long list of health benefits. It is an important aid to digestion that helps to reduce bloating and gas. It is also high in B vitamins and replenishes the friendly bacteria in the intestinal tract that are vital to good health. It is therefore particularly useful if you must take a course of antibiotics. Antibiotics destroy the good bacteria along with the bad, setting the stage for organisms such as *Candida albicans* to overgrow and cause all kinds of health problems.

When purchasing yogurt, be sure to choose a product that is *not* laced with sugar and chemicals. Plain soured dairy products are a better choice. (For more details about yogurt, see Chapter 22.)

PART SEVEN

UNIQUE NUTRITIONAL NEEDS

CHAPTER THIRTY-THREE

NUTRITION FOR CHILDREN

Little Jack Horner sat in a corner, eating a mincemeat pie. He stuck in his thumb, and pulled out a plum and said, "Mom, why do I have to eat this?"

—*Unknown*

The diet of the average American child consists of high-fat and high-calorie foods. Junk food is readily available from fast-food restaurant chains and, too often, is served at home as well. Schoolchildren typically start the day with a breakfast of highly processed breakfast cereals loaded with sugar, or they skip breakfast altogether. For lunch, although school menus have improved, students are still being fed nutritionally unbalanced meals that are much higher in fat and sodium than the recommended dietary allowances (RDAs). A federal government study conducted during the 1998–1999 school year looked at the meals offered to children in more than 1,000 public schools throughout the nation. Researchers found that school cafeteria lunches provided one-third of students' daily needs for calories and nutrients, except in secondary schools, where the needs vary. The school meals all exceeded the recommended daily percentage of calories from fat, saturated fat, and sodium. A majority of the schools had alternative dishes that fell within the recommended guidelines, but they were not as popular with the students.

Innumerable scientific studies have connected fat intake to heart disease and cancer, and sodium intake to high blood pressure. Nearly 3 million children between ages six and seventeen suffer from high blood pressure. Many children of the new millennium are overweight, hyperactive, and deficient in the nutrients they need to grow into healthy adults.

High cholesterol levels also are a problem. The American Heart Association suggests that children as young as two years of age need to limit their fat intake to stave off clogged arteries in adulthood. Guidelines from the American Academy of Pediatrics recommend that children over the age of two get no more than 30 percent of total calories from fat and no more than 10 percent from saturated fat.

Children may be at risk for high cholesterol if they:

- Regularly eat a diet high in fat and low in fiber and vegetables.

- Are overweight.

- Consume a lot of dairy products high in fat.

- Have a family history of high cholesterol.

The National Center for Health Statistics found that more than 11 percent of American children between the ages of six and seventeen are severely overweight. The culprit is consumption of high calorie foods coupled with lack of exercise. Kids are entertained by sedentary pursuits—television, video games, and personal computers. Research shows that children spend an average of fifteen to twenty-five hours a week in front of the television—or some 15,000 hours total by the time they graduate from high school. Nearly two-thirds of American children exercise less than two hours a week. "Couch-potato" kids fatigue more easily than active ones and are more apt to get injured playing sports. They also tend to develop diabetes, high cholesterol, and obesity as adults. Type 2 diabetes, in which the major contributing factor is overweight, is showing up in children at an alarming rate. This condition was once almost exclusively a disease of adults over the age of forty-five. Approximately 20 percent of people diagnosed with Type 2 diabetes are children, compared with 4 percent just a decade ago. If diabetes is not diagnosed and addressed during its early stages, it can lead to high blood pressure and severe hyperglycemia. Left untreated, it can eventually lead to blindness, kidney disease, leg amputations, heart attacks, and stroke. Unfortunately, the early symptoms of excessive thirst, frequent urination, and fatigue are too often overlooked or misdiagnosed. Children with a family history of diabetes are especially at risk.

Even otherwise healthy children can suffer from nutritional deficiencies, especially deficiencies of calcium, zinc, iron, magnesium, selenium, chromium, folic acid, and vitamins A, B_6, B_{12}, and C. These deficiencies may stem from vegetarian or restricted diets, or simply from a refusal to eat foods that provide proper nutrients. Kids tend to eat what they like, not necessarily what is good for them.

Common Nutritional Deficiencies in Children

While we often think of malnutrition as something that happens in faraway developing countries, too many American children are not getting all the nutrients they need for healthy growth and development. According to the *Vitamin Supplement Journal*:

- One in six children is seriously deficient in calcium.
- One in five children is deficient in folate.
- One-third of American children are deficient in iron.
- More than 90 percent of children are deficient in magnesium.
- One in six children lacks sufficient vitamin A.

- Nearly one-third of children are deficient in vitamin B_6.
- One in seven children is deficient in vitamin B_{12}.
- Nearly one-half of children are seriously deficient in vitamin C.
- About one-half of children lack sufficient zinc.

It is a good idea to give children a daily multivitamin and mineral supplement designed for children to prevent and correct such deficiencies and to ensure they are getting the nutrients they need for optimum health and immune function. Studies show that children who take vitamin supplements also tend to perform better on intelligence tests. The appropriate amount and type of supplements will vary, depending on your child's weight and age; discuss this with your child's health-care provider.

In this chapter, we will look at a number of nutritional concerns that are of special relevance for children.

STAGES OF NUTRITIONAL NEEDS

Generally, babies triple their birth weight and increase their birth length by 50 percent in their first year. Thereafter, until they reach their teens, they typically grow two inches and put on nearly six pounds of weight a year. Adolescence brings a growth spurt during which thirty or forty pounds of weight may be added, as well as six to eight inches of height.

Children must have a highly nourishing diet to fuel their rapid development and growth. As they grow and change, so do their nutritional needs, which are somewhat different from those of adults. The amount of food and nutrients a child needs is determined by height, gender, build, and activity level.

To assure that children grow to their full genetic potential, it is essential that women who are planning for pregnancy practice good nutrition before conception as well as during pregnancy. (Detailed information on this subject can be found in Chapter 34.) After birth, the infant will have special nutritional needs of his or her own.

Infant Nutrition

Babies grow faster in the first year of life than at any other time. To support this tremendous growth, infants need sufficient calories, protein, vitamins, and minerals. The American Academy of Pediatrics states that human milk is the ideal food for the full-term infant. It provides complete nutrition for the first six to nine months of life. Newborns, however, are vitamin K deficient because this nutrient is produced in the body by intestinal bacteria that may take several weeks to develop following birth. Vitamin K is needed for blood clotting and bone formation. For this reason, newborns usually are given a vitamin K shot immediately following birth.

Mother's milk contains living cells, hormones, active enzymes, immunoglobulins, and compounds with unique structures that commercially prepared formulas can never duplicate. The antimicrobial properties of breast milk protect babies against viruses, bacteria, and other infectious organisms. Colostrum, the yellowish fluid the breast produces for the first three to four days after birth, is high in protein and antibodies. It gives nursing babies natural immunity and protects their gastrointestinal tract, which is not yet mature enough to handle more complex foods.

More than half of the calories in breast milk come from fat, and babies need lots of calories to supply their energy needs. Restrictions on fat intake are not recommended for babies under two years of age. They need to get 30 to 50 percent of calories from fat to support their growth, especially the proper growth and development of the brain and nervous system. A Danish study reported in the *Journal of the American Medical Association* concluded that breast-fed babies may grow up to score higher on intelligence tests than bottle-fed babies, probably because of the effect of the nutrients in mothers' milk on the developing brain. The close physical and psychological relationship between mother and baby created by breast-feeding also may affect intelligence. The high fat content of breast milk also allows babies to get sufficient calories without consuming an excessive volume of milk, which is important because their small stomach capacity limits the amount of food they can digest.

Nursing mothers should make certain that they are getting enough vitamin B_{12} and that their babies receive at

Sudden Infant Death Syndrome

Sudden infant death syndrome (SIDS) is a situation in which a baby (usually between the ages of two weeks and one year) dies during sleep and no specific cause can be identified. However, current research says that placing babies on their backs to sleep may reduce the risk of SIDS. Other factors that are associated with an increased incidence of SIDS include exposure to secondhand smoke, overwrapping clothing or blankets, and the use of soft bedding.

The exact cause of SIDS is still under study. Most researchers believe it stems from multiple sources. A common belief is that the babies rebreathe the same air over and over when they are on their stomachs, causing carbon dioxide to build up in the blood. This is said to explain why SIDS is uncommon after age one; by that time, the theory goes, children are more capable of turning their heads or moving a blanket if the airway becomes blocked. A newer theory, proposed by British biochemist and researcher Barry Richardson, is that polyvinyl chloride (PVC) in baby mattresses interacts with mildew, a common fungi present in many homes, to produce a toxic gas that causes accidental poisoning. According to this analysis, babies placed on their backs to sleep are less likely to succumb to SIDS because they breathe air from above the zone where the toxic gas is. In support of this theory, Richardson notes that poorer families who use the same mattresses for multiple children over a period of years—mattresses that therefore are more likely to be affected by mildew—have a higher rate of SIDS than families who use new mattresses. Whatever the reason, the number of cases of SIDS has dropped by almost half since the medical community began recommending that parents place sleeping children on their backs.

least two hours total a week of *indirect* exposure to the sun. Vitamin D supplements are recommended for nursing mothers who have limited exposure to the sun. A deficiency of vitamin D can lead to rickets in babies, which causes soft, improperly mineralized bones. Nursing mothers should *avoid* tobacco, caffeine, alcohol, and any medicines (prescription and over the counter) that are not absolutely necessary and prescribed by a health-care professional. All of these substances pass into breast milk and may be harmful to the baby. Spicy or gassy foods can also affect infants of nursing mothers. The mother of a breast-fed baby who has colic should avoid eating yeast breads and vegetables of the Brassica family, such as Brussels sprouts, cauliflower, and cabbage. Trace amounts of pesticide residue have been found in lanolin, a common ingredient in lipsticks, lip glosses, and nipple creams. Nursing mothers should avoid nipple creams containing lanolin, which can be ingested by breast-fed infants, unless the product specifies they are pesticide-free.

Cow's milk, on which most infant formulas are based, is perfect for calves, but must be altered for consumption by human infants. It has three times more protein than human infants need. In addition, it has higher levels of certain minerals than breast milk, which are far more than a baby's kidneys can process. Some babies experience allergic reactions to the protein in cow's milk formula. In fact, milk protein is one of the most common causes of childhood food allergies. Symptoms that may indicate a reaction include vomiting, diarrhea, abdominal pain, recurrent ear infections, and rash. Babies may also develop symptoms of lactose intolerance (lactose is the carbohydrate in cow's milk), such as excessive gas, abdominal distension and pain, and diarrhea. Since there is some overlap between the symptoms of allergy and those of lactose

intolerance, a stool test may be necessary to determine the source of the reaction.

Cow's milk is suspected of causing colic in babies—even in breast-fed babies. Research indicates that colic-causing substances found in cow's milk may make their way into breast milk after a nursing mother consumes dairy products. One study found a higher level of a specific cow's milk antibody present in the mother's milk of colicky babies than in the mother's milk of noncolicky babies. The study suggests that a breast-feeding mother should stop consuming dairy products for seven to ten days to determine if her child's colic is triggered by the cow's antibody. Similarly, a formula-fed baby should be switched to a hydrolyzed casein-based formula, which is made from milk curd and is antibody-free.

Enfamil has a formula bolstered by two fatty acids shown to improve eyesight and brain development in children. Touted to be the "closest formula to breast milk," it is still lacking about forty other ingredients that mothers supply naturally. Doctors still caution that there is nothing comparable to breast milk for a newborn, especially in the first six months.

The main alternative to cow's milk formula is soy formula. The carbohydrates in most soy formulas are sucrose and corn syrup, which are easily digested and absorbed by infants. However, as many as 30 percent of children who have allergic reactions to cow's milk also have reactions to soymilk. The high incidence of reactions to soy may be due to the frequency with which doctors prescribe soy formulas for babies believed unable to tolerate cow's milk. Once considered a wonder food, soy-based infant formulas are now under attack from some scientists and physicians who predict that infants may develop hormonal imbalances due to the presence of soy isoflavones, which act as phytoestrogens (plant-based estrogens). However, many other scientists have stated the opposite. Still, since there are so many alternatives for babies who have problems with milk-based formulas, it might be wiser to stay away from soy-based infant formula. Also, soymilk should not be substituted for soy formula. It does not contain the correct amount of protein, carbohydrates, fat, minerals, and vitamins, and if it is the only food given to an infant, it can pose serious health risks. To make a nutritious soy-based drink for babies, add 1 teaspoon mashed papaya, ¼ teaspoon brewer's yeast, and ½ teaspoon pure blackstrap molasses to 1 quart of plain soymilk. Almond or rice milk can be used in place of soymilk for a baby who has problems with soy. This blend is a good substitute to use when weaning a child from breast milk, and also provides needed iron.

Other alternatives for infants include goat's milk (although the protein in goat's milk is similar to that in cow's milk, so it also can cause allergic reactions), almond milk, or rice milk. If you feed goat's milk to an infant, it is recommended that you dilute it with pure water at a ratio of three parts milk to one part water, and use goat's milk that has been fortified with folic acid and vitamin B_{12}, as it is otherwise deficient in these important vitamins. Rice milk and almond milk, which are available in health food stores, can be used in place of cow's milk. To make almond milk at home, place ½ cup of blanched almonds and ½ cup of pure water in a blender and process on high until the mixture is creamy. If desired, add more water for a thinner consistency.

The American Academy of Pediatrics cautions that, except in very hot weather, infants should not be given water to drink in the first month of life, but should get all the fluid they need from mother's milk or formula. Excess water can dilute sodium levels so much that their body functions may become impaired.

Introducing Solid Foods

Babies are born with sucking reflexes, but without the mechanisms necessary to eat solid foods. Those usually begin developing around the age of six months. Solid foods should not be introduced until babies have good head control, have lost the instinct to push foreign objects out of their mouths with their tongues, and show an interest in solid food. If a baby will not eat solid food on the first attempt, wait a couple of days and try again. Pediatricians commonly recommend that baby's first solid food—introduced as early as three months—be a cereal, usually a rice cereal. Use a cereal made from brown rice rather than white rice, which is stripped of nutrients and is high in starch. Until they are at least one year old, babies do not have the ability to digest starches (starches are not present in breast milk). Feeding starchy foods such as wheat cereals, turnips, and potatoes, and highly processed foods to babies before their digestive systems are able to break them

down, can lead to a variety of childhood illnesses and food allergies. Fresh millet, cooked and mashed, is a good alternative to other grain cereals for baby; it is high in protein and easily digested. Brown rice and millet usually do not cause digestive problems for infants.

Small quantities of bland, nonacidic, organic foods are an ideal way to introduce the baby to solids. Choose from the many organic baby foods available at health food stores and, increasingly, in supermarkets. Earth's Best is one recommended brand. Making your baby's food at home is the surest way to provide the best nutrition available. Before adding seasoning, simply purée a small portion of whatever the family is eating. Food processors and baby food grinders make it easy to create meals from steamed vegetables and fruits. Add tofu for protein. Prepare food in small batches and use it quickly to guard against spoilage. Avoid using nonorganic, commercially processed baby foods. They are less nutritious and may be diluted with cheap fillers and additives. They also may contain traces of pesticide residues.

Introduce each new food separately and wait about a week before feeding the baby a different food to see whether your child has a negative reaction, such as a skin rash, or develops a change in bowel habits. Either may indicate an allergic reaction. After feeding the baby solid food, wait about thirty minutes to nurse so that the food can be digested before liquids are taken.

One special word of caution: Babies should *not* be fed honey in the first year, as it may contain botulism bacteria. The amount of bacteria that can be present in honey is small and poses no threat to adults or older children, but it can be enough to make an infant very ill.

Nutrition for the Growing Years:
Ages One to Twelve

The rapid growth children experience in their first year slows somewhat after that and they begin to experience steady, continuous growth. Their appetite tapers off and varies throughout childhood. Up to age two, fat intake should not be restricted. However, after age two, children should not consume more than 30 percent of their calories from fat and no more than 10 percent of calories from saturated fats.

Children's nutritional needs vary by sex, as well as according to height, weight, and build. For toddlers, the average daily requirement for calories is 1,300. Children aged five through twelve need between 1,700 and 2,700 calories daily to support their more vigorous physical activities and give their bodies stores of nutrients needed for the growth requirements of their coming teenage years.

Calcium and phosphorus are important for developing healthy bones and teeth. During this stage, children's requirements range between 800 and 1,300 milligrams of each daily. Foods abundant in calcium include skim and whole milk; plain low-fat yogurt and cottage cheese; blackstrap molasses; dried beans; dark-green vegetables; tofu made with calcium sulfate; and fortified juices, soymilk, and cereals. Research now indicates that girls should increase their calcium intake to 1,200 milligrams at around age five, instead of at age eleven, as previously recommended. U.S. Department of Agriculture (USDA) researchers believe that the primary prevention of osteoporosis begins before puberty. Vitamin D is necessary for calcium absorption, and, since sunlight triggers the body's manufacture of this essential nutrient, supplementation may be required during dark winter months for children who do not eat any foods fortified with this vitamin. Most foods contain some amount of phosphorus and deficiency of this mineral is rare. Substantial amounts are found in asparagus, bran, corn, dairy products, eggs, fish, dried fruit, legumes, nuts, meats, poultry, and whole grains.

Antioxidant nutrients help to protect children from environmental pollutants, which are present everywhere, from the food we eat to the homes we live in. Since children's bodies are smaller, toxic chemicals pose a greater threat for them. Toxins can slow a child's ability to learn, as well as cause nausea, headaches, and dizziness. Vitamins A, B_2 (riboflavin), B_3 (niacin), C, and E, and the minerals zinc, copper, manganese, sulfur, and selenium are antioxidants that provide a good line of defense against pollutants. A diet sufficient in protein, whole-wheat breads, cereals, fruits, and vegetables can provide most of these nutrients. Good food sources of selenium include wheat germ, tuna, onions, bran, broccoli, and tomatoes.

Magnesium helps the body metabolize essential fatty acids, which in turn produce prostaglandins. These are natural body chemicals that regulate immune function and other body systems. For school-aged children, the RDA for magnesium ranges from 170 to 270 milligrams.

Between the ages of one and three, children are susceptible to iron deficiency because the iron stored during the first months after birth is likely to be depleted. Children who repeatedly hold their breath when upset or angry may be deficient in iron, according to a study reported in the *Journal of Pediatrics*. The best way to provide iron is through a diet that includes iron-rich foods such as raisins, prunes, figs, leafy greens, sea vegetables, winter squash, tofu, grains, kidney beans, millet, rice, and blackstrap molasses. To ensure iron absorption, foods rich in vitamin C should be eaten at the same time. Be aware that while children, especially young children, can develop iron deficiency, taking in too much iron also may be a cause for concern. The *British Medical Journal* reported on a study that indicated that the practice of routinely feeding babies iron to prevent anemia might increase the risk of sudden infant death syndrome (SIDS). If tests show that a child is anemic, he or she should be given iron supplements, but only when and as prescribed by a physician. Taking iron supplements may lead to stomachaches and constipation. Iron drops are difficult to digest. The form of iron known as ferrous fumarate is more easily absorbed and causes less irritation

Fiber Formula

As it is for adults, an adequate intake of fiber is important for children. Use the following simple formula to determine how much fiber a child between the ages of three and eighteen needs daily: Add 5 to the child's age. The total is the number of grams of fiber needed daily. For example, a child of seven should have a daily fiber intake of 12 grams. The maximum daily number of grams should be no more than a child's age plus 10.

to the intestines. As with all medicines, always store iron-containing supplements in childproof bottles and in locations where children cannot reach them. Accidental overdoses of iron-containing supplements are the leading cause of poisoning deaths for children under age six in the United States.

Consuming excessive quantities of fruit juice—more than 8 ounces daily—can cause health problems for young children. Several studies have found that the high levels of sugars in juices, especially fructose and sorbitol, can cause diarrhea, digestive problems, chronic congestion, obesity, and lowered immunity. Also, children who fill up on juice tend not to eat enough of the nutritious foods they need for normal growth and development. It is therefore a good idea to limit a child's intake of fruit juice. In addition, you should not put an infant or small child to bed with a bottle containing juice or any liquid containing sugar—even milk. This increases the risk of tooth decay if a child falls asleep before drinking the entire bottle, as the sugary liquid drips slowly into the child's mouth and collects around the upper teeth, where it can dissolve tooth enamel. If your child falls asleep with a bottle, the National Institute of Dental Research recommends that bedtime bottles be filled with plain, pure water.

Nutrition for the Teen Years: Ages Thirteen to Nineteen

Teenagers grow in huge spurts, seemingly overnight. Usually, children gain 50 percent of their adult body weight between the ages of eleven and seventeen, and their bones lengthen and become denser. This rapid development calls for more nutrients, yet, ironically, teenagers often get less. Activities at school and an expanding social life lead them to eat fewer meals at home, which means that they choose most of what they eat—and they usually do not choose the kind of healthy, nutrient-dense foods their growing bodies need. Studies show that children whose families eat dinner together tend to eat healthier foods.

Teenagers frequently select food brimming with fat, salt, and sugar. A popular choice among teens and preteens are soft drinks. Drinking just one regular soft drink a day can add up to fifteen extra pounds of weight a year—and most American teens drink more than one soft drink a day.

Teenagers require moderate amounts of protein and dietary fiber, adequate amounts of vitamins and minerals, and restricted amounts of fats, salt, and sugar. Calcium is essential for their rapidly growing bones. The optimum daily intake is 1,200 milligrams. Zinc is vital for overall health and growth. It strengthens the immune system and promotes bone health, reproductive system development, clear skin, and joint function. A daily intake of 15 milligrams of zinc is recommended. Pantothenic acid, one of the B vitamins, helps teenaged bodies to cope with the physical stresses of maturing and aids in producing energy. Daily requirements of pantothenic acid range from 80 to 100 milligrams. Food sources of pantothenic acid include beef, brewer's yeast, eggs, fresh vegetables, legumes, liver, mushrooms, nuts, pork, saltwater fish, whole-rye flour, and whole wheat.

Eating disorders such as anorexia and bulimia are on the rise among adolescents, as is obesity. In fact, obesity is often a factor in the development of eating disorders. Parents should be careful not to use food as a reward or form of praise for children. This teaches children to associate success with food, and may predispose them to eating more than they should, resulting in weight gain. Teenage girls are prone to crash dieting, which robs their bodies of vital nutrients. If your child is on a diet, it is important to focus on her becoming healthy, not on the number of pounds lost or sizes dropped. Pointing out amounts will send the wrong message and can subconsciously lead to fad diets or eating disorders. Teenage boys are apt to have vitamin A deficiencies. Nutrient-deficient diets can cause children to turn to alcohol and drugs, and to seek other dangerous activities, in order to make themselves feel better.

ESSENTIAL FATTY ACIDS IN CHILD DEVELOPMENT

The human body needs certain fats in order to properly function. The major components of all fats are known as fatty acids. Two of these types of fatty acids, designated omega-3 and omega-6 essential fatty acids (EFAs), are building blocks for body chemicals that regulate and control critical processes such as normal cell growth, blood clotting, brain development, and cholesterol and fat metabolism. They are classified as essential because the body does not produce them, so they must be obtained from dietary sources. Omega-3 and omega-6 EFAs are polyunsaturated fatty acids (PUFAs) found naturally in vegetables, fish oils, and human milk. A correct balance of omega-3 and omega-6 fatty acids in the body is crucial, as they have different functions and often complement each other. PUFAs are necessary for proper development of a child's brain and nervous system. Pregnant and nursing women should add PUFA-rich foods such as nuts, seeds, soy foods, flaxseeds, cold-water ocean fish, and vegetables to their diets.

Docosahexaenoic acid (DHA), an omega-3 fatty acid, is essential to infant intelligence and vision. During pregnancy, omega-3 fatty acids are conveyed from the mother's blood to the developing fetus by way of the placenta. They are vital for the development of the brain and retina membranes of the fetus. Thus, the amount of DHA the baby receives depends on the mother's dietary intake of omega-3 fatty acids. Following birth, the chief source of DHA available to infants is breast milk, although some American baby food manufacturers have begun adding it to infant formula.

A Purdue University study reported in the *American Journal of Clinical Nutrition* showed a link between low blood levels of essential fatty acids and attention deficit disorder (ADD) in young boys. The affected boys also exhibited the typical symptoms of fatty acid deficiency: frequent thirst and urination, and dry hair and skin. Some 3.5 million children have been diagnosed with ADD or attention deficit hyperactivity disorder (ADHD), which is ADD combined with hyperactive behavior. Many of these children are treated with methylphenidate (Ritalin). This prescription medicine is a central nervous system stimulant, which places it in the same category as amphetamines, which can have numerous detrimental side effects. Research suggests that essential fatty acids could be a natural alternative to this potentially harmful drug. The omega-6 essential fatty acids are usually plentiful in the diet, while omega-3 fatty acids are lacking. This can lead to a detrimental imbalance in a child's diet. Flaxseed oil is a good source of omega-3 fatty acids that aid in balancing the ratio of these two important classes of fats in the body.

THE ROLE OF DIET IN COMMON CHILDHOOD HEALTH PROBLEMS

Many of the disorders that commonly affect children have a dietary component. As a result, dietary modification, along with other natural measures, can be helpful in preventing and alleviating them. Three disorders that are quite common—and whose incidence is rising—in children are asthma, attention deficit disorder, and ear infections. What children eat can play an important part in all three. Another important health threat to children is lead poisoning. Although it cannot be classified as common, it is far *more* common than it ought to be.

Asthma

Asthma is the number one cause of the hospitalization of children. The incidence of asthma has shot up 160 percent since 1980, with asthma specialists speculating that the rising levels of environmental pollution lead to more occurrences of asthma.

It is important that children with asthma get plenty of vitamin C, along with other antioxidant nutrients. Vitamin C also increases the levels of lung enzymes that decrease naturally in people with asthma. Eating fresh fruits and vegetables that contain vitamin C can help to lessen wheezing and coughing. A diet that is high in protein, low in carbohydrates, and contains no refined sugar is best. It is also important to maintain adequate levels of omega-3 essential fatty acids, as studies have shown that this can lessen the severity of attacks and may decrease the frequency of attacks as well.

Quercetin, a phytochemical classified as a flavonoid, can act as an antioxidant and is also beneficial to those who have asthma. It inhibits the release of histamine, the chemical produced by the body in response to allergens that leads to nasal congestion and watery eyes. It also stops the body's output of the compounds that tighten the airway tubes. Quercetin can be found in nuts, berries, apples, garlic, and onions. The herb nettle, which can be taken in tea form, can be helpful in relieving respiratory problems caused by asthma. It is rich in butyric acid, necessary for a healthy metabolism, and in other vitamins and minerals.

Many children with asthma can have attacks triggered by eating certain foods. If you have a child with asthma, keep track of what your child eats and how he or she feels afterward to develop an ongoing list of things that may be triggering asthmatic responses. Then have your child avoid those foods as much as possible.

Attention Deficit Disorder

Although the connection is considered controversial, some experts believe that food allergies may cause behavioral reactions such as those seen in children with attention deficit disorder (ADD) and attention deficit hyperactivity disorder (ADHD). Some of the symptoms are an inability to concentrate, restlessness, learning difficulties, and tiredness. Any food can provoke an allergy in a susceptible individual, but foods that most commonly bring on allergy symptoms include sugar, dairy products, wheat, corn, eggs, citrus fruits, soy, peanuts, shellfish, yeast, and chocolate.

Also implicated in ADD/ADHD are preservatives, sugar, artificial colors and flavors, and other additives in food products. Many parents have found that their children's behavior improves when they eliminate all refined and processed foods from the menu.

Ear Infections

According to research, food allergy is one of the most significant factors at work in children who suffer from chronic ear infections. An allergic reaction causes the eustachian tubes, through which fluid normally drains from the middle ear, to swell. The fluid then builds up and provides a fertile environment for infection. Restricting or stopping a child's consumption of suspected foods can help reduce the incidence of ear infections. Giving children nutritional supplements that boost the immune system, such as vitamins A and C and zinc, can help their bodies resist infections.

A recent Finnish study of more than 300 children between ages four and five found that those who chewed sugar-free gum sweetened with xylitol, a naturally occurring sugar alcohol, had 40 percent fewer ear infections than children who chewed gum containing sugar. The researchers surmised that xylitol impeded the growth of bacteria that cause ear infections.

It is important to know the underlying cause of a child's ear infection. If food allergies are involved, antibiotics may clear up the acute attack, but infections are likely to keep recurring until the allergy problem is addressed. This is important because if antibiotics are given too frequently, there is a chance that the infectious bacteria will become resistant to them and the drugs will no longer be effective if needed to treat more serious illnesses. If an ear infection is caused by a virus, antibiotics will not help at all, since antibiotics fight bacteria only; they have no effect on viruses.

Antibiotics may speed the resolution of ear infections somewhat, though usually by only a matter of days. In fact, most infections will go away on their own if the body's immune system is supported in fighting them. Do not ask for an antibiotic unless the doctor recommends it. Until the infection clears, symptoms can be greatly reduced with natural treatments such as homeopathic remedies. Another good natural remedy for ear infections is garlic. Using an eyedropper, place two to four drops of warm (not hot) liquid garlic extract in each infected ear. Kyolic liquid garlic extract is suitable for this purpose. If both ears are infected, use a clean eyedropper for each ear to avoid spreading the infection, and sterilize the droppers between uses.

Lead Poisoning

Lead is a toxic heavy metal that can be ingested through water and food, as well as inhaled and absorbed through the skin. Children are especially vulnerable to lead poisoning because they absorb as much as 50 percent of the lead they ingest, whereas adults absorb only 5 to 10 percent. Lead poisoning can have a range of effects in children, from nerve damage to brain dysfunctions. A study reported in the *Journal of the American Medical Association* showed that teenagers who had been exposed to high levels of lead in childhood exhibited a substantially higher degree of violent behavior and delinquency.

Because water leaches lead from lead pipes, tap water can be contaminated. If you live in an older home, running the cold water for a few minutes each morning can help reduce the amount of lead in tap water by flushing any lead that may have accumulated in the pipes overnight. Newer pipes are made of hard plastic and most do not contain lead. However, watch out for copper pipes, which also contain toxic substances. It is wise to find out what type of water pipes you have in your home. (See Chapter 15.) However, regardless of what your pipes are made of, it is best to use quality water for cooking, drinking, and even bathing.

Natural Remedies for Children's Health Problems

There are many gentle natural remedies, some of them food-based, some herbal, that can help to soothe childhood illnesses. Following are some examples:

- For abdominal pain, a spoonful of barley malt syrup or rice syrup is helpful.
- For a colicky baby, adding a bit of chamomile, catnip, or fennel tea to juice can help to relieve symptoms.
- To ease constipation, dandelion root and yellow dock tea is useful.
- For a cold, use peppermint and catnip teas to help reduce fever. A catnip tea enema, administered with a baby syringe, can reduce fever quickly. Follow the directions that come with the syringe for the amount to use. Ginger tea aids in loosening up mucus and echinacea extract stimulates immune function.
- Diaper rash can be caused by a number of different things. One possibility is an overly acidic diet on the part of either the mother or the baby. Both the child and the nursing mother should not eat citrus fruits, tomatoes, or anything containing sugar. Calendula cream, applied locally, heals and soothes rashes. Also, homemade plain yogurt promotes healing if applied directly to the area where the problem persists. Be sure to change the diaper often and apply the cream or yogurt with each change. Adding ¼ cup of pure apple cider vinegar to the rinse water when washing cloth diapers may help to resolve the problem as well.
- For diarrhea, warm nettle tea is helpful.
- For a soothing massage to help relieve gas, add one drop of essential oil of peppermint to one tablespoon of vegetable oil. Place the baby on his or her stomach, position your hand underneath, and gently massage the abdomen with the mixture.
- For a teething baby, catnip and chamomile tea are soothing. You can also buy a teething solution to apply directly to the gums; look for a product that contains garlic and clove oils. Or make your own by mixing 5 drops each of clove, anise oil, and liquid garlic extract (such as Kyolic) oil with 2 tablespoons of pure virgin olive oil. Rub a drop of the mixture on your baby's gums every four hours. Store the solution in a cool place.

There are also many premade herbal combinations specifically designed to meet the needs of children. Herbs for Kids, a line of alcohol-free, organic tinctures has products that are gentle, safe, effective, and tasty. If you give an herbal tea to a child, it is important to determine the appropriate dosage, which is based on the average adult dose of one cup. To figure the correct dosage for a child, divide the child's weight by 150 to give the approximate percentage of the adult dosage. For example, for a child who weighs 50 pounds, divide by 150 to get 0.33 percent—or one-third—of the adult dosage. If you are nursing your baby, you can take a cup of tea yourself, and the benefits of the herb will be passed on to your child in your milk. Do not give teas to an infant under six months old.

To protect against the absorption of lead and to help remove it from the body, children need sufficient amounts of zinc, iron, copper, calcium, chromium, B-complex vitamins, vitamin C, and fiber. A diet that is rich in whole grains and fresh fruits and vegetables is the best way to ensure this. If you cannot be sure your child is getting enough vitamins and minerals from food, a good multivitamin and mineral supplement that is designed for children is a good insurance policy. Discuss this with your child's health-care provider.

SETTING A GOOD DIETARY EXAMPLE

To guide children in developing healthy eating habits, parents must set a good example for them. Don't tell them not to eat sugary junk foods and then polish off a quart of ice cream. Children must learn there are good treats and bad treats. Keep lots of fresh fruits on hand for snacks, such as grapes, bananas, peaches, melons, apples, and other favorites. British researchers found that children who ate at least one or two pieces of fresh fruit daily had better lung function and fewer incidences of colds and flu.

Have convenient foods to eat in a hurry that are good sources of nutrients, such as organic, farm-fed skinless turkey or chicken breast; water-packed tuna; bean dips and bean, potato, and coleslaw salads prepared ahead of time; homemade fruit gelatin; yogurt with fruit; nut butters; scrubbed and sliced vegetables ready to snack on and/or serve with dip; fresh fruits; and whole-wheat bread or crackers. For a way to entice kids to eat more vegetables, try Just Veggies, a packaged snack of crunchy bits of dried corn, carrots, peas, bell peppers, and tomatoes—kids can eat it like popcorn. Also keep a supply of fresh raw seeds and nuts on hand (always purchase them in sealed packages and avoid nuts from heated showcases or bulk bins), as well as plenty of pure unpasteurized fruit juice, and homemade iced tea and lemonade to keep children from grabbing a soft drink. Cola beverages contain phosphoric acid and are high in sugar, which research shows is a significant cause of hypocalcemia, abnormally low blood calcium, in children. It is best not to even have such products in the house.

Set aside the time to have at least one meal a day together as a family. Serve plenty of nutrient-rich food in a relaxed, pleasant atmosphere. Nourishing children from the beginning gives them the head start they need to become healthy adults.

GREAT RECIPES FOR KIDS—AND GROWN-UPS

FROZEN YOGURT POPS

> 3 cups plain yogurt
> 1 cup fruit juice concentrate (apple juice is good)

In a medium mixing bowl, blend the yogurt and juice concentrate together well. Pour the mixture into three ice cube trays, cover the trays with plastic wrap and stand up a wooden Popsicle stick in the center of each cube, and freeze.

FROZEN FRUIT POPS

> Unsweetened fruit juice (use watermelon for weight loss)

Fill an ice cube tray with fruit juice and place in the freezer. When the juice is almost frozen, stand up a wooden Popsicle stick in the center of each cube and return to the freezer.

KIDS' GRAHAM TREATS

> Graham crackers to form a single layer on a cookie sheet
> ½–1½ teaspoons fresh peanut, almond, or cashew butter for each graham cracker
> 1–2 bananas, sliced (optional)
> ½–1 cup carob chips
> ¼ cup crushed nuts (optional)

1. Preheat the oven to 300°F.
2. Place the graham crackers or cookies on the cookie sheet. Top each with a ¼"–½" layer of nut butter. If desired, top with a layer of banana slices.
3. Sprinkle with carob chips and, if desired, crushed nuts.
4. Bake just until the carob chips melt. Serve immediately.

CRISPY BARS

> 3 cups puffed or crispy rice cereal
> ¾ cup pecan butter or other nut butter
> ⅓ cup honey or brown rice syrup
> ⅓ cup crushed pecans or other nuts (optional)
> Fructose (optional; as desired to make the bars softer or sweeter)

1. Lightly oil a six-inch by ten-inch baking pan.
2. In a mixing bowl, thoroughly combine all ingredients with oiled hands.
3. Press the mixture into the pan and refrigerate until firm. Cut into squares and serve.

CHILI PIE

> 1 package Arrowhead Mills Multigrain Corn Bread Mix
> ¼ cup nonhydrogenated margarine, melted
> 1 tablespoon taco seasoning (optional)
> 3 cups homemade chili or canned organic vegetarian chili
> ½ cup chopped onion
> ¼ cup chopped green pepper
> ½ cup shredded cheese of your choice

1. Preheat the oven to 450°F and oil an eight-inch by eight-inch by two-inch cake pan or baking dish.
2. Prepare the corn bread mix, adding melted margarine and, if desired, taco seasoning to the mix. Pour the batter into the pan.
3. Spoon the chili into the center of corn bread batter. Sprinkle chopped onion and pepper over the chili and top with the cheese.
4. Bake until the corn bread is done, about twenty-five to thirty minutes (a toothpick inserted into the center should come out clean). Do not overbake or it will dry out. Serve immediately.

Variations: (1) Instead of baking in a single dish, divide the batter and toppings into single-serving size dishes (reduce the baking time accordingly). When the pies are done, allow them to cool, then freeze for later use or serve immediately. (2) Top the pie with fresh avocado and tomato slices before serving.

"SODA POP"

> ¾ cup sparkling water
> ¼ cup of any of the following: cranberry, apple, or cherry juice concentrate; fresh lemon, lime, or any other fruit juice
> Barley malt or other sweetener to taste

Pour the water into a glass or pitcher, add the fruit juice and sweetener, and stir to blend. If desired, add the cinnamon or sassafras and stir again. Serve immediately.

Variation: Instead of using fruit juice or fruit juice concentrate, soak two cinnamon sticks or one piece of sassafras bark in the sparkling water overnight. Add a sweetener and, if desired, ½ teaspoon pure vanilla extract.

BANANA-NUT SPREAD

> ½ ripe banana
> 2 tablespoons almond or sesame butter
> 2 teaspoons tofu mayonnaise
> 1 tablespoon soft raisins

In a medium bowl, mix all of the ingredients together. Serve in a pita pocket, on whole-grain bread, or with crackers.

VEGGIE-TAHINI SPREAD

3 tablespoons tahini
1 tablespoon grated carrot
1 tablespoon chopped green pepper
1 teaspoon miso
1 tablespoon minced onion
1 tablespoon tamari sauce

In a medium bowl, mix all of the ingredients together. Serve with whole-grain bread or crackers.

CHICKPEA SPREAD

4 cups chickpeas, cooked until tender
¾ cups brown rice
2½ tablespoons Dijon mustard
½ green or red pepper, chopped
1 teaspoon grated horseradish
1 sprinkling of garlic granules
1 dash of sea salt

Mix all of the ingredients together until smooth. Refrigerate for two hours or longer to allow flavors to blend. Serve in a pita pocket with vegetables such as sliced cucumbers, tomatoes, and alfalfa sprouts.

KID-FRIENDLY POCKET SANDWICH IDEAS

For a healthy snack, fill a whole-grain pita pocket bread (or mini-pita) with any of the following:

- Almond butter and sliced bananas

- Soy cream cheese or mashed tofu and nut butter

- Nut butter and chopped, diced dates

- Jelly and sliced bananas

- Soy cream cheese, pineapple rings, and chopped nuts

For a more substantial meal, spread any of the following in a pita pocket:

- Chicken salad

- Tuna salad

- Egg salad

- Eggless egg salad

- Hummus

- Nut loaf

Add sprouts or lettuce and tomato slices and serve. (Before using sprouts, please read Chapter 23.) For a hot lunch, fill a pita pocket with tofu hot dogs, top with Tofutti grated cheese, and place under the broiler for a minute or two, until the cheese is melted. Serve immediately.

CHAPTER THIRTY-FOUR

SPECIAL WISDOM FOR WOMEN

Women's health has emerged as both a powerful political platform and a dynamic public health issue. It has long been recognized that women have worse health than men, despite the fact that women live longer. Overall, women have more acute symptoms, chronic conditions and short- and long-term disabilities resulting from health problems.

—*The American Dietetic Association*

The expanding roles of women over the past fifty years make diet and nutrition a more critical concern than ever. Women today have increased demands placed on their time, energy, and physical stamina. In addition to protecting and maintaining their own bodies, women are generally gatekeepers of their families' health and diet.

New ailments that didn't even exist (or have names) many years ago further add to the threats to women's health. Anorexia nervosa, bulimia, chronic fatigue syndrome, fibromyalgia, HIV/AIDs (women make up 24 percent of new cases of AIDS, as compared with just 6.7 percent two decades ago), and complications from such things as body piercing, breast implants, diet pills and other prescription drugs, liposuction, and many others have all taken their toll.

When Superwoman finally does hang up her cape and retire, new demands are often made on her health and energy. Longer life spans mean that increasing numbers of older adults are outliving their retirement funds and ability to care for themselves. As a result, a growing group of sixty and seventy year olds are providing daily care for their parents. And most of these caregivers are women who, much to their dismay, are also experiencing age-related problems of their own.

There appear to be no immediate societal solutions for the increasingly heavy load that women are shouldering in the new millennium. There is excellent support, however, available through dietary, nutritional, and lifestyle choices that can nourish, sustain, and prevent—and in some cases cure—many of the health problems that commonly affect women. This chapter offers information on how women can use diet and nutrition to stay strong, active, and healthy at every age. It also suggests dietary cures for physical problems that are unique to being female or that disproportionately affect women.

NUTRITION FOR THE CHILDBEARING YEARS

During their twenties and thirties, women's levels of sex hormones are at their peak. Metabolism also is at its peak, as the body continues to build both fat and muscle. Throughout the childbearing years, women require more iron than men do to replace losses due to menstruation. Good food sources of iron include blackstrap molasses, figs, grains, kidney beans, leafy greens, millet, prunes, raisins, rice, sea vegetables, tofu, and winter squash. Women who have especially heavy periods and/or short menstrual cycles may be susceptible to anemia even with the healthiest diet, however. These women may need to take iron supplements. However, because too-high levels of iron pose dangers of their own (an excess of free radicals in the body and an increased risk of cardiovascular disease), you should not take supplemental iron unless your doctor diagnoses anemia by means of a blood test *and* prescribes supplements for you.

This is the time of life to build up your bones, with a view toward preventing osteoporosis later in life. There are two key aspects to this. First, the body must have an adequate supply of bone-building minerals. Our bodies cannot make essential minerals, so they must come from the diet. Key minerals are, first and foremost, calcium, but also magnesium (which is necessary to balance with calcium), plus iodine, manganese, and zinc. Adequate amounts of vitamins D and K also are required, since calcium cannot be absorbed properly without them. Second, regular exercise that stresses the bones, such as brisk walking, prompts the body to add mass to the bones of the legs, hips, and spine.

To support sexual vitality and function, which can be weakened by stress, allergies, and the consumption of too much sugar, the adrenal glands need adequate levels of vitamins A, C, and E; B vitamins; and essential fatty acids.

Birth Control Pills (Be Sure to Read This!)

Many women of childbearing age who do not wish to become pregnant are encouraged to take oral contraceptives, or birth control pills, to prevent pregnancy. They are considered to be the most effective form of birth control, and many women like them because they are easy, neat, and discreet to use. There are substantial risks associated with these drugs, however.

Research indicates that women who are infected with transmitted human papilloma virus (HPV), a common sexually transmitted virus associated with the development of cervical cancer, have an even higher risk of cancer if they have taken birth control pills for more than five years. Gynecologists have suspected for some time that there is a causal connection between birth control pills and cervical cancer.

Dangerous blood clots are another potential complication with birth control pills. Scientists have confirmed that women taking the so-called third-generation contraceptive pills are more likely to develop life-threatening blood clots in the deep veins of the legs or the pelvis. And more and more studies are linking birth control pills with breast cancer. Clearly, finding safer, less invasive ways to control reproduction should be a priority goal for those who care about women's health.

Prepregnancy Nutrition

Before conception, a healthy diet is crucial to ensure adequate nutrition for the developing fetus. During the first several weeks after conception, the embryo's mass increases dramatically. At this critical growth stage, many women do not know they are pregnant. Unless they are already eating a well-balanced diet, mothers-to-be could unintentionally ignore this essential stage of the baby's development. Women who are underweight when they conceive risk giving birth prematurely to low-birth-weight babies. Babies who weigh five and one-half pounds or less at birth are twenty times more apt to die during their first month of life. Women who are obese when they conceive are at risk for developing high blood pressure and diabetes during pregnancy. Their children are more likely to become overweight or have high blood sugar. Whatever your weight, however, dieting while you are trying to become pregnant is not recommended. A body that is losing weight might be unable to provide sufficient nourishment for a newly conceived fetus.

Folic acid, one of the B vitamins, is a nutrient of special importance in the months before and during the earliest weeks of pregnancy. Deficiency is linked to such neurological birth defects as spina bifida and anencephaly. It can be difficult to get enough folic acid from the diet, so if you are considering becoming pregnant, it is wise to take 400 micrograms of supplemental folic acid daily before you conceive. (See "The Importance of Folic Acid in Pregnancy" on page 259.)

Women of childbearing age, and particularly those who are trying to become pregnant, should be cautious about using prescription or over-the-counter drugs as well. One especially dangerous drug is isotretinoin (Accutane), a drug that is prescribed for cystic acne. Although a derivative of vitamin A, this drug poses a great risk of birth deformities. Doctors generally will not prescribe it to a woman unless she agrees to use two forms of birth control and to have monthly pregnancy tests for as long as she is on the drug.

Nutrition During Pregnancy

A healthy diet is crucial for both the mother-to-be and for her developing child. The best sources of nutrients are high-quality, unprocessed (or minimally processed) foods like whole grains, fresh vegetables and fruits, legumes, fish, soy products, and some fresh low-fat yogurt and cottage cheese.

Women who are a healthy weight before conceiving should gain between twenty-five and thirty-five pounds during pregnancy. In part, the amount of weight a pregnant woman gains determines her baby's birth weight, and a baby's weight at birth is very important for future good health. The desirable, healthy weight range for babies at birth is not less than six and one-half pounds and not more than nine pounds.

Most women need to consume an extra 300 calories a day during the last six months of pregnancy to gain the weight necessary to nourish the developing fetus. These should not be empty calories, however, as growing fetuses receive their nutrition directly from their mothers. They should be quality nutrient-dense foods such as those listed above. Additionally, high-fiber foods such as grains, vegetables, fresh and dried fruits, and fruit juices have a natural laxative effect that helps to ease the constipation that often accompanies pregnancy. Eating five or six small meals a day instead of three larger ones can help offset digestive problems and heartburn, which are also common during pregnancy, especially during the last few months.

Although protein needs increase during pregnancy, they can be met adequately by plant sources. Pregnant women who desire meat and other animal products should eat only organic, range-fed meat and free-range poultry and eggs to avoid ingesting pesticide residues and other contaminants. Make sure all meat is well cooked and take special care in handling the meat before it is cooked; wash hands, utensils, and preparation areas very well.

If you do eat meat while you are pregnant, consume it in moderation only. Some studies indicate that excessive protein consumption could be detrimental to the fetus, resulting in premature birth or slowed growth. Also, consuming too much protein can stress the kidneys and lead to calcium loss through the urine.

A pregnant woman should eat at least three servings of calcium-rich foods daily. Pregnant women and nursing mothers require 40 percent more calcium each day than nonpregnant women. However, it is advisable to avoid milk as a calcium source because the phosphorus and protein it contains can interfere with calcium absorption. Instead, select nondairy foods that provide abundant calcium, such as green, leafy vegetables; sardines; shellfish; canned salmon with the bones; citrus fruits; dried peas and beans; soy foods; and dried figs, dates, and almonds. That said, however, pregnant and nursing women should eat fish no more than twice weekly because of the possibility of heavy metal contamination. Avoid eating game fish such as swordfish, shark, king mackerel, and tilefish, which tend to contain high levels of mercury. Mercury can harm an unborn child's developing nervous system. Farm-raised fish generally contain lower levels of mercury and are a better choice than wild-caught fish.

Folic acid continues to be important during pregnancy, and supplements are a good idea to ensure that you are getting enough of this nutrient. Supplements containing iron, however, should be approached with caution during pregnancy. Avoid taking supplemental iron beyond the recommended levels, as excess iron in the system can be damaging. In addition, both vitamins A and D can be toxic if taken at levels higher than the recommended daily allowance. Such levels are rarely reached through food intake alone; however, women taking dietary supplements need to be aware of this risk and monitor their intake. Women who take nutritional supplements should discuss with a health-care professional which vitamins and minerals are safe to continue taking during pregnancy.

Finally, pregnant women should avoid substances that place the fetus in danger, including raw or undercooked meat or seafood, sugar and fried foods, caffeine, cigarettes (a four-year study conducted in Europe confirmed that smoking during pregnancy increases the risk of sudden infant death syndrome [SIDS]), alcohol, and any drugs other than those that are absolutely necessary and are prescribed by a health-care professional.

MIDLIFE AND MENOPAUSE

Women and their hormones have a lifelong connection, and many of the chronic health problems that affect women are hormone related. Monthly menstruation depletes iron reserves. Childbirth taxes the nutritional reserves of even healthy women. When a woman is in her thirties and forties, her levels of the sex hormones estrogen and progesterone begin falling. With declining fertility and hormone levels, a woman may experience fluctuations in moods and body functions, uncomfortable symptoms such as hot flashes and night sweats, and a host of other unwelcome changes. For some women, especially those with nutritional deficiencies, menopause can seem like round-the-clock PMS. Additionally, many doctors overlook the

---

The Importance of Folic Acid in Pregnancy

Would-be mothers, as well as pregnant women, need to consider increasing their intake of folic acid, a B vitamin, through either diet or supplementation. Folic acid (also sometimes called folate or folacin) is essential for the formation of healthy red blood cells, especially during the first weeks of pregnancy when the brain and other vital organs of the fetus form. Folic acid deficiency in the mother can lead to neural tube defects in the child, including spina bifida (failure of the spinal column to close properly) and anencephaly (the formation of little or no brain tissue.) It is especially important that women get sufficient folic acid *before* they become pregnant, as the neural tube develops during the twenty-eight days after conception—well before most are aware of having conceived. The U.S. Public Health Service therefore recommends that all women of childbearing age who are capable of conceiving consume 400 micrograms of folic acid daily. Pregnant women and nursing mothers need 800 micrograms daily. Taking extra folic acid reduces a woman's chance of having a child with spina bifida and other abnormalities of the spine and brain. Experts estimate that if every woman capable of having a baby took the appropriate amounts of folic acid, 75 percent of neural defects could be prevented.

Folic acid has been found to be so essential to preventing birth defects, as well as helping to protect against cervical cancer and heart disease, that the U.S. Food and Drug Administration (FDA) now requires manufacturers to add it to enriched grain products. Foods that are naturally good sources of folic acid include brewer's yeast, lentils, dry beans, barley, brown rice, salmon, tuna, mushrooms, broccoli, asparagus, spinach, split peas, toasted wheat germ, most berries, most breakfast cereals, romaine lettuce, Brussels sprouts, peas, peanuts, beets, avocados, and citrus fruit.

Taken in excess of 1,000 micrograms (1 milligram) per day, however, folic acid can mask the symptoms of pernicious anemia, a condition caused by vitamin B_{12} deficiency that can lead to nerve damage. It is possible that folic acid can delay the anemia, but leave the neurological damage unchecked. If you take folic acid supplements, take them with vitamin B_{12}, especially if you are a vegetarian.

Hormone Replacement Therapy: Proceed with Caution!

For many years now, physicians have been prescribing hormone replacement therapy (HRT) for their menopausal patients to relieve symptoms such as hot flashes. More recently, long-term HRT has been touted as a preventive for osteoposis, heart disease, and even aging itself. Now, though, experts are having second thoughts. As an article in the Harvard Medical School publication *Women's HealthWatch* reported, "Experts advise extreme caution in seeking a hormonal remedy for aging. In the complicated balance of our endocrine systems, boosting the level of one hormone could have unanticipated effects on others. Supplementary hormones are delivered in ways considerably different from their normal patterns of release. Moreover, there may be good reasons for age-related hormone declines—say, reducing the growth of hormone-dependent tumors." Those active in this field counsel patience, saying that more research is needed. Yet they concede that our relationship with estrogen, which began with high hopes, has been tempered by unexpected downsides and lowered expectations as evidence has come in.

Researchers who conducted a study reported in the *Journal of the National Cancer Institute* concluded that women using estrogen replacement therapy had a 43 percent increased risk of ovarian cancer, while those using combination estrogen and progestin therapy had a 54 percent increased risk. Meanwhile, the component of a major study evaluating the benefits of HRT for preventing cardiovascular disease was discontinued when preliminary results showed that HRT not only had no benefit, but might actually add to the risk. The American Heart Association has now released guidelines recommending that HRT *not* be prescribed for the prevention of strokes and heart disease, whether a woman has a history of heart disease or not. Clearly, finding other ways to ease hormonal symptoms associated with aging is necessary and important for women.

importance of thyroid testing at this stage of a woman's life. Thyroid disorders can not only cause many of the same symtoms but can also make menopausal symptoms unbearable. For this reason, it is a good idea to have your thyroid function tested.

The good news is that a healthy diet can help to minimize menopausal discomforts and make for an easier transition. One of the best things you can do during this time is to be sure to drink plenty of quality water—at least 2 quarts daily. Drinking water replaces fluids lost to perspiration during hot flashes and can even prevent or minimize the hot flashes themselves. You should also eat plenty of mineral- and fiber-rich foods such as whole grains and fresh vegetables (raw if possible) to replace minerals lost to perspiration and prevent constipation, a common complaint. Equally important, avoid or strictly limit your consumption of animal products, except for marine fish and fresh plain yogurt. For protein, emphasize soy foods and fish. Japanese women, who eat a great deal more soy and fish than American women, are known to experience fewer unpleasant symptoms at menopause than their American counterparts. Soy contains phytoestrogens (plant estrogens), which may help to compensate for a woman's own declining estrogen. Marine fish contain valuable omega-3 essential fatty acids, which help to combat inflammation, keep the skin supple, and protect the cardiovascular system. Also, avoid alcohol, caffeine, sugar, spicy foods, and hot soups and drinks, which can trigger hot flashes and aggravate mood swings. Sugar, dairy products, and alcohol have been reported to cause severe hot flashes.

Estro-Logic, a natural estrogen-balancing formula produced by Wakunaga of America Company, is an herbal product containing extracts of astragalus, black cohosh, chaste tree berry, motherwort, sage, and wild yam, and it also includes isoflavones. It has been shown to reduce menopausal symptoms.

THE POSTMENOPAUSAL YEARS (SIXTY AND BEYOND)

By the year 2020, women will account for 85 percent of persons aged sixty-five and older who live alone. The number of women aged 100 years or older will double in the next ten years. Nutrition is more important than ever to women who want to enjoy these quality years when they are "seasoned" veterans of life.

Women, who are still the primary caregivers for spouses, family, friends, and grandchildren, are not always rewarded economically. More than three-quarters of older adults with incomes below the poverty line are women. Those who receive pensions and retirement benefits often receive less than men because, traditionally, women earn less money and take time off from work to bear and raise children. However, even as they look to financial priorities and planning, women should remember that healthy eating can enhance both the quality and length of life. There are also beneficial short-term effects, such as increasing your resistance to disease, hastening healing, and preventing dehydration (a problem for many older people). Preparing fresh food from scratch, rather than relying on processed, nutritionally empty foods that are high in salt, fat, and sugar, will help women to stay healthy and cut grocery costs. Meals made from even the highest-cost fruits, vegetables, and whole grains still are priced much lower per pound than most meat products and packaged foods.

Aging promotes a loss of lean muscle tissue, body water, and bone mineral mass (density), and favors an increase in the proportion of body fat. As people age, their appetites

DHEA

The most abundant hormone in the bloodstream, dehydroepiandrosterone (DHEA), is produced by the adrenal glands. It is produced abundantly in youth, peaking around age twenty-five, when production starts to wane. The age-related drop in DHEA levels parallels the development of a number of common degenerative syndromes, such as atherosclerosis, osteoporosis, declining immunity, and depression, and is associated with an increased risk of cancer. In older women, the production of DHEA declines and that of cortisol, a stress hormone, rises. People with low levels of DHEA and high levels of cortisol are more likely to suffer dementia.

Taking DHEA seems to have the ability to improve the overall sense of well-being of postmenopausal women. DHEA is a precursor necessary for the production of both androgens and estrogen, and may help to fight osteoporosis. Women who use DHEA supplementation report higher energy levels, an improved state of well-being, and an increased ability to cope with stress. However, DHEA supplements should be taken with caution. Taking high doses can damage the liver and may suppress the body's natural ability to synthesize the hormone. If you choose to try DHEA replacement therapy, it is best to do so under the guidance of a knowledgeable health-care provider and to be sure to take supplements of the antioxidants vitamins C and E and selenium to prevent oxidative damage to the liver. A supplement called 7-Keto (DHEA), produced by Enzymatic Therapy, acts to balance levels of estrogens and androgens in the body. It is safe and has no known side effects.

and energy decline, but their nutritional needs do not. Seniors tend to need more calcium, magnesium, vitamin B_{12}, vitamin K, boron, and vitamin D than they get because they generally drink less milk and get less exposure to sunlight. In addition, many older people cannot absorb vitamin B_{12} properly. They are also prone to decreased nutrient absorption, metabolism, and excretion; a lessened sense of taste and smell; decline in salivary secretions and swallowing function; decreased gastric functioning; and a decline in liver function. Because blood glucose levels increase more quickly as women get older, they should consume products containing sugar more sparingly.

Studies have found that vitamin B_{12} and folic acid can have very positive effects for older women. Folic acid helps to protect against heart disease, stroke, Alzheimer's disease, and colon cancer. It is especially important for people with declining mental function—including dementia—or at a high risk of cardiovascular disease. Rich sources of folic acid include asparagus, avocado, bananas, broccoli, pinto beans, orange juice, spinach, and enriched grains, cereals, and breads. Vitamin B_{12} is found primarily in meat and other animal products. Deficiencies of both of these nutrients are common in older adults. Taking supplements, in amounts of 2,000 to 5,000 micrograms each daily, is a good way to ensure an adequate supply. They should be taken together, because taking folic acid alone can hide symptoms of B_{12} deficiency.

A diet rich in grains, vegetables, and fruit but low in saturated fat and highly processed food will provide the nutrition most postmenopausal women need. Water intake also becomes important, as it is common for the ability to sense thirst to decrease with age. Drink eight 8-ounce glasses of quality water every day to avoid dehydration and constipation. Select nutritionally dense foods that are low in calories and fat, so that eating less will still provide the needed nutrients. Everyone should take multivitamin and calcium supplements (bone health is a primary concern). This will help you to maintain generally adequate nutrient levels and pre-

vent continued bone loss. Also remember that exercise stimulates bone formation. If your cholesterol levels are normal, eating an egg or two a day should not be a problem. Eggs are a relatively inexpensive source of high biological value protein that is easy to prepare, chew, and digest.

Prevention, screening, and early testing are critical to women's health care as well, and, in the final outcome, will save precious dollars. (For a list of medical tests that are recommended for older women, see the inset on page 262.)

THE ROLE OF DIET IN WOMEN'S COMMON HEALTH PROBLEMS

Many of the disorders that commonly affect women have a dietary component. As a result, dietary modification, along with other natural measures, can be helpful in preventing and alleviating them. The following sections look at disorders that are either unique to women or that disproportionately affect them for one reason or another.

ALZHEIMER'S DISEASE

Alzheimer's affects 10 percent of Americans over the age of sixty-five and as many as 50 percent of those over eighty-five. It is not limited to women, of course, but the risk of developing Alzheimer's disease rises with age, and the majority of the oldest American adults are women.

The precise cause or causes of this condition are unknown, but research is pointing, more and more, at nutritional deficiencies. Alzheimer's disease is far more than simple memory loss. It is a brain disease characterized by a gradual, permanent tangling of the nerve fibers that surround the memory center of the brain and a death of cells, which leads to dementia and, eventually, to death.

Some experts believe that the death of brain cells may be a result of immune-system malfunction or free-radical activity that might be neutralized with antioxidants. One study of men and women aged seventy-five and older

Medical Tests and Procedures Recommended for Women in Midlife and Beyond

It really is true that an ounce of prevention (or early detection) can be worth many pounds of cure. The following are health maintenance and diagnostic procedures recommended for women in midlife and beyond. This is not an exhaustive list, and individual needs and symptoms may require other and/or more frequent testing of various types.

Test/Procedure	Age	Recommended Frequency
Bone mineral density test	50 and older	Baseline at perimenopause; thereafter every three years or as recommended by physician.
Chest x-ray	50 and older	As recommended by physician.
Cholesterol screening	50 and older	As recommended by physician.
Colonoscopy	50 and older	Every ten years.
Colorectal examination	50 and older	Every one to three years, depending on risk.
Complete physical, including height, weight, and blood pressure measurement; breast, pelvic, rectovaginal, skin, and thyroid examinations	50 and older	Once a year.
Dental examination and cleaning	50 and older	Twice a year.
Electrocardiogram	50 and older	As recommended by physician.
Eye examination with glaucoma test	50 and older	Every year for high-risk women; every three years for others.
Fasting glucose test	50 and older	Every three years.
Fecal occult blood test	50 and older	Once a year.
Hearing test	60 and older	Every three years.
Influenza vaccine	50 and older	Every year.
Mammogram	45 and older	Once a year.
Pap smear	50 and older	Every one to three years, depending on risk (may be discontinued after age sixty-five if all previous tests have been normal).
Pneumococcal (pneumonia) vaccine	65 and older	Every three years.
Sigmoidoscopy	50 and older	Every five years.
Tetanus-diphtheria vaccine booster	50 and older	Every ten years.
Thyroid function screening	At perimenopause	Every three years or as recommended by physician.
Thyroid-stimulating hormone	50 and older	As recommended by physician.

found that those with low levels of vitamin B_{12} and folate, which are key to the production and maintenance of body cells, were twice as likely to develop Alzheimer's disease as those with normal levels of these nutrients. Vitamin B_{12} is found almost exclusively in animal products, including meat, fish, eggs, and milk. If you are a vegetarian, you should supplement your diet with vitamin B_{12}. (Vegetarian forms of vitamin B_{12}, extracted from algae, are available.)

Folate, also known as folic acid and folacin, occurs naturally in leafy green vegetables, beans and peas, and citrus fruits. Many cereals are fortified with folic acid.

Although various studies have come to many different conclusions about the causes of and potential treatments for Alzheimer's disease, one thing they all seem to agree on is the importance of exercise. There is plenty of evidence that regular exercise helps to protect against neurological decline of all types. *Mental* exercise, such as reading and doing word and/or math puzzles, also seems to have a positive effect on cognitive functioning as we age.

CANCER

The second leading cause of death in women is cancer. A complex myriad of genetic, environmental, and hormonal factors place women at greater risk for different types of cancer than ever before. Surprisingly, lung cancer now kills more women in the United States than breast cancer. It is well established that the leading cause of lung cancer is cigarette smoking. Smoking is a major cause of cancers of the bladder, mouth, and throat as well. It is also the major cause of heart disease.

Both animal and human research have connected breast and colon cancer with a diet high in sugar, fat, and highly processed foods—the typical American diet. High-fat diets are also directly linked to obesity, and, according to the American Cancer Society, overweight women have a 55 percent greater chance of dying from cancer than those of normal weight. Birth control pills, which brought an end to women's fears of unwanted pregnancy and botched abortions, have turned out to be a double-edged sword. The latest research shows that women who take oral contraceptives over long periods of time increase their risk of developing breast cancer by 58 percent as compared with those who have never taken contraceptive pills. Women who continue taking birth control pills past the age of forty-five have a 144 percent higher risk of breast cancer. While early detection and treatment have greatly increased cancer survival rates, the number of women who are expected to develop some form of cancer in their lifetimes is staggering—and rising. And the incidence of cancer rises with age. Over half the cases of ovarian cancer in the United States are detected in women over the age of sixty-five.

Researchers from the National Cancer Institute have found that women who eat the most fruits, vegetables, whole grains, low-fat dairy products, lean meat, and fish have a 30 percent lower death rate than those who eat the smallest amounts of these foods. There is also a strong association between higher blood levels of ascorbic acid (vitamin C) from dietary sources and a lower mortality from all causes.

CARDIOVASCULAR DISEASE

Many people are surprised to learn that the number-one cause of death among American women today is not breast cancer but cardiovascular disease, a category of disorders that includes high blood pressure, coronary artery disease, heart failure, and heart attacks, among others. In fact, cardiovascular disease is responsible for the deaths of more American women than all other diseases combined. Further, there has been a shocking rise in the rate of sudden cardiac death in young women, which jumped by an alarming 30 percent between 1989 and 1996. Experts calculate that one of every two women will die of some cardiovascular complication. Heart disease, once predominantly a male problem, has now moved to the top of the list of women's diseases, and more women than men now have some form of cardiovascular disease. Unfortunately, many physicians, who were not trained to think of cardiovascular disease as a major threat to women, do not look for (or fail to correctly interpret) cardiovascular symptoms in their female patients, nor do they offer information about preventative measures, further adding to the problem. Additionally, women are less likely than men to experience the crushing chest pressure or pain that is typically associated with a heart attack. More commonly, women experience vague chest discomfort accompanied by shortness of breath or nausea. They may also notice a numbness or aching feeling in the left arm. Because women mainly experience these vague sensations, and are also more likely than men to have what are called "silent" heart attacks (ones with no noticeable symptoms), they frequently remain untreated.

Heredity is a huge factor in heart disease, but so is diet. Dietary factors that are known to be related to diseases of the heart and blood vessels are excessive consumption of salt, sugar, and nonessential fats. Women who smoke are two to six times more likely to develop heart disease than nonsmokers. Sedentary lifestyles, overweight, high cholesterol levels, diabetes, and stress are other factors involved in cardiovascular disease. Many women today are full-time members of the workforce, in addition to raising children and maintaining households. This has created an exponential increase in women's average daily stress levels, which now meet or surpass those of working men. Far exceeding working men's stress levels are those of single mothers, who must work outside the home and face alone the responsibilities and daily strife of providing for a family.

You can lower your chances of getting cardiovascular disease by choosing the foods you eat with care. Eat less fat, especially in the form of foods of animal origin, including meat (especially red meat), milk, cheese, and butter, and also avoid plant-based saturated fats (palm and coconut oils). Make the fats that you do consume good fats—monounsaturated fats such as those in olive oil, canola oil, and marine fish. Cut down on salt. Consume fewer calories. Eating more calories than the body can use results in excess weight. Get more fiber from fresh fruits and vegetables, whole grains, and beans and legumes.

DIABETES

Type 2 diabetes strikes twice as many women as men over the age of forty-five. At about this age, levels of women's sex hormones start to decrease and menopausal symptoms begin, adding to the problem. In people with type 2 diabetes, by far the more common form of the condition, the pancreas produces insufficient quantities of the hormone insulin to process glucose (sugar), or blood glucose, the chief source of energy for all of the body's cells. The cells also may become resistant to the effects of what little insulin there is in the bloodstream. Obesity is the most significant risk factor for this condition, followed by lack of exercise and heredity. Studies show that depression and stress play a significant role in women's eating habits. Sugar and fatty foods, the type of foods most often craved, cause an increase in brain chemicals that temporarily make you feel good. These are the types of foods that lead to both obesity and diabetes.

Diet is critical to the prevention and management of type 2 diabetes. It is important to limit your consumption of sugar and white flour. If possible, try to avoid foods that contain them altogether. Concentrated sources of simple carbohydrates such as honey, fruit juices, and dairy products such as butter, cheese, and ice cream block insulin activity. These foods too should be avoided or strictly limited.

Increasing your intake of fiber is a key part of combating diabetes, as it helps to slow the release of sugar into the bloodstream. Eat plenty of fresh whole vegetables, fruits, beans, and whole grains. Drinking plenty of water is also important. Keep your protein levels steady with servings of fish, poultry, low-fat cheeses, and beans and legumes. Keeping blood sugar and protein levels on an even keel helps to reduce cravings for sweets, a common problem for women with type 2 diabetes. If you have unbearable cravings for sugar, use stevia instead. This is an herbal-based sweetener that tastes as good as sugar and does not disturb the body's blood sugar or insulin levels.

MACULAR DEGENERATION

Poor eyesight contributes to tripping, falling, car and kitchen accidents, and being more vulnerable to strangers and criminals. The most common cause of visual impairment in people over the age of fifty-five, age-related macular degeneration (AMD) causes an incurable, progressive loss of vision that starts in the center of the visual field and gradually expands toward the peripheral vision. As with Alzheimer's disease, this is not a disorder limited to women, but it is one that becomes more likely with age—and gets worse with age unless proper preventive measures are taken.

Studies suggest that damage caused by free radicals may be the culprit behind AMD, and that it may be possible to prevent this type of damage by increasing the intake of carotenoid antioxidants (see Chapter 6), as well as other targeted nutrients, amino acids, and minerals. The carotenoids lutein, lycopene, and zeaxanthin, in combination, work better than single compounds to protect the eyes. Wonderful sources of these carotenoids, as well as beta-carotene, are carrots, tomatoes, Brussels sprouts, orange juice, kale, collard greens, spinach, Swiss chard, parsley, mustard greens, red pepper, celery, broccoli, and romaine lettuce. Lycopene is released when cooked, so use cooked tomato products such as tomato paste and pasta sauces. Bilberry extract, derived from an herb related to the blue-

berry, has been found to protect eye cells and membranes from free-radical damage as well.

OSTEOPOROSIS

Osteoporosis affects more than 25 million women over the age of forty-five in the United States and Canada. This disorder—which cannot be cured, only prevented or delayed—results when the bones lose minerals that give them their strength, rendering them increasingly porous, fragile, and vulnerable to fracture. Half of postmenopausal women have some degree of undetected bone loss.

We have long been aware of the importance of calcium in building strong bones and teeth. Calcium has many other benefits as well. It is important for maintaining muscle tone and elasticity, and is involved in muscle growth, contraction, and relaxation (including that of the body's most vital muscle, the heart). It helps to prevent muscle cramping and is necessary for the absorption of vitamin B_{12}, which fosters healthy nerves. You might be tempted to think, therefore, that preventing osteoporosis would be as simple as getting megadoses of calcium. This is not necessarily the case, however, and can even lead to deficiencies in magnesium, because calcium and magnesium levels in the body must be in proper balance. Furthermore, osteoporosis in women is not so much caused by a failure to get enough calcium as by a failure to absorb and maintain the calcium they do get. Older adults also may lack vitamins D and K, which are needed for calcium absorption and strong bones. Food choices that rob the body of calcium and should be avoided are sugar, caffeine, and soft drinks that contain phosphates. Phosphates cause the body to eliminate calcium, even if calcium must be leached from the bones to do this.

Milk and other dairy products are frequently spoken of as sources of dietary calcium, but studies have shown that consuming large quantities of dairy foods may actually end up robbing the body of calcium. Fortunately, there are many healthy nondairy sources of calcium that you can incorporate into your diet. These sources will provide variety and give you enough calcium to build up the necessary bone density to prevent or slow the progression of osteoporosis.

The Best Dietary Calcium Sources

Getting enough calcium is important for women of all ages. It is best to get as much of your calcium requirement as possible from food. The following is an extensive list of the best sources of dietary calcium:

- Vegetables: Dark-green and leafy vegetables (including broccoli, collard greens, dandelion greens, kale, parsley, raw spinach, turnip greens, and watercress); aparagus; kelp, dulse, and other sea vegetables; globe artichokes; okra; green snap beans; and tomatoes.

- Fruits: Dried figs and prunes, raisins, dates, ripe olives, and oranges.

- Legumes: Soybeans and soy foods, such as tofu, and cooked dried peas and beans.

- Nuts and seeds: Almonds, chestnuts, English walnuts, pecans, hazelnuts, Brazil nuts, sunflower seeds, pumpkinseeds, squash seeds, sesame seeds, and tahini (sesame butter).

- Grains: Amaranth, wheat bran, wheat germ, raw buckwheat, and oats.

- Seafood: Flounder, oysters, salmon, sardines (with the bones), and shrimp.

- Miscellaneous: Brewer's yeast, blackstrap molasses, buttermilk, carob, corn tortillas (with lime), fortified soy and rice beverages, orange juice, whey, and yogurt.

Calcium Supplements

It is important to get as much calcium from food sources as possible, but since calcium is one of the hardest minerals for the body to absorb, supplementation is often necessary. There are different forms of calcium available, so it is important to look at the amount of *elemental calcium* a given supplement contains, rather than the amount of the whole compound.

The National Academy of Sciences recommends an intake of 1,000 to 1,200 milligrams per day of elemental calcium, plus 200 to 400 international units (IUs) of vitamin D (600 IUs after age seventy) to promote calcium absorption. If you are unsure of getting enough calcium from food, supplementation is recommended. Different supplement products contain different forms of calcium, some of which are better than others. *Calcium carbonate* contains 40 percent elemental calcium, and is a form of calcium that needs to be acted on by stomach acid to be absorbed. If you take a supplement containing calcium carbonate, take it with food, preferably toward the end of a meal. *Calcium citrate* doesn't require stomach acid for absorption so it can can be taken any time. It is 21 percent elemental calcium, so it may take more tablets to meet the daily needs. Other available forms of calcium include *calcium lactate* (13 percent elemental calcium) and *calcium gluconate,* (9 percent elemental calcium), both of which contain lower percentages of calcium and are usually more expensive. Taking calcium supplements made from bone meal, unrefined oyster shells, or dolomite is *not* recommended, as they are a potential source of contaminants. A USP symbol or the word "purified" on the label indicates a safer product.

How to Take Calcium

When choosing a calcium supplement, look for the "serving size" (the number of pills or capsules that makes up the specified dosage) and amount of elemental calcium the dose contains. A recommended daily intake of calcium is at least 1,000 to 1,200 milligrams of elemental calcium. However, the body can absorb only about 500 milligrams of calcium at a time, so take it in divided doses with various meals during the day. Taken at bedtime, calcium helps with sleep. Because calcium and magnesium have to be in the proper balance, make sure to get at least 320 milligrams of magnesium each day. Try to get magnesium from the foods you eat—good dietary sources include vegetables (especially leafy green), fruits, tofu, whole grains, almonds, and cashews—but if that is not possible, it is wise to take a supplement.

To check the absorbability of the calcium in a given supplement, put the tablet in 4 ounces of white vinegar. If it does not dissolve within thirty minutes, it probably will not dissolve in your stomach, either, so you should choose a different product.

Iron and zinc supplements interfere with calcium absorption, so if you are taking those minerals in supplement form, take them several hours apart from the calcium supplement. Also, calcium supplements can interfere with the effects of verapamil (Calan, Isopta), a calcium-channel blocker often prescribed for heart problems and high blood pressure, and decrease the effectiveness of tetracycline or quinolone antibiotics, thyroid hormone, certain anticonvulsants, and steroids, so if you must take these drugs, put off taking your calcium supplement for two to four hours after taking the medication.

OVERWEIGHT

One-third to one-half of American women, depending on age, are currently overweight.

Excess pounds take a large toll on women's health. It is a major contributing factor to both cardiovascular disease and diabetes. In addition, obesity increases a women's chance of breast cancer. Studies have found that women who gain too much weight during pregnancy face increased risks of breast cancer later in life.

Women who have fought the weight battle all their lives face another hurdle at menopause. One survey indicated that 65 to 75 percent of women gain weight involuntarily during menopause. This may be due to a lack of progesterone—estrogen that is not balanced by an adequate amount of progesterone can cause weight gain. Another cause could be that during the first ten days to two weeks of the menstrual cycle, women's bodies use up a significant number of calories in ovulation. When a woman enters menopause and her periods cease, she no longer ovulates and so these calories are no longer burned.

If you have a problem keeping your weight under control, whether before menopause or after, eat smaller portions at meals, avoid second helpings, stay away from fried foods, and eat more fruits and vegetables.

Exercise is another important factor in weight control. A study of more than 40,000 women over a seven-year period found that women in their fifties and sixties who exercised regularly had up to a 40 percent reduced chance of dying prematurely. The more active the women were and the

Stress and Your Hair

Can stress make your hair fall out? Maybe. A study at Tuft's University School of Medicine reveals that skin cells contain receptors for corticotrophin-releasing hormone (CRH), which is sometimes released in the skin in response to stress. CRH can cause inflammation that interrupts the growth of hair follicles and destroys the roots. Evidently, when a woman is under stress, her scalp produces more CRH receptors, allowing more of the hormone to bind to them and cause inflammation.

more intense the activity they engaged in, the lower their risk of dying. Even infrequent moderate activity has a beneficial effect. An article in *The New England Journal of Medicine* reported that women who walked just three hours a week had a 30 to 40 percent lower risk of having a heart attack than those who do not, and women who walked more than five hours a week had a 50 percent lower risk. The combination of proper nutrition and exercise is the maintenance women require to sustain high levels of optimum health. Incorporating some form of regular exercise fights aging and many associated diseases, and can improve your quality of life at any age.

PREMENSTRUAL SYNDROME

At least 150 symptoms have been linked to premenstrual syndrome (PMS), among them acne breakouts and oily skin, breast tenderness, cramps, depression, fatigue, fluid retention and bloating, irritability, moodiness, sugar cravings, and tension. Symptoms are often amplified by an unhealthy diet. Essential fatty acids (the omega-6 linoleic acid and omega-3 linolenic) play a big role in soothing PMS symptoms. These essential fatty acids are required for normal development and functioning of the reproductive tract. They are also necessary for the synthesis of prostaglandins (hormonelike chemicals) that help reduce menstrual cramps. To maintain adequate levels of essential fatty acids, eat raw seeds and nuts, salmon, tuna, trout, and halibut. Evening primrose oil, which contains the essential gamma-linolenic acid (GLA), can also help. Women with PMS tend to have abnormally low levels of GLA.

Eating high-carbohydrate foods such as pasta, cereal, and rice, trigger an increase in the production of serotonin, a natural brain chemical, which can help with anger, tension, and depression. The dense carbohydrates found in fruits, vegetables, and grains are a healthy alternative to the sugar women may crave. Vitamin E, found in wheat germ, beet greens, apples, turnip greens, Brussels sprouts, and sweet potatoes, also helps to fight irritability, depression, and anxiety.

Calcium is helpful for cramps and associated pain. (See pages 264–65 for detailed information about calcium.)

Vitamin A, which helps to stave off premenstrual acne and oily skin, is found in carrots, butternut and Hubbard squash, salmon, dandelion greens, and sweet potatoes. Salmon, chicken, tuna, and soybeans are a good source of vitamin B_6, which helps to ward off irritability, mood swings, fluid retention, breast tenderness, bloating, sugar cravings, and fatigue. Fight stress with vitamin C, found in significant concentrations in sweet red peppers, collard greens, sorrel, kale, strawberries, oranges, and grapefruit. Eating six small meals rather than three, with a ratio of 60 percent complex carbohydrates, 20 percent protein, and 20 percent fat, helps some women to feel better during a "hormone crisis."

Foods that aggravate the symptoms associated with PMS are salt, red meat, and dairy products. Caffeine-containing beverages and foods, fruit juice, alcohol, and refined sugar also can make PMS symptoms worse. All of these foods should be avoided. For coffee, substitute grain-based drinks, ginger tea (a good stimulant), and mineral water with lemon.

STRESS AND DEPRESSION

When the hand that rocked the cradle started bringing home the bacon as well, new influences (many of them negative) began to affect women's health. Stress levels climbed right up the career ladder with them, as workloads and responsibilities expanded to outside as well as inside the home. Women's dual roles as breadwinners and homemakers have created stress levels that are even higher than those of many men. The number of women suffering from depression is also on a steady rise.

According to Mark Hyman, M.D., a specialist in women's health and integrative and preventive medicine, "Stress [in women] is the epidemic of the twenty-first century." Stress increases the risk of heart disease, osteoporosis, and stroke. It can even affect hair growth. (See "Stress and Your Hair" on this page.) Stress also goes hand in hand with depression. The National Institute of Mental Health (NIMH) has launched a study that will monitor stress hormones and bone loss in 160 women between the ages of twenty-one and forty-five who have been diagnosed with depression. Depression is a disease not just of the soul and mind, but also of the body, according to NIMH researcher Giovanni Cizza, M.D., Ph.D., but, he continues, "The question is if there is something intrinsic to depression that might affect bones." One idea is that cortisol, the "fight-or-flight" hormone, levels of which are elevated in depressed people, may contribute to bone loss. Depression is also associated with decreased levels of estrogen and human growth hormone. This also may weaken bones. People with depression tend to have low levels of eicosapentaenoic acid (EPA), an essential fatty acid. Eating oily fish, which contain EPA, or taking fish oil supplements, may therefore help to ease depression.

Perhaps in response to the new, higher levels of stress they are experiencing, many women have learned to relax just like the "good old boys." Alcoholism and nicotine addiction have become women's health issues. Joining the workforce full time has placed huge additional draws on women's health and nutritional "banks," which often are already depleted by hormonal fluctuations associated with menstrual cycles, childbearing, nursing, and menopause. As a result, diseases that once primarily threatened men, such as high blood pressure and coronary artery disease, are now equally threatening to many women.

THYROID DISORDERS

The thyroid gland is the body's internal thermostat, regulating the temperature by secreting two hormones that control how quickly the body burns calories and uses energy. Too high a level of thyroid hormones is known as *hyperthyroidism;* too low a level is known as *hypothyroidism.*

Women between the ages of thirty and fifty are the most prone to developing thyroid conditions. Hyperthyroidism is rare, but it is estimated that one in eight women will develop hyperthyroidism at some point in her lifetime. The symptoms of hyperthyroidism include fatigue, loss of appetite, inability to tolerate cold, slow heart rate, weight gain, painful premenstrual problems, a milky discharge from the breasts, fertility problems, muscle weakness, muscle cramps, dry and scaly skin, a yellow-orange coloration in the skin (particularly on the palms of the hands), yellow

bumps on the eyelids, hair loss (including the eyebrows), recurrent infections, migraines, hoarseness, respiratory infections, constipation, depression, difficulty concentrating, slow speech, goiter, and drooping, swollen eyes. If you are experiencing any combination of these symptoms, you can perform the following simple self-test to evaluate your thyroid function: Keep a thermometer right by your bed. As soon as you wake up in the morning, before doing *anything* else, place the thermometer under your arm and keep it there for fifteen minutes. Remain still and quiet, as any motion can upset your temperature reading. A temperature of 97.6°F or lower may indicate an underactive thyroid. Keep a temperature log for five days. If your readings are consistently low, consult your health care provider.

Doctors tend to prescribe synthetic thyroid hormone preparations for people with hypothyroidism, but correcting underlying mineral and vitamin imbalances can do much to correct thyroid function without using drugs. If you suspect you may have a thyroid imbalance, eat foods rich in B vitamins, such as wheat germ, whole grains, nuts, seeds, dark-green leafy vegetables, and legumes. Brewer's yeast is another natural source. Kelp, dulse, Irish moss, and other sea vegetables, as well as natural iodized sea salt, are good sources of sodium and iodine, which the thyroid needs. If symptoms continue despite dietary changes, see a health-care practitioner to have your thyroid function tested and discuss additional treatment.

CHAPTER THIRTY-FIVE

VEGETARIAN NUTRITION

Nothing will benefit human health and increase the chances for survival of life on Earth as much as the evolution to a vegetarian diet.

—*Albert Einstein, physicist and Nobel laureate*

There are many different reasons to consider a vegetarian diet. Some people are concerned about the use of hormones and antibiotics (also sprayed on feed) in livestock, as well as potential threats such as mad cow disease. Health, animal welfare, religion and spirituality, and a concern for our planet's resources are just a few of the reasons people think of trying a vegetarian diet. The big question is, "Can I get all the nutrition I need to be healthy if I become a vegetarian?" The answer is a resounding *yes!* It is even possible that adopting a well-balanced vegetarian diet can improve your health.

APPROACHES TO VEGETARIANISM

Deciding to become a vegetarian leaves room for different interpretations and degrees of strictness, as well as choices. Celebrities like Paul McCartney and Fred (Mr.) Rogers, both vegetarians, may enjoy very different diets. The following are some of the different types of vegetarians:

- *Semivegetarians* eat dairy products, eggs, chicken, and fish, but no other animal flesh.

- *Pescovegetarians* eat dairy products, eggs, and fish, but no other animal flesh.

- *Lacto-ovo-vegetarians* eat dairy foods and eggs, but no animal flesh.

- *Lactovegetarians* eat dairy products but do not eat eggs or animal flesh.

- *Ovo-vegetarians* eat eggs but no dairy products or animal flesh.

- *Vegans* (pronounced VEE-gan, with a hard G) eat no animal products of any type.

Which approach you decide on depends on what your personal reasons for pursuing vegetarianism are, issues such as food allergies and intolerances, and, to some extent, your individual tastes.

A HEALTHY VEGETARIAN DIET

Just because a diet is vegetarian does not mean it is healthy. There can be significant amounts of sugar, fat, salt, and preservatives in "vegetarian" food products. In fashioning a nutritious diet, cutting out meat is not as important as eating foods that are nutritionally charged, such as fresh fruits and vegetables, whole grains, and healthy, nonhydrogenated fats and oils. As with any diet, vegetarian menus take planning to provide adequate nutrition. With some simple adjustments, however, a vegetarian diet does offer many health benefits.

Many vegetarians, especially ovo-vegetarians, explore the creative use of soy products, which offer good plant-based substitutes for meat, milk, mayonnaise, sour cream, cheese, hamburgers, yogurt, and even ice cream. (See Chapter 24.) Soy foods are high in protein, fiber, and complex carbohydrates. They are good sources of many vitamins and minerals, including calcium and iron; are low in saturated fat; and can help to lower blood cholesterol. There are plenty of delicious soy products, such as those made by the Tofutti company, which produces "ice cream," cheeses, and other substitutes for dairy products that do not contain casein and caseinate, which are derivatives of dairy products.

VEGETARIANISM AND SPECIFIC HEALTH PROBLEMS

A good vegetarian diet offers a number of health benefits. Indeed, this is one of the reasons many people decide to become vegetarians. The following sections look at a number of specific disorders that may be prevented or helped through a vegetarian diet.

Cancer

It is well documented that eating red meat is a risk factor for colon cancer (chicken and fish are not risk factors unless contaminated). A diet that includes plenty of fruits, vegetables, and fiber, on the other hand, is associated with a significantly lower than average risk of some types of cancer, including colorectal cancer and breast cancer. Eating a combination of different types and colors of vegetables each day provides the most protection. (See Chapter 6.)

Cardiovascular Disease

The incidence of coronary artery disease has long been known to be lower in vegetarians than in nonvegetarians. Studies show that vegetarians are 24 percent less likely than the general public to die of coronary artery disease. This is likely due at least in part to their lower intake of saturated fats and cholesterol, which translates into lower levels of total blood cholesterol. In addition, vegetarians generally consume more of the key antioxidants—vitamins C and E, and phytochemicals such as carotenoids—that are known to help protect against heart disease. There are definitely cardiovascular benefits to a vegetarian diet. Dr. William Castelli, one of the researchers with the renowned Framingham Heart Study in Massachusetts, once remarked, in reference to a group of macrobiotic vegetarians in Boston that, hypothetically at least, "vegans have cholesterol levels so low, they'd never get a heart attack."

Diabetes

Vegetarians who follow a well-balanced diet have a *90 percent lower* than average risk of developing type 2 diabetes. The connection is not completely understood, but it is possible that people who choose to be vegetarians are more health-conscious than average to begin with and so may be more likely to exercise regularly, and to avoid drinking and smoking—all key factors in the prevention of diabetes. Vegetarians also are less prone to obesity, which has a strong link to the development of type 2 diabetes.

Obesity

Vegetarian diets are generally lower in calories and fat and higher in fiber than a meat-based diet, which make them more conducive to weight loss and maintenance. However, if you already eat a healthy diet and simply eliminating meat is the goal, don't expect a large weight loss. On the other hand, if your current diet is high in saturated fat but low in vegetables, fruits, and whole grains, you can reasonably expect to lose weight if you become a vegetarian. This is simply because the foods vegetarians eat tend to be nutrient-dense but not calorie-dense.

A FEW WORDS OF PRUDENCE

A well-balanced vegetarian diet can meet the nutritional requirements of virtually anyone, from babies to senior citizens, and including athletes, pregnant women, and nursing mothers. The body's daily requirements for protein, calcium, fat, vitamins, and minerals can all be met with well-planned vegetarian menus. Just remember, however, that you cannot remove animal-based sources of these nutrients from a nonvegetarian diet without replacing them with plant-based sources. Also, be aware that children and infant vegetarians need greater amounts of nutrients than adults, and careful planning is necessary to ensure they get a balanced diet. Children have small stomachs and vegetarian dishes can be so high in bulk that it is difficult for them to eat enough to meet their growth and energy needs. If you are raising a young vegetarian, it may be a good idea to consult with a professional dietitian or nutritional counselor.

There are some nutritional concerns of particular importance for all vegetarians, regardless of age. These are principally the need to ensure an adequate intake of protein, iron, and vitamin B_{12}.

Protein

Vegetarians can receive all the protein their bodies need by combining the right two or three vegetables at each meal. Eliminating some animal-based foods from the diet, however, does make it necessary to replace them with other foods to get all the nutrients needed to maintain health. For example, combine beans or legumes with corn, nuts, rice, seeds, or wheat. Soy foods, such as tofu, by themselves are excellent vegetarian protein sources. (For detailed information about this topic, see Chapter 19.)

Iron

Many vegetarian foods are rich in iron, but it is not as easily absorbed as the iron in meat. Vitamin C increases the absorption of iron from plant foods, so consume vitamin C–rich foods with meals. Dark-green leafy vegetables, strawberries, potatoes, and watermelon are good sources of both vitamin C and iron. Iron is also found in lentils, garbanzo beans, sesame seeds, almonds, and blackstrap molasses.

Vitamin B_{12}

One particular nutritional concern for vegetarians is vitamin B_{12}, which is needed for the formation of red blood cells, proper utilization of iron, digestion and absorption of nutrients from foods, and the health of the nervous system, among other vital functions. This vitamin is present almost exclusively in foods of animal origin, so people who do not consume any such foods are susceptible to deficiencies. Consequently, vegetarians—especially vegans—should take particular care to obtain the equivalent of 2,000 to 4,000 micrograms of vitamin B_{12} daily. The few good vegetarian food sources of this vitamin include tempeh, sea vegetables such as dulse and kombu, nutritional (or brewer's) yeast, tofu, and yogurt. Include these foods in your diet. There are also vegetarian vitamin B_{12} supplements (made from algae) available. Taking care to nourish the intestinal tract is also important. If there are enough friendly intestinal bacteria, the body can manufacture vitamin B_{12}.

MAKING THE CHANGE TO A VEGETARIAN DIET

If you are considering any type of vegetarian diet, first make sure to be armed with enough information to ensure a successful change. Foods that you may have never eaten before might become your best sources of nutrients formerly derived from meat, eggs, dairy products, or fish. Be open to new possibilities.

In order to enjoy this new way of eating, it is important to find (or create) recipes for dishes you like that are not meat-centered. Many of the recipes in this book are vegetarian or have vegetarian options. Your local library and bookstore are good sources for more information and recipes.

Appendix A: Recognizing and Correcting Nutritional Deficiencies

Nutritional deficiencies are more common than you might think, even in developed countries where food is abundant. Use the table below to learn the recommended intake of basic nutrients, what the signs of deficiency are, and which foods are good sources of these nutrients. If you suspect you are deficient in one or more nutrients, increase your consumption of foods that supply them. Note that any given symptom may or may not be a sign of a particular deficiency. Also, the symptoms are listed in alphabetical order, not in the order of likelihood. If you have any questions about symptoms you are experiencing, consult with your health-care practitioner.

KEY TO ABBREVIATIONS:

RDI = reference daily intake (formerly the recommended dietary allowance, or RDA); the necessary daily intake for the average adult as established by the Food and Nutrition Board of the U.S. Institute of Medicine, part of the National Academy of Sciences

UL = upper limit officially considered safe

ODI = optimum daily intake (recommended by many nutritionists and researchers)

IU = international unit (a measure of potency)

mg = milligram (a measure of weight)

mcg = microgram (a measure of weight, equal to 1/1000 mg)

NUTRIENT	DAILY INTAKE	POSSIBLE SYMPTOMS OF DEFICIENCY	FOOD SOURCES
VITAMINS			
Vitamin A (and beta-carotene, which is converted into vitamin A in the liver)	RDI: 700–900 mcg (2,300–3,000 IU) UL: 3,000 mcg (10,000 IU) ODI: 1,500 mcg (5,000 IU)	Abscesses in the ears, cancer, dry hair, dry skin, dry eyes, fatigue, frequent colds and other respiratory infections, insomnia, nerve deterioration, night blindness, pneumonia, premature aging, reproductive problems, sinusitis, skin disorders (including acne), stunted growth, weight loss.	Best: fish liver oil, mangoes, sweet potatoes, yellow squash, pumpkin. Good: tomatoes, eggs, dairy products, leafy greens, carrots, sea vegetables, spinach, red peppers, apricots, papaya, cantaloupe.
Vitamin B$_1$ (thiamine)	RDI: 1.1–1.2 mg UL: not established ODI: 5–10 mg	Beriberi; constipation; edema; enlarged liver; fatigue or general weakness; forgetfulness; gastrointestinal disturbances; heart changes; irritability; labored breathing; loss of appetite; nervousness; numbness of the hands and feet; pain and sensitivity; poor coordination; severe weight loss; tingling sensations; weak, sore muscles; muscle atrophy.	Best: eggs, legumes, whole grains, most nuts. Good: fish, brown rice, peas, rice bran, wheat germ, brewer's yeast, potatoes, dulse, kelp, oatmeal, prunes, raisins, spirulina, leafy greens.
Vitamin B$_2$ (riboflavin)	RDI: 1.1–1.3 mg UL: not established ODI: 15–50 mg	Cracks and sores at the corners of the mouth, dermatitis, dizziness, eye disorders, hair loss, inflammation of the mouth and tongue, insomnia, light sensitivity, poor digestion, retarded growth, skin lesions, slowed mental response.	Best: cheese, egg yolks, legumes, spinach, leafy greens, nuts. Good: fish, milk, whole grains, yogurt, asparagus, avocados, broccoli, Brussels sprouts, currants, dandelion greens, dulse, kelp, mushrooms, blackstrap molasses.

NUTRIENT	DAILY INTAKE	POSSIBLE SYMPTOMS OF DEFICIENCY	FOOD SOURCES
VITAMINS			
Vitamin B₃ (niacin)	RDI: 14–16 mg UL: 35 mg ODI: 15–50 mg	Canker sores, dementia, depression, diarrhea, dizziness, fatigue, halitosis, headaches, indigestion, inflammation, insomnia, limb pains, loss of appetite, low blood sugar levels, muscular weakness, pellagra, skin eruptions.	Best: brewer's yeast, dates, eggs, fish, wheat germ, whole-wheat products. Good: dandelion greens, cheese, bran, milk, potatoes.
Vitamin B₆ (pyridoxine)	RDI: 1.3–1.7 mg UL: 100 mg ODI: 50–100 mg	Acne, anemia, anorexia, arthritis, carpal tunnel syndrome, conjunctivitis, convulsions, depression, dizziness, fatigue, flaky skin, hair loss, headaches, hearing problems, hyperirritability, impaired memory or memory loss, impaired wound healing, learning difficulties, nausea, vomiting, numbness, tingling sensations, oily facial skin, sore tongue, cracks and sores on mouth and lips, inflammation of mouth and gums, stunted growth.	Best: brewer's yeast, fish, peas, spinach, beans. Good: carrots, eggs, sunflower seeds, nuts, wheat germ, avocado, bananas, blackstrap molasses, broccoli, brown rice, potatoes.
Vitamin B₁₂ (cobalamin)	RDI: 2.4 mcg UL: not established ODI: 200–400 mcg	Abnormal gait, bone loss, chronic fatigue, drowsiness, depression, digestive disorders, constipation, dizziness, enlargement of the liver, eye disorders, hallucinations, headaches (including migraine), inflammation of the tongue, irritability, moodiness, labored breathing, memory loss, nervousness, neurological damage, palpitations, pernicious anemia, ringing in the ears, spinal cord degeneration.	Best: brewer's and nutritional yeast, shellfish, seafood, legumes, nuts, fortified grains. Good: fortified vegetarian products, eggs, dairy products.
Biotin	RDI: 30 mg UL: not established ODI: 400–800 mg	Anemia, depression, hair loss, high blood sugar levels, inflammation or pallor of the skin and mucous membranes, insomnia, loss of appetite, muscular pain, nausea, soreness of the tongue.	Best: brewer's yeast, cooked egg yolks, milk, mushrooms, cruciferous vegetables. Good: saltwater fish, bananas, avocado, wheat bran, whole grains, legumes, nuts.
Choline	RDI: not established UL: not established ODI: 50–200 mcg	Cardiac symptoms, fatty buildup in the liver, gastric ulcers, high blood pressure, inability to digest fats, kidney and liver impairment, neurological and psychiatric disorders, stunted growth.	Best: brewer's yeast, eggs, legumes, wheat germ, cauliflower. Good: lecithin, liver, fish, milk, soybeans, cabbage.
Folate (folic acid)	RDI: 400 mcg UL: 1,000 mcg ODI: 400–800 mcg	Anemia; apathy; birth defects in offspring; digestive disturbances; fatigue; graying hair; growth impairment; insomnia; labored breathing; memory problems; paranoia; sore, red tongue; weakness.	Best: brewer's yeast, leafy greens, dried beans, legumes, whole grains. Good: dates, asparagus, lentils, oranges, blackberries, kiwi, strawberries, split peas, wheat germ.
Inositol	RDI: not established UL: not established ODI: 50–200 mg	Constipation, depression, hair loss, heart disease, high blood cholesterol, irritability, liver disease, mood swings, panic or anxiety attacks, skin eruptions.	Best: brewer's yeast, lima beans, cabbage, grapefruit, cantaloupe, raisins, wheat germ. Good: brown rice, lecithin, legumes, lentils, dried beans, bananas, oranges, unrefined molasses, whole grains, nuts.
Pantothenic acid	RDI: 5 mg UL: not established ODI: 50–100 mg	Fatigue, headache, nausea, tingling in hands.	Best: saltwater fish, nuts, legumes, whole-rye flour, whole wheat. Good: fresh vegetables, blackstrap molasses, sunflower seeds, mushrooms, milk, brewer's yeast, eggs, wheat germ, royal jelly.
Para-amino-benzoic acid (PABA)	RDI: not established UL: not established ODI: 10–50 mg	Depression, fatigue, gastrointestinal disorders, graying hair, irritability, nervousness, patchy areas of white skin.	Best: eggs, molasses, wheat germ, brown rice, brewer's yeast. Good: mushrooms, whole grains, sunflower seeds, lecithin, yogurt.
Vitamin C (ascorbic acid)	RDI: 75–90 mg UL: 2,000 mg ODI: 1,000–3,000 mg, depending on tolerance	Adrenal malfunction; anemia; asthma; cancer; gums that bleed when brushed; increased susceptibility to infection, especially colds and bronchial infections; joint pain; fragile bones and joints; lack of energy; poor digestion; prolonged wound healing time; scurvy; stiff joints; tendency to bruise easily; tooth loss.	Best: strawberries, blackberries, leafy greens, lemons, oranges, grapefruit, avocados. Good: broccoli, Brussels sprouts, snow peas, sweet peppers, sweet potatoes, rose hips, plantain, persimmons, papaya, mangoes, cantaloupe, pineapple, summer squash, watermelon, honeydew, kiwi, tomatoes.
Bioflavonoids (although not true vitamins, bioflavonoids are partners with vitamin C and are sometimes referred to as vitamin P)	RDI: not established UL: not established ODI: 200–500 mg	Alkalosis, allergies, colitis, heart disorders, heel and bone spurs, hemorrhoids, immune deficiency, infections, tendency to bruise easily, varicose veins.	Best: lemons, oranges, grapefruit. Good: cherries, grapes, blackberries, plums, black currants, buckwheat, apricots, papayas, peppers, rose hips, tomatoes.

NUTRIENT	DAILY INTAKE	POSSIBLE SYMPTOMS OF DEFICIENCY	FOOD SOURCES
VITAMINS			
Vitamin D	RDI: 200–600 IU UL: 600 IU ODI: 400 IU	Bone diseases, burning sensation in mouth and throat, cataracts, diarrhea, gum disease, hair loss, insomnia, loss of appetite, osteomalacia in adults, rickets in children, visual problems, weight loss.	Exposure to sunshine causes the body to manufacture vitamin D, and is the optimum source. Best: cod liver oil, egg yolks, butter, halibut. Good: milk, salmon, tuna, oatmeal.
Vitamin E	RDI: 15 mg (23 IU) UL: 1,000 mg (1500 IU) ODI: 120–180 mg (180–270 IU)	Cardiovascular/circulatory disorders, hot flashes, impotence, infertility in both men and women, menstrual problems, neuromuscular impairment, premature aging, shortened red blood cell life span, spontaneous abortion (miscarriage), uterine degeneration, weakened immune system.	Best: almonds, nuts, seeds, cold-pressed vegetable oils, whole grains, eggs. Good: wheat germ, leafy greens, mangoes, corn, avocados, olives, soybeans.
Vitamin K	RDI: 90–120 mcg UL: not established ODI: 100–500 mcg	Abnormal and/or internal bleeding, such as nosebleeds, bleeding gums, heavy menstruation, hemorrhagic anemia, and lack of clot formation; bone disorders; colitis and intestinal/colon disorders; diverticulitis; easy bruising; hemorrhoids; leg ulcers; liver disorders; multiple sclerosis.	Best: leafy greens, egg yolks, whole wheat, alfalfa, cheese. Good: cruciferous vegetables, dried beans and peas, oats, asparagus, tomatoes, avocados, soybeans, butter, yogurt.
MINERALS			
Boron	RDI: not established UL: 3 mg ODI: 1–3 mg	Arthritis, bone disorders, calcium loss, postmenopausal osteoporosis.	Fruits, vegetables, raisins, prunes, nuts.
Calcium	RDI: 1,000–2,000 mg UL: 2,500 mg ODI: 1,500–2,000 mg	Aching joints, brittle nails, cognitive impairment, convulsions, delusions, depression, eczema, elevated blood cholesterol, heart palpitations, hyperactivity, hypertension (high blood pressure), insomnia, muscle cramps/spasms, nervousness, numbness in the arms and/or legs, pasty complexion, rheumatoid arthritis, rickets, tooth decay.	Best: almonds, leafy greens, carob, broccoli, kelp, yogurt, goat's milk. Good: filberts, sesame seeds, sunflower seeds, salmon with bones, anchovies, sardines, dried figs, raisins, watercress, oranges, legumes, Brussels sprouts, figs, blackstrap molasses, tofu.
Chromium	RDI: 20–35 mcg UL: not established ODI: 150–400 mcg	Anxiety, atherosclerosis, depressed growth rate, fatigue, glucose intolerance (particularly in people with diabetes), inadequate metabolism of amino acids, memory loss, muscle loss, weight problems.	Best: whole grains, corn oil, potatoes with skins, brown rice, brewer's yeast, dried beans. Good: wheat germ, dairy products, eggs, broccoli, spinach, blackstrap molasses, mushrooms, seafood.
Copper	RDI: 900 mcg UL: 10 mg ODI: 2–3 mg	Anemia, arthritis, hair loss, diarrhea, general weakness, heart disorders, impaired respiratory function, increased blood fat levels, osteoporosis, skin sores, ulcers.	Best: raisins, legumes, seafood/oysters, whole grains, nuts, eggs, meat. Good: prunes, shellfish, brewer's yeast, potatoes, cherries, leafy greens, lentils, mushrooms, soybeans, blackstrap molasses.
Iodine	RDI: 150 mcg UL: 1,100 mcg ODI: 100–225 mcg	Breast cancer, dry skin and hair, fatigue/low vitality, goiter, irritability, mental retardation in children, neonatal hypothyroidism, obesity, weight gain.	Best: seafood (fish, shellfish, sea vegetables), sea salt, iodized salt, garlic, onions. Good: whole grains, leafy greens, dairy products.
Iron	RDI: premenopausal women: 18 mg; all others: 8 mg UL: 45 mg ODI: 18–30 mg	Anemia, brittle hair, difficulty swallowing, digestive disturbances, dizziness, fragile bones, hair loss, headaches, heart palpitations, inflammation of the tissues of the mouth, irritability, listlessness and fatigue, nails that are spoon-shaped or have lengthwise ridges, nervousness, obesity, pallor, slowed mental reactions.	Best: beets, figs, asparagus, raisins, blackstrap molasses. Good: fish and shellfish, eggs, breads and cereals (whole grain or enriched with iron), leafy vegetables, broccoli, prunes, dried fruit, almonds, brewer's yeast, dulse, kelp, kidney beans, lima beans, lentils, millet, pumpkinseeds.
Magnesium	RDI: women: 310–420 mg; men: 400–420 mg UL: not established ODI: 750–1,000 mg	Asthma, cardiac arrhythmia and cardiac arrest, chronic fatigue, chronic pain, confusion, depression, hypertension, insomnia, irritability, irritable bowel syndrome, kidney stones, poor digestion, pulmonary disorders, rapid heartbeat, seizures, tantrums, tooth grinding (bruxism), tremors and convulsions.	Best: whole grains, figs, fish and seafood, nuts, tofu, soybeans, seeds, dried apricots. Good: raisins, millet, lima beans, dried beans, legumes, bananas, brown rice, leafy greens, dairy products.
Manganese	RDI: 1.8–2.3 mg UL: 11 mg ODI: 3–10 mg	Atherosclerosis, breast ailments, confusion, convulsions, eye problems, hearing problems, heart disorders, high cholesterol levels, hypertension, irritability, memory loss, muscle contractions, pancreatic damage, profuse perspiration, rapid pulse, tooth grinding (bruxism), tremors.	Best: whole grains, egg yolks, leafy greens, nuts, seeds, avocados, kelp, blueberries. Good: blackberries, raspberries, beets, broccoli, pineapples, dried peas, cabbage, Brussels sprouts, legumes, sweet potatoes, honey.

NUTRIENT	DAILY INTAKE	POSSIBLE SYMPTOMS OF DEFICIENCY	FOOD SOURCES
MINERALS			
Molybdenum	RDI: 45 mg UL: 2,000 mg ODI: 30–100 mg	Anemia, cancer, decreased ability to metabolize carbohydrates and fats, decreased growth, impotence in older men, loss of appetite, mouth and gum disorders.	Best: wheat grass, spirulina, sea vegetables, whole grains, leafy greens, legumes. Good: green beans, sunflower seeds, potatoes, buckwheat, yams, wheat germ.
Phosphorus	RDI: 700 mg UL: 4,000 mg (3,000 mg for people aged 70 and older) ODI: 1,200 mg	Anxiety; bone pain; fatigue/weakness; irregular breathing; irritability; memory loss; numbness; skin sensitivity; slowed hair, nail, and bone growth; trembling; weakness; weight changes.	Best: whole grains, dairy products, eggs, fish. Good: nuts, seeds, garlic, asparagus, artichokes, dried beans, legumes, lentils, bran, corn, brewer's yeast, mushrooms, potatoes.
Potassium	RDI: not established UL: not established ODI: 99–500 mg	Abnormally dry skin, acne, chills, cognitive impairment, constipation, depression, diarrhea, diminished reflex function, edema/water retention, fluctuations in heartbeat, glucose intolerance, growth impairment, headaches, high cholesterol levels, insatiable thirst, insomnia, muscular fatigue and weakness, nausea and vomiting, nervousness, proteinuria (protein in the urine), respiratory distress, salt retention.	Best: dairy products, fish, legumes, nuts, avocados, raisins. Good: leafy greens, beets, bok choy, bananas, whole grains, potatoes, apricots, dried beans, blackstrap molasses, pomegranates, dates, figs, mushrooms, dried fruit, tomatoes, broccoli, Brussels sprouts.
Selenium	RDI: 55 mcg UL: 400 mcg ODI: 100–200 mcg	Cancer, exhaustion, growth impairment, heart disorders, high cholesterol levels, infections, liver impairment, pancreatic insufficiency, premature aging, sterility.	Best: tuna, salmon, seafood, brewer's yeast, garlic, brown rice, Brazil nuts. Good: bran and germ cereals, broccoli, onions, mushrooms, cucumbers, dairy products, oatmeal.
Zinc	RDI: 8–11 mg UL: 40 mg ODI: 30–50 mg	Acne; delayed sexual maturation; fatigue; growth impairment; hair loss; high cholesterol levels; impaired night vision; impotence; increased susceptibility to infection; infertility; loss of the senses of taste and smell; memory impairment; propensity to diabetes; prostate trouble; recurrent colds and flu; skeletal abnormalities; skin lesions; slow wound healing; thin, peeling nails that may develop white spots.	Best: fish and seafood, pumpkinseeds, soybeans, eggs, legumes, whole grains, wheat germ, wheat bran, brewer's yeast. Good: lima beans, lentils, green peas, dairy products, kelp, dulse, buckwheat, sardines, sunflower seeds, nuts.

Appendix B: Nourishing Every Part of the Body Beautiful

All healthful foods are beneficial, but certain foods are particularly nourishing for specific organs, systems, and structures within the body. The table below indicates which vegetables, fruits, nuts, grains, and seeds are especially good for "preventive maintenance" of a number of vital parts of the body.

BODY PART	VEGETABLES	NUTS, GRAINS, AND SEEDS	FRUITS	OTHER
Adrenal glands Two triangular shaped glands located just above the kidneys, the adrenals are responsible for the excretion of very important hormones and steroid hormones. The hormones epinephrine (adrenaline) and norepinephrine are involved in the body's natural reaction to stressors (fight or flight).	Best: asparagus, all leafy greens. Good: legumes, lima beans, mushrooms, okra, olive oil, onions, red peppers, sea vegetables, soybeans, sprouts.	Brewer's yeast, brown rice, almonds, cereals, flaxseed, millet, blackstrap molasses, pumpkinseeds, whole grains, wheat bran, wheat germ, wild rice.	Blueberries, coconut, figs, gooseberries, grapefruit, lemons, oranges, prunes, strawberries.	Deepwater ocean fish, such as tuna or salmon, is very beneficial. Fats, fried food, pork, processed foods, red meat, sodas, sugar, and white flour put unnecessary stress on adrenal glands and should be avoided. Coenzyme A reduces stress on the adrenals, and coenzyme Q_{10} carries oxygen to the glands. Pantothenic acid and vitamin C aid in reducing stress on the adrenals.
Bladder A small, hollow balloon-shaped organ below the kidneys connected by two ureters. As urea (liquid waste) and water drain out of the kidneys, they are stored in the bladder until nerves in the bladder communicate to the brain that draining is needed.	Best: celery. Good: broccoli, cauliflower, cabbage, green beans, lettuce, potato skins, red and green peppers, spinach.	Almonds, brown rice, flaxseed, blackstrap molasses, oats, soybeans, sunflower seeds, wheat bran, wheat germ.	Best: cranberries, watermelon. Good: acerola cherries, apples, blueberries, cantaloupe, grapefruit, lemons, strawberries.	Unsweetened cranberry juice prevents bacteria from adhering to the lining of the bladder, prohibiting infection. Coffee, black tea, carbonated sodas, and alcohol are irritating to the bladder and should be avoided. Drinking at least 8 glasses of quality water each day promotes a healthy urinary tract. If you must take antibiotics for a bladder infection, use acidophilus to replace friendly bacteria. For a natural antibiotic, use colloidal silver or goldenseal.

BODY PART	VEGETABLES	NUTS, GRAINS, AND SEEDS	FRUITS	OTHER
Blood vessels (veins and arteries) The circulatory system, driven by the heart muscle, delivers oxygen and nutrients while picking up wastes and toxins to be eliminated. The blood vessels—arteries, veins, and capillaries—provide the pathways. Arteries have thick elastic walls and swell when the heart pumps blood in. Veins are thin-walled and return blood back to the heart. Capillaries are small vessels that connect arteries and veins, feed tissues, and collect waste and carry it to the lungs, liver, or kidneys for elimination.	All leafy greens, asparagus, beets, cabbage, carrots, celery, cucumbers, dandelion greens, olives, endive, kelp, legumes, lettuce, mushrooms, okra, onions, parsnips, potato skins, spinach, turnips, watercress.	Flaxseed, whole grains, almonds, barley, brewer's yeast, buckwheat, chestnuts, blackstrap molasses, oatmeal, pignolia nuts, pumpkinseeds, soybean, sunflower seeds, walnuts, wheat germ.	Apricots, blackberries, black cherries, blueberries, cranberries, dates, figs, gooseberries, grapefruit, oranges, peaches, prunes. NOTE: Eat foods low in cholesterol and fat, as well as high-fiber foods, such as fruits, vegetables, and whole grains, for healthy circulation.	If arteries lose their elasticity, harden, and have calcium deposits, it is arteriosclerosis. Atherosclerosis is a similar condition except that the deposits are fatty substances. One-quarter of deaths in the U.S. occur from heart attacks and most are attributed to these causes. Drinking 1–4 cups of green tea each day can lower cholesterol and lipid levels, decreasing chances of atherosclerosis. Pure cold–pressed olive oil or unrefined canola oil provide essential fatty acids (also found in fresh deepwater fish, fish oil, and walnut oil) that may aid in lowering cholesterol. Vitamin E improves circulation. Good sources include dark-green leafy vegetables, legumes, nuts, seeds, soybeans, wheat germ, and whole grains. Lecithin is good for veins and arteries. See also the entry for Heart.
Bones Composed of minerals and collagen, the body's 206 bones are the framework that supports and provides protection for vital organs.	Best: leafy greens, collards, raw spinach, kale, Swiss chard, Brussels sprouts, most beans, tofu, chickpeas, kelp, sea vegetables. Good: broccoli, turnip greens, cauliflower, cabbage, green beans, potato skins, red and green peppers.	Best: almonds, amaranth flour, oats, oatmeal, wheat bran, wheat germ, raw buckwheat, chestnuts. Good: pecans, hazelnuts, sunflower seeds, filberts, flaxseeds, blackstrap molasses, oats, rice, sesame seeds, soybeans.	Best: dried figs and prunes, raisins, dates, oranges. Good: apples, acerola cherries, bananas, blueberries, cantaloupe, figs, gooseberries, grapefruit, kiwi, lemons, pineapple, peaches, prunes, red grapes, strawberries.	Primary to prolonged bone health is abundant calcium that can be absorbed. Calcium is a key mineral to maintain muscle tone and elasticity and is also needed for muscle growth, contraction, and relaxation. The healthiest diet for bones is "greens and beans." Poultry, red meat, and dairy products leech calcium from the bones and encourage its passage into the urine—plant protein in beans, grains, and vegetables, does not. Sugar, salt, alcohol, caffeine, and soft drinks eliminate calcium from the body and should be avoided. If you take calcium supplements, calcium citrate is a good form to supplement with and is easily assimilated. Calcium in bone meal, unrefined oyster shells, or dolomite are potential sources of contaminants. A USP symbol or the word "purified" indicates a safer product.

BODY PART	VEGETABLES	NUTS, GRAINS, AND SEEDS	FRUITS	OTHER
Brain The brain is the body's onboard computer. It is the center for all thought, as well as the command center for all senses.	Best: all leafy greens, beans, broccoli. Good: cabbage, cauliflower, chickpeas, corn, dry peas, green beans, kelp, legumes, lentils, lettuce, mushrooms, potatoes, spinach, sprouts, red and green peppers, reishi mushrooms, soybeans, tomatoes, yams.	Almonds, barley, brewer's yeast, brown rice, flaxseed, millet, blackstrap molasses, oats, peanuts with skins and peanut butter, pecans, rice bran, rye, sesame seeds, soybeans, sunflower seeds, wheat bran, wheat germ, whole grains, wild rice.	Best: avocado, bananas, blackberries, black cherries, blueberries. Good: cantaloupe, coconut, figs, gooseberries, grapefruit, guava, oranges, pineapple, prunes, strawberries.	Fatty acids from dietary fats are used to nourish the cells involved in thought and emotion. Essential fatty acids from flaxseed, fish, or borage oil are important for proper brain function. Glucose from carbohydrates becomes fuel and creates energy. Micronutrients from fruits and vegetables are antioxidants that protect cells from damage. Amino acids from proteins create neurotransmitters for cell networking and communication. People with Alzheimer's disease tend to have low levels of vitamin B_{12}, zinc, and the antioxidant vitamins A and E. Vitamin B_{12} deficiency alone can cause symptoms similar to those of Alzheimer's disease.
Breasts/mammary glands The human breast is a gland that contains milk ducts, lobes, fatty tissue, and a network of lymphatic vessels. In women, they are responsible for lactation; in men, they are normally undeveloped and have no function. Estrogen promotes the growth of the gland and ducts, and progesterone stimulates growth of milk-producing cells.	Asparagus, beets, broccoli, cabbage, celery, kelp, leafy greens, lettuce, okra, onions, parsnips, radishes, spinach, tomatoes. A daily glass of juice made from fresh organic broccoli, cauliflower, carrots, kale, dark leafy greens, and apple is high in phytochemicals and may combat breast cancer.	Flaxseed oil, almonds, barley, brown rice, oats, oatmeal, millet, soybeans, sunflower seeds, wheat, wheat bran.	Apples, cherries, plums, apricots, black figs, cranberries, dates, gooseberries, prunes, strawberries.	
Bronchi and lungs The lungs are the body's largest internal organs. Air enters through the trachea (windpipe), which connects to the bronchi, the breathing tubes that lead into the air sacs in the lungs, where the air is exchanged for carbon dioxide.	Best: all leafy greens. Good: asparagus, broccoli, cabbage, cauliflower, corn, dry peas, green beans, green vegetables, lentils, mushrooms, onions, potatoes, red and green peppers, rutabaga, sprouts, tomatoes.	Almonds, barley, millet, blackstrap molasses, oats, peanuts with skins, pecans, rice bran, sesame seeds, soybeans, sunflower seeds, wheat bran, wheat germ, whole grains, wild rice.	Apples, avocados, blackberries, black cherries, blueberries, cranberries, gooseberries, grapefruit, peaches, prunes, strawberries.	Dairy products, processed foods, sugar, sweet fruits, and white flour promote mucus formation and should be avoided. Bronchitis is an infection or irritation of the bronchi, and pneumonia is an infection or irritation of the lungs. Antibiotics do not help most cases of bronchitis and pneumonia—these drugs have no effect on viral infections. The natural approach to treating bronchitis and pneumonia involves stimulating processes that expel mucus and strengthen the immune system to deal with viral infection.
Ears Ears are direct links to the mind. They are the external organs involved in the hearing function. Composed of three sections—the outer, middle, and inner ear—they are highly specialized tools with sophisticated systems that work together to provide sound.	Best: all leafy greens. Good: beans, broccoli, cabbage, carrots, cauliflower, chickpeas, leeks, lettuce, onions, pumpkin, sea vegetables, spinach, sprouts, squash, sweet peppers, sweet potatoes, tomatoes, watercress.	Almonds, barley, flaxseed oil, oats, pumpkinseeds, rye, soybeans, sunflower seeds, wheat bran, wheat germ, whole grains.	Apricots, blueberries, cantaloupe, cranberries, dates, figs, peaches, prunes, strawberries.	The Mayo clinic advises that people not clean their ears with cotton-tipped swabs—they do not remove the problem wax and can easily damage the ear canal or eardrum.

BODY PART	VEGETABLES	NUTS, GRAINS, AND SEEDS	FRUITS	OTHER
Eyes The eyes are indeed the windows to the soul. They act as emissaries between the light reflected from objects in the surrounding world and the mind, which interprets that light. Light enters the eye through the cornea, passes across the aqueous humor (liquid behind the cornea), passes through the pupil, and then passes through the lens. The lens grows continuously with age, and new cells are added on the outside in layers.	Carrots, collard greens, kale, broccoli, turnip greens, mustard greens, sea vegetables, cabbage, dandelion greens, dry peas, kelp, mushrooms, sprouts, sweet potatoes, spinach, tomatoes.	Almonds, flaxseeds, millet, oats, peanuts with skins, pecans, rice bran, sesame seeds, soybeans, sunflower seeds, wheat bran, wheat germ, whole grains, wild rice.	Best: kiwi, grapes, avocados, bananas, dates, figs, cantaloupe, apricots. Good: blueberries, cherries, cranberries, gooseberries, peaches, pineapples.	Proper amounts of vitamins A, C, and E; the B vitamins; and the minerals selenium and zinc are important to eye health. With age, dead cells degenerate and "yellow" the lens. Crystallization of the inner lens may occur (cataracts), blocking vision. Foods rich in the phytochemicals lutein and zeaxanthin (broccoli, greens, kale, egg yolks, corn, spinach, and turnip greens) may help to prevent age-related cataracts and reduce the risk of age-related macular degeneration (AMD). Raspberry leaf tea compresses can be used to soothe red and irritated eyes.
Female reproductive organs The ovaries, about the size and shape of almonds, produce female hormones and eggs. All other reproductive organs exist to transport and care for the egg or developing fetus. The egg makes a five-day journey through the fallopian tubes (where fertilization may occur) on its way to the uterus, where a fertilized egg becomes implanted and grows into a fetus. The ovaries, fallopian tubes, and uterus are all part of the female hormonal system. These structures are interconnected and their health is interrelated. The uterus is very sensitive to the effects of hormones. The vagina extends from the cervix to the vulva and receives the penis and semen during sexual intercourse.	Best: all leafy greens. Good: asparagus, beans, broccoli, beet greens, beets, Brussels sprouts, cabbage, carrots, cauliflower, celery, cucumbers, kelp, lettuce, mushrooms, onions, parsnips, potato skins, red peppers, soybeans, spinach, sea vegetables, sprouts, tomatoes, watercress.	Best: flaxseeds, soybeans, tofu. Good: almonds, barley, black currant seed oil, brewer's yeast, blackstrap molasses, nuts, oats, pumpkinseeds, sunflower seeds, wheat, wheat bran, wheat germ, whole-grain cereals.	Acerola cherries, apples, apricots, black cherries, blackberries, cantaloupe, cranberries, figs, gooseberries, grapefruit, oranges, prunes, raspberries, strawberries.	Salt, red meat, sugar, and dairy aggravate PMS symptoms and should be avoided. Uterine fibroids are very common—three out of ten women develop them, usually between their late thirties and early forties. A diet high in fiber and soy products (especially miso and tempeh) and low in animal fat and fried foods is recommended for women with fibroids.
Gallbladder A small, pear-shaped organ directly under the liver, which acts as a bile reservoir, concentrating the bile that digests fats. Bile contains cholesterol, bile salts, lecithin, and other substances. Bile ducts connected to the liver and small intestine may become blocked by hard, crystalline structures called gallstones.	Broccoli, cauliflower, carrots, lettuce, radishes, red and green peppers, spinach, sweet potatoes, tomatoes.	Flaxseeds, oats, olive oil, sunflower seeds, wheat, wheat germ.	Best: apples. Good: beets, blackberries, lemons, pears, pineapple.	Gallstones are approximately 80 percent cholesterol. Gallbladder attacks frequently occur after a large, fatty meal following a period of fasting. During an acute attack, apply hot compresses over the gallbladder until pain subsides. Drinking 1 tablespoon of apple cider in a glass of apple juice will help relieve the pain. After an attack, drinking pure apple juice for five days cleanses the system.
Gums and teeth	Best: leafy greens. Good: bok choy, broccoli, cabbage, cauliflower, carrots, kale, legumes, lettuce, mushrooms, red and green peppers, spinach, wheatgrass.	Almonds, brown rice, flaxseed oil, millet, sesame seeds, wheat bran, wheat germ, whole grains.	Apricots, apples, bananas, blackberries, cherries, cranberries, elderberries, figs, gooseberries, raspberries, strawberries, papaya, prunes.	Periodontal disease is the second most prevalent infectious ailment in the U.S. In advanced stages, it causes tooth loss, mouth abscesses, halitosis, and bleeding and painful gums. Problems in the mouth may also signal a vitamin deficiency or other underlying disorders in the body.

BODY PART	VEGETABLES	NUTS, GRAINS, AND SEEDS	FRUITS	OTHER
				Use a new toothbrush each month and clean brush between uses to keep periodontal disease in check.
				Taking coenzyme Q$_{10}$ and coenzyme A daily, or applying them directly to the gums, can improve periodontal disease.
Hair and scalp	Best: brewer's yeast, cabbage, green peas. Good: asparagus, beans, lentils, broccoli, carrots, cauliflower, dandelion greens, lettuce, watercress, red and green peppers, kelp, sea vegetables, spinach, sweet potatoes, tomatoes.	Best: flaxseed oil or other sources of essential fatty acids, brown rice, lentils, oats. Good: alfalfa, almonds, brown rice, flaxseeds, millet, mushrooms, nuts, rye flour, sesame seeds, soy products and tofu, sunflower seeds, wheat, wheat germ, walnuts.	Apples, avocado, bananas, cranberries, cantaloupe, dates, grapefruit, grapes, gooseberries, oranges, prunes, raisins.	Consuming flaxseed oil, primrose oil, or salmon oil can help to prevent dry, brittle hair. Massaging sesame oil into the scalp can relieve an itchy, flaky scalp and moisturizes and conditions hair. Specific vitamins, minerals, and amino acids are crucial to metabolic pathways involved in producing keratin, the protein that makes up hair. Deficiencies of zinc, copper, manganese, or iron can affect hair growth and loss. Folic acid and vitamin B$_{12}$ deficiencies can cause hair loss as well. Conversely, too-high levels of selenium and/or copper can cause hair loss, as can megadoses of vitamins A and E. Biotin and inositol are vital to hair health. Good sources of these nutrients are brewer's yeast, lima beans, cabbage, grapefruit, cantaloupe, raisins, wheat germ, and brown rice. Natural biotin shampoo is also good. Apple cider vinegar or sage tea rinses help to promote hair growth.
Heart This strong, muscular pump is only a little larger than a fist. It expands or contracts (beats) 100,000 times a day and, on the average, pumps about 2,000 gallons of blood. There are two upper chambers and two lower chambers. Blood moves through the chambers aided by four heart valves, which close and open in only one direction. Cardiovascular disease is a general term encompassing heart attack, stroke, and other disorders of the heart and blood vessel system and is the leading health problem in the Western world.	Best: artichoke, asparagus, broccoli. Good: cabbage, carrots, cauliflower, eggplant, kale, kelp, lettuce, olive oil, onions, parsnips, peas, potato skins, potato skin broth, spinach, sweet potatoes, yams, tomatoes, watercress, yellow squash.	Best: flaxseeds. Good: almonds, barley, brown rice, buckwheat, millet, blackstrap molasses, oats, oat bran, olive oil, psyllium seed, rice bran, rye, sesame seeds, soybeans, sunflower seeds, wheat germ.	Apples, apricots, avocado, bananas, black cherries, blueberries, dates, figs, kiwi, papaya, peaches, red grapes, tomatoes.	One study found that men who ate five or more servings of fruits and vegetables a day had a 39 percent lower risk of stroke than those who did not. Coffee and tea, including green tea, increase stress hormones and the risk of heart disease. Anyone with heart disease should avoid these drinks. Also avoid tobacco, alcohol, chocolate, sugar, butter, red meats, fats, fried foods, processed and refined foods, soft drinks, spicy foods, white-flour products, and all sources of sodium. Coenzyme Q$_{10}$ increases oxygenation and has been shown to prevent recurrences of a heart attack. Calcium and magnesium are important to proper functioning of the heart.

BODY PART	VEGETABLES	NUTS, GRAINS, AND SEEDS	FRUITS	OTHER
Intestines The small and large intestines are around 15 feet long. They have five layers of tissue: the serosa, the outermost layer; the circular muscle and the longitudinal muscle responsible for the muscular contraction of smooth muscle (peristalsis); the submucosa and the mucosa, with around 4 million microscopic fingerlike projections called intestinal villi, shaped to increase the surface area for digestion and absorption of nutrients. Once food is reduced to tiny particles, it is absorbed through the walls of the small intestine and nutrients enter the bloodstream.	Best: beans, beets, carrots, cabbage. Good: artichokes, chard, cucumbers, kohlrabi, leafy greens, lentils, lettuce, okra, olives, onions, parsnips, peas, romaine, spinach, tomatoes, turnips.	Best: flaxseeds, all beans. Good: almonds, brown rice, millet, oat bran, oatmeal, pumpkinseeds, rice, rice bran, psyllium, soybeans, wheat germ.	Best: apples, prunes, figs, all berries. Good: bananas, cantaloupe, grapefruit, papaya, peaches, pineapple, prunes.	Constipation arises from insufficient amounts of fiber and fluids in the diet. Fiber is a nutrient with certain components that cannot be absorbed by the human body. It is found in plant foods such as whole grains, fruits, and vegetables. An average stool is 75 percent water. The remainder is made up of fiber, dead cells, and bacteria. If a laxative is necessary, take acidophilus to replace "friendly" bacteria in the intestines. Try Naturalax 2 from Nature's Way for a gentle laxative. Aloe vera juice cleanses and soothes the digestive tract. Drink ½ cup morning and night. Mix with herbal tea for flavor.
Joints A joint is where two bones meet. The joints are responsible for nearly every mobile function of the body. For joint movements to stay smooth and flexible, there must be a layer of lubrication and a cushion between the bones. The layer is made of shock-absorbing tissue called cartilage, combined with a natural fluid called synovial fluid. This layer has to stay healthy for joints to be able to move fluidly.	Beans, beets, cabbage, carrots, celery, collards, cucumbers, dandelion greens, lentils, lettuce, olives, olive oil, onions, okra, parsnips, peas, spinach, sea vegetables, turnips. The nightshade vegetables (potatoes, tomatoes, peppers) may contribute to osteoarthritis, so they should be consumed in moderation.	Best: flaxseeds, almonds. Good: lentils, oats, pumpkinseeds, brown rice, raw nuts, rice bran, soybeans, wheat, wheat bran, wheat germ.	Best: pineapple. Good: bananas, blueberries, coconut, cranberries, figs, gooseberries, grapefruit, lemons, peaches, prunes, strawberries, watermelon.	Good nutrition and healthy lifestyle support joints, which deteriorate with age and may become stiffer. A diet high in vegetables, fruit, nuts, and fish provides essential fatty acids to support joint structure. Caffeine, sugar, fried fats, red meat, preservatives, and processed foods promote inflammation and should be avoided, particularly if you have arthritis. Glucosamine and chondroitin sulfate are compounds produced by the body that contribute to the natural cushioning effect of cartilage. MSM (methylsufonyl-methane), another naturally occurring organic sulfur compound, helps the body manufacture collagen to repair cartilage, tendons, ligaments, and muscles. Various combinations of these nutrients can help to restore flexibility and ease joint pain for some people. Proper exercise can be a profound protector against arthritis, a common joint disease.
Liver Located below the diaphragm in the upper right of the abdomen, the liver is a vital organ. It removes or neutralizes poisons (toxins) in the blood, creates immune agents to fight infection, and removes bacteria and germs from blood. It processes nutrients and drugs absorbed from the digestive tract into forms that are easily assimilated. It also creates bile, which is stored in the gallbladder and released as necessary for digestion.	Best: leafy greens, artichoke leaf. Good: asparagus, beets, spinach, radishes, Brussels sprouts, cabbage, carrots, celery, cucumbers, dandelion greens, endive, green beans, okra, onions, potato skins, reishi mushrooms, string beans, turnips, watercress.	Almonds, barley, brown rice, corn germ, lentils, oats, oat bran, peanuts, rice, soybeans, sunflower seeds, wheat bran, wheat germ.	Apples, blackberries, black cherries, figs, gooseberries, grapefruit, oranges, papaya, peaches, prunes, strawberries.	Alcohol, drugs, fatty foods, and cigarettes overload the liver with toxins and should be avoided.

BODY PART	VEGETABLES	NUTS, GRAINS, AND SEEDS	FRUITS	OTHER
Lymphatic system This is a system of organs (the spleen, thymus, tonsils, and lymph nodes) and fluid, called lymph, which circulates through lymphatic vessels in the body and bathes the body's cells. It provides continuous cleansing at a cellular level. Fluid from the spaces between cells is drained, washing away waste products, toxins, and other tissue debris. Part of the immune system, lymph nodes in the neck, underarms, and groin produce antibodies that fight off intruders.	Best: asparagus, beets, barley grass, cabbage, kelp. Good: carrots, celery, collards, cucumbers, dandelion greens, horseradish, kale, kohlrabi, okra, olives, onions, potato skins, sea vegetables, string beans, turnips.	Best: flaxseed. Good: almonds, brown rice, oats, oatmeal, pumpkinseeds, sunflower, wheat, wheat germ.	Best: apples, all berries. Good: bananas, black figs, figs, peaches, prunes, watermelon.	Liver health is the key to lymphatic health as it produces the majority of lymph. Maitake, reishi, and shiitake mushrooms (or mushroom extracts) build immunity and fight viral infections. Spicy foods like natural salsas, cayenne, horseradish, and ginger can boost the lymphatic system. Coenzyme Q_{10} and coenzyme A are nutrients that support the lymphatic system.
Male reproductive organs The male pelvis, which holds the reproductive organs, is narrower, deeper, and has thicker, stronger bones than the female pelvis. The male reproductive glands, testes, lie within the scrotum, which is outside the body, between the legs. The testes produce sperm and male hormones. From the testes, sperm pass into a coiled tube called the epididymis where they mature and are stored until ejaculation through the urethra or until reabsorbed by the body. The prostate is a walnut-sized gland that surrounds the urethra at the point where it leaves the bladder. It produces prostatic fluid, which makes up part of the male ejaculate and nourishes and transports sperm. It is the most common site of disorders in the male genitourinary system. Nearly every man over age forty-five has some form of prostate enlargement, which can cause urinary problems.	Asparagus, beets, broccoli, cabbage, celery, kelp, leafy greens, lettuce, okra, onions, parsnips, peas, parsley, radishes, spinach, tomatoes.	Best: flaxseed oil, flaxseeds, pumpkinseeds. Good: almonds, barley, brown rice, millet, oats, oatmeal, sunflower seeds, wheat, wheat bran, wheat germ, whole-grain cereals.	Best: all berries, watermelon. Good: apricots, bananas, coconut, dates, figs, kiwi, prunes.	Essential fatty acids aid in the formation of sperm and seminal fluid in the prostate. Iodine is a component of the thyroid hormone and necessary for development of reproductive organs. Kelp is a good source of this mineral. Lycopene, a phytonutrient found in tomatoes and watermelon, may be the most important antioxidant for male sexual health. The testicles contain more lycopene than any other part of the body; impotent men have very low levels of lycopene. Vitamin C helps to boost testosterone levels. Zinc is important for male reproductive health. Eating 1–4 ounces of raw pumpkinseeds daily will supply this necessary mineral. Drinking cranberry juice can protect against urinary tract infection, which has been linked to some forms of prostatitis. Daily meat consumption triples the risk of prostate enlargement. Regular milk consumption doubles the risk. Both should be avoided. Alcohol decreases the body's ability to produce testosterone and may cause the hormonal equivalent of menopause in men. It should be consumed in moderation or avoided altogether.

BODY PART	VEGETABLES	NUTS, GRAINS, AND SEEDS	FRUITS	OTHER
Muscles Ordinarily, a muscle contracts when it is used, then stretches out when the motion is completed. If a muscle contracts without stretching out again, the pain of a muscle cramp is often the result. Cramping is often caused by an imbalance in the body's electrolytes—minerals such as potassium, calcium, and magnesium—or a vitamin-E deficiency.	Best: all leafy greens, kelp. Good: asparagus, beans, beets, cabbage, lentils, lettuce, onions, parsnips, radishes, reishi mushrooms, spinach, tomatoes.	Best: brewer's yeast, cornmeal. Good: almonds, barley, brown rice, flaxseeds, mushrooms, oats/oatmeal, sesame seeds, soy beans, sunflower seeds, wheat, wheat bran, wheat germ.	Apricots, black figs, cranberries, dates, gooseberries, prunes, strawberries.	Cramping of the legs and feet during the night may be a sign of calcium and, especially, magnesium deficiency. Drinking a large glass of quality water every three hours during the day flushes out toxins stored in the muscles and relieves aches.
Nails The nails protect nerve-rich fingertips and tips of the toes from injury. They are a substructure of the epidermis (outer skin) and are composed mainly of keratin, a type of protein. Healthy nail beds are pink, indicating a rich blood supply.	Asparagus, beets, bok choy, cabbage, kelp, lettuce, onions, parsnips, radishes, sea vegetables, spinach, soybeans, tomatoes.	Best: flaxseeds, legumes. Good: almonds, barley, brown rice, oats, sesame seeds, sunflower seeds, tofu, wheat bran, wheat germ.	Cherries, coconut, cranberries, dates, figs, gooseberries, plums, prunes, strawberries.	A diet with plenty of quality protein, grains, legumes, oatmeal, nuts, and seeds is best. Changes or abnormalities in the nails are often the result of nutritional deficiencies or an underlying disorder. A lack of protein, folic acid, and vitamin C causes hangnails. White bands across the nails are also an indication of protein deficiency. For split nails and/or hangnails, take 2 tablespoons of brewer's yeast or wheat-germ oil daily. Cuts and cracks in nails may indicate a need for more liquids. Taking acidophilus internally inhibits bacteria that cause fungal infection of the nails. Fungal infections can be treated using a cotton swab to apply equal parts of vinegar and water.
Pancreas A 5- to 6-inch-long leaf-shaped gland behind the lower part of the stomach extending downward toward the spleen and left kidney, the pancreas produces digestive enzymes that break down proteins, fat, and carbohydrates in the small intestine. It also releases the hormones glucogen and insulin, which together regulate blood sugar levels.	Artichokes, asparagus, leafy greens, beets, bok choy, cabbage, celery root, green beans, kale, kohlrabi, okra, onions, parsnips, peas, radishes, spinach, sea vegetables, tomatoes, turnips, watercress.	Flaxseed oil or essential fatty acids, almonds, barley, brown rice, all grains, oats, oatmeal, pumpkinseeds, sunflower seeds, wheat bran, wheat germ.	Apples, apricots, all berries, bananas, black figs, cranberries, dates, gooseberries, papaya, pineapple, prunes, strawberries.	Sugar overworks the pancreas and should be avoided. Stevia is a wise substitute. In general, eating a diet low in fat and sugar and avoiding alcohol in any form is recommended. Pancreatitis (inflammation of the pancreas), especially if it is chronic, often leads to glucose intolerance (diabetes) and digestive difficulties. Pancreatitis can result if digestive enzymes build up inside the pancreas and begin to attack it. Symptoms of pancreatitis include sudden, severe pain around the area of the navel and radiating to the back. This is an extremely serious condition that requires immediate medical attention.

BODY PART	VEGETABLES	NUTS, GRAINS, AND SEEDS	FRUITS	OTHER
Pituitary gland A small gland the size of a peanut that is located behind the eyes at the base of the brain, the pituitary gland is often called the "master" gland. It secretes hormones that control other glands (thyroid, adrenal, testicles, and ovaries) as well as growth. It secretes thyroid-stimulating hormone (TSH), which helps control thyroid function. The pituitary gland also secretes human growth hormone (HGH).	Best: asparagus, beets, broccoli, cabbage, kelp. Good: carrots, legumes, lettuce, onions, parsnips, radishes, sea vegetables, soybeans, sprouts, spinach, tomatoes, watercress.	Barley, flaxseeds, oat bran, millet, pumpkinseeds, walnuts, wheat bran, wheat germ, whole-grain cereals.	Apples, apricots, blackberries, coconut, cranberries, dates, figs, prunes, gooseberries, grapefruit, pineapple, strawberries.	Para-aminobenzoic acid (PABA) and lecithin, together with vitamins C and E, help to normalize the pituitary gland. Acetylcholine and serine improve proper pituitary function.
Skin The skin is the body's largest organ. It has two main layers: the epidermis outside and the dermis inside. The epidermis serves as a "barrier" and the inner dermis contains the sweat glands, hair follicles, and nerve endings, which respond to heat, cold, pressure, itch, and pain.	Best: all leafy greens, kelp. Good: beets, broccoli, carrots, celery, cucumbers, kale, kidney beans, lentils, pumpkin, sea vegetables, spinach, squash, sweet potatoes.	Best: flaxseed oil. Good: brown rice, brewer's yeast, millet, oat bran, pumpkinseeds, rice bran, soybeans, wheat germ.	Best: apples, apricots, avocados. Good: bananas, blueberries, cantaloupe, cherries, figs, prunes, lemons, papaya, peaches, red grapes, strawberries, watermelon.	Primrose oil and black currant seed oil are healing for dermatitis, acne, and other skin disorders. Avocado can be mashed to use as a facial. Wash it off when it dries.
Spine The spine is composed of the cervical vertebrae (neck area), thoracic vertebrae (chest with ribs attached), and lumbar vertebrae below the last thoracic bone and the top of the sacrum. Sacral vertebrae are caged within the bones of the pelvis. The coccyx is the terminal vertebrae (vestigial tail).	Asparagus, beets, Brussels sprouts, cabbage, carrots, cauliflower, celery, collards, cucumbers, dandelion greens, kale, legumes, lima beans, okra, olives, peas, potato skins, soybeans, string beans, turnips.	Almonds, barley, brewer's yeast, brown rice, chestnuts, nuts, oatmeal, pignolia nuts, sunflower seeds, walnuts, wheat germ, whole-grain cereals.	Apricots, blackberries, black cherries, blueberries, coconut, cranberries, dates, figs, gooseberries, grapefruit, oranges, peaches, prunes, raisins.	Some experts recommend taking the structural raw materials such as glucosamine, chondroitin, and MSM in supplement form to support a healthy spine. See also the entry for Bones.
Thymus The thymus gland orchestrates the work of the immune system. It is located in the upper chest, behind the breastbone, and has two lobes that join in front of the trachea. Each lobe is made of lymphoid tissue, consisting of tightly packed white blood cells and fat. It transforms lymphocytes (white blood cells developed in the bone marrow) into T cells (cells developed in the thymus). These cells are then transported to various lymph glands, where they play an important part in fighting infections and disease.	Best: all leafy greens. Good: beets, Brussels sprouts, cabbage, carrots, cauliflower, lettuce, onions, parsnips, potato skins, spinach, tomatoes.	Barley, brown rice, cereals, corn germ, millet, oats, wheat bran, wheat germ, wheatgrass, whole wheat.	Apricot, blackberries, black cherries, cranberries, figs, gooseberries, prunes, strawberries.	A diet of fresh fruits and vegetables (preferably raw), plus nuts, seeds, grains, and other high-fiber foods nurture the immune system. Coenzyme Q_{10} and coenzyme A support the immune system and increase energy. Essential fatty acids are necessary for a healthy immune system. Green drinks and spirulina protect the immune system. Zinc is needed for proper thymus function; 15–30 milligrams of zinc per day may help to restore thymus function in adults aged forty and older (thymus function decreases power with age).

BODY PART	VEGETABLES	NUTS, GRAINS, AND SEEDS	FRUITS	OTHER
Thyroid This small butterfly-shaped endocrine gland just below the larynx and above the trachea is the body's internal thermostat. Thyroid hormone affects all metabolic processes. An under-active thyroid is known as hypothyroidism; an overactive thyroid is known as hyper-thyroidism. Thyroid conditions affect five times more women than men. An underactive thyroid results in immune deficiency.	Best: kelp, dulse, leafy greens, parsley. Good: asparagus, beets, Brussels sprouts, cabbage, carrots, cauliflower, celery, cucumbers, dandelion greens, okra, onions, potato skins, sea vegetables, turnips, yellow corn.	Best: brewer's yeast, pumpkin-seeds, flaxseeds. Good: almonds, barley, coconut, chestnuts, blackstrap molasses, nuts, oatmeal, pignolia nuts, soybeans, sunflower seeds, walnuts, wheat germ, whole-grain cereals, yeast.	Apples, apricots, all berries, black cherries, dates, figs, gooseberries, grapefruit, oranges, peaches, prunes.	A diet high in processed sugars can increase thyroid problems and should be avoided. Some doctors recommend natural coconut for their patients with thyroid problems—it has strong antiviral properties and is soothing fuel for the glandular system. Some experts believe that hormones in meat and the use of aspartame (Nutra-Sweet) are factors that may affect thyroid function.

Appendix C: Dietary Prescriptions

> Formerly, when religion was strong and science weak, men mistook magic for medicine; now, when science is strong and religion weak, men mistake medicine for magic.
>
> —*Thomas Szasz, M.D., psychiatrist and author*

Americans spent $155 billion on prescription drugs in 2001. The most profitable business on the annual Fortune 500 list, year after year, is the pharmaceutical industry. While the overall profits of "500" companies declined an average of 53 percent in 2001, the top ten U.S. drug manufacturers increased profits by an average of 33 percent. The same year, 2.9 billion prescriptions were filled in the United States—that's 9.9 prescriptions for every man, woman, and child in the country.

Pharmaceutical companies spent $2.5 billion in 2000 promoting prescription drugs, an increase of nearly 45 percent over 1999. These advertisements contribute to rising costs by inducing consumer demand for newer, higher-priced drugs, when the older ones may work just as well. Pharmaceutical companies have migrated toward becoming more marketing than research and development organizations, according to Nancy Chockley, president of the National Institute for Health Care Management.

These trendy new drugs, though often requested by consumers, are not time-tested, and therefore can reasonably be considered much riskier than natural approaches with long-standing histories. An analysis of 548 drugs approved from 1975 through 1999 showed that 56 (10 percent) were later given serious side effect warnings or taken off the market for safety reasons. According to Karen E. Lasser, who wrote a study reported in the *Journal of the American Medical Association (JAMA)*, only half of all serious adverse reactions are detected seven years after a drug enters the market, exposing millions of people to potentially unsafe drugs each year. The Associated Press reported in 2002 that an estimated 2 million Americans are hospitalized annually from drug side effects, and that 100,000 of them die. The American Medical Association published research in 2000 that linked birth control pills manufactured before 1975 with an elevenfold increase in the risk of breast cancer. In 2002, one component of a landmark study on the effects of estrogen plus progestin therapy on 16,608 women was halted after the National Heart, Lung, and Blood Institute found that participants had a markedly higher risk of breast cancer, heart attacks, stroke, and blood

clots. Remember the Dalkon Shield? This intrauterine birth control device caused sterility and pelvic inflammatory disease, and maimed the reproductive organs of 400,000 women who sued for, and won, nearly $3 billion in a class-action lawsuit. More recently, Baycol, a type of cholesterol-lowering drug known as a statin was taken off the market after being linked to deaths worldwide. Glucophage, one of several drugs used to treat many of the 17 million Americans with diabetes, is potentially life-threatening, according to another study in *JAMA*. And the list goes on. Redux. Fen-Phen. Propulsid. Latronex. Rezulin. Seldane. Hismanal. All were pulled from the market because of serious side effects or harm to users.

Prescription drugs are not the only source of concern. Dr. Barbara Starfield of the Johns Hopkins School of Hygiene and Public Health reported other ways in which the conventional health-care system in the United States contributes to poor health, including:

- 12,000 deaths per year due to unnecessary surgery.

- 7,000 deaths per year due to medication errors in hospitals.

- 20,000 deaths per year from hospital errors.

- 80,000 deaths per year due to infections in hospitals.

- 106,000 deaths per year due to nonerror, negative effects of drugs.

Antibiotic use (and, especially, overuse) is creating another threat to public health in this country. These drugs, which are effective only against bacteria, are useless against viruses, worms, parasites, and fungi, yet they are often overprescribed by physicians. In addition, 70 percent of the antibiotics used in the United States each year are fed to healthy pigs, chickens, and cattle to speed growth and prevent disease. When low doses of antibiotics are given to animals, only some of the bacteria are killed and the more resistant survive, multiply, and pass on their strength to future generations of bacteria. Many types of bacteria have now become resistant to antibiotics, rendering them ineffective when they are truly needed. This raises the specter of formerly minor infections that can no longer be treated successfully.

Then there is the matter of drug costs. Older adults, many of them living on fixed incomes, are hardest hit by the rising cost of prescription drugs. According to a report by Families USA, a consumer health organization, older adults make up 13 percent of the population but account for 34 percent of all prescriptions dispensed and 42 percent of all prescription spending. Prices for the fifty drugs most commonly used by seniors rose by more than three times the rate of inflation from January 2000 to January 2001.

The rising cost of drugs, financially and physically, has inspired many consumers to seek alternative sources of healing. Internet sites sell drugs prescribed by online doctors after "cyberexaminations," often at lower prices for both services. Folks travel to, or join, groups filling prescriptions in Canada and Mexico, where government price controls keep costs down.

At times, prescription drugs, surgery, or hospitalization

are necessary and the most appropriate treatment for illness, especially when health is in crisis. There are, however, natural, time-tested ways to maintain health and even prevent serious illness. The easiest, cheapest, and most drastic change people can make to improve every existing and future health condition involves *diet*. Nutritional deficiencies are at the root of most physical ailments, as well as some types of mental illness, including depression. Chronic diseases like diabetes, cancer, heart disease, and even aging can often be helped or cured by low-cost "pharmafoods" that have been healing naturally, without deadly side effects, for thousands of years. The natural prescriptions of pharmafoods provide age-old, as well as cutting-edge, resources for safe, alternative, paths to achieve optimal health. Other natural healing alternatives are medicinal herbs. For detailed information on using herbs and on interactions between drugs and herbs (an important concern), consult *Prescription for Herbal Healing* (Avery/Penguin Putnam, 2000). Use the table below to identify some of the many foods that can be used for healing.

TYPE OF DRUG	THERAPEUTIC ALTERNATIVE	COMMENTS
Antibiotics	Foods: garlic (a natural broad-spectrum antibiotic), onions, cinnamon (but not during pregnancy), orange peel, orange oil, horseradish, lemon.	Many types of bacteria are now antibiotic resistant. Taking antibiotics for long periods of time can upset natural intestinal flora. Antibiotics are useless against viruses, fungi, worms, and parasites. Frequent use may depress the immune system, contribute to allergies, and even damage major organs. If you must take antibiotics, eat fresh plain yogurt (with live cultures) to restore healthy intestinal bacteria, but do not eat it within two hours of taking the antibiotics.
Antifungals	Foods: onions, garlic. Seasonings: oregano oil, oregano juice.	
Antihistamines and decongestants	Foods: lemon. Seasonings: capsicum (cayenne), horseradish. Nutrients: bioflavonoids.	
Anti-inflammatories	Foods: cabbage, deepwater marine fish, flaxseeds, flaxseed oil, garlic, lemon, papaya, pineapple, reishi mushrooms. Seasonings: oregano oil, oregano juice, turmeric. Nutrients: vitamin C.	The anti-inflammatory effects of fish and flaxseeds are due to the omega-3 essential fatty acids they contain.
Antioxidants	Foods: alfalfa sprouts, all berries (especially blueberries, blackberries, and strawberries), bananas, broccoli, beets, Brussels sprouts, carrots,	

TYPE OF DRUG	THERAPEUTIC ALTERNATIVE	COMMENTS
	cherries, garlic, green tea, kale, kelp, kiwi, onions, oranges, pink grapefruit, plums, red grapes, red bell peppers, reishi mushrooms, rose hips, spinach, tomatoes. Nutrients: the amino acids cysteine and glutathione, coenzyme Q_{10}, lipoic acid, the fatty acid gamma-linoleic acid, vitamin A, vitamin C (in high amounts), vitamin E.	
Antiviral	Foods: cranberries, onions, prunes, plums, shiitake mushrooms, strawberries. Seasonings: capsicum (cayenne), clove oil, oregano oil.	
Blood purifiers	Foods: beets, beet greens, blackberries, black cherries, coconut, dandelion greens, garlic, parsley, radishes, wheatgrass juice and other green juices.	
Estrogen blockers	Foods: buckwheat, citrus fruits, cruciferous vegetables, flaxseeds, whole wheat.	
Estrogen promoters	Foods: flaxseeds, soybeans, soy products. Seasonings: anise, fennel, fenugreek, sage.	Plant estrogens help to relieve menopausal symptoms and decrease the risk of heart disease and osteoporosis, without promoting breast cancer. If you are taking an estrogen blocker such as tamoxifen, you should not use estrogen promoters.

TYPE OF DRUG	THERAPEUTIC ALTERNATIVE	COMMENTS
Immune boosters	Foods: alfalfa, barley grass, pearl barley, cruciferous vegetables (raw), fruits (raw), carrots, flaxseeds, garlic, legumes, oily fish, maitake and shiitake mushrooms, onions, sprouted seeds, sea vegetables (kelp, dulse, agar-agar, nori, arame), wheatgrass juice and other green drinks, yogurt. Nutrients: coenzyme Q_{10}, vitamin C, zinc.	
Muscle relaxants	Foods: kudzu root. Seasonings: fenugreek. Nutrients: magnesium.	
Steroids (natural)	Foods: reishi mushrooms. Nutrients: beta-sitosterol, s-adenosylmethionine (SAMe).	
Tranquilizers	Nutrients: SAMe.	

There are also certain foods, nutrients, and dietary recommendations that are helpful for specific disorders. The table below summarizes some of the most important of these.

DISORDER	DIETARY RECOMMENDATIONS
Acne/skin disorders	Foods: apples, cabbage, cauliflower, cucumber, carrots, leafy greens, primrose oil. Seasonings: basil. Nutrients: zinc. Avoid: alcohol, caffeine, chocolate, cocoa, dairy products, fried foods, iodized salt, pineapples, saturated fats, sea vegetables, soft drinks, all forms of sugar. Other: A juice fast is very beneficial for the skin, which is the body's largest organ.
Allergies/hay fever	Foods: lemons. Nutrients: bioflavonoids, bromelain, quercetin, vitamin C. Avoid: any foods known to cause reactions.
Anal itching or burning	Foods: potato peel broth made by simmering the skins of 3 potatoes in 2 quarts of quality water for 30 minutes (strain out the peelings before drinking it), umeboshi plums (eat two plums every four hours for two days). Other: Investigate food allergies and omit suspect foods from the diet. Use the acid and alkaline self-test in Chapter 19 to see if hyperacidity is a problem.
Anxiety disorders	Foods: apricots, asparagus, avocados, bananas, broccoli, blackstrap molasses, brewer's yeast, brown rice, dried fruits, figs, fish, garlic, leafy greens, legumes, raw nuts and seeds, reishi mushrooms, soy foods, whole grains. Seasonings: cayenne pepper. Nutrients: calcium, magnesium, potassium, selenium, B-complex vitamins, vitamin C, vitamin E, zinc. Avoid: baking powder; canned food and beverages; cheese; chocolate; corn; dairy products; eggs; foods containing additives; fried, junk, and processed foods; saturated fats; tap water; wheat. Other: Eat a diet high in complex carbohydrates. When you feel nervous, consume more complex carbohydrates.

DISORDER	DIETARY RECOMMENDATIONS
Arthritis	Foods: apples, black cherries, celeriac, dandelion greens, fish oil, flaxseed oil, garlic, kelp, leafy greens, lemons, papaya, parsley, pineapple, watercress. Seasonings: cayenne pepper, ginger root, turmeric. Nutrients: chondroitin, folic acid, glucosamine. Avoid: caffeine, citrus fruits (except lemon), dairy products, eggplant, eggs, fried foods, peppers, potatoes, processed foods, red meat, saturated fats, cooked or juiced spinach, sugar, tobacco, tomatoes.
Asthma/bronchitis/ emphysema	Foods: all leafy greens, apples, carrots, cranberries, flaxseed oil, parsley, rutabaga, turnips. Seasonings: cayenne pepper, fennel seed, fenugreek, ginger root, peppermint leaf. Avoid: animal fats; caffeine; dairy products; food additives, especially BHA, BHT, FD&C yellow #5 dye, and MSG; gas-producing foods such as beans, broccoli, cabbage, cauliflower; pork; poultry; processed foods; red meat; salt; saturated fats; sugar; tobacco and smoke; white-flour products. Other: Follow a hypoglycemic diet (see the entry for Hypoglycemia). Investigate allergies and avoid allergens, including allergenic foods.
Attention deficit disorder (ADD)/attention deficit hyperactivity disorder (ADHD)	Foods: beans and legumes; borage oil, flaxseed oil, or primrose oil; all fresh fruits (but not fruit juices); all fresh vegetables; herring; oats; rice; salmon; tuna; whole grains (except for corn and wheat). Nutrients: calcium, gamma-aminobutyric acid (GABA), magnesium. Avoid: all artificial colorings, flavorings, and sweeteners; apple cider vinegar; carbonated beverages; chocolate; corn; hot dogs; luncheon meat; margarine; salt; soy sauce; sausage; tea. Other: Investigate food allergies and avoid allergenic foods (chocolate, dairy products, eggs, oranges, peanuts, and wheat are common culprits). Choose complex carbohydrates over starches.
Back pain (lower)	Foods: alfalfa sprouts. Nutrients: boron, calcium, magnesium, manganese, vitamin C, zinc. Other: Use periodic cleansing enemas to relieve pressure and pain.
Bladder infection/urinary burning, itching, frequency, urgency	Foods: collards, cranberries, cranberry juice (unsweetened), garlic, parsley, pineapple, pineapple juice (unsweetened), rose hips, watermelon. Seasonings: celery seed. Nutrients: calcium, magnesium, selenium, vitamin A, vitamin C, vitamin E, zinc. Avoid: alcohol, caffeine, chocolate, citrus fruits, fats, pepper, processed foods, spicy foods, sugar. Other: Limit your consumption of dairy products, red meat, and shellfish. If you have a bladder infection, drink at least one 8-ounce glass of quality water every hour. Use acidophilus and take hot sitz baths.
Breast soreness/ fibrocystic breasts	Nutrients: vitamin A; B-complex vitamins, plus extra vitamin B_6; vitamin C; vitamin E. Avoid: caffeine, colas, chocolate, coffee. Other: Eat a low-fat, high-fiber diet.
Bruising (frequently or easily)	Foods: beans, cheese, dark leafy greens, egg yolks, garlic, kelp, lemons, oats, peas, whole wheat. Nutrients: bioflavonoids, vitamin C, vitamin K.

DISORDER	DIETARY RECOMMENDATIONS
Bruxism (tooth-grinding)	Foods: kelp. Nutrients: calcium; magnesium; B-complex vitamins, especially pantothenic acid. Avoid: any form of sugar, especially before bedtime. Other: Eat a hypoglycemic diet. (See the entry for Hypoglycemia.)
Cancer and HIV/AIDS	Foods: beans and legumes; blueberries; carrots; cherries; cruciferous vegetables; flaxseeds; garlic; kelp; all leafy greens; maitake, reishi, and shiitake mushrooms; millet; papaya; peaches; red grapes; vegetables; soy foods; wheatgrass. Seasonings: ginger root. Nutrients: folic acid, omega-3 fatty acids, selenium. Avoid: alcohol; animal protein; caffeine; dairy products; all saturated and hydrogenated fats; food additives; fried and junk food; hydrogenated oils; peanuts; processed foods; salt; salt-cured, smoked, or nitrate-cured meats; sugar; tobacco. Other: Drink plenty of water (steam-distilled only) and juices. Eat a diet of soft foods.
Candidiasis	Foods: garlic, leafy greens, onions, rutabaga, spirulina, turnips, wheatgrass, live-culture yogurt (with no form of sugar added). Nutrients: caprylic acid, monolaurin. Avoid: alcohol, all cheeses, butter, chocolate, citrus and dried fruits, fermented foods, all fruit juices, all forms of gluten, ham, honey, mushrooms, nuts, pickles, soy and tamari sauces, all forms of sugar, yeast products. Other: Eat a diet high in complex carbohydrates, protein, and fiber.
Canker sores	Foods: garlic, onions. Nutrients: folic acid, iron, lysine, vitamin B_{12}. Avoid (until healed): acidic fruits and other acidic foods, fish, meat, and hard-to-chew foods. Other: Use the acid and alkaline self-test in Chapter 19 to see if hyperacidity is a problem.
Cardiovascular disease	Foods: canola oil, carrots, eggplant, fish oils, flaxseed oil, flaxseeds, garlic, green tea, all leafy greens, lecithin, olive oil, onions, parsley, potato skins, red grapes, shiitake mushrooms, soybeans, sunflower seeds, wheat germ. Seasonings: cayenne pepper, fenugreek, ginger root. Nutrients: L-Carnitine, coenzyme Q_{10}, omega-3 and omega-6 essential fatty acids, vitamin E. Avoid: alcohol, all fats, baking soda, butter, caffeine, canned vegetables, coconut oil, dairy products, diet sodas, fried foods, meat tenderizers, mold inhibitors, MSG, palm oil, preservatives, processed foods, red meat, refined foods, salt, soft drinks, softened or tap water, spicy foods, sugar, tobacco, white-flour products.
Carpal tunnel syndrome	Foods: garlic, kelp, parsley, primrose oil. Seasonings: cayenne pepper. Nutrients: coenzyme Q_{10}; vitamin A; B-complex vitamins, especially vitamins B_1 and B_6; vitamin C; vitamin E; all minerals.

DISORDER	DIETARY RECOMMENDATIONS
Chronic fatigue/lack of energy and/or endurance	Foods: garlic, spirulina, wheat germ, wheat-germ oil. Nutrients: calcium, chromium, coenzyme Q_{10}, magnesium, potassium, vitamin A, B-complex vitamins (especially vitamins B_6 and B_{12}), zinc. Avoid: alcohol, dairy products, fried and junk foods, soft drinks, all forms of sugar, tobacco, animal protein, caffeine, chemicals, chocolate, tap water, hydrogenated oils, MSG, peanuts, preservatives, processed foods, soybeans. Other: Eat complex carbohydrates for energy, plus protein.
Circulatory problems	Foods: garlic. Seasonings: cayenne pepper, ginger root. Nutrients: bioflavonoids, calcium, coenzyme Q_{10}, magnesium, vitamin C, vitamin E. Avoid: alcohol, all animal fats, baking soda, caffeine, canned vegetables, coconut oil, colas, dairy products, diet sodas, fast and fried foods, meat tenderizers, mold inhibitors, MSG, palm oil, preservatives, processed foods, red meat, refined foods, salt, saturated fats, soft drinks, spicy foods, all forms of sugar, tobacco, softened or tap water, white-flour products. Other: Get regular exercise.
Cold/flu/persistent fever	Foods: catnip tea, garlic, plantain leaves. Nutrients: vitamin A, vitamin C, zinc. Avoid: all forms of sugar. Other: Drink hot liquids, including turkey or chicken soup and steam-distilled water with lemon juice added every two hours. Use catnip tea in enemas for fever.
Colic (in infants)	Foods: chamomile tea, fennel seed tea, ginger tea, savory tea, slippery elm bark tea, papaya (mashed and added to expressed breast milk or formula). Other: Switch a formula-fed baby to soy- or rice-based formula (avoid cow's milk).
Colitis, irritable bowel syndrome (IBS)	Foods: alfalfa sprouts, aloe vera juice, dandelion greens, flaxseed oil, ground flaxseeds, kelp, papaya, reishi mushrooms. Seasonings: ginger root. Nutrients: glutamine. Avoid: dairy products, saturated fats, whole grains, meat, nuts, processed foods, seeds, and sugar until healed. Daily bowel movements are important to avoid toxic buildup. Other: Drink plenty of quality water and juices. Eat a diet of soft foods.
Constipation	Foods: aloe vera juice, dandelion greens, flaxseeds, oat bran. Seasonings: fennel seed. Nutrients: calcium, magnesium, vitamin C, and zinc. Avoid: caffeine, dairy products, fried foods, processed foods, sugar, yeast products, potentially allergenic foods. Other: Drink plenty of quality water and fresh juices. Eat a high-fiber diet. Use periodic cleansing enemas with the juice of one lemon to relieve pressure and pain, but do not abuse them. Get regular exercise.

DISORDER	DIETARY RECOMMENDATIONS
Cough (persistent) laryngitis	Foods: honey with a bit of lemon juice added. Nutrients: bioflavonoids, vitamin A, vitamin C, zinc.
Crohn's disease	Foods: alfalfa sprouts; aloe vera juice; nonacidic fresh or cooked vegetables such as broccoli, Brussels sprouts, cabbage, carrots, celery, garlic, kale, spinach, and turnips; ground flaxseeds; kelp; papaya; reishi mushrooms. Nutrients: calcium, glutamine, magnesium, omega-3 fatty acids. Seasonings: ginger root. Avoid (until healed): alcohol, animal products, caffeine, chocolate, corn (including popcorn), dairy products, eggs, saturated fats, fried foods, meat, nuts, seeds, processed foods, refined carbohydrates, sodas, spicy foods, sugar, tobacco, white-flour products, yeast products, whole grains. Other: Drink plenty of quality water and juices. Eat a diet of soft foods. Daily bowel movements are important to avoid toxic buildup.
Depression	Foods: salmon, turkey. Nutrients: tyrosine (unless you are taking MAO inhibitors), B-complex vitamins. Avoid: alcohol, fried and junk foods, allergenic foods, baker's and brewer's yeast, caffeine, cheese, chocolate, dairy products, herring, meat tenderizers, phenylalanine, saturated fats and oils, soy sauce, all forms of sugar, yeast extracts.
Diabetes	Foods: brewer's yeast. Nutrients: alpha-lipoic acid, chromium, B-complex vitamins. Avoid: caffeine, canned foods, saturated and hydrogenated fats and oils, fish oil capsules, fried foods, processed foods, salt, soft drinks, all forms of sugar, white-flour products. Other: Eat a diet that is high in fiber and complex carbohydrates and low in protein (less than 40 grams of protein per day). Keep your weight down.
Diarrhea	Foods: apples, bananas, blackberries, well-cooked brown rice, carrot juice, carob, leafy greens, papaya. Seasonings: fennel seed. Avoid: barley, oats, rye, wheat, fats, nuts, seeds, alcohol, apple juice, caffeine, dairy products, low-fat soured products (yogurt), processed foods, spicy foods. Other: Drink plenty of quality water and fresh juices. Avoid all foods except for those listed for twenty-four hours. If diarrhea persists, investigate food allergies.
Edema/swelling of abdomen, ankles, feet, hands, or legs	Foods: alfalfa, bananas, carob, celery, garlic, kelp, parsley, rose hips, watercress, watermelon. Nutrients: B-complex vitamins, especially vitamin B_6. Avoid: alcohol, animal protein and fat, caffeine, chocolate, dairy products, fried foods, gravies, olives, pickles, salt, shellfish, soy sauce, tobacco, white flour, refined sugar. Other: Drink at least 8 glasses of quality water daily, but do not drink a lot at any one time. Investigate the possibility of food allergies.

DISORDER	DIETARY RECOMMENDATIONS
Food poisoning	Foods: papaya. Seasonings: ginger. Avoid: processed foods, sugar. Other: Drink plenty of quality water and juices. Eat a diet of soft foods.
Gas/bloating	Foods: papaya. Seasonings: fennel. Avoid: processed foods, sugar. Other: Drink plenty of quality water and juices. Eat a diet of soft foods.
Glaucoma	Foods: blackberries, blueberries, cherries, raspberries, rose hips. Nutrients: B-complex vitamins (but avoid excessive amounts of vitamin B_3 [niacin]), vitamin C, vitamin E. Avoid: alcohol, caffeine, excessive amounts of vitamin B_3 (niacin).
Gout	Foods: apples, black cherries, blueberries, brown rice, garlic, leafy greens, kelp, lemons, millet, parsley, pears, pineapple, strawberries. Seasonings: cayenne pepper, turmeric. Nutrients: pantothenic acid. Avoid: alcohol, anchovies, asparagus, broth, cauliflower, consommé, desserts, dried beans, fats, gravies, herring, legumes, mackerel, mushrooms, oil-rich foods, organ meats, peas, poultry, processed foods, red meat, sardines, shellfish, refined sugar, sweetbreads. Other: Avoid eggplant, peppers, potatoes, and tomatoes until healed. Eat a diet of 50 percent raw vegetables and whole grains. Limit yeast products.
Gum disease	Nutrients: bioflavonoids, calcium, coenzyme Q_{10}, vitamin A, vitamin C, vitamin E.
Headache	Foods: celery. Seasonings: rosemary. Other: Drink an 8-ounce glass of quality water every two hours. Investigate food allergies and avoid potentially allergenic foods.
Hemorrhoids and varicose veins	Foods: alfalfa sprouts, aloe vera juice, flaxseed oil. Avoid: fried foods, tobacco.
Hyperacidity	Foods: umeboshi plums (eat two every four hours for two days), potato peel broth made by simmering the skins of 3 potatoes in 2 quarts of quality water for 30 minutes (strain out the peels before drinking it).
Hyperthyroidism	Foods: broccoli, Brussels sprouts, cabbage, kale, mustard greens, peaches, pears, spinach, turnips. Avoid: carbonated soft drinks, coffee, dairy products, processed and refined foods, iodized salt, tap water.
Hypoglycemia	Foods: avocado, beet greens, beets, dandelion greens, flaxseeds, garlic, kale, parsley, spirulina, turnip greens, turnips. Seasonings: cayenne pepper. Avoid: alcohol, dairy products (except soured), fats, fried foods, gravies, ham, instant potatoes, instant rice, junk food, processed foods, sausage, all forms of sugar, sweet fruits, white-flour products. Other: Eat high-fiber foods, especially in the morning. Eat five small meals of complex carbohydrates and protein each day. Investigate food allergies.

DISORDER	DIETARY RECOMMENDATIONS
Hypothyroidism	Foods: apples, apricots, grapes, leafy greens, parsley, primrose oil, rose hips, watercress.
	Seasonings: rosemary.
	Nutrients: essential fatty acids.
	Avoid: all processed and refined foods, iodized salt, tap water.
	Other: Consume broccoli, Brussels sprouts, cabbage, kale, mustard greens, peaches, pears, and spinach in moderation only.
Impotence	Foods: borage oil, flaxseed oil, pumpkinseeds.
	Nutrients: coenzyme Q_{10}, copper, selenium, vitamin C, vitamin E, zinc.
	Avoid: alcohol, dairy products, saturated and hydrogenated fats, meat, sugar, tobacco, yeast.
Indigestion	Foods: alfalfa sprouts, aloe vera juice, artichokes, chamomile tea, dandelion greens, fennel, fennel seed tea, okra, papaya leaf tea.
	Seasonings: fenugreek, ginger root, peppermint, rosemary.
	Nutrients: bromelain, calcium.
	Avoid: dairy products, fats, fried foods, grains, meats, nuts, seeds, spicy foods.
	Other: Avoid lying on your right side after eating.
Infertility, female	Nutrients: vitamin A; B-complex vitamins, especially para-aminobenzoic acid.
	Avoid: caffeine.
	Other: Do not douche.
Infertility, male	Foods: pumpkinseeds.
	Nutrients: manganese, selenium, vitamin A, vitamin C, vitamin E.
	Avoid: alcohol, saturated and hydrogenated fats, sugar, tobacco.
Insomnia	Nutrients: calcium, magnesium, vitamin C.
	Avoid: alcohol; baking powder; caffeine; canned food and beverages; cheese; chocolate; citrus fruits and juices; corn; cured meats; dairy products; eggs; foods containing additives; fried, junk, and processed foods; saturated fats; all forms of sugar; tap water; tobacco; wheat.
Memory problems	Foods: blueberries, garlic, kelp, spinach and other leafy greens.
	Seasonings: cayenne pepper, ginger root.
	Nutrients: choline, coenzyme Q_{10}, glutamine, glutathione, lecithin, B-complex vitamins with extra vitamin B_{12} and folic acid, serine, zinc.
	Avoid: alcohol, baking powder, canned food and beverages, cheese, chocolate, corn, dairy products, eggs, foods containing additives, fried foods, junk food, all forms of sugar, tobacco, wheat.
Menopause-related problems	Foods: alfalfa sprouts, all berries, amaranth, blackstrap molasses, broccoli, chickweed, dandelion greens, garlic, kelp, maitake mushrooms, papaya, parsley, pineapple, primrose oil, salmon with bones, sardines, sea vegetables, soy foods, watercress, white fish.
	Seasonings: aniseed, ginger root, sage.
	Nutrients: calcium, magnesium, B-complex vitamins (especially vitamin B_6), vitamin D, vitamin E.

DISORDER	DIETARY RECOMMENDATIONS
	Avoid: alcohol, all animal products (meat and dairy products), all forms of caffeine, saturated and hydrogenated fats, fried foods, junk foods, soft drinks, all forms of sugar.
	Other: Eat a diet of 50 percent raw foods and take a protein supplement to help stabilize blood sugar levels.
Migraine	Foods: almonds, almond milk, cherries, fennel, parsley, garlic, fresh pineapple, watercress.
	Seasonings: cayenne pepper.
	Nutrients: calcium, magnesium, quercetin.
Nausea	Foods: aloe vera juice.
	Nutrients: calcium, vitamin B_6.
	Seasonings: ginger root, peppermint
	Other: Drink a glass of quality water every hour to help rid the body of toxins.
Obesity	Foods: borage oil, celery, cucumber, dandelion greens, garlic, grapefruit, kale, kelp, lemon, parsley, primrose oil, spirulina, strawberries, watercress, watermelon.
	Seasonings: ginger root.
	Nutrients: bromelain, chromium, glutamine.
	Avoid: all animal fats, artificial sweeteners, chocolate, dairy products, junk and fast foods, nuts, olives, pastries, processed foods, salt, salty foods, soft drinks, sugar, white-flour products.
	Other: Drink at least 8 glasses of quality water daily. Consume in moderation high-calorie foods such as corn, hominy, figs, grapes, green peas, pears, pineapple, sweet potatoes, white rice, bananas, cherries, avocados, coconut, nuts, and seeds. Consume an abundance of raw vegetables and live juices. Use a fiber source such as psyllium a half-hour before meals. If necessary, use a moderate amount of a natural sweetener such as rice malt or barley malt. Get plenty of exercise, such as walking and/or stretching.
Osteoporosis	Foods: apples, blueberries, red grapes, leafy greens, bok choy, broccoli, collard greens, dulse, garlic, kale, kelp, parsley, primrose oil, rose hips, spirulina, turnip greens, turnips.
	Nutrients: boron, calcium, iron, magnesium, omega-3 fatty acids, silica, vitamin A, vitamin C, vitamin D, vitamin K.
	Avoid: alcohol, animal products (meat and dairy products), any food containing sugar, caffeine, chocolate, cocoa, salt, saturated fats, soft drinks, tobacco.
	Other: Eat a diet that supplies quality (vegetable) protein, calcium, iron, magnesium, phosphorus, and vitamins A, C, D, and E. Limit your intake of almonds, beet greens, cashews, chard, citrus fruits, rhubarb, spinach, and tomatoes. Get regular exercise. If you take calcium supplements, do not take them at the same time as you eat whole grains.
Pain	Foods: fresh papaya juice.
	Seasonings: cayenne pepper.
	Other: Drink a glass of quality water every four hours. Go on a juice fast (unless you have diabetes).
Parasites/worms	Foods: fig juice, papaya seeds, raw pumpkinseeds.
	Other: Have a child with pinworms eat a heavily salted diet for one week. Use cleansing enemas.

DISORDER	DIETARY RECOMMENDATIONS
Pneumonia	Foods: alfalfa sprouts; flaxseed oil; garlic; green drinks; lemon juice; maitake, reishi, or shiitake mushrooms; raw fruits and vegetables; rose hips.
	Seasonings: fenugreek, ginger.
	Nutrients: bromelain, B-complex vitamins, cysteine, selenium, vitamin A, vitamin C, zinc.
	Other: Eat plenty of protein and drink quality water often.
Premenstrual syndrome (PMS)	Foods: cucumber, garlic, leafy greens, kale, parsley, pineapple, primrose oil, watermelon.
	Seasonings: ginger root, sage.
	Nutrients: B-complex vitamins, especially vitamin B6.
	Avoid: alcohol, caffeine, dairy products, saturated and hydrogenated fats, fried foods, junk foods, processed foods, red meat, salt, soft drinks, sugar, tobacco.
	Other: Drink 8 glasses of quality water daily.
Skin rash	Nutrients: vitamin A, vitamin C, zinc.
	Avoid: alcohol, caffeine (chocolate, cocoa, coffee, tea), dairy products, fried foods, iodine (including iodized salt), pineapples, saturated fats, sea vegetables, soft drinks, all forms of sugar.
	Other: Eat a yeast-free and sugar-free diet.
Stress	Foods: spirulina.
	Nutrients: calcium, magnesium, B-complex vitamins, vitamin C.
	Avoid: alcohol, allergenic foods, baker's and brewer's yeast, caffeine, cheese, chocolate, dairy products, fried and junk foods, herring, meat tenderizers, phenylalanine, saturated fats and oils, soy sauce, all forms of sugar, tobacco, yeast extracts.
	Other: Practice breathing slowly and deeply often during the day; exercise; get a massage; enjoy music or reading; take warm baths to break the stress cycle.
Sweating (excessive)	Foods: alfalfa sprouts, garlic, kelp, pomegranates, spirulina.
	Seasonings: sage.
	Nutrients: potassium.
	Avoid: alcohol, dairy products, fat, all forms of sugar, tobacco.
	Other: Drink 8–10 glasses of quality water daily. Use a juice fast to cleanse the body of toxins (unless you have diabetes).
Swollen lymph nodes	Foods: garlic, parsley.
	Nutrients: selenium, vitamin A, vitamin C, vitamin E, zinc.
	Other: Drink a glass of quality water with lemon juice first thing each morning to revitalize lymph. Go on a three-day juice fast (unless you are pregnant or nursing, or have diabetes).

DISORDER	DIETARY RECOMMENDATIONS
Tuberculosis (TB)	Foods: apples, barley grass, carrots, cantaloupe, collards, garlic, kale, kefir, kelp, leafy greens, lemon, papaya, wheat germ, wheatgrass, yogurt.
	Nutrients: beta-carotene, cysteine, selenium, vitamin C, vitamin E.
	Avoid: alcohol, animal products, caffeine, dairy products, fried foods, junk foods, all processed foods, red meat, salt, saturated fats, soft drinks, all forms of sugar, tap water, tobacco and smoke, white-flour products.
	Other: Eat a diet of 50 percent raw live juices and raw foods. Consume only steam-distilled water. If you eat reishi mushrooms, dip them in boiling water before using them. Rest, sunshine, and fresh air are vital. Use acidophilus.
Ulcer	Foods: almond milk, aloe vera juice, blue grapes, buttermilk, cabbage, cabbage juice, carrots, kefir, leafy greens, okra, parsley, rutabaga, soymilk, watercress, yogurt.
	Seasonings: ginger root.
	Avoid: alcohol, caffeine, carbonated drinks, chocolate, dairy products, decaffeinated coffee, fried foods, salt, saturated fats, spicy foods, tobacco.
	Other: Consume small, frequent meals. Fiber and plenty of quality water are important.
Vaginal discharge	Foods: aloe vera juice, garlic, garlic juice.
	Nutrients: B-complex vitamins.
	Avoid: alcohol, butter, all cheeses, chocolate, citrus and dried fruits, fermented foods, fruit and soft drinks, all forms of gluten, ham, honey, junk foods, mushrooms, nuts, pickles, soy sauce, all forms of sugar, tamari sauce, yeast products.
	Other: Use acidophilus.
Weight loss (unexplained)	Foods: apples, blackberries, brewer's yeast, garlic, spirulina, wheat germ.
	Seasonings: fenugreek,
	Nutrients: all nutrients, particularly B-complex vitamins and iron.
	Avoid: alcohol, coffee, fried foods, junk food, soft drinks, yeast products.
	Other: Eat a diet high in complex carbohydrates and protein.

Appendix D: Live Juice Therapy: Powerful Nutritional Combinations

The world of dietary healing includes the use of live juices made from fresh vegetables and juices. As with whole foods, certain juices are particularly beneficial for certain health problems. In some cases, the power of these dietary healers can be boosted with the addition of certain herbal extracts. Use the table below to identify some of the many juices that can be used for healing.

DISORDER	VEGETABLE JUICES	FRUIT JUICES	OTHER ADDITIONS
Acne/skin disorders	Best: all leafy greens, cauliflower, cucumber, carrot. Good: beet green, cabbage, alfalfa, green pepper, onion, potato, reishi mushroom, Swiss chard.	Best: apple. Good: apricot, blackberry, blueberry, kiwi, lemon, raspberry, strawberry.	Best: dandelion root, burdock root, milk thistle, goldenseal, red clover (herbal extracts). Also, primrose oil. Good: alfalfa, basil, barberry, coltsfoot, echinacea, Oregon grape root, yellow dock root (herbal extracts).
Alzheimer's disease	Best: all leafy greens, watercress, kale. Good: alfalfa, beet green, cabbage, carrot, dandelion green, onion, pepper, reishi mushroom, sea vegetables, Swiss chard, turnip.	Best: banana, blueberry, lemon, peach, papaya. Good: apple, apricot, cherry, grape, pineapple, prune.	Best: butcher's broom, ginkgo biloba, gotu kola, turmeric, Siberian ginseng (herbal extracts). Good: blessed thistle, cayenne, garlic, ginger, valerian root (herbal extracts). Also, borage oil, coenzyme Q10, N,N-Dimethylglycine (DMG), primrose oil.
Arthritis	Best: all leafy greens, celery root, kelp, watercress. Good: asparagus, barley grass, beet green, carrot, celery, cucumber, cabbage, green bean, kale, onion, wheatgrass, sea vegetables, sea cucumber.	Good: apple, black cherry, lemon, papaya, pineapple. Good: grape, pear.	Best: alfalfa, boswellia, garlic, dandelion, horsetail, turmeric, yucca (herbal extracts). Also, omega-3 oil. Good: borage, cat's claw, cayenne, ginger, juniper, olive leaf extract, parsley, pau d'arco (herbal extracts). Also, primrose oil.
Asthma/bronchitis/emphysema	Best: all leafy greens, barley grass, carrot, horseradish root, rutabaga, turnip, turnip green. Good: broccoli, celery, collard, onion, spinach, watercress, wheatgrass.	Best: apple, cranberry. Good: lemon, mango, papaya, grape, grapefruit, kiwi, pineapple.	Best: eucalyptus, chickweed, ephedra (ma huang), garlic, lobelia, mullein, myrrh, pau d'arco (herbal extracts). Also, flaxseed oil. Good: astragalus, bayberry, calendula flower, cayenne, echinacea, fennel seed, fenugreek, ginger root, ginkgo biloba, horehound, Iceland moss, licorice root, marshmallow, peppermint leaf, parsley, skullcap (herbal extracts). Also, primrose oil.
Attention deficit disorder (ADD)/ attention deficit hyperactivity disorder (ADHD)	All fresh vegetable juices.	No fruit juices.	Best: ginkgo biloba, valerian root (herbal extracts). Good: catnip, chamomile, gotu kola, hops, lemon balm, licorice (herbal extracts). Also, borage oil, flaxseed oil, primrose oil.
Bladder infection/urinary burning, itching, frequency, urgency	Best: collard. Good: carrot, celery, kale, spinach, wheatgrass.	Best: cranberry, pineapple. Good: blueberry, watermelon.	Best: alfalfa, astragalus, bilberry, buchu, parsley, uva ursi (herbal extracts). Good: birch leaves, dandelion, echinacea, ginger, goldenseal, juniper berry, marshmallow, rose hip (herbal extracts). Also, apple cider vinegar, colloidal silver, spirulina.

DISORDER	VEGETABLE JUICES	FRUIT JUICES	OTHER ADDITIONS
Cancer and HIV/AIDS	Best: all cruciferous vegetables, all leafy greens, black radish, cabbage, carrot, dandelion green, reishi and shiitake mushroom, sea vegetables, wheatgrass. Good: asparagus, kale, kohlrabi, onion, spinach, Swiss chard, watercress.	Best: blueberry, cherry, papaya, peach, red grape. Good: apple, apricot, citrus fruits, cantaloupe, pineapple, plum, strawberry.	Best: alfalfa, astragalus, bilberry, burdock root, garlic, milk thistle, pau d'arco, red clover, schisandra, suma, yellow dock (herbal extracts). Also, Essiac tea. Good: echinacea, ginger root, ginseng, goldenseal, green tea, marshmallow, mistletoe (herbal extracts). Also, chlorella, spirulina.
Candidiasis	Best: all leafy greens, cabbage, carrot. Good: beet green, broccoli, celery, kale, onion, rutabaga, turnip, wheatgrass.	No fruit juices.	Best: garlic, pau d'arco (herbal extracts). Also, grapefruit seed extract, primrose oil. Good: barberry bark, black walnut, dong quai, echinacea, goldenseal, red clover (herbal extracts). Also, bee propolis, chlorophyll, spirulina.
Cardiovascular disease	Best: all leafy greens, carrot, celery, kale, onion. Good: bok choy, beet green, cabbage, cucumber, eggplant, green pepper, kelp, mustard green, potato skins (cut out the eyes), red pepper, sea vegetables, shiitake mushroom, spinach, Swiss chard, turnip, turnip green, wheatgrass.	Best: apple, banana, apricot, cantaloupe, grapefruit, lemon, papaya, red grape. Good: avocado, grapefruit, pomegranate, strawberry, watermelon.	Best: cayenne, chickweed, garlic, ginkgo biloba, green tea, hawthorn berry, valerian root (herbal extracts). Also, flaxseed oil, lecithin. Good: alfalfa, bilberry, butcher's broom, fenugreek, ginger root, horsetail, parsley, motherwort, suma, yarrow (herbal extracts). Also, apple pectin, borage oil, chlorophyll, primrose oil, psyllium seed, salmon oil.
Chronic fatigue/lack of energy and/or endurance	Best: all leafy greens, carrot, dandelion green, wheatgrass. Good: beet green, bok choy, broccoli, cabbage, celery, onion, potato (with skin), reishi and shiitake mushroom, turnip, watercress.	In moderation only. Best: apple, avocado, lemon, papaya. Good: apricot, banana, blueberry, cantaloupe, peach, red grape.	Best: astragalus, cayenne, echinacea, garlic, pau d'arco, suma (herbal extracts). Good: burdock, dandelion, ginseng, ginkgo biloba, licorice, parsley, milk thistle, olive leaf, red clover, St. John's wort (herbal extracts). Also, bee propolis, coenzyme 1 (ENADA), omega-3 oil, primrose oil.
Depression	Best: all leafy greens, broccoli, dandelion green. Good: beet green, cabbage, carrot, green pepper, kale, onion, kelp, spinach, watercress, wheatgrass.	Apple, banana, blueberry, cranberry, lemon, papaya, peach, pineapple.	Best: alfalfa, flaxseed oil, garlic, St. John's wort (herbal extracts). Also, S-adenosylmethionine (SAMe), spirulina. Good: cat's claw, ginkgo biloba, gotu kola, parsley, Siberian ginseng, slippery elm (herbal extracts). Also, aloe vera juice, gamma-aminobutyric acid (GABA), lecithin, selenium, zinc.
Diabetes	Best: all leafy greens, Brussels sprouts. Good: asparagus, broccoli, celery, green bean, green pepper, kale, kohlrabi, spinach, turnip green.	No fruit juices.	Best: dandelion root, garlic, huckleberry, parsley (herbal extracts). Good: buchu leaves, cat's claw, dandelion, ginger root, ginseng, juniper berry, licorice root, uva ursi (herbal extracts). Also, aloe vera juice, alpha-lipoic acid, brewer's yeast, chromium, primrose oil, spirulina.
Diarrhea	Best: all leafy greens, carrot. Good: beet green, cabbage, kelp.	Best: apple, banana, blackberry, papaya. Good: peach.	Best: blackberry root, raspberry leaf (herbal extracts). Also, acidophilus. Good: cayenne, chamomile, garlic, ginger root, Irish moss, marshmallow root, peppermint, parsley, slippery elm bark (herbal extracts). Also, psyllium seed.

DISORDER	VEGETABLE JUICES	FRUIT JUICES	OTHER ADDITIONS
Edema/swelling of abdomen, ankles, feet, hands, or legs	Best: celery, watercress. Good: all leafy greens, cucumber, kelp, spinach, Swiss chard.	Best: banana, watermelon. Good: apple, blueberry, peach.	Best: alfalfa, cornsilk, garlic, parsley, uva ursi (herbal extracts). Good: butcher's broom, dandelion root, horsetail, juniper berry, rose hip (herbal extracts). Also, carob powder.
Gout	Best: all leafy greens, kelp. Good: beets, carrot, celery, kale, watercress, wheatgrass.	Best: black cherry, lemon. Good: apple, blueberry, pear, pineapple, strawberry.	Best: dandelion root, garlic (herbal extracts). Good: alfalfa, boswellia, burdock root, cayenne, devil's claw, horsetail, juniper, parsley, turmeric, yucca (herbal extracts). Also, psyllium seed.
Hyperthyroidism	Best: broccoli, Brussels sprouts, cabbage, kale, mustard green, spinach, turnip. Good: alfalfa, beet green, carrot, celery, green pepper, watercress.	Best: peach, pear. Good: apple, apricot, cranberry, grapefruit, grape, pineapple.	Barberry, black cohosh, goldenseal, skullcap, parsley, white oak bark (herbal extracts).
Hypoglycemia	Best: beet green, beet, kale, turnip, turnip green. Good: bok choy, cabbage, green pepper, mustard green, parsnip, spinach, kelp.	Best: avocado. Good (but must be unsweetened): apple, blueberry, cranberry, grapefruit, kiwi, lemon (drink mixed with an equal amount of water or herbal tea).	Best: artichoke leaf, astragalus, dandelion root, gentian, gotu kola, licorice root (herbal extracts). Also, spirulina. Good: alfalfa, bilberry, cayenne, dandelion, garlic, goldenseal, juniper berry, parsley, wild yam (herbal extracts). Also, bee pollen, flaxseed, royal jelly.
Hypothyroidism	Best: all leafy greens, watercress. Good: beet green, carrot, celery, green pepper, kelp, sea vegetable, sprout.	Best: apple, apricot, grape. Good: cranberry, grapefruit, pineapple, prune.	Best: alfalfa, bayberry, rosemary (herbal extracts). Good: black cohosh, gentian, ginkgo biloba, goldenseal, licorice, parsley, rose hip (herbal extract). Also, primrose oil.
Insomnia	Best: all leafy greens, watercress, kale. Good: alfalfa, beet green, cabbage, carrot, dandelion green, onion, pepper, reishi mushroom, sea vegetables, Swiss chard, turnip.	Best: banana, lemon, peach, papaya, blueberry. Good: apple, apricot, cherry, grape, pineapple, prune.	Best: butcher's broom, ginkgo biloba, gotu kola, turmeric, Siberian ginseng (herbal extracts). Good: blessed thistle, cayenne, garlic, ginger, primrose oil, valerian root (herbal extracts). Also, borage oil, primrose oil.
Memory problems	Best: all leafy greens, watercress, kale. Good: alfalfa, beet green, cabbage, carrot, dandelion green, onion, pepper, reishi mushroom, sea vegetables, Swiss chard, turnip.	Best: banana, lemon, peach, papaya, blueberry. Good: apple, apricot, cherry, grape, pineapple, prune.	Best: butcher's broom, ginkgo biloba, gotu kola, turmeric, Siberian ginseng (herbal extracts). Good: blessed thistle, cayenne, garlic, ginger, valerian root (herbal extracts). Also, borage oil, coenzyme Q_{10}, N,N-dimethylglycine (DMG), primrose oil.
Menopause-related problems	Best: broccoli, kelp. Good: all leafy greens, alfalfa, beet, cabbage, carrot, celery, collard, cucumber, dandelion green, kale, spinach, Swiss chard.	Best: all berries, papaya, pineapple. Good: apple, apricot, banana, blackberry, fig, grape, lemon, orange.	Best: black cohosh, garlic, licorice, raspberry leaf, sarsaparilla, Siberian ginseng (herbal extracts). Good: aniseed, buchu, chasteberry, dong quai, ginger root, gotu kola, parsley, passionflower, squawvine, valerian root (herbal extracts). Also, primrose oil.
Obesity	Best: celery, cucumber, kale, kelp, watercress. Good: all leafy greens, broccoli, cabbage, carrot, green bean, radish, spinach, shiitake mushroom, tomato, turnip, turnip green.	Best: grapefruit, lemon, pineapple, strawberry, watermelon. Good: tart apple, cranberry, papaya.	Best: chickweed, cornsilk, parsley (herbal extracts). Also, bromelain, seawrack, spirulina. Good: cascara sagrada, chickweed, dandelion, garlic, ginger root, ginseng, nettle (herbal extracts). Also, borage oil, primrose oil, psyllium seed.

DISORDER	VEGETABLE JUICES	FRUIT JUICES	OTHER ADDITIONS
Osteoporosis	Best: all leafy greens, bok choy, broccoli, collard, kale, kelp, turnip, turnip green, watercress. Good: cabbage, carrot, cauliflower, celery, dandelion green, dulse, shiitake mushroom, Swiss chard.	Best: apple, blueberry, red grape. Good: banana, cherry, fig, lemon, papaya, pineapple, prune, raisin.	Best: alfalfa, horsetail, nettle (herbal extracts). Also, omega-3 oil, primrose oil. Good: dandelion, garlic, Irish moss, oat straw, parsley, red clover, rose hip (herbal extracts). Also, silica, spirulina.
Premenstrual syndrome (PMS)	Best: all leafy greens, cucumber, kale, kelp. Good: broccoli, cabbage, celery root, spinach, turnip, turnip green.	Best: pineapple, watermelon. Good: apple, cherry, fig, grape, kiwi, lemon, papaya, raspberry, red grape.	Best: dong quai, parsley, sarsaparilla, squawvine (herbal extracts). Good: blessed thistle, chasteberry, dong quai, garlic, ginger root, licorice, valerian, raspberry leaves, sage (herbal extracts).
Tuberculosis (TB)	Best: all leafy greens, barley grass, carrot, kelp, kale, collard, wheatgrass. Good: alfalfa, beet, beet green, broccoli, celery, green pepper, onion, reishi mushroom, watercress.	Best: apple, cantaloupe, lemon, papaya. Good: all berries, cranberry, grapefruit, grape, pineapple, rose hip.	Best: echinacea, garlic, goldenseal (herbal extracts). Good: astragalus, bayberry, horsetail, mullein, myrrh, pau d'arco, rose hip, St. John's wort (herbal extracts). Also, primrose oil, wheat germ.
Ulcer	Best: all leafy greens, cabbage, okra, rutabaga, watercress. Good: carrot, celery, kale, potato, red pepper.	Best: blue grape. Good: apple, banana, cantaloupe, papaya, blueberry, raisin.	Best: peppermint (herbal extract). Also, aloe vera juice. Good: bilberry, chamomile, ginger root, goldenseal, marshmallow, parsley (herbal extracts). Also, psyllium seed.

Resources

Below are the manufacturers and distributors of some of the brand-name products mentioned in this book, plus their addresses and phone numbers. This information is provided to enable you to contact these companies to order or to obtain further information about their products. None of the manufacturers or distributors mentioned has had any connection with the production of this book. Rather, I list these companies because I believe their products to be effective and of high quality. Be aware that addresses and telephone numbers are subject to change.

Aerobic Life Industries
23025 North 15th Avenue, Suite B106
Phoenix, AZ 85027
800–798–0707
www.aerobiclife.com
Aerobic Bulk Cleanse (ABC).

Arrowhead Mills
c/o The Hain Celestial Group
734 Franklin Avenue, #444
Garden City, NY 11530
806–364–0730
www.arrowheadmills.com
Grains and flours; multigrain corn bread mix.

Avalon Natural Products
1105 Industrial Avenue
Petaluma, CA 94952
800–227–5120 or 707–769–5120
Fax: 707–769–0868
www.avalonnaturalproducts.com
Un-Petroleum natural petroleum jelly substitute.

Barlean's Organic Oils
4936 Lake Terrell Road
Ferndale, WA 98248
360–384–0485
www.barleans.com
Organic oils sold in Bio-Electron Process modified atmospheric packaging.

CMServices & Evert-Fresh Bags
P.O. Box 76238
St. Petersburg, FL 33734–6238
800–372–3610 or 727–527–9084
www.greenbags.com
Evert-Fresh produce storage bags.

Earth's Best
Consumer Affairs
734 Franklin Avenue, Suite 444
Garden City, NY 11530
800–434–4246
www.earthsbest.com
Organic baby foods.

Earthrise Nutritionals, Inc.
424 Payran Street
Petaluma, CA 94952
800–949–7473
Fax: 707–778–9028
www.earthrise.com
Spirulina products.

Eclectic Institute
14385 SE Lusted Road
Sandy, OR 97055
800–332–4372
www.eclecticherb.com
Herbal extracts and other products.

Econugenics
2208 Northpoint Parkway
Santa Rose, CA 95407
800–308–5518
www.econugenics.com
Modified Citrus Pectin, MycoCeutics Ten Mushroom Combination, MycoCeutics MycoPhyto Complex.

EcoWater Systems
P.O. Box 64420
St. Paul, MN 55164
800–808–9899
www.ecowater.com
Reverse osmosis water purification systems.

Eden Foods, Inc.
701 Tecumseh Road
Clinton, MI 49236
888–424–EDEN (888–424–3336) or 517–456–7424
Fax: 517–456–6075
www.edenfoods.com
Grains and flours.

Environmental Protection Agency Safe Drinking Water Hotline
800–426–4971
Toll-free phone number to help locate the nearest office or lab that performs certified water testing.

Enzymatic Therapy
825 Challenger Drive
Green Bay, WI 54311
800–783–2286 or 414–469–1313
www.enzy.com
Esberitox echinacea formula.

Flora Manufacturing & Distributing, Ltd.
P.O. Box 73
805 East Badger Road
Lynden, WA 98264
800–446–2110 or 360–354–2110
Fax: 360–354–5355
www.florahealth.com
Herbal extracts and other products.

Follow Your Heart
P.O. Box 9400
Canoga Park, CA 91309–0400
818–348–3240
Fax: 818–348–1509
www.followyourheart.com
Veganaise soy mayonnaise.

Fruitsource
1803 Mission Street, Suite 404
Santa Cruz, CA 95060
408–464–9891
Fruitrim sweetener.

Gerber Products Company
445 State Street
Fremont, MI 49413–0001
800–4–GERBER (800–443–7237)
www.gerber.com
Tender Harvest organic baby foods.

Gourmet Mushroom Products
P.O. Box 515 IP
Graton, CA 95444
800–789–9121 or 707–829–7301
Fax: 707–823–9091
www.gmushrooms.com
Fresh and dried gourmet mushrooms; kits for cultivating mushrooms.

Grassland Beef
R.R. 1, Box 20
Monticello, MO 63457
877–383–0051
Fax: 573–767–8337
www.grasslandbeef.com
Organically raised, grass-fed beef.

Hain's
c/o The Hain Celestial Group
734 Franklin Ave, #444
Garden City, NY 11530
www.hain-celestial.com
Brown gravy mix, dry soup mixes, salad dressing mixes, soft safflower margarine.

Health Valley
c/o The Hain Celestial Group
734 Franklin Ave, #444
Garden City, NY 11530
www.hain-celestial.com
Canned soups.

Heartland Mill, Inc.
Route 1, Box 2
Marienthal, KS 67863
800–232–8533 or 316–379–4472
www.heartlandmill.com
Grains and flours.

Herbs, Etc.
1345 Cerrillos Road
Santa Fe, NM 87501
888–694–3727
www.herbsetc.com
Herbal extracts and other products.

Herbs for Kids
c/o Botanical Laboratories, Inc.
1441 West Smith Road
Ferndale, WA 98248
360–384–5656
Fax: 360–384–1140
www.herbsforkids.com
Alcohol-free organic herbal extracts designed for children.

Himalaya USA
10440 Westoffice Drive
Houston, TX 77042
800–869–4640 or 713–863–1622
Fax: 800–577–6930 or 713–863–1686
www.himalayausa.com
ImmunoCare.

Hodgson Mill, Inc.
Hodgson Mill, Inc.
1203 West Niccum Avenue
Effingham, IL 62401
800–347–0105
www.hodgsonmill.com
Grains and flours.

Hulman & Company
c/o Clabber Girl, Inc.
P.O. Box 150
Terre Haute, IN 47808–0150
812–232–9446
Fax: 812–232–2397
www.bakewithlove.com
Rumford brand aluminum-free baking powder.

JHS Natural Products
P.O. Box 50398
Eugene, OR 97405
888–330–4691 or 541–344–1396
www.jhsnp.com
Medicinal mushrooms, extracts, and supplements.

King Arthur Flour
Norwich, VT 05055
800–827–6836
www.kingarthurflour.com
Grains and flours.

Knudsen. See R.W. Knudsen Family.

Life Sprouts
P.O. Box 150
Paradise, UT 84328
800–241–1516
Sprouters and organic seeds.

Lumen Foods
409 Scott Street
Lake Charles, LA 70601
800–256–2253 or 337–436–6748
Fax: 337–436–1769
www.soybean.com
Heartline Meatless Meats, a textured-protein product made from soybeans that works well in casseroles, stews, and soups.

Lundberg Family Farms
5370 Church Street
P.O. Box 369
Richvale, CA 95974–0369
530–882–4551
Fax: 530–882–4500
www.lundberg.com
Grains and flours.

Maine Coast Sea Vegetables
3 Georges Pond Road
Franklin, ME 04634
207–565–2907
Fax: 207–565–2144
www.seaveg.com
Organic sea vegetables, including Sea Pickles, made from fresh, undried kelp.

Maitake Products, Inc.
P.O. Box 1354
Paramus, NJ 07653
800–747–7418
Fax: 201–229–0585
www.maitake.com
Grifron Maitake D-fraction capsules and Grifron Maitake caplets.

Mayacamas Fine Foods
1206 MacArthur
Sonoma, CA 95476
800–826–9621
Fax: 707–996–4501
Brown gravy mix; dry soup mixes.

Miracle Exclusives
64 Seaview Boulevard
Port Washington, NY 11050
800–645–6360 or 516–621–3333
www.miracleexclusives.com
Miracle Soy Wonder Soymilk Machine.

M.D. Labs
P.O. Box 27688
Tempe, AZ 85285
800–88–DETOX (800–883–3869)
www.mdlabs.com or www.dailydetox.com
Daily Detox.

Nasoya
c/o Vitasoy-USA, Inc.
400 Oyster Point Boulevard, Suite 201
South San Francisco, CA 94080
800–VITASOY (800–848–2769)
www.nasoya.com
Nayonaise Dijon-style soy mayonnaise.

National Testing Laboratories, Ltd.
6555 Wilson Mills Road, Suite 102
Cleveland, OH 44143
800–426–8378 or 800–458–3330 or 440–449–2525
Fax: 440–449–8585
Water testing by mail order (note this is contact information for corporate headquarters; call or write for testing laboratory locations; do not send water samples to the above address).

Natren
3105 Willow Lane
Westlake Village, CA 91361
800–992–3323
Acidophilus and other probiotic supplements.

Nature's Answer, Inc.
75 Commerce Drive
Hauppauge, NY 11788
800–439–2324
Fax: 631–231–8391
www.naturesanswer.com
Herbal extracts and other products.

Nature's Plus
c/o Natural Organics, Inc.
548 Broadhollow Road
Melville, NY 11747–3708
800–937–0500 or 631–293–0030
Fax: 631–293–0349
www.naturesplus.com
Herbal extracts and other products.

Nature's Way
10 Mountain Springs Parkway
Springville, UT 84663
801–489–1500
Fax: 801–489–1700
www.naturesway.com
Naturalax 2, Primadophilus.

NSF International
789 North Dixboro Road
Box 130140
Ann Arbor, MI 48113–0140
800–NSF–MARK (800–673–6275) or 734–769–8010
Fax: 734–769–0109
http://www.nsf.org/
Information on EPA-recommended maximum contaminant levels for water, water purification systems, and other water-quality issues.

Omega Nutrition
6515 Aldrich Road
Bellingham, WA 98226
800–661–FLAX (800–661–3529) or 360–384–1238
Fax: 360–384–0700
Organic oils sold in Omegaflo modified atmospheric packaging.

Omega-Life, Inc.
15355 Woodbridge Road
Brookfield, WI 53005
800–328–3529 or 414–786–2070
Fortified Flax.

Peruvian Rainforest Botanicals
212 North US Highway 1, Suite 17
Tequesta, FL 33469
800–742–2529
Herbal extracts and other products.

Pure Water, Inc.
P.O. Box 83226
Lincoln, NE 68501
800–875–5915 or 402–467–9300
Fax: 402–467–9393
www.purewaterinc.com
Water distillation systems for the home.

RainSoft
Division, Aquion Partners LP
2080 East Lunt Avenue
Elk Grove Village, IL 60007
800–860–7638 or 847–437–9400
Reverse osmosis water purification systems.

Rumford. See Hulman & Company.

R.W. Knudsen Family
P.O. Box 369
Speedway Avenue
Chico, CA 95927
530–899–5000
Chili Veggie juice; Very Veggie juice.

Solgar Vitamin and Herb Company, Inc.
500 Willow Tree Road
Leonia, NJ 07605
877–765–4274 (for consumers)
800–645–2246 (for retail stores)
www.solgar.com
Reishi Shiitake Maitake Mushroom Extract Vegicaps.

Soy Wonder. See Miracle Exclusives; Tree of Life, Inc.

Spectrum Organic Products, Inc.
1304 South Point Boulevard, Suite 280
Petaluma, CA 94954
707–778–8900
Fax: 707–765–8470
www.spectrumnaturals.com
Spectrum Spread; Spectrum Naturals organic oils sold in Spectra-Vac modified atmospheric packaging.

Suburban Water Testing Labs
4600 Kutztown Road
Temple, PA 19560–1548
800–433–6595 or 610–929–2920
www.h2otest.com
Water testing by mail order.

Sweet Wheat, Inc.
P.O. Box 187
Clearwater, FL 33757
888–227–9338 or 727–442–5454
www.sweetwheat.com
Sweet Wheat freeze-dried wheatgrass.

Taste Adventure
Will-Pak Foods, Inc.
Harbor City, CA 90710
800–874–0883 or 310–325–3504
Fax: 310–325–7038
www.tasteadventure.com
Pinto bean flakes.

The Sproutpeople
311 South Main Street
Viroqua, WI 54665
887–777–6887
www.sproutpeople.com
Sprouters and seeds, including a special mix for birds. The Web site offers a great deal of information about sprouting as well.

TofuttiBrands, Inc.
50 Jackson Drive
Cranford, NJ 07016
908–272–2400
Fax: 908–272–9492
Soy-based foods, including cream cheese, ice cream, sour cream, cheese slices, frozen macaroni, hot dogs, cheese, and others (including frozen dishes).

Trace Minerals Research
1990 West 3300 South
Ogden, UT 84401
800–624–7145 or 801–731–6051
www.traceminerals.com
ConcenTrace trace mineral drops.

Tree of Life, Inc.
P.O. Box 9000
St. Augustine, FL 32085–9000
800–260–2424 or 904–940–2100
www.treeoflife.com
Soy Wonder soy nut butter.

Un-Petroleum. See Avalon Natural Products.

Wakunaga of America Company, Ltd.
23501 Madero
Mission Viejo, CA 92691
800–421–2998 or 949–855–2776
Fax: 949–458–2764
www.kyolic.com
Dairy-free acidophilus; Kyo-Dophilus; Kyo-Green; Kyolic Aged Garlic Extract; Probiata.

Water Quality Association
4151 Naperville Road
Lisle, IL 60532
630–505–0160
Fax: 630–505–9637
www.wqa.org
Information on EPA-recommended maximum contaminant levels for water, water purification systems, and other water-quality issues.

Waterwise
3608 Parkway Boulevard
P.O. Box 494000
Leesburg, FL 34749–4000
800–874–9028 or 352–787–5008
Fax: 352–787–8123
www.waterwise.com
Reverse osmosis water purification and distillation units for the home.

Westbrae Foods
c/o The Hain Celestial Group
734 Franklin Ave, #444
Garden City, NY 11530
800–434–4246
www.westbrae.com
Organic sauces and condiments.

White Wave, Inc.
1990 North 57th Court
Boulder, CO 80301
303–443–3470
www.whitewave.com
Silk cultured soy (nondairy yogurt), Silk soymilk, Soylatte.

Zumbro, Inc.
82241 250th Avenue
Hayfield, MN 55940
800–631–0655
Jerusalem artichoke flour.

Index

About the Author

Phyllis Balch is a certified nutritional consultant who received her certification from the American Association of Nutritional Consultants and was a leading nutritional counselor for more than two decades. Ms. Balch experienced firsthand the benefits of using diet as a remedy for illness when, in the 1970s, she and her children suffered from undiagnosed or misdiagnosed illnesses. Although they had expert medical knowledge close at hand, maladies continued to disrupt their lives. Ms. Balch felt that there was something missing in the typical approach that treated the symptoms rather than the cause of illness.

Her first introduction to the relationship between nutrition and well-being was through the late Paavo Airola, a well-known naturopath and writer. She then pursued her own intensive research into the science of nutrition and, by making radical changes in diet, was able to transform her health and the health of her children. She became convinced that nutrition was, in many cases, the answer to regaining and maintaining health.

In 1979, she published *Nutritional Outline for the Professional and the Wise Man*—now known as *Prescription for Nutritional Healing*—to share her knowledge with a broader audience. Now in its third revised edition from Avery/Penguin, this book has had millions of readers in many countries (it has been translated into seven foriegn languages) and continues to be the authoritative classic in its field. In 2002, Ms. Balch published the definitive book on medicinal herbs, *Prescription for Herbal Healing*.

As a pioneering nutritional counselor and advocate of alternative health care, Ms. Balch has traveled widely and worked tirelessly researching to find the elusive answers to how the body maintains good health and which alternative methods best promote natural healing. In her writings, which have also included numerous newspaper columns and magazine articles, and at her nutritional center, she has consistently emphasized the importance of people taking responsibility for their own health. Her writings have convinced many traditionally schooled medical practitioners to incorporate dietary methods of restoring health into their treatments. She is highly sought after as a visiting lecturer and also appears on television and radio programs throughout Canada and the United States.

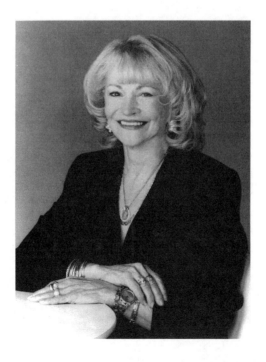

BOOKS BY PHYLLIS A. BALCH, CNC

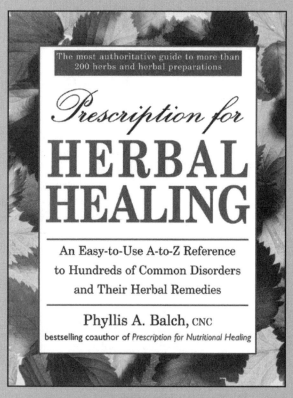

The most authoritative guide to more than 200 herbs and herbal preparations

Prescription for
HERBAL HEALING

An Easy-to-Use A-to-Z Reference
to Hundreds of Common Disorders
and Their Herbal Remedies

Phyllis A. Balch, CNC
bestselling coauthor of *Prescription for Nutritional Healing*

ISBN 0-89529-869-4

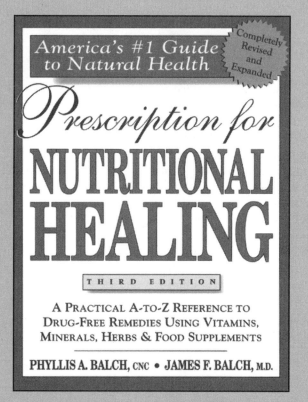

America's #1 Guide
to Natural Health

Completely
Revised
and
Expanded

Prescription for
NUTRITIONAL HEALING

THIRD EDITION

A PRACTICAL A-TO-Z REFERENCE TO
DRUG-FREE REMEDIES USING VITAMINS,
MINERALS, HERBS & FOOD SUPPLEMENTS

PHYLLIS A. BALCH, CNC • JAMES F. BALCH, M.D.

ISBN 1-58333-077-1

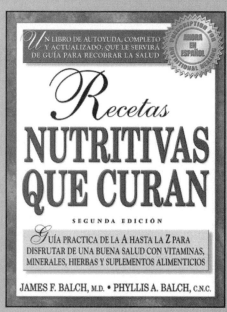

UN LIBRO DE AUTOYUDA, COMPLETO
Y ACTUALIZADO, QUE LE SERVIRÁ
DE GUÍA PARA RECOBRAR LA SALUD

AHORA
EN
ESPAÑOL

Recetas
NUTRITIVAS QUE CURAN

SEGUNDA EDICIÓN

GUÍA PRACTICA DE LA A HASTA LA Z PARA
DISFRUTAR DE UNA BUENA SALUD CON VITAMINAS,
MINERALES, HIERBAS Y SUPLEMENTOS ALIMENTICIOS

JAMES F. BALCH, M.D. • PHYLLIS A. BALCH, C.N.C.

ISBN 1-58444-010-0

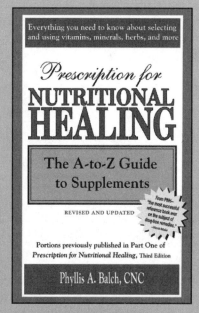

Everything you need to know about selecting
and using vitamins, minerals, herbs, and more

Prescription for
NUTRITIONAL HEALING

The A-to-Z Guide
to Supplements

REVISED AND UPDATED

Portions previously published in Part One of
Prescription for Nutritional Healing, Third Edition

Phyllis A. Balch, CNC

ISBN 1-58333-143-3

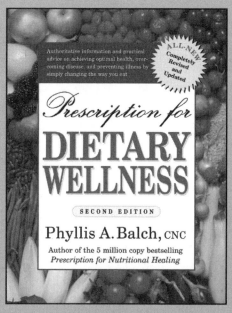

Authoritative information and practical
advice on achieving optimal health, over-
coming disease, and preventing illness by
simply changing the way you eat

ALL-NEW
Completely
Revised
and
Updated

Prescription for
DIETARY WELLNESS

SECOND EDITION

Phyllis A. Balch, CNC
Author of the 5 million copy bestselling
Prescription for Nutritional Healing

ISBN 1-58333-147-6

natural remedies that work!